CEREBRAL CORTEX

Volume 6
Further Aspects of
Cortical Function,
Including Hippocampus

CEREBRAL CORTEX
Edited by Edward G. Jones and Alan Peters

Advisory Committee
J. C. Eccles, *Ça a la Gra, Switzerland*
H. H. Jasper, *Montreal, Canada*
V. B. Mountcastle, *Baltimore, Maryland*
W. J. H. Nauta, *Cambridge, Massachusetts*
S. L. Palay, *Boston, Massachusetts*
F. Plum, *New York, New York*
R. D. Terry, *La Jolla, California*
P. Ulinski, *Chicago, Illinois*

CEREBRAL CORTEX

Volume 6
Further Aspects of
Cortical Function,
Including Hippocampus

Edited by

EDWARD G. JONES
California College of Medicine
University of California, Irvine
Irvine, California

and

ALAN PETERS
Boston University College of Medicine
Boston, Massachusetts

Plenum Press · New York and London

Library of Congress Cataloging in Publication Data

(Revised for vol. 6)

Cerebral cortex.

Vol. 2,   edited by Edward G. Jones and Alan Peters.
Includes bibliographies and indexes.
Contents: v. 1. Cellular components of the cerebral cortex—v. 2. Functional
properties of the cortical cells—[etc.]—v. 6. Further aspects of cortical function, in-
cluding hippocampus.
1. Cerebral cortex—Collected works. I. Peters, Alan, 1929-   .II. Jones, Ed-
ward G., 1939-   . [DNLM: 1. Cerebral Cortex—anatomy and histology. 2.
Cerebral Cortex—physiology. WL 307 C4136]
QP383.C45   1984   612′.825   84-1982
ISBN 0-306-42503-3

© 1987 Plenum Press, New York
A Division of Plenum Publishing Corporation
233 Spring Street, New York, N.Y. 10013

Printed in the United States of America

Contributors

Robert W. Baughman   Department of Neurobiology, Harvard Medical School, Boston, Massachusetts 02115

J. DeFelipe   Department of Anatomy and Neurobiology, University of California, Irvine, California 92717. *Present address:* Unidad de Neuroanatomia, Instituto Cajal, CSIC, 28006 Madrid, Spain

Felix Eckenstein   Department of Neurobiology, Harvard Medical School, Boston, Massachusetts 02115. *Present address:* Department of Neurology, Oregon Health Sciences University, Portland, Oregon 97201

James H. Fallon   Department of Anatomy and Neurobiology, University of California, Irvine, California 92717

S. H. C. Hendry   Department of Anatomy and Neurobiology, University of California, Irvine, California 92717

E. G. Jones   Department of Anatomy and Neurobiology, University of California, Irvine, California 92717

Donald A. Kristt   Stanford University Medical Center, Division of Neuropathology, Stanford, California 94305. *Present address:* Department of Pathology, Division of Neuropathology, University of Maryland School of Medicine, Baltimore, Maryland 21201

Sandra E. Loughlin   Department of Anatomy and Neurobiology, University of California, Irvine, California 92717

Alan L. Mueller   Department of Neurological Surgery, University of Washington, Seattle, Washington 98195. *Present address:* Abbott Laboratories, Abbott Park, Illinois 60064

vi

CONTRIBUTORS

Penelope Clare Murphy   Department of Physiology, University College, Cardiff CF1 1XL, United Kingdom

Alan Peters   Department of Anatomy, Boston University School of Medicine, Boston, Massachusetts 02118

Douglas L. Rosene   Department of Anatomy, Boston University School of Medicine, Boston, Massachusetts 02118

Philip A. Schwartzkroin   Department of Neurological Surgery and Department of Physiology and Biophysics, University of Washington, Seattle, Washington 98195

Adam Murdin Sillito   Department of Physiology, University College, Cardiff CF1 1XL, United Kingdom

George G. Somjen   Department of Physiology, Duke University, Durham, North Carolina 27710

Gary W. Van Hoesen   Departments of Anatomy and Neurology, University of Iowa College of Medicine, Iowa City, Iowa 52242

Preface

Volume 6 of *Cerebral Cortex* is in some respects a continuation of Volume 2, which dealt with the functional aspects of cortical neurons from the physiological and pharmacological points of view. In the current volume, chapters are devoted to the catecholamines, which for a number of reasons were not represented in the earlier volume, and to acetylcholine and the neuropeptides, about which much new information has recently appeared.

Volume 6 deals in part with the structure and function of cholinergic and catecholaminergic neuronal systems in the cerebral cortex and with new aspects of the cortical peptidergic neurons, notably the almost universal propensity of the known cortical peptides for being colocalized with classical transmitters and with one another. It thus completes our coverage of the major cortical neurotransmitter and neuromodulatory systems. Other chapters in this volume deal with data pertaining to the proportions of different types of cells and synapses in the neocortex and the physiology of the cortical neuroglial cells. These latter are topics that rarely receive separate treatment and the current chapters serve again to continue discussions of subjects that were introduced in Volume 2.

The previous volumes have all been devoted to the neocortex but the present one introduces the subject of the archicortex. To this end, separate chapters are devoted to the physiology and anatomy of the hippocampal formation.

We are extremely grateful, as always, for the efforts of the contributors to this volume and we know that the high quality of their articles will speak for itself. The staff of Plenum Press have once again done an excellent job of producing the volume and we thank them also.

Edward G. Jones
Alan Peters

Irvine and Boston

Contents

Chapter 3

Cholinergic Innervation in Cerebral Cortex

Felix Eckenstein and Robert W. Baughman

Chapter 4

The Cholinergic Modulation of Cortical Function

Adam Murdin Sillito and Penelope Clare Murphy

Chapter 5

Acetylcholinesterase in the Cortex

Donald A. Kristt

Chapter 6

**GABA–Peptide Neurons of the Primate Cerebral Cortex: A Limited
Cell Class**

E. G. Jones, S. H. C. Hendry, and J. DeFelipe

Chapter 7

Number of Neurons and Synapses in Primary Visual Cortex

Alan Peters

Chapter 8

Electrophysiology of Hippocampal Neurons

Philip A. Schwartzkroin and Alan L. Mueller

Chapter 9

The Hippocampal Formation of the Primate Brain: A Review of Some Comparative Aspects of Cytoarchitecture and Connections

Douglas L. Rosene and Gary W. Van Hoesen

Functions of Glial Cells in the Cerebral Cortex

GEORGE G. SOMJEN

1. Introduction

In the introductory chapter to the printed proceedings of a conference, Windle (1958) wrote that neuroglia is like the weather: everyone talks about it, but no one does anything about it. Today, little over a quarter century later, this can no longer be said. Instead of a scarcity, today's reviewer is faced with an over-abundance of data. The great activity in research into the nature of neuroglia is attested in a number of reviews, monographies, and anthologies (Glees, 1955; Windle, 1958; De Robertis and Carrea, 1965; Kuffler and Nicholis, 1966; Kuf-fler, 1967; Lasansky, 1971; Watson, 1974; Somjen, 1975, 1981b; Orkand, 1977; Schoffeniels *et al.*, 1978; Varon and Somjen, 1979; Hertz, 1979; Treherne, 1981; Roitbak, 1983; Walz and Hertz, 1983a).

The topic of this chapter is the functional role of glial cells in the cortex of adult mammals. Defining its limits helps in reducing the material to manageable size. For this reason there will be no discussion of the myelination of central axons, nor of the repair of cerebral wounds or the role of embryonal glia in development. It would, however, be a mistake to avoid all reference to experiments on glial cells in tissues other than the adult cortex, because so many of the recent investigations have been carried out on systems considered to be "models" of the mammalian brain. Such "models" include the central nervous systems of lower vertebrates and of invertebrates, as well *in vitro* systems, such

GEORGE G. SOMJEN • Department of Physiology, Duke University, Durham, North Carolina, 27710.

as cultured cells and gradient-separated cell fractions. Moreover, the glial cells in parts of the mammalian nervous system other than the cortex deserve attention. The proper title of this chapter should therefore be, not "Physiology of Cortical Glia," but "Physiology *Relevant to* Cortical Glia."

Because of the limits just defined, this chapter will mainly deal with the functions of protoplasmic astrocytes. The interfascicular oligodendrocytes need not be considered, because their function has clearly been identified with the production of the myelin sheaths of axons (Bunge, 1968; Wood and Bunge, 1984). The status of del Rio Hortega's "type 1" oligodendrocyte (see Wood and Bunge, 1984), found near neuron somata and blood vessels in gray matter, is, however, somewhat uncertain (see also Peters *et al.,* 1970). To some authors it had seemed that the oligodendrocytes lying in the proximity of neuron somata are satellites living in symbiosis with their neuron neighbors. Among others, the work of Hydén and collaborators (e.g., Hamberger and Hydén, 1963; Hydén, 1973) is based on this premise. Wood and Bunge (1984), however, take the position that perineuronal oligodendrocytes are probably also myelin-forming cells that just happen to be near a neuron cell body. In cell cultures the membrane potential of oligodendrocytes was influenced by K^+ ions in a manner similar to that of astrocytes (Kettenmann *et al.,* 1983b; see also section 2.1). However, the one identified oligodendrocyte from which Kelly and Van Essen (1974) had obtained intracellular recordings differed from the astrocytes in that it did not respond to visual stimulation. There was, similarly, among the glial cells from which Picker *et al.* (1981) made intracellular recordings, one oligodendrocyte that, unlike the astrocytes, did not respond to electrical stimulation.

While much has been learned from "model" systems such as cell cultures or dissociated cells, such results should, whenever possible, be reconciled with observations of intact brains. For example, oligodendrocytes were seen to form electrically patent gap junctions in cell cultures, albeit less frequently than astrocytes (Kettenmann *et al.,* 1983a). By contrast, freeze-fracture studies of cat white matter revealed no gap junctions between oligodendrocytes, although many were found between astrocytes (Massa and Mugnaini, 1982). To be sure, no comparable study has as yet been published of oligodendrocytes in gray matter, and therefore their status is still unresolved.

In all, it must be said that, in spite of the rapidly accumulating body of data, unresolved questions of quite fundamental nature still outnumber those that have satisfactorily been answered. In fact, an even better title for this chapter could be "The *Suspected* Functions of Glial Cells in Cerebral Cortex."

2. The Electrophysiology of Cortical Glial Cells

2.1. Ion Distribution and Membrane Potential

The membrane potential of living cells is generated by a combination of (1) diffusion potentials augmented by the highly selective permeability of cell membranes for different ion species, and (2) active electrogenic transport of ions. In the case of neurons, the first of these two mechanisms dominates. Knowledge of the distribution of ions between cell interior and exterior is essential for an understanding of the potential across the membrane. Compared to the amount of attention paid to the electrophysiology of neurons, that of glial cells was largely neglected until the 1960s, apparently having been regarded as irrelevant, uninteresting, inaccessible, or all three. Interest in the ionic composition of glial cells was aroused at first not as a problem of electrophysiology, but in connection with the problem of the extracellular space of the brain.

The first electron micrographs made of brain tissue showed very little space between cellular elements. From these pictures it seemed that the interstitial space cannot occupy more than 3 to 5% of the total volume of the CNS. Cerebral tissue was, however, known to contain a substantial amount of Na and Cl, and the problem arose where these ions could be located, if there was no interstitium; hence the idea that glial cells contain a high concentration of Na^+ and should be viewed as part of the "functional" extracellular space of the brain (Gerschenfeld *et al.*, 1959; Katzman, 1961; Horstmann, 1962; Koch *et al.*, 1962; De Robertis 1965).

Measurements of cerebral extracellular space based on indicator distribution ("inulin space") or electric conductivity of the tissue yielded, however, values very different from those derived from electron micrographs. These methods showed the interstitium to occupy about 15% or slightly more of the total volume (Davson and Bradbury, 1956; Van Harreveld, 1966; Rall and Fenstermacher, 1971). Van Harreveld (1966) reconciled the two methodologies by making electron micrographs prepared from specimens fixed by freeze-dry substitution, instead of the conventional perfusion techniques. On electron micrographs prepared from rapidly frozen tissues, in which cells did not have a chance to swell due to anoxia in the agonal period, there appeared to be ample interstitial space between the cell membranes. The most recent measurement, based on the diffusion of nonpermeant ions in the cerebellar cortex, yielded a figure slightly in excess of 20% of the total volume (Nicholson and Phillips, 1981). In comparing values obtained by different investigators, it should be realized that the size of the interstitial space is smaller in white matter than in gray, and within the gray matter smaller in nuclear layers than in neuropil. Furthermore, it makes a difference whether an estimate includes the volume of intracerebral blood vessels, or is limited to the interstitium in the strict sense. But whichever of the more recent estimates is taken as the basis for calculations, it now is clear that most of the Na^+ and Cl^- has a place in the interstitial fluid of the brain, and the smaller fraction that still has to be accounted for is probably distributed approximately evenly among neurons and glial cells.

The K^+ content of leech glia has been analyzed by microchemical techniques (see Kuffler and Nicholls, 1966). Radiochemical methods have been used to estimate ion distributions in cultured glial ganglionic satellite cells (Brown and Shain, 1977). Direct measurement of intracellular free potassium concentration ($[K^+]_i$) became possible with the introduction of ion-selective electrodes with ultrafine tip diameter. In glial cells of leech (Schlue and Wuttke, 1983), frog (Buhrle and Sonnhoff, 1983), and olfactory cortex of guinea pig (Grafe *et al.*, 1987), high values of $[K^+]_i$ were found that were comparable to those of neurons.

It is in keeping with the high $[K^+]_i$ of glial cells that their membrane potential is similar to that of neurons, or even greater (Tasaki and Chang, 1958; Orkand *et al.*, 1966; Kuffler and Nicholls, 1966; Karahashi and Goldring, 1966; Krnjević and Schwartz, 1967; Kelly *et al.*, 1967). Moreover, the membrane potential is dependent on the extracellular concentration of potassium ($[K^+]_o$). According to Kuffler and his colleagues (Kuffler *et al.*, 1966; Orkand *et al.*, 1966; Kuffler and Nicholls, 1966; Kuffler, 1967), the dependence of the membrane potential on the concentration of K^+ ions was so strong that they compared the glial membrane to a "good K^+-electrode." By this they meant that the membrane potential closely followed the Nernst equation for potassium:

$$V_m = RT/F \ln ([K^+]_o/[K^+]_i)$$

which, at 37.5°C, works out to be, approximately:

$$V_m = 61 \log_{10} ([K^+]_o/[K^+]_i$$

where V_m is the membrane potential, $[K^+]_o$ and $[K^+]_i$ are the external and internal potassium concentrations, and R, T, and F have their usual meaning. Parenthetically, it should be pointed out that the use of concentrations instead of ion activities is valid only if the activity coefficient of K^+ is the same in the cytoplasm as it is in the extracellular fluid, an assumption that seems reasonable, but has never been experimentally proven. In perusing the literature, it should furthermore be borne in mind that, while ion-selective electrodes sense ion activity, they usually are calibrated in terms of concentration. Therefore, the numbers reported by most investigators refer to concentration, even if the title of the article mentions activity. There are, however, exceptions, because some workers prefer to calculate activity, based on an assumed activity coefficient; therefore, it is necessary to consult the small print of the Methods section of each paper to find the real meaning of the reported values.

As far as mammalian glial cells are concerned, it seemed at first that their membrane potential does not follow the Nernst equation as closely as does the membrane potential of leech and *Necturus* glial cells. Dennis and Gerschenfeld (1969) working on rat optic nerve *in vitro* and Pape and Katzman (1972) and Ransom and Goldring (1973a) recording from glial cells in cerebral cortex superfused with solutions of varying K^+ concentration found that the influence of changing $[K^+]_o$ on the glial membrane potential was less than predicted by the Nernst equation. Later, however, Lothman and Somjen (1975) found that the membrane potential of spinal glial cells does indeed resemble a good K^+-electrode (Fig. 1). Futamachi and Pedley (1976) found the same to be true for cortical glia, but only when the $[K^+]_o$ was steady or slowly changing. During fast transients the Nernst equation did not seem to hold. There were technical differences between these studies. Superfusing the cerebral cortical surface with a solution containing high $[K^+]$ sets up a gradient of concentration across the pia-glial membrane as well as within the tissue, and it also causes a change of the extracellular potential (e.g., see Gardner-Medwin, 1983a). If these two factors are ignored, the change of glial membrane potential will be underestimated and the change of $[K^+]_o$ overestimated, both resulting in a seemingly too low slope of the dependency of membrane potential on log $[K^+]_o$. In cultured astrocytes, Sugaya *et al.* (1979) confirmed the Nernstian dependence of membrane potential on $[K^+]$ in the bathing solution. Picker *et al.* (1981) examined glial cells *in vitro* in tissue slices cut from surgical specimens of human brains. Normal glial cells in these slices responded to changing $[K^+]_o$ as predicted by the Nernst equation, but reactive fibrillary astrocytes and glioma cells responded less, probably because of a higher permeability to Na^+ ions.

An assumption, stated or implied, in all these studies was that $[K^+]_i$ remains unchanged in the face of changing $[K^+]_o$. There have, however, been a number of studies showing uptake of K^+ ions into glial cells *in vitro* under the influence of raised $[K^+]_o$ (e.g., Bourke *et al.*, 1970; Hertz, 1978; Franck *et al.*, 1978). In some instances the influx of K^+ ions was accompanied by anions and water so that the concentration of K^+ in the cytoplasm was not expected to change; in others, K^+ seemed to have been exchanged for Na^+. Recent measurements of $[K^+]_i$ with intracellular ion-selective microelectrodes in the glial elements of the bee eye (Coles and Tsacopoulos, 1979), in glial cells of the leech (Schlue and Wuttke, 1983), in cultured mouse oligodendrocytes (Kettermann *et al.*, 1983b), and in glial cells in guinea pig olfactory cortex slices *in vitro* (Grafe *et al.*, 1987)

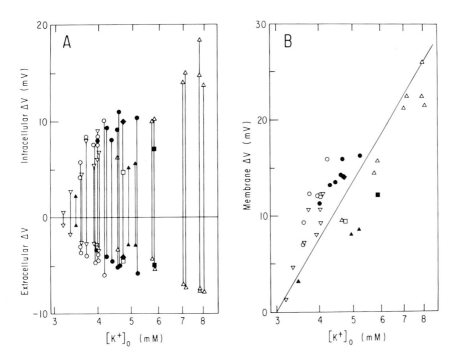

Figure 1. The correlation of the depolarization of glial cells and the concentration of potassium in the vicinity of the glial cell. (A) The potential shifts recorded inside and outside glial cells, referred to a distant ground electrode. Recordings made with an intracellular electrode, and a double-barreled ion-selective electrode fixed to lie about 50 μm proximal of the intracellular tip. Each symbol a different cell; each cell stimulated by different pulse trains applied to an afferent nerve. The vertical lines connect corresponding simultaneously made measurements. Measurements from recordings similar to those of Fig. 6A, except that $[K^+]_o$ was also recorded. (B) Transmembrane potential shift, calculated as the sum of intra- and extracellular potential shifts from data shown in A. The straight line shows the Nernst function of 37.5°C. Reproduced from Lothman and Somjen (1975) by permission.

suggest, however, that the internal concentration of K^+ is influenced by its external concentration. Walz and Hertz (1983a) come to the same conclusion concerning mouse astrocytes in primary culture, based on a comparison of the effects of changing external ion levels on membrane potential, and radiotracer flux measurements.

If $[K^+]_i$ changed under the influence of $[K^+]_o$, then glial cells could not behave as "perfect K^+-electrodes." In fact, Kettenmann *et al.* (1983b) report that the Nernst equation correctly defines the membrane potential of oligodendrocytes if and only if both $[K^+]_o$ and $[K^+]_i$ are taken into account. It is then puzzling that in other instances, entering changes of $[K^+]_o$ in the Nernst equation correctly predicted changes of the membrane potential of astrocytes. The disparate findings could be reconciled if the deviation from the Nernst function caused by changing $[K^+]_i$ was compensated for by an opposite effect. Such a spurious compensation could be supplied by electrogenic transport of cations, especially of Na^+, out of the cell. Whether or not glial ion pumps are stimulated by raised $[K^+]_o$, or whether they require raised $[Na^+]_i$ in order to be activated; and if they are activated, whether the pump is electrogenic, are other unresolved questions (Henn *et al.*, 1972; Ransom and Goldring, 1973c; Hertz, 1978; Tang *et al.*, 1980; Walz and Hertz, 1983a,b). Differences in findings may be due to differences in species, or in methodology. We shall return to some of these questions once more when discussing the role of glial cells cells in potassium homeostasis (Section 3).

Which of these findings will turn out to be most similar to the behavior of glial cells of the intact mammalian brain is not clear at present. It cannot be doubted, however, that astrocytes in the mammalian cortex are cells with high internal K^+ activity, and that their membrane sustains a strongly inside-negative potential that is greatly influenced by the $[K^+]_o$.

2.2. Ion Channels of Glial Membranes

Orkand (1977) estimated the relative permeability of squid axon membranes to a number of cations, and compared it to *Necturus* glial cell membranes. Since the neuronal and glial membranes appeared to pass cations in similar manner, he concluded that they might contain similar ion channels. Kettenmann (manuscript submitted) confirmed this relationship in cultured mammalian glial cells.

Somewhat surprisingly, the patch clamp technique also revealed that the K^+ channels of glial membranes are voltage dependent: whole-cell current (Bevan and Raff, 1985) as well as single channel opening probability (Kettenmann *et al.*, 1984c; Sonnhoff, 1987) increase with depolarization. Gardner-Medwin (1985) pointed out that, so far, the nonlinearity of the current–voltage relationship was detected only in cultured glial cells, and he raised the question as to why it has not been noticed in electrophysiological studies of glial cells *in situ*.

Several investigators asked whether glial membranes are significantly permeable to ions other than K^+. Many of these studies relied on changes of membrane potential caused by ion substitution in the bathing solution while several others used radiotracer flux measurements. Generally, normal glial membranes were not significantly permeable to any of the ions commonly found in biological fluids, other than K^+ (e.g., Wardell, 1966; Kuffler and Nicholls, 1966; Moonen and Nelson, 1978; Gibson, 1980; Kettenmann *et al.*, 1983b; Walz and Hertz, 1983a,b). Moreover, Tang *et al.* (1979) found no binding of saxitoxin to glial membranes, nor other evidence of the presence of significant numbers of Na^+ channels. Walz and Hertz (1983b) did find Na^+ and Cl^- flux into cultured astrocytes that could be blocked by furosemide but, since changing the concentration of these ions did not change the membrane potential significantly, they consider these fluxes minor compared to that of K^+.

Recently, however, Sonnhoff (1987) reported that the membrane of cultured astrocytes contains voltage-dependent Cl^- channels and Grafe *et al.* (1987) found that $[Cl^-]_i$ of glial cells increases if $[K^+]_o$ is elevated. It also became apparent that, under the influence of certain treatments, glial membranes can become permeable to Na^+ and to Ca^{2+} in a voltage-dependent manner. Bowman *et al.* (1984) report that cultured astrocytes treated with veratridine show Na^+-dependent and tetrodotoxin (TTX)-sensitive "anode break" excitation, somewhat reminiscent of nerve membranes. TTX-sensitive Na^+ conductance of cultured glial cells has also been demonstrated by Reiser *et al.* (1983), but only after treatment with a combination of both veratridine and scorpion toxin. MacVicar (1984) showed that after blocking the normal K^+ permeability of the glial membrane by tetraethyl ammonium, cultured glial cells generated Ca^{2+}-dependent action potentials, not unlike those fired by the dendritic membrane of some central neurons. These treatments bring out latent functional characteristics of the glial membrane that demonstrate that nerve and glial membranes are in some very basic sense related. Whether or not these latent functions ever become manifest in the course of the normal function of cortical glia or, what is more likely, during pathological conditions, remains to be seen.

2.3. Responses of the Membrane Potential of Glial Cells

Tasaki and Chang (1958) had reported that strong current pulses applied directly to the membrane of glial cells in cat cerebral cortex evoked slow action potential-like responses. Based on observations made on cultured glial cells, Wardell (1966) argued, however, that what Tasaki and Chang (1958) had seen was dielectric breakdown of the cell membrane and that glial cells are, essentially, electrically inexcitable. These conclusions of Wardell (1966) were not challenged until quite recently, as mentioned in the preceding section (see Bowman *et al.*, 1983; Reiser *et al.*, 1983; MacVicar, 1984).

Sugaya *et al.* reported in 1964 that what they called "idle" cells of the cerebral cortex were not completely inactive, but did show slow depolarizing shifts of the membrane potential during intense activation of the neurons that surround them. In this early report, the authors were uncertain whether their "idle cells" were glial elements, nonspiking neurons, or distal neuronal dendrites. The same uncertainty was expressed in a later paper by Karahashi and Goldring (1966). Figure 2 is reproduced from their paper. Similar recordings were obtained by Grossman and Hampton (1968) who proved that the "inexcitable cells" from which they were recording in fact were glia by marking the cell with dye ejected from the intracellular electrode and subsequently identifying the cell in stained histological sections.

At about the same time when these investigations on cortical glial cells were conducted, Kuffler and associates (Kuffler *et al.*, 1966; Orkand *et al.*, 1966; Kuffler and Nicholls, 1966; Kuffler, 1967) made their observations on glial cells of leech and *Necturus*. They found that repeated activation of neuronal elements is accompanied by depolarization of the glial cells among them. They also determined that the K^+ released from neurons mediated the effect. Krnjević and Schwartz (1967) observed that iontophoretically released K^+ causes depolarization of cortical "unresponsive" cells, and Kelly *et al.* (1967) proved by dye deposition that these "unresponsive" cells were glia.

The depolarizing responses of cortical glial cells mentioned so far were either evoked by electrical stimulation, or they were associated with seizure discharges (as also reported by Somjen, 1970; Ransom and Goldring, 1973b,c; Ransom, 1974). An indication that cortical glial cells respond also in conjunction with more normal, physiological activation came in a report by Kelly and Van Essen (1974). They recorded depolarization of glial cells in cat visual cortex during photic stimulation. The glial response had a receptive field, and was selective for stimulus orientation and stimulus movement, in the same manner as that of neurons found in the same column of cortical cells (Fig. 3). As the other investigators, Kelly and Van Essen (1974) also attributed the depolarization of the glial membrane to elevated $[K^+]_o$, caused by the release of K^+ ions from neurons.

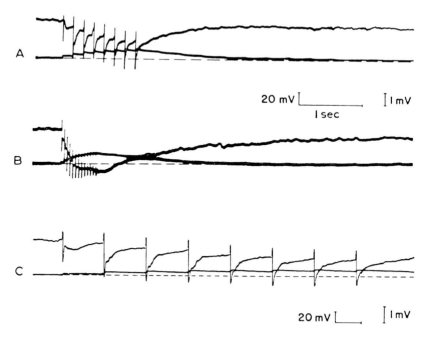

Figure 2. Responses of a cortical glial cell to direct stimulation of the cortical surface. In each recording (A–C) the upper trace is the cortical surface potential and the lower trace the intracellular potential of the glial cell. All tracings with positive plotted upward. The time calibration of C is 0.1 sec. Reproduced from Karahashi and Goldring (1966) by permission.

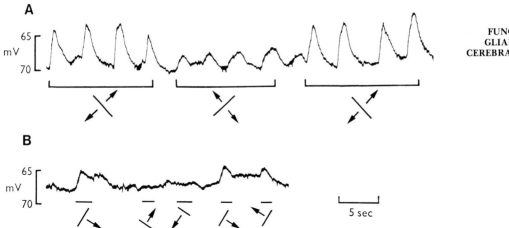

Figure 3. Visually evoked responses of glial cells. A and B are intracellular recordings made from two cells. The insets show the orientation and the direction of movement of the visual stimulus, which was a slit of light projected on a screen in front of the (anesthetized) cat's eye. Reproduced from Kelly and Van Essen (1974) by permission.

Realization that glial cell membranes undergo substantial potential changes raised the possibility that glia could contribute to the electric signals recorded from the surface of the cortex. Experiments designed to test this suggestion will be discussed in the next section.

2.4. Contribution by Glia to Electrocorticographic Signals

There were scattered early suggestions that glial cells might be responsible for the slowest of the potential changes that can be recorded from the cortex with DC coupled amplifiers (reviewed in Somjen, 1973). A precise theory, based on experiments, as to how glial tissue might add to surface potentials was proposed by Kuffler's group (Orkand *et al.*, 1966; Kuffler and Nicholls, 1966; Kuffler, 1967). These investigators found, besides the $[K^+]_o$-dependent depolarization of glial cells already described, that glial cells are electrically connected one to another. Because of these electrically patent junctions, if one glial cell is depolarized, it will inject current into all its neighbors. From a group of depolarized glial cells, electric charge will be displaced through chains of adjacent cells and the current so created must find a return path through the interstitial space among and around these cells. Current flowing in the extracellular volume conductor creates a gradient of extracellular potential (Figs. 4 and 5), and this might be picked up by extracellular electrodes. Cohen (1970) demonstrated that, in fact, the fraction of the glial depolarizations that can be recorded from the surface of a *Necturus* optic nerve *in vitro* is comparable to the fraction of nerve fiber action potentials similarly recorded. This work opened the possibility, but did not prove, that the slow potential responses that can be recorded from the cerebral cortex may in part or whole be generated by glial cells.

Repetitive stimulation of the cortical surface, or of an afferent fiber pathway of the cortex, evokes a sustained potential (SP) shift that can be recorded either from the surface of the brain or from the interstitial spaces. When glial depolarization and extracellular SP shifts are recorded simultaneously, the two have opposite polarity and remarkably similar (though not identical) time course (Karahashi and Goldring, 1966; Castellucci and Goldring, 1970; Sugaya *et al.*, 1971) (see also Fig. 2). In the spinal cord, Somjen (1970) found a close correlation between the amplitudes of the depolarizing responses of glial cells and the SP shifts recorded simultaneously near the cell. This correlation held when twin electrodes were moved through the tissue and the same stimulus was repeatedly delivered (Fig. 6), and also when the electrodes were held stationary and the stimulus parameters were varied. When depressant drugs were administered, extracellular SP shifts and depolarizing responses of spinal glial cells were depressed to the same degree (Strittmatter and Somjen, 1973).

If the agent mediating the influence of neuronal activity upon the glial membrane potential is potassium, then there should be a correlation between $\log [K^+]_o$ and glial depolarization. If, furthermore, SP shifts are of glial origin, then SP shifts should also be correlated with changes of $[K^+]_o$. This dual prediction could be tested after the introduction of K^+-selective microelectrodes into the instrumentation of neurophysiology laboratories. Krnjević and Morris (1972) and Vyklický *et al.* (1975) have remarked on the similarity of SP shifts and on the changes of $[K^+]_o$ induced in different parts of the central gray matter by stimulation of afferent pathways. Lothman and Somjen (1975) demonstrated the three-way correlation between changes of $[K^+]_o$, extracellular SP shift, and depolarization of glial cells, by recording all three variables simultaneously with

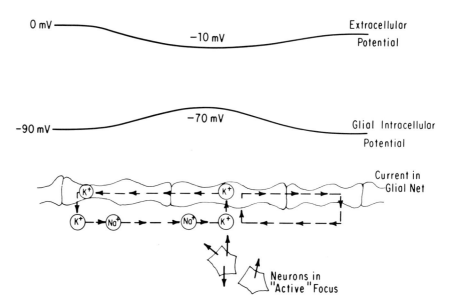

Figure 4. Diagrammatic representation of the current generated by an electrotonic network of glial cells, and the potential gradients associated with it. Near the center of the glial cells, neurons have released an excess of K^+ ions into the interstitial fluid. This causes depolarization of adjacent glial cells, which results in current flow. Compare the hypothetical profile of intra- and extracellular potentials with the experimental results represented in Fig. 6B. Reproduced from Somjen (1981b) by permission.

microelectrodes in cat spinal cord (Fig. 1). Figure 7 suggests that in cortex, as in spinal cord, there is a correlation of the spatial distribution ("laminar profile") of SP shifts and of $[K^+]_o$ responses evoked by various modes of stimulation (Cordingley and Somjen, 1978). Figure 8 demonstrates the closeness of this correlation, when the recording electrode is held stationary and the stimulus is varied.

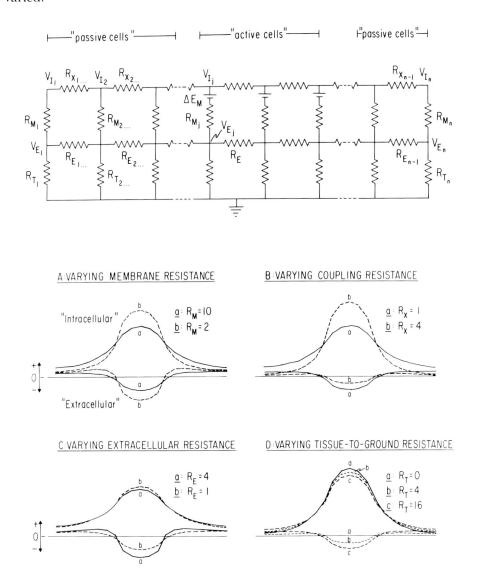

Figure 5. Computer simulation of the glial network represented in Fig. 4. The upper diagram is the electric equivalent circuit; the lower four diagrams (A–D) show the results of the computations. "Active cells" are those exposed to elevated $[K^+]_o$, that are depolarized by the excess K^+; "passive cells" those exposed to normal $[K^+]_o$ but depolarized by current injected from the active cells. V_I represents the intracellular potential of glial cells; R_X the resistance of the junctions coupling cells to one another; R_M the membrane resistances; V_E the extracellular potentials; R_E the extracellular resistances; R_T the resistance of the tissue to ground. A–D show how voltage profiles change when these parameters are altered one by one. Computation by R. Joyner; reproduced from Somjen (1973) by permission.

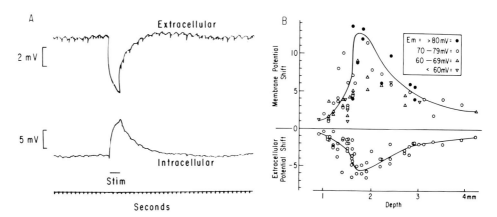

Figure 6. Distribution of glial responses and of sustained potential shifts evoked by trains of afferent stimuli in spinal cords of cats. (A) Sample recordings made with twin microelectrodes fastened so that the tips should lie not more than 50 μm apart. (B) Amplitude of the responses evoked by stimulating with identical trains of pulses numerous cells in seven cats. The abscissa shows the recording depth relative to the dorsal surface of the cord. Inset shows the resting potential of the cells. Reproduced from Somjen (1970) by permission.

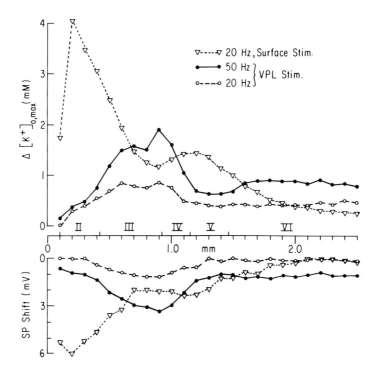

Figure 7. The amplitude of the sustained potential shifts and of the responses of extracellular potassium evoked in the cerebral cortex of a cat by trains of pulses applied directly to the cortical surface and to the VPL nucleus of the thalamus. The abscissa shows the depth from the cortical surface, and also the cytoarchitectonic layer. Reproduced from Cordingley and Somjen (1978) by permission.

Much that has been inferred about the behavior of glial cells is based on such extracellular measurements. If, during an experimental manipulation, the changes of $[K^+]_o$ and SP shifts are correlated both in spatial extension and in magnitude, then, on the basis of the experimental findings and theoretical reasoning just outlined, it can be assumed that glial cells have contributed a major fraction of the current generating the SP shift. It is clear, however, that in a tissue where neurons are active, neuronal responses must contribute to a variable degree to voltage changes recorded with extracellular electrodes. Thus, for example in Fig. 2, the upper traces of recordings A–C seem to be the composite of brief transients, attributable to neuronal responses, and a sustained shift of the potential "baseline" interpreted as probably mainly glial in origin. Sustained changes of membrane potential do, however, also occur in nerve cells. Depending on the details of cytoarchitectonics, and on the values of the tissue resistances represented schematically in Fig. 5, the relative contributions of glia and neurons to extracellular potentials may vary in different tissues and even in the same tissue under different circumstances.

Figure 8 shows that, for a given change of $[K^+]_o$, the SP shift is larger in spinal cord than in cortex. From this it seems that the influence of glial depolarization on extracellular potential is less in cortex than in spinal cord. Several theoretical reasons could be found to explain the difference and the available data are insufficient to choose between them. In spinal cord the administration of a barbiturate caused a depression of extracellular SP shifts and of glial depolarizations in equal proportion (Strittmatter and Somjen, 1973), but in cortex barbiturate caused an enhancement of SP shifts while it did depress both glial

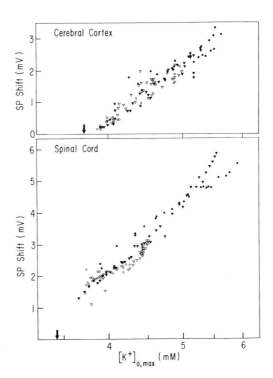

Figure 8. The correlation of the sustained potential shift and the responses of extracellular potassium concentration, recorded simultaneously, from a single site in the cortex, and from a single site in the spinal cord, in two different cats. Responses in cortex evoked by stimulating VPL nucleus of the thalamus; in the spinal dorsal horn by stimulating the dorsal root. Different symbols used to denote varying different stimulus parameters. Experiment by G. Cordingley; figure reproduced from Somjen (1978) by permission.

depolarization and responses of $[K^+]_o$ (Ransom *et al.*, 1977). Apparently, a nonglial potential that makes a contribution to the cortical SP shift is potentiated by this drug. GABA-mediated inhibitory potentials are known to be enhanced by some of the barbiturates. The mixed generation of cortical SP shifts associated with seizure discharges was emphasized by Heinemann *et al.* (1979). And, recently, we have found that SP shifts associated with paroxysmal discharges in the fascia dentata and in hippocampal cortex are independent of changes of $[K^+]_o$ and seem to be predominantly generated by depolarization of the somata of granule cells and of pyramidal cells (Somjen *et al.*, 1985).

In spite of these exceptions to the general rule, predictions of the theory of a substantial contribution by glial cells to the generation of SP shifts, schematically represented in Figs. 4 and 5, have thus been borne out by experimental observations. The one missing piece of information is the direct experimental demonstration of electrically conductive junctions between glial cells in the mammalian cortex. As already mentioned, such junctions have been shown to exist in neural tissues of lower forms (e.g., Kuffler and Nicholls, 1966; Cohen, 1970). Mammalian glial cells readily form electrically patent gap junctions in culture (Moonen and Nelson, 1978; Kettenmann *et al.*, 1983a). Immature cells are insulated one from another when they are first placed in the culture dish, but they become coupled as they mature (Fischer and Kettenmann, 1985). Dennis and Gerschenfeld (1969) failed to demonstrate electric coupling between oligodendrocytes of rat optic nerve, but attribute their failure to technical difficulty. Gap junctions between astrocytes can be seen on electron micrographs of cortical tissue (Brightman and Reese, 1969; Landis and Reese, 1981; Massa and Mugnaini, 1982). In surviving isolated tissue slices cut from cerebral cortex, Gutnick *et al.* (1981) demonstrated the passage of intracellularly injected dyes from one astrocyte to its neighbors. Connors *et al.* (1984) have also shown that this so-called "dye-coupling" is abolished when the tissue slices are made acidotic by exposure to a high concentration of CO_2. In other tissues it has been found that the conductance of intercellular electric junctions is a function of the prevailing pH (Spray *et al.*, 1981). All these observations taken together make it quite plausible that astrocytes in cerebral cortex are electrically interconnected. Measurement of the glial junctional conductance would, nevertheless, be necessary in order to estimate the contribution of glial depolarization to extracellular current flow (see Fig. 5 and Somjen, 1973).

3. Neuroglia and Ion Homeostasis

The two main extracellular fluids of the CNS are the cerebrospinal fluid (CSF) and the interstitial fluid of the tissue. The two are separated from the blood plasma, and therefore also from all the other extracellular fluids of the body, by two systems of insulation known as the blood–brain and blood–CSF barriers. In the choroid plexus the specialized ependymal cells that secrete the CSF are joined by complete seams of tight junctions, and these are considered to be the structure that forms the blood–CSF barrier (Bradbury, 1979; see also

Fig. 9A). If it is accepted that ependymal cells are a species of glia, then the blood–CSF barrier is formed by specialized glial cells.

Golgi was the first to call attention to the glial endfeet that are found around cerebral capillaries, and also to the fact that parts of neurons are almost never near blood vessels. Golgi had thought that nutrients are extracted by glial endfeet from the bloodstream, transported through glial processes, and then supplied to neurons. Lugaro (1907) interpreted the relationship of glia to capillaries differently. He suggested that glial endfeet form a sieve that filters and processes the materials that are exchanged between blood and cerebral tissue. More in general, it was Lugaro's idea that glia keeps the interstitial fluid fit for neurons to live in and to function properly. How this idea came to be elaborated into the theory that pericapillary glia is the blood–brain barrier, and how that theory came to be refuted, has been reviewed repeatedly (e.g., Katzman and Pappius, 1973; Bradbury, 1979) and will not be discussed here. It is interesting to note that, nevertheless, the idea is not without merit. In some classes of animals, for example in elasmobranch fish, glial cells indeed form the blood–brain barrier (Bundgaard and Cserr, 1981). In mammals, however, the capillary wall itself is the barrier. In the CNS of mammals and of most other vertebrates, the endothelium of the capillaries in brain has a fine structure different from capillaries elsewhere (Bradbury, 1979). One specialized feature is the presence of tight

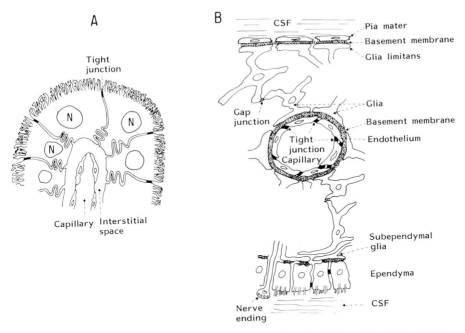

Figure 9. Schematic representation of the cell layers separating the fluids of the CNS. (A) The specialized ependyma investing the choroid villi. Note the tight junctions between the ependymal cells. The interstitial fluid of the choroid plexus is not different from interstitial fluid elsewhere in the body. (B) The relationship of glial cells to pia mater, cerebral capillaries, and the ependyma lining the cerebral ventricles. Note tight junctions between capillary endothelial cells. Reproduced from Somjen (1983) by permission.

junctions, which join endothelial cells of CNS capillaries, and seal the gaps between them. Another is the unusual abundance of mitochondria and of transport enzymes such as Na^+, K^+-activated ATPase in these endothelial cells, consonant with their supposed functions in transporting solutes.

Even though the blood–brain barrier itself is formed by the capillary endothelium, it is noteworthy that glial endfeet are an ever-present feature not only around capillaries but also at the interfaces between CNS parenchyma and CSF (Fig. 9B), and that neuronal elements are rare at these boundary layers. This does seem to confirm that glial cells may have a special role in blood–brain as well as in brain–CSF exchanges. Glial cells seem to be the ones that get first chance to sample all material that enters the parenchyma of the CNS, and also to exert some control over that which leaves the CNS. Landis and Reese (1981) described a specialized structure in the glial membrane that could possibly be related to such specialized transport function. In electron micrographs of freeze-fractured cerebral tissue samples, they found that the plasma membrane of astrocytes contains orthogonal "assemblies" of intramembrane particles, but only in the surfaces that face either capillaries or the subependymal and subpial basement membranes. These unusual particle aggregates are readily distinguishable from the ones believed to represent gap junctions. The particle arrays of gap junction are numerous in glial membranes within the brain parenchyma as well as at the cerebral surface, wherever astrocytes face one another. While the gap junctions are believed to be functional connections between glial cells, the newly discovered orthogonal arrays may represent a submicroscopic organelle that moves material in or out of the pericapillary, subependymal, and subpial spaces (see also Somjen, 1981a).

3.1. The Role of Glial Cells in the Regulation of Potassium Levels

It is well known that the concentration of K^+ in the CSF and in the interstitial fluid of the CNS is about 3.0 mM, about 50% lower than in blood plasma and the other extracellular fluids of the mammalian organism (reviewed in Katzman and Pappius, 1973; Somjen, 1979; Varon and Somjen, 1979). There is good evidence that K^+ ions are actively transported from CSF and from the cerebral interstitium into blood, and this transport is credited with keeping cerebral $[K^+]_o$ below the body average (Bradbury, 1979). The reason for this difference between the somatic and the cerebral *milieu interieur* is not unequivocally known, but evidence is accumulating that the 3.0 mM level of $[K^+]_o$ represents an optimum for the functioning of central synapses (e.g., King and Somjen, 1981; Somjen, 1984a; Balestrino *et al.*, 1986).

Transport of K^+ ions from CNS into blood plasma may take care of the overall long-term regulation of $[K^+]_o$ in brain, but each time a neuron is activated it releases some K^+ into the restricted volume of the interstitial fluid. Neuronal activity can thus perturb $[K^+]_o$, on a time scale of milliseconds to seconds, and such transient fluctuations of $[K^+]_o$ probably cannot be compensated by transport of K^+ between CNS and blood. K^+ ions that have been lost from neurons must, in time, be restored to the cells that lost them, or the brain could not continue to function for very long. Measurements made with ion-selective microelectrodes show, clearly, however, that when neuron assemblies are activated, $[K^+]_o$ does rise transiently (see Section 2.3 and reviews by Somjen, 1979; Varon and Somjen, 1979; Syková, 1983; Walz and Hertz, 1983a). It is during these transient periods, while the neuronal ion pumps cannot quite keep pace with ion displacements, that glial cells might keep the rising tide of $[K^+]_o$ within the bounds compatible with normal neuronal function. There are several ways in which glial tissue might perform its function.

Ranck (1964; see also in: Galambos, 1964) had first formulated a detailed theory of the manner in which glial cells may regulate interstitial $[K^+]$. His scheme, called the *"glial potassium sponge,"* was based on the notion that astrocytes contain high $[Na^+]_i$ (Gerschenfeld *et al.,* 1959; Katzman, 1961; Koch *et al.,* 1962; De Robertis, 1965; see also Section 2.1). Ranck's (1964) own work and that of Van Harreveld (1966) indicated that glial cells swell at the expense of the interstitial space during spreading depression, a condition in which K^+ is released from cells (Grafstein, 1956; Brinley *et al.,* 1960). Ranck suggested that glial cells take up and temporarily sequester the K^+ released by activated neurons. If, as Ranck believed, glial cells contain unusually large amounts of Na^+, then excess K^+ could be taken up from interstitial fluid in exchange for Na^+. Ranck also thought that additional K^+ ions are taken up in cotransport with Cl^-. Such cotransport would have to be accompanied by the uptake of water to maintain osmotic balance and hence it would lead to the swelling of glial cells at the expense of interstitial space.

With the discovery that glial cells do not contain unusually high $[Na^+]_i$, Ranck's "glial sponge" theory lost favor, and then was replaced by the *"spatial buffer"* or *spatial dispersal* theory. Kuffler and associates (Orkand *et al.,* 1966; Kuffler, 1967) suggested that whenever one part of an electronic network of glial cells is exposed to high $[K^+]_o$ and another region is not, a net displacement of K^+ must occur (Fig. 4). The force driving the ion current is the potential gradient that is created by the depolarization of glial cells in high-$[K^+]_o$ neighborhoods. Since the glial membrane allows the passage of K^+ but of no other ion, both the inward membrane current responsible for depolarization at the site of high $[K^+]_o$, and the corresponding outward current at the site of normal $[K^+]_o$ must be carried by K^+ ions. As a result, $[K^+]_o$ will be lowered where it initially had been high, and it will be raised somewhat where it had been normal. Kuffler (1967) believed, however, that the current generated in such glial nets is weak and therefore the amount of ions dispersed by it small. This conclusion was based on his estimate of the specific membrane resistance of glial cells, which, in the leech, was found to be quite high.

In contrast to the sparing permeability of leech glia, Trachtenberg and Pollen (1970) found the specific membrane resistance of mammalian glial cells to be lower than that of neurons (see also Trachtenberg *et al.,* 1972; and tabulation of other published values in Somjen, 1975). According to Trachtenberg and Pollen (1970) the displacement of K^+ ions through the network of glial cells, from areas of high $[K^+]_o$ to low, is one of the main mechanisms regulating $[K^+]_o$ in the mammalian CNS. While the magnitude of transglial migration of K^+ ions has still not precisely been determined, calculations suggest that it is not negligible (Somjen, 1981c; Gardner-Medwin, 1983b). The nonlinear behavior of K^+ channels (mentioned earlier; see Bevan and Raff, 1985; Kettenmann *et al.,* 1984c) may have a functional role here: increasing $[K^+]_o$ depolarizes glial cells, causing more K^+ channels to open, thus favoring their dispersal by way of the glial network. But, as Gardner-Medwin (1985) pointed out, if the threshold for channel opening is a depolarization of 40 mV, it would operate only under pathological conditions and have no role in the normal functioning of the tissue.

There are also new experimental data confirming that transglial displacement of K^+ ions is actually taking place. Gardner-Medwin (1983a) and Gardner-Medwin and Nicholson (1983) have shown that if an electric potential gradient is imposed upon cortical tissue, it drives a current of which a substantial fraction is carried by K^+ ions. So much K^+ could not have migrated, unless a substantial part of the current has passed through cells instead of flowing through interstitial spaces. In a detailed theoretical treatment, Gardner-Medwin (1983b) comes to two important conclusions. The first is that no matter whether driven by a chemical or by an electric potential gradient, migrating K^+ ions will pass through cell membranes. The second point is that glial cells need not necessarily be joined by electrically conductive junctions in order to disperse K^+ ions. For the dispersal mechanism to work, it is sufficient that (1) the processes of individual glial cells should be long enough so that each be exposed to a significant gradient of $[K^+]_o$, and (2) that processes of successive glial cells should be closely apposed.

Other experimental data come not from cortical glia, but from Müller cells of retinas maintained *in vitro*. Müller cells are glial elements that span virtually the entire thickness of the retina and that have endfeet abutting the vitreous. Using live cells separated by microdissection from the retinas of amphibia, Newman (1984) and Newman *et al.* (1984) have demonstrated that K^+ deposited by microiontophoresis anywhere along a Müller cell is taken up by the cell, and then released preferentially from the terminal that normally faces the vitreous. They also have shown that the properties of the membrane of the Müller cell are not uniform over the entire cell surface. The membrane has a much lower resistance at the endfoot than elsewhere. These experiments support the idea that whenever $[K^+]_o$ rises in the retinal interstitium, Müller cells channel the excess toward the vitreous where excess K^+ can do no harm. In the mouse the membrane of Müller cells differs from that in amphibia in that specialized points of high K^+ permeability exist not only at the vitreal endfeet but also at the endings of processes that, *in situ*, would lie near capillaries (Newman, 1987). These findings may be viewed in conjunction with the discovery of structural membrane specializations at the astrocytic endfeet around capillaries and near the cerebral surfaces (Landis and Reese, 1981; see preceding section and refer to Fig. 9). It does not seem farfetched to suggest for astrocytes a function similar to that of Müller cells. Astroglia might channel excess K^+ ions from the cerebral interstitium toward the CSF through the pial and the ependymal surfaces, or toward the bloodstream by releasing the excess in pericapillary spaces (see also Somjen, 1981a).

Schemes such as the one illustrated in Fig. 4 consider only the movements of K^+ and Na^+. A more complete accounting for the dislocations of various ions caused by accumulating K^+ has been given by Dietzel *et al.* (1980, 1982) that is reproduced in Fig. 10. They argue that, under the influence of a potential gradient in interstitial fluid, not only cations, but also anions will be moving.

Since only the cation K^+ is believed to cross the glial membrane, a net osmotic imbalance will be created and this will cause water to flow as well. Thus, cells should swell at the expense of the interstitial space where $[K^+]_o$ is high, whereas cells should shrink in the zone of normal $[K^+]_o$ that surrounds the active focus. The shrinking of cells in the surround should be less noticeable than their swelling in the focus, because the former occurs in a much larger volume of tissue than the latter. Dietzel *et al.* (1980, 1982) obtained experimental evidence of changes in interstitial volume in conjunction with ion concentration changes in areas of intense neuronal activity.

Granted that of the K^+ ions released by neurons, some find their way into glial cells, but how important, for the functioning of neurons, is this glial uptake? Grossman and Seregin (1977) attempted to answer this question by, essentially, reversing the process. Injection of Na^+ ions into the cytoplasm of a glial cell is expected to cause the release of K^+ ions from the cell. In the experiments of Grossman and Seregin (1977), such intracellular injection of Na^+ into glial cells did indeed cause excitation of neurons lying nearby.

Both the glial sponge and the glial dispersion theories postulated passive mechanisms by which K^+ would flow downhill along electrochemical gradients created as a by-product of neuronal excitation. There have, however, also been suggestions that energy-demanding active transport by the glial membrane may

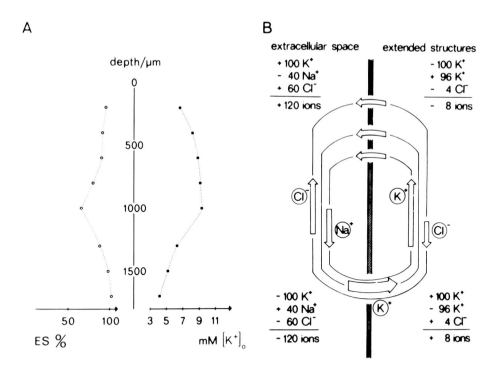

Figure 10. The movement of ions, and the changes of the interstitial space, evoked by afferent stimulation in the cerebral cortex. (A) Experimental data; (B) calculated changes, and direction and relative magnitude of ion movements. The "extended structures" are probably glial cells. Reproduced from Dietzel *et al.* (1982) by permission.

play a part in $[K^+]_o$ regulation (Hertz, 1966, 1978; Henn *et al.*, 1972; review by Walz and Hertz, 1983a). There is of course no disputing the fact that glial cells actively accumulate K^+ ions against a concentration gradient. The outstanding question is whether the K^+ transport is used for purposes other than maintaining the status quo of a high $[K^+]_i$ in the glial cells themselves. As with the passive processes, there are, in principle, two ways in which glial tissue could temporarily relieve a flood of K^+ ions. It could boost the dispersal of K^+, by assisting and accelerating the already discussed passive dispersal process, utilizing metabolic energy to do so. Alternatively, glial cells could take up K^+ ions and temporarily store them; this would be a variant on the glial sponge theory, differing from it by postulating an energy-consuming active mechanism. Uptake into glial cells would have obvious limits: if the influx of K^+ would be balanced by an outflux of Na^+, then the process would come to an end when the intracellular store of Na^+ was exhausted. If entering K^+ ions would take with them Cl^-, then water would have to accompany these ions and this would be limited by the swelling of the cell.

That K^+ is actually taken up by glial cells has been shown by Coles and Tsacapoulos (1979) who measured $[K^+]_i$ in cells of the retina of the honeybee. The increase of $[K^+]_i$ in such glial cells during photic stimulation could only in small part be accounted for by exchange for Na^+, and therefore an additional uptake mechanism must exist (Coles and Orkand, 1985). For mammalian glial cells, Bourke *et al.* (1970; see also Kimelberg, 1979, 1981; Kimelberg and Bourke, 1982) have shown two different uptake mechanisms of K^+ and Cl^-, one with and one without swelling of the cells. These processes may, however, be initiated only at pathologically high $[K^+]_o$, and not be part of physiological regulation (Kimelberg, 1979). There have been numerous other attempts to determine whether moderately elevated $[K^+]_o$ leads to accelerated active transport of K^+ ions by glial cells. The results of these experiments differed, depending on the "model" system used and perhaps also on the experimental protocol (e.g., Hertz, 1966, 1978; Orkand *et al.*, 1973; Coles and Tsacopoulos, 1979; Walz and Hertz, 1982; Tang *et al.*, 1980; review by Walz and Hertz, 1983a). As far as the intact mammalian cortex is concerned, the matter cannot be considered to be decided.

3.2. Glia and pH

There are slightly more free protons in the extracellular fluids of the brain than in those of the remainder of the body, resulting in a pH between 7.3 and 7.35 for CSF and for the cortical interstitium (Katzman and Pappius, 1973; Mutch and Hansen, 1984). The relative acidity is associated with a lower $[HCO_3^-]_o$. The excess of H^+ may be the product of the cerebral cellular metabolism, which could set up a gradient from cells to ISF, then to CSF and to blood. Intracellular pH of glial cells and neurons of leach has been measured by Schlue and Deitmer (1987). The pH_i of these cells was found more acid than that of the surrounding fluid, but not acid enough to be explained by a passive distribution of H^+ across the cell membrane. The authors suggest that a dual active regulation maintains pH_i of glial cells and neurons. Active transport of HCO_3^- and of H^+ across the blood–brain barrier may be a factor also in the regulation of pH_o of the mammalian brain (Held *et al.*, 1964; Katzman and Pappius, 1973; Kimelberg and Bourke, 1982; Mutch and Hansen, 1984). As with K^+, the average, steady-state, long-term level of pH is presumably maintained by the active transports across the blood–CSF and blood–brain barriers, but transient changes due to localized activation of neuronal metabolism (Urbanics *et al.*, 1978; Kraig *et al.*, 1983; Somjen, 1984b) must be buffered by cerebral tissue elements. As with K^+, there is good reason to believe these cellular elements are glial.

Giacobini established in 1962 that most or all of the carbonic anhydrase in cerebral tissue is contained in glial cells. Since this enzyme is usually associated with pH regulation in other tissues, it is natural to assume that it has this function in the CNS as well. If so, then CO_2 produced by neurons that found its way into glial cells would there be hydrated to carbonic acid, which then dissociated into HCO_3^- and H^+ ions. In erythrocytes this reaction is followed by an exchange of HCO_3^- against Cl^- across the cell membrane: the so-called chloride shift. In erythrocytes much of the H^+ formed in the reaction is buffered by hemoglobin. What buffers, besides the carbonic acid/bicarbonate system, are available in brain cells is not known. It is at least possible that transport through the network of glial cells toward capillaries is a method of getting rid of an excess of either ion. The available data, many derived from observations made on *in vitro* models, do not permit the formulation of a definitive, quantitative, theory. The literature has been reviewed by Kimelberg and Bourke (1982) and Fig. 11 is borrowed from their article.

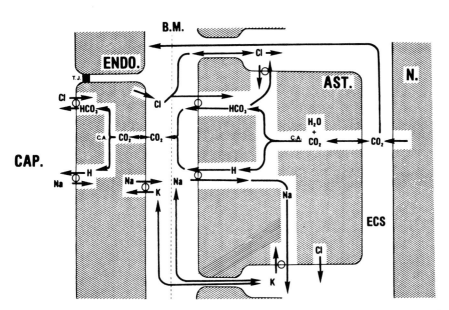

Figure 11. Hypothetical scheme of the transport systems in endothelial cells and astrocytes, moving ions and regulating pH. CAP., capillary; T.J., tight junction; ENDO., endothelial cell; C.A., carbonic anhydrase; B.M., basement membrane; AST., astrocyte; ECS, interstitial space; N., neuron. Reproduced from Kimelberg and Bourke (1982) by permission.

4. Glia and Transmitter Substances

Lugaro wrote in 1907 that glial processes around "neural articulation" (read: synapses) could serve to remove and to break down the chemical substances that transmit excitation from one nerve cell to another. Considering the date it was made, this is a most remarkable proposition indeed. Peters and Palay (1965; also Peters *et al.,* 1970) described the glial envelopes that surround presynaptic terminals. They suggested that the glial septa are barriers that prevent the spilling of transmitter substance into the surrounding interstitial fluid. A barrier to the dispersal of transmitter released at synaptic sites could solve two problems at once: it could prevent transmitter from acting on receptors at sites outside the one synapse where it was released, and by the same token it would favor the buildup of a sufficient concentration at the target site.

During the last decade or two, the hypothetical possibility of a functional relationship between neuroglia and transmitter substances has been discussed from these and also from other points of view. Several sets of fact support such a relationship, at least in a general sense. Glial receptors have been described that specifically bind transmitters, and the glial membrane potential was found to respond to certain transmitters. Glial cells appear to be able to accumulate some transmitters by high-affinity uptake systems, and they contain certain enzyme systems that either make or break transmitter molecules. These observations have been taken to confirm that glial cells have a role in terminating synaptic action by removing spent transmitter, as well as acting as scavengers of neuroactive substances outside synaptic sites, guarding the purity of interstitial fluid. But, in addition, the same observations also resulted in a revival of Nageotte's (1910) belief that glia is an endocrine organ. In the contemporary version, this hypothesis predicts that glial cells not only remove neuroactive agents from the extracellular medium, but also release them and so influence neuronal activity in their neighborhood. Finally, there also are modern revisions of Golgi's theory that glia and neurons live in symbiosis, complementing one another's biochemical processes.

4.1. Amino Acid Transmitters

4.1.1. The Glutamine/Glutamate/GABA System

In 1969 Van den Berg *et al.* measured the incorporation of radioactive label from different precursors into glutamine and glutamate in brain tissue. They came to the conclusion that there are two "pools" of glutamate in cerebral tissues: a smaller one, in contact with a fast-turning tricarboxylic acid cycle that accepts acetate as well as glucose as substrate and produces glutamine as well as glutamate; and a larger pool, in contact with a slow-turning tricarboxylic acid cycle utilizing glucose only, which produces glutamate that then can be turned into GABA. A theoretical model incorporating various components of these two interacting systems, and taking account of the experimentally determined concentrations and conversion rates of component compounds, has been proposed by Van den Berg and Garfinkel (1971).

Shortly thereafter, Benjamin and Quastel (1972) examined the pharmacology of the release of glutamate and glutamine from cerebral tissue slices. They assumed that if the release of a substance can be accelerated by protovertarine and suppressed by tetrodoxin (TTX), then it is the product of neurons; whereas the source of a compound the release of which is unaffected by these drugs is most probably mainly glia. After experiments in which these agents were applied singly and in combination with others, they came to the conclusion that glutamine is principally released from glial cells. Glutamate, on the other hand, seemed to seep from both neurons and glia, but its major pool was in neurons and the small pool in glial cells. Benjamin and Quastel (1972) proposed

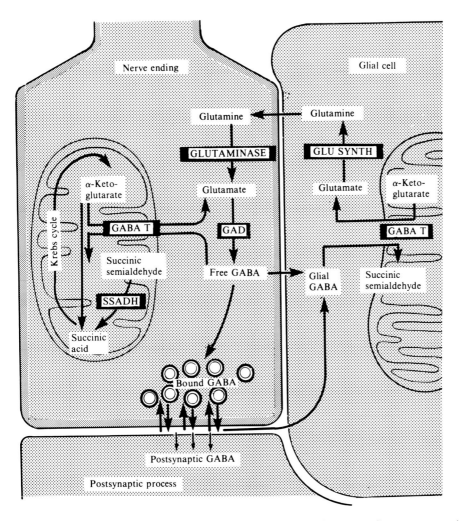

Figure 12. Schematic diagram showing the relationship of a GABAergic nerve ending, a postsynaptic neuron process, and a perisynaptic glial process. Enzymes are shown in black rectangles, intermediates in white. Reproduced from McGeer and McGeer (1981) by permission.

that glutamate released from neurons is taken up by glial cells and converted into glutamine, which is made available to neurons again. The neurons then recycle the glutamine into gutamate and reuse it as transmitter. A number of reports support this scheme, or some modification thereof (e.g., Hamberger *et al.*, 1979a,b; Norenberg and Martinez-Hernandez, 1979; Turský *et al.*, 1979; Ramaharobandro *et al.*, 1982).

A synthetic summary of the conclusions of various investigators is presented in Fig. 12, taken from McGeer and McGeer (1981). It should be noted that perisynaptic astrocytes are supposed to serve the needs of both glutaminergic excitatory and GABAergic inhibitory nerve endings. The presence or absence

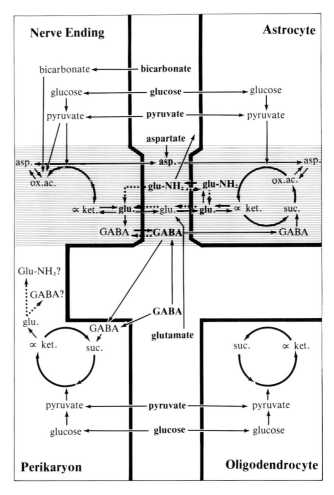

Figure 13. Hypothetical scheme of the biochemical interaction between neurons and glial cells. The shaded area indicates the "small compartment" of glutamate, which is assumed to be shared by astrocyte and presynaptic nerve terminal. The perisomatic oligodendrocyte is not believed to be directly interacting with the neuron; the perisynaptic astrocyte is. glu-NH$_2$, glutamine; glu., glutamate; asp., aspartate; ox. ac., oxaloacetate. Reproduced from Hertz (1979) by permission.

of glutamic acid decarboxylase (GAD) determines whether a presynaptic terminal manufactures excitatory or inhibitory transmitter. In both cases the spent transmitter is believed to be taken up by the perisynaptic glia for reprocessing into glutamine.

A different synthesis has been presented by Hertz (1979), and is reprinted in Fig. 13. His diagram shows cell body and synaptic ending of a neuron as separate systems, each with its own, different, satellite glial cell. The axon is shown as being mainly a passive conveyor of material between soma and synaptic terminal. Van den Berg and colleagues' (1969) "large pool" is shown as located in the neuron soma, while the "small pool" is shown as being a shared function of the axon terminal and its perisynaptic astrocyte.

The picture is further clouded by the fact that ammonia can be utilized to aminate intermediates of the tricarboxylic acid cycle. Ammonia is a toxic product of metabolism. It has been suggested that its detoxification is one of the principal functions of the tricarboxylic acid of glial cells (Norenberg and Martinez-Hernandez, 1979).

4.1.2. The Role of Neuroglia in Regulating GABA Levels

In 1972 Neal and Iversen reported that GABA administered from an external source is taken up, in the retina, preferentially by Müller (glial) cells, not by the neuronal elements or the photoreceptors. Similarly, in sympathetic ganglia and also in sensory dorsal root ganglia, the satellite glial cells accumulate GABA by preference (Bowery and Brown, 1972; Schon and Kelly, 1974, 1975). The affinity constant of the uptake process was comparable to that determined for GABAergic nerve terminals elsewhere in the CNS, but the rate constant was slower (Iverson and Kelly, 1975). The glial uptake process was Na^+-dependent, and selectively inhibited by β-alanine. Kelly and Dick (1978) surveyed electron microscopic autoradiograms statistically and demonstrated that glial cells (both astrocytes and oligodendrocytes) of the cerebral and of the cerebellar cortex accumulated more of microinjected β-alanine than could be expected by chance. If we accept β-alanine to be a marker of glial GABA transport, then this demonstrates that glial cells in the central gray matter also are capable of accumulating GABA (see also discussion in Varon and Somjen, 1979).

That glial cells can release the GABA that they have accumulated was also shown in several *in vitro* systems. Raising $[K^+]$ in the solution bathing a dorsal root ganglion to between 15 and 64 mM causes the dose-dependent release of GABA from previously loaded satellite cells (Minchin and Iversen, 1974), and a similar effect was noted in retinal Müller cells (Sarthry, 1983). In both tissues the release was Ca^{2+}-dependent. Vargas *et al.* (1977) found, however, that the release of transmitters from glial cells of the filum terminale of the spinal cord, under the influence of high $[K^+]_o$, was Ca^{2+}-independent. Bowery *et al.* (1975) used β-alanine or other competing substances to block the influx of GABA into satellite cells of the sympathetic ganglion. The consequent increase of the net outflow of endogenous GABA was sufficient to cause a depolarization of the neurons in the ganglion. This experiment shows that even without preloading there is enough GABA in satellite cells to influence neuronal function, if the cells are provoked to discharge their content. Not answered by any of the foregoing experiments is the question whether in normal tissue physiologic stimuli ever act to cause such release.

It is thus a well-documented fact that glial elements can make GABA, they can take it up from their environment, and they also can release it. GABA is, however, not only a neurotransmitter, but also an intermediate in metabolic processes, and it therefore need not necessarily be utilized in relation to neuronal signaling. One fact that especially gives reason to pause is the accumulation of GABA in the glial cells of ganglia and of some parts of the CNS that do not contain any GABAergic synapses. In places where there are no GABAergic synapses, the GABA-uptake system of glial cells could neither regulate nor support synaptic transmission. An alternative function has been suggested by Bowery *et al.* (1979). They noticed that for glial cells to accumulate GABA, the concentrations of GABA must exceed 10^{-6} M. Below that level, glial cells release more GABA than they take up; above the critical concentration, uptake exceeds outflow. This critical level is lower than what is found in rat plasma, which normally contains 10^{-5} M. Very similar results have been obtained by Schrier and Thompson (1974) in experiments on cultured glioma cells. According to both Schrier and Thompson (1974) and Bowery *et al.* (1979), the uptake system of satellite glial cells might regulate the GABA concentration in the interstitial fluid. For the neurons to function optimally, the concentration of GABA may have to be kept below that in blood, but above a certain minimal level.

In a review of the mechanism of clearing GABA from the CNS interstitium, Lodge *et al.* (1978) distinguished high-affinity and low-affinity uptake systems. They argued that in order to be of use at synapses, uptake should reach maximal velocity only at relatively high concentration. During synaptic transmission the concentration of transmitter in the synaptic cleft is probably quite high and an uptake system adapted to low substrate concentrations would therefore saturate before it could do its job. The uptake systems that regulate GABA concentration in the interstitial spaces should, on the other hand, be maximally effective at the low concentrations expected outside synaptic regions. In a study of enkephalin-degrading peptidases, Horsthemke *et al.* (1983) also concluded that glial cells serve to remove neuroactive peptides from interstitial fluid outside synaptic regions and not to terminate enkaphalinergic transmission at synapses.

One way to test whether the active uptake of GABA into either nerve endings or glial cells actually influences the effectiveness of applied GABA is to compare the effect of GABA in the absence and in the presence of uptake blockers. In sympathetic ganglia Brown and Galvan (1977) and in dorsal root ganglia Gallagher *et al.* (1983) found that blocking glial uptake of GABA enhances the depolarization of neurons by applied doses of GABA. Using a slightly modified technical approach, Desarmenien *et al.* (1980) obtained negative effects: uptake blockers did not alter the effectiveness of applied GABA. In central gray matter this type of experimental approach is complicated by the fact that GABAergic neurons mingle with glial cells, and both accumulate GABA actively. To distinguish between the two systems in the olfactory cortex, Brown *et al.* (1980) used several selective blockers. They found that only those that selectively blocked neuronal uptake had any effect; those working mainly on glial cells had none.

They concluded that the glial uptake system had no function in regulating GABA levels in this tissue.

4.1.3. Effects of GABA and Glutamate on the Membrane of Glial Cells

Krnjević and Schwartz (1967) applied both glutamate and GABA iontophoretically to glial cells in the cerebral cortex. They found no effect by the former, but GABA caused depolarization of some but not all the cells they tested. Krnjević and Schwartz (1967) pointed out that these effects could have been indirectly mediated through an action of the drugs on neighboring neurons. Based on experiments on cell cultures, Hösli *et al.* (1977, 1981) concluded that membrane responses of glial cells to GABA and excitatory amino acids are caused indirectly, by the K^+ ions released by neurons coexisting with glial cells in the culture dish. More recently, however, Kettenmann *et al.* (1984a,b) have shown that aspartate, glutamate, and GABA can depolarize astrocytes as well as oligodendrocytes in cultures that are free of neurons. Whether or not the required concentration of amino acid is realized at the membrane of glial cells *in situ* and, if so, what the functional significance is of their depolarization, are questions yet to be answered.

4.2. Other Transmitters and Glial Cells

4.2.1. Monoamines

In their iontophoretic study of glial cells of the cerebral cortex, Krnjević and Schwartz (1967) found that adrenaline had no effect on the glial membrane potential. They also stated, however, that this drug was tested on only a few cells. Quite recently, several independent studies showed that α-adrenergic agents cause depolarization of cultured glial cells (Hösli *et al.*, 1982; Hirata *et al.*, 1983; Kimelberg *et al.*, 1983). The report of Hösli *et al.* (1982) is especially interesting because they also found that β-adrenergic agents cause hyperpolarization of some glial cells and in a few cases the two opposite responses could be demonstrated by delivering two different drugs to the same glial cell. In each case the appropriate blocking agent selectively inhibited the effect. Hösli *et al.* (1982) have furthermore demonstrated binding of catecholamines to glial cells by autoradiography. Again, the question of the functional significance of these observations may be raised. In this context it may be relevant that activation of β-adrenergic receptors causes the release of taurine from glial cells (Shain and Martin, 1984).

Of the other monoamines, 5-hydroxytryptamine apparently causes hyperpolarization of glial cells, at least in leech ganglia (Walz and Schlue, 1982). The effect is mediated by an increase of potassium conductance of the membrane. In homogenates of mammalian brain, tritiated 5-hydroxytryptamine binds with high affinity to synaptosomes, and with low affinity to glial membranes (Fillion *et al.*, 1983).

References to a possible glial clearing of monoamine transmitters are fewer than those dealing with the clearing of amino acid transmitters. According to

Hösli and Hösli (1976), glial cells from cerebellum, maintained *in vitro*, do not take up noradrenaline, even though they avidly accumulate GABA. Haber *et al.* (1978), however, have shown that the glial cells of the filum terminale of frogs are capable of accumulating not only GABA but also 5-hydroxytryptamine. In the same paper they also report that cells cultured from a glioma cell line do take up norepinephrine and dopamine as well. More recently, Schoepp and Azzaro (1983) reported that, following lesions made by microinjection of kainic acid, the monoamine oxidase content of the striatum increases in proportion to the proliferation of reactive glial cells. The authors suggest that glial cells may take up and oxidize dopamine, or other monoamines.

It is not clear which of these findings that show some effect of monoamines on glial cells in various model systems are relevant to the functions of glial cells in the mammalian cortex. It is worth remembering, however, that many monoaminergic fibers terminate in the cortex in a string of varicosities without forming definitive synapses with individual neurons. These fibers are probably able to raise the concentration of noradrenaline or of dopamine in interstitial fluid and so influence numerous cells in their neighborhood. It is at least possible that among their cellular targets there are glial cells as well as neurons. Some older findings also come to mind. Working with the cultured cell lines derived from gliomas, Gilman and Nirenberg (1971), Clark and Perkins (1971), and Schubert *et al.* (1976) reported that exposure to β-adrenergic agents caused elevation of cAMP levels. By contrast, in an immunocytochemical study, Chan-Palay and Palay (1979) found that in the normal cerebellum cAMP is contained in neurons, cGMP in glial cells. Superfusing the cerebellar cortex with solutions containing either glutamate or noradrenaline resulted in correlated changes of neuronal activity and the amount of cGMP in glia. It is thus possible that exposure to catecholamines influences the biochemical activity of glial cells, but the exact nature and significance of these changes are not clear.

4.2.2. Acetylcholine

Krnjević and Schwartz (1967) also reported that iontophoretically applied acetylcholine causes depolarization of cortical glial cells but, as with GABA, it is likely that this effect is mediated by acetylcholine causing the release of K^+ from nearby neurons. There is, however, the earlier observation by Cavanagh *et al.* (1954) and by Koelle (1954) that the pseudocholinesterase of the cortex is contained in glia rather than in neurons. The functions of this enzyme in the CNS are still unknown. Desmedt and LaGrutta (1957) have, however, reported that inhibition of pseudocholinesterase, but not of true cholinesterase, caused cerebral arousal and they thought that this effect is mediated by glia. Neither the observation nor the inference has either been challenged or confirmed in the decades that have elapsed since.

In an extensive series of experiments pursued over several years, Villegas (1978) has shown that acetylcholine influences the Schwann cells surrounding the giant axon of squids. As before, we have to repeat that the significance of this finding for the mammalian nervous system has not been clarified.

5. Pathophysiology of Cortical Glia

5.1. Seizures

Epilepsy is a frequent sequela of head trauma, tumors, or infarction of cortical tissue. Opinions remain divided as to whether it is the direct damage to the nervous tissue, or its scarification that makes damaged cortex prone to development of seizure discharges. Loss of neuronal elements could be epileptogenic if there were a selective loss of inhibitory interneurons, or if partial deafferentation of the cortex would lead to denervation supersensitivity. The scar tissue, formed in part or in whole by glial cells, could conceivably cause seizures by mechanical or by chemical means. Cortical scars tend to shrink, and this has been considered to be an irritant (e.g., Ward, 1961). It is said that scars that contain many fibroblasts contract more than those entirely composed of glia (Penfield, 1927). It seems, however, that the mechanical theory of epileptogenesis has been abandoned or, at the least, it has received little attention in recent years.

Chemical theories of a glial origin of epilepsy are rooted in the idea that glial tissue controls the milieu in which neurons live, and that the malfunction of the glial controller could result in excessive excitability of neurons or of synapses. For example, if glial cells regulate the level of excitatory and inhibitory amino aids in interstitial fluid, then their malfunction could give rise to abnormal irritability of the cortex either by allowing the level of the former to rise, or by allowing the latter to decline. If, furthermore, one of the functions of glial cells is the detoxification of ammonia (Norenberg and Martinez-Hernandez, 1979), then failure of this function could also lead to seizures. Excess ammonia (or ammonium ions, it is not clear which) causes seizures, probably because it interferes with synaptic inhibition (Deisz and Lux, 1982). These possible links between glial function and seizures are, however, entirely hypothetical.

Perhaps the most discussed of the chemical theories is the idea that disturbed regulation of $[K^+]_o$ by neuroglia is the cause, or one of several possible causes, of the eruption of seizures. I have reviewed the literature dealing with potassium and epilepsy in some detail earlier (Somjen, 1980, 1984a), and only a condensed summary will be given here.

It has been known for a long time that excess K^+ can induce seizures (e.g., Feldberg and Sherwood, 1957) and the accumulation of this ion has been blamed for the generation of seizure discharges by several authors (e.g., Fertziger and Ranck, 1970). The accumulation of K^+ in epileptogenic scars was explicitly linked to a malfunction of the glial dispersion of K^+ by Pollen and Trachtenberg (1970). Attempts at testing this theory revolved around two questions. One was whether the functions of the reactive astroglial cells that form epileptogenic scar tissue are degraded in some way compared to astrocytes in healthy cortical tissue. The other question was whether in or near epileptogenic foci the clearing of excess K^+ ions from interstitial fluid is deficient.

Numerous investigators reported the depolarization of glial cells during experimentally induced seizure discharges (e.g., Sugaya *et al.*, 1964, 1971; Glötzner and Grüsser, 1968; Sypert and Ward, 1971; Dichter *et al.*, 1972; Futamachi and Pedley, 1976; Greenwood *et al.*, 1981). These depolarizations were, however, apparently caused by the rise of $[K^+]_o$, which in turn was the consequence of the seizure discharge of neurons. Generally, both glial depolarization and extracellular SP shifts were during penicillin-induced seizures of the same magnitude as in nonconvulsing tissue, when $[K^+]_o$ was equally elevated (Lothman and Somjen, 1976; Futamachi and Pedley, 1976). Greenwood *et al.* (1981) found, however, that the rise of $[K^+]_o$ associated with electrically provoked spreading paroxysmal afterdischarge caused a less than normal amount of glial depolarization. They too found, however, no indication that this disruption of the usual correlation between $[K^+]_o$ and glial membrane potential had a deleterious effect, nor that the secondary rise of $[K^+]_o$ would be instrumental in triggering the spread of the seizure.

Grossman and Rosman (1971; see also Grossman, 1972) and Pollen and Richardson (1972) recorded the membrane potential of glial cells in and near artificially induced epileptogenic foci in cat cortex. Although their results were not decisive, both teams felt that glial cells in the foci may be pathologically altered, and may handle K^+ ions inefficiently. Glötzner (1973), on the other hand, was of the opinion that if there was a significant change, it was such as to enable reactive glia in scar tissue to handle excess K^+ ions more rather than less efficiently. Picker *et al.* (1981) made intracellular recordings in cortical tissue removed from human patients in the course of surgical treatment of partial epilepsy and also from specimens of glial tumors. They found the membrane of reactive and neoplastic glia to be more than normally permeable to ions other than K^+. They also found, however, that cortex that was electrographically epileptogenic but histologically normal, contained glial cells with normal membrane characteristics. This dissociation of seizure activity from glial pathology casts some doubt on the importance of failed handling of K^+ by glia in the generation of seizures.

The clearing of K^+ in and near focal gliotic tissue was gauged with K^+-selective electrodes by Pedley *et al.* (1976), who found it to be within normal limits, and by Lewis *et al.* (1977), who found it abnormally slow. Lewis *et al.* (1977) concluded that, since the resting level of $[K^+]_o$ was not elevated in the gliotic scar, the initiation of seizures could not be blamed on the faulty clearing of K^+ ions, but since the clearing rate was slow, this could contribute to the positive feedback that is believed to favor the progression of paroxysmal discharges. The problem was reinvestigated by Heinemann and Dietzel (1984) who found no evidence indicating that abnormal handling of K^+ ions could explain the epileptogenesis of gliotic scars.

In summary, the weight of the evidence is against defective clearing of K^+ being the cause of the generation of seizure discharges near glial scar tissue.

5.2. Glia and Spreading Depression of Leão

During episodes of Leão's depression, both glial cells and neurons are severely depolarized (Collewijn and Van Harreveld, 1966; Higashida *et al.*, 1974; Sugaya *et al.*, 1975, 1978). Associated with the cell depolarization is a strong negative shift of the extracellular potential (Leão, 1951) and a massive release of K^+ ions into interstitial space (Vyskočyl *et al.*, 1972; Lothman *et al.*, 1975; reviewed by Somjen, 1975, 1979). The depolarization of glial cells associated with the activation of neurons by electrical stimulation in normal cortex and with seizure discharges is attributed to the rise of $[K^+]_o$ due to the release of K^+ ions from neurons. Measured levels of $[K^+]_o$ and of glial membrane potentials are compatible with this explanation (see Sections 2.1, 2.3, and 5.1). During spreading depression, however, the glial membrane potential declines to within a few millivolts of zero (e.g., see Higashida *et al.*, 1974). The question is whether in this state, as in seizures, the membrane of glial cells behaves passively, responding to the elevated $[K^+]_o$ without participating actively in the process. Sugaya *et al.* (1978) report that the input impedance of glial cells does not change during spreading depression, but this finding alone is not sufficient to exclude a role of glial cells in bringing about the depressed state.

Sugaya *et al.* (1975, 1978) made the remarkable discovery that Leão's depression can be provoked by local application of KCl to cortex that has been treated with TTX. Moreover, a wave of depression, once started, will propagate unhindered through TTX-treated cortex. TTX prevents neurons from firing action potentials; therefore, the depressive process does not depend on nerve impulses. It could, still, be related to nonimpulsive neuronal processes. Sugaya *et al.* (1978) suggest, however, that glial cells can mediate Leão's depression. This is based on the observation that edema induced by intracarotid injection of sesame oil causes the selective loss of glial cells, and with their demise the cortex loses the ability to produce depressive episodes. Indeed, Walker and Hild (1971) have reported earlier that potential changes like those seen in cortical spreading depression can be induced in cultures of glial cells that contain no neurons at all.

In conclusion, there is still no solid evidence that failing function of glial cells is the cause, or even that it is a contributing cause in the pathophysiology of epilepsy. There are strong indications that neuroglia is in some manner involved in bringing about Leão's spreading depression.

6. Closing Remarks

Writing a chapter in a book, unlike writing an article for a periodical, one would wish to end with well-founded conclusions that have a chance to stand for at least a few years to come. With neuroglia as the subject, I am not sure that, today, this is possible. I have concentrated on two aspects of glial function, those for which the pieces of the puzzle best seemed to fit together. It now seems well established that K^+ ions traverse glial cells when $[K^+]_o$ is locally elevated. Still not clear is whether the dispersion of K^+ is an important component in maintaining homeostasis of the cerebral interstitial fluid, or whether failure of the dispersal results in disturbed neuronal function. Also well established is the intense involvement of glia in the turnover of neuroactive amino acids, but here again the significance of this activity is obscure.

There are many other intriguing leads that had to be neglected here. Do glial cells change shape as they perform their function in the adult brain (e.g., Salm *et al.*, 1983)? Are they involved in the storing of memory traces and in the strengthening of temporary connections that enable the formation of conditional reflexes (e.g., Hydén, 1973; Roitbak, 1983; also discussion in Varon and Somjen, 1979)? Is K^+ a signal by which neurons communicate to glial cells (e.g., Pentreath and Kai-Kai, 1982, also discussion in Varon and Somjen, 1979)? Or do glia and neurons mutually influence one another through adrenergic receptors (e.g., Maderspach and Fajszi, 1983)? Indeed, as in an overdone mystery story, there are too many diverging footprints in the snow. Not only are we at a loss, which trail to follow, we do not even know what it is we have set out to find. Could glia be the key to unlock some of the mysteries of the brain? Or is it, as Dr. Kuffler used to say when warding off all too insistent questioners, just holding nerve cells together?

7. References

Balestrino, M., Aitken, P. G., and Somjen, G. G., 1986, The effects of moderate changes of extracellular K^+ and Ca^{2+} on synaptic and neural function in the CA1 region of the hippocampal slice, *Brain Res.* **377:**229–239.

Benjamin, A. M., and Quastel, J. H., 1972, Locations of amino acids in brain slices from the rat, *Biochem. J.* **128:**631–646.

Bevan, S., and Raff, M., 1985, Voltage-dependent potassium currents in cultured astrocytes, *Nature* **315:**229–232.

Bourke, R. S., Nelson, K. M., Nauman, R. A., and Young, O. M., 1970, Studies of the production and subsequent reduction of swelling in primate cerebral cortex under isomotic conditions in vivo, *Exp. Brain Res.* **10:**427–446.

Bowery, N. G., and Brown, D. A., 1972, Gamma-amino butyric acid uptake by sympathetic ganglia, *Nature New Biol.* **238:**89–91.

Bowery, N. G., Brown, D. A., Collins, G. G. S., Galvan, M., Marsh, S., and Yamini, G., 1975, Indirect effects of amino acids on sympathetic ganglion cells mediated through the release of gamma-aminobutyric acid from glial cells, *Br. J. Pharmacol.* **57:**73–91.

Bowery, N. G., Brown, D. A., White, R., and Yamini, G., 1979, ^{3}H-gamma-amino butyric acid uptake into neuroglial cells of rat superior cervical sympathetic ganglia, *J. Physiol. (London)* **293:**51–74.

Bowman, C. L., Kimelberg, H. K., Frangakis, M. V., Berwald-Netter, Y., and Edwards, C., 1984, Astrocytes in primary culture have chemically activated sodium channels, *J. Neurosci.* **4:**1527–1534.

Bradbury, M., 1979, *The Concept of a Blood–Brain Barrier*, Wiley, New York.

Brightman, M. W., and Reese, T. S., 1969, Junctions between intimately apposed cell membranes in the vertebrate brain, *J. Cell Biol.* **40:**648–677.

Brinley, F. J., Kandel, E. R., and Marshall, W. H., 1960, Potassium outflux from rabbit cortex during spreading depression, *J. Neurophysiol.* **23:**246–256.

Brown, D. A., and Galvan, M., 1977, Influence of neuroglial transport on the action of gamma-amino butyric acid on mammalian ganglion cells, *Br. J. Pharmacol.* **59:**373–378.

Brown, D. A., and Shain, W., 1977, Cation concentration gradients in cultured sympathetic neuroglial cells, *J. Physiol. (London)* **269:**45P–46P.

Brown, D. A., Collins, G. G. S., and Galvan, M., 1980, Influence of cellular transport on the interaction of amino acids with gamma-amino butyric acid (GABA)-receptors in the isolated olfactory cortex of the guinea pig, *Br. J. Pharmacol.* **68:**251–262.

Bührle, C. P., and Sonnhof, U., 1983, Intracellular ion activities and equilibrium potentials in motoneurones and glial cells of the frog spinal cord, *Pfluegers Arch.* **396:**144–153.

Bundgaard, M., and Cserr, H., 1981, A glial blood–brain barrier in elasmobranchs, *Brain Res.* **226:**61–73.

Bunge, R. P., 1968, Glial cells and the central myelin sheath, *Physiol. Rev.* **48:**197–251.

Castellucci, V. F., and Goldring, S., 1970, Contribution to steady potential shifts of slow depolarization in cells presumed to be glia, *Electroencephalogr. Clin. Neurophysiol.* **28**:109–118.

Cavanagh, J. B., Thompson, R. H., and Webster, G. R., 1954, The localization of pseudocholinesterase activity in nervous tissue, *Q. J. Exp. Physiol.* **39**:185–197.

Chan-Palay, V., and Palay, S. L., 1979, Immunocytochemical localization of cyclic GMP: Light and electromicroscopic evidence for involvement of neuroglia, *Proc. Natl. Acad. Sci. USA* **76**:1485–1488.

Clark, R. B., and Perkins, J. P., 1971, Regulation of adenosine 3′, 5′-cyclic monophosphate concentration in cultured human astrocytoma cells by catecholamines and histamine, *Proc. Natl. Acad. Sci. USA* **68**:2757–2760.

Cohen, M. W., 1970, The contribution by glial cells to surface recordings from optic nerve of an amphibian, *J. Physiol. (London)* **210**:565–580.

Coles, J. A., and Orkand, R. K., 1985, Changes in sodium activity during light stimulation in photoreceptors, glia and extracellular space in drone retina, *J. Physiol. (London)* **362**:415–435.

Coles, J. A., and Tsacopoulos, M., 1979, Potassium activity in photoreceptors, glial cells and extracellular space in the drone retina: Changes during photic stimulation, *J. Physiol. (London)* **290**:525–549.

Collewijn, H., and Van Harreveld, A., 1966, Membrane potential of cortical cells during spreading depression and during asphyxia, *Exp. Neurol.* **15**:425–436.

Connors, B. W., Benardo, L. S., and Prince, D. A., 1984, Carbon dioxide sensitivity of dye coupling among glia and neurons of the neocortex, *J. Neurosci.* **4**:1324–1330.

Cordingley, G. E., and Somjen, G. G., 1978, The clearing of excess potassium from extracellular space in spinal cord and cerebral cortex, *Brain Res.* **151**:291–306.

Davson, H., and Bradbury, M., 1956, The extracellular space of the brain, *Prog. Brain. Res.* **15**:124–134.

Beisz, R. A., and Lux, H.-D., 1982, The role of extracellular chloride in hyperpolarizing post-synaptic inhibition of crayfish stretch receptor neurones, *J. Physiol. (London)* **326**:123–138.

Dennis, M. J., and Gerschenfeld, H. M., 1969, Some physiological properties of identified mammalian neuroglial cells, *J. Physiol. (London)* **203**:211–222.

De Robertis, E. D., 1965, Some new electron microscopical contributions to the biology of neuroglia, *Prog. Brain. Res.* **15**:1–11.

De Robertis, E. D. P., and Carrea, R., 1965, *Progress in Brain Research Vol. 15.*

Desarmenien, M., Feltz, P., and Headley, P. M., 1980, Does glial uptake affect GABA responses? An intracellular study on rat dorsal root ganglion neurones in vitro, *J. Physiol. (London)* **307**:163–182.

Desmedt, J. E., and LaGrutta, G., 1957, The effect of selective inhibition of pseudocholinesterase on the spontaneous and evoked activity of the cat's cerebral cortex, *J. Physiol. (London)* **136**:20–40.

Dichter, M. A., Herman, C. J., and Seizer, M., 1972, Silent cells during interictal discharges and seizures in hippocampal seizure foci: Evidence for the role of extracellular K^+ in the transitions from the interictal state to seizures, *Brain Res.* **48**:173–183.

Dietzel, I., Heinemann, U., Hofmeier, G., and Lux, H.-D., 1980, Transient changes in the size of the extracellular space in the sensorimotor cortex of cats in relation to stimulus-induced changes in potassium concentration, *Exp. Brain Res.* **40**:432–439.

Dietzel, I., Heinemann, U., Hofmeier, G., and Lux, H.-D., 1982, Stimulus-induced changes in extracellular Na and Cl concentration in relation to changes in the size of the extracellular space, *Exp. Brain Res.* **46**:73–84.

Feldberg, W., and Sherwood, S. L., 1957, Effects of calcium and potassium injected into the cerebral ventricles of the cat, *J. Physiol. (London)* **139**:408–416.

Fertziger, A. P., and Ranck, J. B., 1970, Potassium accumulation in interstitial space during epileptiform seizures, *Exp. Neurol.* **26**:571–585.

Fillion, G., Beaudoin, D., Fillion, M.-P., Rousselle, J.-C., Robant, C., and Netter, Y., 1983, 5-Hydroxytryptamine receptors in neurones and glia, *J. Neural Transm. Suppl.* **18**:307–317.

Fischer, G., and Kettenmann, H., 1985, Cultured astrocytes form a syncytium after maturation, *Exp. Cell Res.* **159**:273–279.

Franck, G., Grisar, T., Moonen, G., and Schoffeniels, E., 1978, Potassium transport in mammalian astroglia, In: *Dynamic Properties of Glia Cells* (E. Schoffeniels, G. Franck, L. Hertz, and D. B. Tower, eds.), Pergamon Press, Elmsford, N.Y., pp. 315–325.

Futamachi, K., and Pedley, T. A., 1976, Glial cells and potassium: Their relationship in mammalian cortex, *Brain Res.* **109**:311–322.

Galambos, R., 1964, Glial cells, *Neurosci. Res. Program Bull.* **2**:1–63.

Gallagher, J. P., Nakamura, J., and Shinnick-Gallagher, P., 1983, Effects of glial uptake and desensitization on the activity of gamma-aminobutyric acid (GABA) and its analogs at the rat dorsal root ganglion, *J. Pharmacol. Exp. Ther.* **226:**876–884.

Gardner-Medwin, A. R., 1983a, A study of the mechanism by which potassium moves through brain tissue, *J. Physiol. (London)* **335:**353–374.

Gardner-Medwin, A. R., 1983b, Analysis of potassium dynamics in mammalian brain tissue, *J. Physiol. (London)* **335:**393–426.

Gardner-Medwin, A. R., 1985, Potential challenge from glia, *Nature* **315:**181.

Gardner-Medwin, A. R., and Nicholson, C., 1983, Changes in extracellular potassium activity induced by electric current through brain tissue in the rat, *J. Physiol. (London)* **335:**375–392.

Gerschenfeld, H. M., Wald, F., Zadunaisky, J. A., and De Robertis, E. D. P., 1959, Function of astroglia in the water and ion metabolism of the central nervous system, *Neurology* **9:**412–425.

Giacobini, E., 1962, A cytochemical study of the localization of carbonic anhydrase in the nervous system, *J. Neurochem.* **9:**169–177.

Gibson, J. L., 1980, Glial membrane potential and input resistance in chloride substituted solution, *Neurosci. Lett. Suppl.* **5:**S433.

Gilman, A. G., and Nirenberg, M. W., 1971, Effects of catecholamines on the $3':5'$-cyclic adenosine monophosphate concentration of clonal satellite cells of neurons, *Proc. Natl. Acad. Sci. USA* **68:**2165–2168.

Glees, P., 1955, *Neuroglia: Morphology and Function,* Thomas Springfield, Ill.

Glötzner, F. L., 1973, Membrane properties of neuroglia in epileptogenic gliosis, *Brain Res.* **55:**159–171.

Glötzner, F., and Grüsser, O.-J., 1968, Membranpotential und Entladungsfolgen corticaler Zellen, EEG und corticales DC-Potential bei genralisierten Krampfanfallen, *Arch. Psychiat. Z. Ges. Neurol.* **210:**313–339.

Grafe, P., Ballanyi, K., and ten Bruggencate, G, 1987, Ion activities in glial cells of guinea pig olfactory cortex slices, *Can. J. Physiol. Pharmacol.* in press.

Grafstein, B., 1956, Mechanisms of spreading cortical depression, *J. Neurophysiol.* **19:**154–171.

Greenwood, R. S., Takato, M., and Goldring, S., 1981, Potassium activity and changes in glial and neuronal membrane potentials during initiation and spread of after discharge in cerebral cortex of cat, *Brain Res.* **218:**279–298.

Grossman, R. G., 1972, Alterations in the microphysiology of glial cells and neurons and their environment in injured brain, *Clin. Neurosurg.* **19:**69–83.

Grossman, R. G., and Hampton, T., 1968, Depolarization of cortical glial cells during electrocortical activity, *Brain Res.* **11:**316–324.

Grossman, R. G., and Rosman, L. J., 1971, Intracellular potentials of inexcitable cells in epileptogenic cortex undergoing fibrillary gliosis after local injury, *Brain Res.* **28:**181–201.

Grossman, R. G., and Seregin, A., 1977, Glial–neuronal interaction demonstrated by the injection of Na^+ and Li^+ into cortical glia, *Science* **195:**196–198.

Gutnick, M. J., Connors, B. W., and Ransom, B. R., 1981, Dye-coupling between glial cells in the guinea pig neocortical slice, *Brain Res.* **213:**486–492.

Haber, B., Suddith, R. L., Pacheco, M., Gonzalez, A., Ritchie, T. L., and Glusman, S., 1978, Model systems for the glial transport of biogenic amines and GABA: Clonal cell lines and the filum terminale of the frog spinal cord, in: *Dynamic Properties of Glial Cells* (E. Schoffeniels, G. Franck, L. Hertz, and D. B. Tower, eds.), Pergamon Press, Elmsford, N.Y., pp. 193–206.

Hamberger, A., and Hydén, H., 1963, Inverse enzymatic changes in neurons and glia during increased function and hypoxia, *J. Cell Biol.* **16:**521–525.

Hamberger, A. C., Chiang, G. H., Nylen, E. S., Scheff, S. W., and Cotman, C. W., 1979a, Glutamate as a CNS transmitter. I. Evaluation of glucose and glutamine as precursors for the synthesis of preferentially released glutamate, *Brain Res.* **168:**513–530.

Hamberger, A., Chiang, G., Sandoval, E., and Cotman, C. W., 1979b, Glutamate as a CNS transmitter. II. Regulation of synthesis in the releasable pool, *Brain Res.* **168:**531–541.

Heinemann, U., and Dietzel, I., 1984, Changes in extracellular potassium concentration in chronic alumina cream foci of cats, *J. Neurophysiol.* **52:**421–434.

Heinemann, U., Lux, H.-D., Marciani, M. G., and Hofmeier, G., 1979, Slow potentials in relation to changes in extracellular potassium activity in the cortex of cats, in: *Origin of Cerebral Field Potentials* (E. J. Speckmann and H. Caspers, eds.), Thieme, Stuttgart, pp. 33–48.

Held, D., Fencl, V., and Pappenheimer, J. R., 1964, Electrical potential of cerebrospinal fluid, *J. Neurophysiol.* **27:**942–959.

Henn, F. A., Haljamäe, H., and Hamberger, A., 1972, Glial cell function: Active control of extracellular K⁺ concentration, *Brain Res.* **43**:437–443.

Hertz, L., 1966, Neuroglial localization of potassium and sodium effects on respiration in brain, *J. Neurochem.* **13**:1373–1387.

Hertz, L., 1978, An intense potassium uptake into astrocytes, its further enhancement by high concentrations of potassium, and its possible involvement in potassium homeostasis at the cellular level, *Brain Res.* **145**:202–208.

Hertz, L., 1979, Functional interactions between neurons and astrocytes. I. Turnover and metabolism of putative amino acid transmitters, *Prog. Neurobiol.* **13**:277–323.

Higashida, H., Mitarai, G., and Watanabe, S., 1974, A comparative study of membrane potential changes in neurons and neuroglial cells during spreading depression in the rabbit, *Brain Res.* **65**:411–425.

Hirata, H., Slater, N. T., and Kimelberg, H. K., 1983, Alpha-adrenergic receptor mediated depolarization of rat neocortical astrocytes in primary culture, *Brain Res.* **270**:358–362.

Horsthemke, B., Hamprecht, B., and Bauer, K., 1983, Heterogeneous distribution of enkephalin-degrading peptidases between neuronal and glial cells, *Biochem. Biophys. Res. Commun.* **115**:423–429.

Horstmann, E., 1962, Was wissen wir uber den intercellularen Raum im Zentralnervensystem?, *World Neurol.* **3**:112–116.

Hösli, E., and Hösli, L., 1976, Autoradiographic studies of the uptake of ³H-noradrenaline and ³H-GABA in cultured rat cerebellum, *Exp. Brain Res.* **26**:319–324.

Hösli, L., Andrés, P. F., and Hösli, E., 1977, Action of GABA on neurones and satellite glial cells of cultured rat dorsal root ganglia, *Neurosci. Lett.* **6**:79–83.

Hösli, L., Hösli, E., Landolt, H., and Zehnter, C., 1981, Efflux of potassium from neurones excited by glutamate and aspartate causes depolarization of cultured glial cells, *Neurosci. Lett.* **21**:83–86.

Hösli, L., Hösli, E., Zehnter, C., Lehmann, R., and Lutz, T. W., 1982, Evidence for the existence of alpha and beta adrenoceptors on cultured glial cells, *Neuroscience* **7**:2867–2872.

Hydén, H., 1973, Changes in brain protein during learning. Nerve cells and their glia: Relationships and differences, in: *Macromolecules and Behaviour* (G. B. Ansell and P. B. Bradley, eds.), Macmillan & Co., London, pp. 3–75.

Iversen, L. L., and Kelly, J. S., 1975, Uptake and metabolism of gamma-aminobutyric acid by neurones and glial cells, *Biochem. Pharmacol.* **24**:933–938.

Karahashi, Y., and Goldring, S., 1966, Intracellular potentials from "idle" cells in cerebral cortex of cat, *Electroencephalogr. Clin. Neurophysiol.* **20**:600–607.

Katzman, R., 1961, Electrolyte distribution in mammalian central nervous system: Are glia high sodium cells?, *Neurology* **11**:27–36.

Katzman, R., and Pappius, H. M., 1973, *Brain Electrolytes and Fluid Metabolism*, Williams & Wilkins, Baltimore.

Kelly, J. P., and Van Essen, D. C., 1974, Cell structure and function in the visual cortex of the cat, *J. Physiol. (London)* **238**:515–547.

Kelly, J. S., and Dick, F., 1978, GABA in glial cells of the peripheral and central nervous system, in: *Dynamic Properties of Glia Cells* (E. Schoffeniels, G. Franck, L. Hertz, and D. B. Tower, eds.), Pergamon Press, Elmsford, N.Y. pp. 183–192.

Kelly, J. S., Krnjević, K., and Yim, G. K. W., 1967, Unresponsive cells in cerebral cortex, *Brain Res.* **6**:767–769.

Kettenmann, H., Orkand, R. K., and Schachner, M., 1983a, Coupling among identified cells in nervous system culture, *J. Neurosci.* **3**:506–516.

Kettenmann, H., Sonnhof, U., and Schachner, M., 1983b, Exclusive potassium dependence of the membrane potential in cultured mouse oligodendrocytes, *J. Neurosci.* **3**:500–505.

Kettenmann, H., Backus, K. H., and Schachner, M., 1984a, Aspartate, glutamate and gamma-amino butyric acid depolarize cultured astrocytes, *Neurosci. Lett.* **52**:25–29.

Kettenmann, H., Gilbert, P., and Schachner, M., 1984b, Depolarization of cultured oligodendrocytes by glutamate and GABA, *Neurosci. Lett.* **47**:271–276.

Kettenmann, H., Orkand, R. K., and Lux, H.-D., 1984c, Some properties of single potassium channels in cultured oligodendrocytes. *Pfluegers Arch.* **400**:215–221.

Kimelberg, H. K., 1979, Glial enzymes and ion transport in brain swelling, in: *Neural Trauma* (A. J. Popp, ed.), Raven Press, New York, pp. 137–153.

Kimelberg, H. K., 1981, Active accumulation and exchange transport of chloride in astroglial cells in culture, *Biochim. Biophys. Acta* **646**:179–184.

Kimelberg, H. K., and Bourke, R. S., 1982, Anion transport in the nervous system, in: *Handbook of Neurochemistry*, 2nd ed. (A. Lajtha, ed.), Vol. 1, Plenum Press, New York, pp. 31–67.

Kimelberg, H. K., Bowman, C. L., Hirata, H., Edwards, C., Bourke, R. S., and Slater, N. T., 1983, Norepinephrine induced depolarization of astrocytes in primary culture, *Soc. Neurosci. Abstr.* **9:**449.

King, G. L., and Somjen, G. G., 1981, Effects of variations of extracellular potassium activity on synaptic transmission and calcium responses in hippocampal tissue in vitro, *Neurosci. Soc. Abstr.* **7:**439.

Koch, A. R., Ranck, J. B., and Newman, B. L., 1962, Ionic content of neuroglia, *Exp. Neurol.* **6:**186–200.

Koelle, G. B., 1954, The histochemical localization of cholinesterases in the central nervous system of the rat, *J. Comp. Neurol.* **100:**211–236.

Kraig, R. P., Ferreira-Filho, C. R., and Nicholson, C., 1983, Alkaline and acid transients in cerebellar microenvironment, *J. Neurophysiol.* **49:**831–850.

Krnjević, K., and Morris, M. E., 1972, Extracellular K^+ activity and slow potential changes in spinal cord and medulla, *Can. J. Physiol. Pharmacol.* **50:**1214–1217.

Krnjević, K., and Schwartz, S., 1967, Some properties of unresponsive cells in the cerebral cortex, *Exp. Brain Res.* **3:**306–319.

Kuffler, S. W., 1967, Neuroglial cells: Physiological properties and a potassium mediated effect of neuronal activity on the glial membrane potential, *Proc. R. Soc. London Ser. B* **168:**1–21.

Kuffler, S. W., and Nicholls, J. G., 1966, The physiology of neuroglial cells, *Ergeb. Physiol.* **57:**1–90.

Kuffler, S. W., Nicholls, J. S., and Orkand, R. K., 1966, Physiological properties of glial cells in the central nervous system of amphibia, *J. Neurophysiol.* **29:**768–787.

Landis, D., and Reese, T., 1981, Membrane structure in mammalian astrocytes, *J. Exp. Biol.* **95:**35–48.

Lasansky, A. 1971. Nervous function at the cellular level: Glia, *Annu. Rev. Physiol.* **33:**241–256.

Leão, A. A. P., 1951, The slow voltage variation of cortical spreading depression of activity, *Electroencephalogr. Clin. Neurophysiol.* **3:**315–321.

Lewis, D. V., Mutsuga, N., Schuette, W. H., and Van Buren, J., 1977, Potassium clearance and reactive gliosis in the alumina gel lesion, *Epilepsia* **18:**499–506.

Lodge, D., Johnston, G. A. R., and Curtis, D. R., 1978, In vivo correlates of in vitro GABA-uptake inhibition in cat CNS, in: *Iontophoresis and Transmitter Mechanisms in the Mammalian Central Nervous System* (R. W. Ryall and J. S. Kelly, eds.), Elsevier, Amsterdam, pp. 378–380.

Lothman, E. W., and Somjen, G. G., 1975, Extracellular potassium activity, intracellular and extracellular potential responses in the spinal cord, *J. Physiol. (London)* **252:**115–136.

Lothman, E. W., and Somjen, G. G., 1976, Functions of primary afferents and responses of extracellular K^+ during spinal epileptiform seizures, *Electroencephalogr. Clin. Neurophysiol.* **41:**253–267.

Lothman, E. W., LaManna, J., Cordingley, G., Rosenthal, M., and Somjen, G., 1975, Responses of electrical potential, potassium levels and oxidative metabolic activity of the cerebral neocortex of cats, *Brain Res.* **88:**15–36.

Lugaro, E., 1907, Sullie funzioni della nevroglia, *Riv. Patol. Nerv. Ment.* **12:**225–233.

McGeer, P. L., and McGeer, E. G., 1981, Amino acid transmitters, in: *Basic Neurochemistry*, 3rd ed. (G. J. Siegel, R. W. Albers, B. W. Agranoff, and R. Katzman, eds.), Little Brown, Boston, pp. 233–253.

MacVicar, B. A., 1984, Voltage-dependent calcium channels in glial cells, *Science* **226:**1345–1347.

Maderspach, K., and Fajszi, C., 1983, Development of beta-adrenergic receptors and their function in glia–neuron communication in cultured chick brain, *Dev. Brain Res.* **6:**251–257.

Massa, P., and Mugnaini, E., 1982, Cell junctions and intramembrane particles of astrocytes and oligodendrocytes: A freeze-fracture study, *Neuroscience* **7:**523–538.

Minchin, M. C. W., and Iversen, L. L., 1974, Release of [^{3}]gamma-aminobutyric acid from glial cells in dorsal root ganglia, *J. Neurochem.* **23:**533–540.

Moonen, G., and Nelson, P. G., 1978, Some physiological properties of astrocytes in primary cultures, in: *Dynamic Properties of Glial Cells* (E. Schoffeniels, G. Franck, L. Hertz, and D. B. Tower, eds.), Pergamon Press, Elmsford, N.Y., pp. 389–393.

Mutch, W. A. C., and Hansen, A. J., 1984, Extracellular pH changes during spreading depression and cerebral ischemia: Mechanisms of brain pH regulation, *J. Cerebr. Blood Flow Metab.* **4:**17–27.

Nageotte, J., 1910, Phenomenes de secretion dans le protoplasma des cellules neurogliques de la substance grise, *C.R. Soc. Biol.* **68:**1068–1069.

Neal, M. J., and Iversen, L. L., 1972, Autoradiographic localization of ^{3}H-GABA in rat retina, *Nature New Biol.* **235:**217–218.

Newman, E. A., 1984, Regional specialization of retinal glial cell membrane, *Nature* **309**:155–157.

Newman, E. A., 1987, Regulation of potassium levels by Müller cells in the vertebrate retina, *Can. J. Physiol. Pharmacol.* in press.

Newman, E. A., Frambach, D. A., and Odette, L. L., (1984), Control of extracellular K^+ levels by retinal glial cell K^+-siphoning, *Science* **225**:1174–1175.

Nicholson, C., and Phillips, J. M., 1981, Ion diffusion modified by tortuosity and volume fraction in the extracellular microenvironment of the rat cerebellum, *J. Physiol. (London)* **321**:225–257.

Norenberg, M. D., and Martinez-Hernandez, A., 1979, Fine structural localization of glutamine synthetase in astrocytes of rat brain, *Brain Res.* **161**:303–310.

Orkand, P. M., Bracho, H., and Orkand, R. K., 1973, Glial metabolism: Alteration by potassium levels comparable to those during neuronal activity, *Brain Res.* **55**:467–471.

Orkand, R. K., 1977, Glial cells, in: *The Nervous System, Handbook of Physiology,* 2nd ed., Section 1, Vol. 1, Part 2 (J. M. Brookhart, V. B. Mouncastle, and E. R. Kandel, eds.), American Physiological Society, Bethesda, Md., pp. 855–875.

Orkand, R. K., Nicholls, J. G., and Kuffler, S. W., 1966, Effect of nerve impulses on the membrane potential of glial cells in the central nervous system of amphibia, *J. Neurophysiol.* **29**:788–806.

Pape, L. G., and Katzman, R., 1972, Responses of glia in cat sensorimotor cortex to increased extracellular potassium, *Brain Res.* **38**:71–92.

Pedley, T. A., Fisher, R. S., and Prince, D. A., 1976, Focal gliosis and potassium movement in mammalian cortex, *Exp. Neurol.* **50**:346–361.

Penfield, W., 1927, The mechanism of cicatrical contraction in the mammalian brain, *Brain,* **50**:499–517.

Pentreath, V. W., and Kai-Kai, M. A., 1982, Significance of the potassium signal from neurones to glial cells, *Nature* **295**:59–61.

Peters, A., and Palay, S. L., 1965, An electron microscopic study of the distribution and patterns of astroglial processes in the central nervous system, *J. Anat.* **99**:419P.

Peters, A., Palay, S. L., and Webster, H. D., 1970, *The Fine Structure of the Nervous System,* Harper & Row, New York.

Picker, S., Pieper, C. F., and Goldring, S., 1981, Glial membrane potentials and their relationship to $[K^+]_o$ in man and guinea pig, *J. Neurosurg.* **55**:347–363.

Pollen, D. A., and Richardson, E. P., Jr., 1972, Intracellular microelectrode studies at the border zone of glial scars developing after penetrating wounds and freezing lesions of the sensorimotor area of the cat, in: *Recent Contributions to Neurophysiology* (J. P. Cordeau and P. Gloor, eds.), Elsevier, Amsterdam, pp. 28–41.

Pollen, D. A., and Trachtenberg, M. C., 1970, Neuroglia: Gliosis and focal epilepsy, *Science* **167**:1252–1253.

Rall, D. P., and Fenstermacher, J. D., 1971, Volume of cerebral extracellular fluids, in: *Ion Homeostasis of the Brain* (B. K. Siesjo and S. C. Sorensen, eds.), Academic Press, New York, pp. 113–133.

Ramaharobandro, N., Borg, J., Mandel, P., and Mark, J., 1982, Glutamine and glutamate transport in cultured neuronal and glial cells, *Brain Res.* **244**:113–121.

Ranck, J. B., 1964, Specific impedance of cerebral cortex during spreading depression, and an analysis of neuronal, neuroglial and interstitial contributions, *Exp. Neurol.* **9**:1–16.

Ransom, B. R., 1974, The behavior of presumed glial cells during seizure discharge in cat cerebral cortex, *Brain Res.* **69**:83–99.

Ransom, B. R., and Goldring, S., 1973a, Ionic determinants of membrane potential of cells presumed to be glia in cerebral cortex of cat, *J. Neurophysiol.* **36**:855–868.

Ransom, B. R., and Goldring, S., 1973b, Slow depolarization in cells presumed to be neuroglia in cerebral cortex of cat, *J. Neurophysiol.* **36**:869–878.

Ransom, B. R., and Goldring, S., 1973c, Slow hyperpolarization in cells presumed to be glia in cerebral cortex of cat, *J. Neurophysiol.* **36**:879–892.

Ransom, B. R., Greenwood, R. S., Goldring, S., and Letcher, F. S., 1977, The effect of barbiturate and procaine on glial and neuronal contributions to evoked cortical steady potential shifts, *Brain Res.* **134**:479–499.

Reiser, G., Löffler, F., and Hamprecht, B., 1983, Tetrodotoxin-sensitive ion channels characterized in glial and neuronal cells from rat brain, *Brain Res.* **261**:335–340.

Roitbak, A. I., 1983, *Neuroglia, Eigenschaften, Funktionen, Bedeutung,* Fischer, Jena.

Salm, A. K., Smithson, K. G., and Hatton, G. I., 1983, Lactation-associated glial plasticity in the supraoptic nucleus of the rat, *Soc. Neurosci. Abstr.* **9**:451.

Sarthry, P. V., 1983, Release of [^{3}H]gamma-aminobutyric acid from glial (Muller) cells of rat retina: Effects of K^+, veratridine and ethylenediamine, *J. Neurosci.* **3**:2494–2503.

Schlue, W. R., and Deitmer, J. W., 1987, Direct measurement of intracellular pH in identified glial cells and neurons of the leech central nervous system, *Can. J. Physiol. Pharmacol.* in press.

Schlue, W. R., and Wuttke, W., 1983, Potassium activity in leech neuropil glial cells changes with external potassium concentration, *Brain Res.* **270:**368–372.

Schoepp, D. D., and Azzaro, A. J., 1983, Effects of intrastriatal kainic acid injection on [^{3}H]dopamine metabolism in rat striatal slices: Evidence for postsynaptic glial cell metabolism by both type A and B forms of monoamine oxidase, *J. Neuroschem.* **40:**1340–1348.

Schoffeniels, E., Franck, G., Hertz, L. and Tower, D. B. (eds.), 1978, *Dynamic Properties of Glia Cells,* Pergamon Press, Elmsford, N.Y.

Schon, F., and Kelly, J. S., 1974, Autoradiographic localisation of [3H]-GABA and [^{3}H]-glutamate over satellite glial cells, *Brain Res.* **66:**275–288.

Schon, F., and Kelly, J. S., 1975, Selective uptake of [^{3}H] beta-alanine by glia: Association with the glial uptake system for GABA, *Brain res.* **86:**243–257.

Schrier, B. K., and Thompson, E. J., 1974, On the role of glial cells in the mammalian nervous system: Uptake, excretion and metabolism of putative neurotransmitters by cultured glial tumor cells, *J. Biol. Chem.* **249:**1769–1780.

Schubert, D., Tarikas, H., and LaCorbiere, M., 1976, Neurotransmitter regulation of adenosine 3′-5′-monophosphate in clonal nerve, glia and muscle cell lines, *Science* **192:**471–472.

Shain, W. G., and Martin, D. L., 1984, Activation of beta-adrenergic receptors stimulates taurine release from glial cells, *Cell. Mol. Neurobiol.* **4:**191–196.

Somjen, G. G., 1970, Evoked sustained focal potentials and membrane potential of neurons and of unresponsive cells of the spinal cord, *J. Neurophysiol.* **33:**562–582.

Somjen, G. G., 1973, Electrogenesis of sustained potentials, *Prog. Brain. Res.* **1:**199–237.

Somjen, G. G., 1975, Electrophysiology of neuroglia, *Annu. Rev. Physiol.* **37:**163–190.

Somjen, G. G., 1978, Metabolic and electrical correlates of the clearing of excess potassium in cortex and spinal cord, in: *Studies in Neurophysiology* (R. Porter, ed.), Cambridge University Press, Cambridge, pp. 181–201.

Somjen, G. G., 1979, Extracellular potassium in the mammalian central nervous system, *Annu. Rev. Physiol.* **41:**159–177.

Somjen, G. G., 1980, Influence of potassium and neuroglia in the generation of seizures and their treatment, in: *Antiepileptic Drugs: Mechanisms of Action* (G. H. Glaser, J. K. Penry, and D. M. Woodbury, eds.), Raven Press, New York, pp. 155–167.

Somjen, G. G., 1981a, Neuroglia and spinal fluids, *J. Exp. Biol.* **95:**129–133.

Somjen, G. G., 1981b, Physiology of glial cells, in: *Physiology of Non-excitable Cells, Adv. Physiol. Sci.,* Vol. 3 (J. Salanki, ed.), Akademiai Kiado/Pergamon Press, pp. 23–43.

Somjen, G. G., 1981c, The why and how of measuring the activity of ions in extracellular fluid of spinal cord and cerebral cortex, in: *The Application of Ion-Selective Microelectrodes* (T. Zeuthen, ed.), Elsevier, Amsterdam, pp. 175–193.

Somjen, G. G., 1983, *Neurophysiology: The Essentials,* Williams & Wilkins, Baltimore.

Somjen, G. G., 1984a, Interstitial ion concentration and the role of neuroglia in seizures, in: *Electrophysiology of Epilepsy* (H. V. Wheal and P. A. Schwartzkroin, eds.), Academic Press, New York, pp. 303–341.

Somjen, G. G., 1984b, Acidification of interstitial fluid in hippocampal formation caused by seizures and by spreading depression, *Brain Res.* **311:**186–188.

Somjen, G. G., Aitken, P. G., Giacchino, J. L., and McNamara, J. O., 1985, Sustained potential shifts and paroxysmal discharges in hippocampal formation, *J. Neurophysiol.* **53:**1079–1097.

Sonnhof, U., 1987, Single voltage-dependent K^+ and Cl-channels in cultured astrocytes, *Can. J. Physiol. Pharmacol.* in press.

Spray, D. C., Harris, A. L., and Bennet, M. V. L., 1981, Gap junctional conductance is a simple and sensitive function of intracellular pH, *Science* **211:**712–715.

Strittmatter, W. J., and Somjen, G. G., 1973, Depression of sustained evoked potentials and glial depolarization in the spinal cord by barbiturates and by diphenylhydantoin, *Brain Res.* **55:**333–342.

Sugaya, E., Goldring, S., and O'Leary, J. L., 1964, Intracellular potentials associated with direct cortical response and seizure discharge in cat, *Electroencephalogr. Clin. Neurophysiol.* **17:**661–669.

Sugaya, E., Karahashi, Y., Sugaya, A. and Haruki, F., 1971, Intra- and extracellular potentials from "idle" cells in cerebral cortex of cats, *Jpn. J. Physiol.* **21:**149–157.

Sugaya, E., Takato, M., and Noda, Y., 1975, Neuronal and glial activity during spreading depression in cerebral cortex of cat, *J. Neurophysiol.* **38:**822–841.

Sugaya, E., Takato, M., Noda, Y., and Sekiya, Y., 1978, Glial cells and spreading depression, in: *Dynamic Properties of Glia Cells* (L. Schoffeniels, G. Franck, L. Hertz, and D. B. Tower, eds.), Pergamon Press, Elmsford, N. Y., pp. 305–314.

Sugaya, E., Sekiya, Y., Kobori, T., and Noda, Y., 1979, Glial membrane potential and extracellular potassium concentration in cultured glial cells, *Exp. Neurol.* **66**:403–408.

Syková, E., 1983, Extracellular K$^+$ accumulation in the central nervous system, *Prog. Biophys. Mol. Biol.* **42**:135–189.

Sypert, G. W., and Ward, A. A., 1971, Unidentified neuroglial potentials during propagated seizures in neocortex, *Exp. Neurol.* **33**:239–255.

Tang, C. M., Strichartz, G. R., and Orkand R. K., 1979, Sodium channels in axons and glial cells in the optic nerve of Necturus maculosa, *J. Gen. Physiol.* **74**:629–642.

Tang, C. M., Cohen, M. W., and Orkand, R. K., 1980, Electrogenic pump in axons and neuroglia and extracellular homeotasis, *Brain Res.* **194**:283–286.

Tasaki, I., and Chang, J J., 1958, Electric response of glia cells in cat brain, *Science* **128**:1209–1210.

Trachtenberg, M. C. and Pollen, D. A., 1970, Neuroglia: Biophysical properties and physiologic function, *Science* **167**:1248–1252.

Trachtenberg, M. C., Kornblith, P. L., and Hauptil, J., 1972, Biophysical properties of cultured human glial cells, *Brain Res.* **38**:279–298.

Treherne, J. E. (ed.), 1981, *Glial–Neurone Interactions, J. Exp. Biol.* **95.**

Turský, T., Ruščak, M., Laššanova, M., and Ruscakova, D., 1979, [^{14}C]-amino acid formation from labelled glucose and/or acetate in brain cortex slices with experimentally elicited proliferation of astroglia: Correlation of biochemical and morphological changes, *J. Neurochem.* **33**:1209–1215.

Urbanics, R., Leniger-Follert, E., and Lubbers, D. W., 1978, Time course of changes of extracellular H$^+$ and K$^+$ activities during and after direct electrical stimulation of the brain cortex, *Pfluegers Arch.* **378**:47–53.

Van den Berg, C. J., and Garfinkel, D., 1971, A simulation study of brain compartments: Metabolism of glutamate and related substances in mouse brain, *Biochem. J.* **123**:211–218.

Van den berg, C. J., Krzalic, L. J., Mela, P., and Waelsch, H., 1969, Compartmentation of glutamate metabolism in brain, *Biochem. J.* **113**:281–290.

Van Harreveld, A., 1966, *Brain Tissue Electrolytes*, Butterworths, Washington.

Vargas, F., Erlij, D., and Glusman S., 1977, Transmitter release by glial cells in the frog spinal cord, *Fed. Proc.* **36**:553.

Varon, S. S., and Somjen, G. G., 1979, Neuron–glia interactions, *Neurosci. Res. Program Bull.* **17**:1–239.

Villegas, J., 1978, Cholinergic properties of satellite cells in the peripheral nervous system, in: *Dynamic Properties of Glia Cells* (E. Schoffeniels, G. Franck, L. Hertz, and D. B. Tower, eds.), Pergamon Press, Elmsford N.Y., pp. 207–215.

Vyklický, L., Syková, E., and Křiž, N., 1975, Slow potentials induced by changes of extracellular potassium in the spinal cord of the cat, *Brain Res.* **87**:77–80

Vyskočyl, F., Křiž, N, and Bureš, J., 1972, Potassium-selective microelectrodes used for measuring the extracellular brain potassium during spreading depression and anoxic depolarization in rats, *Brain Res.* **39**:255–259.

Walker, F. D., and Hild, W. J., 1971, Spreading depression in tissue culture, *J. Neurobiol.* **3**:223–235.

Walz, W., and Hertz, L., 1982, Ouabaine-sensitive and ouabaine-resistant net uptake of potassium into astrocytes and neurons in primary cultures, *J. Neurochem.* **39**:70–77.

Walz, W., and Hertz, L., 1983a, Functional interactions between neurons and astrocytes. II. Potassium homeostasis at the cellular level, *Prog. Neurobiol.* **20**:133–183.

Walz, W., and Hertz, L., 1983b, Electrophysiology of astrocytes in primary cultures, *Neurosci. Soc. Abstr.* **9**:447.

Walz, W., and Schlue, W. R., 1982, Ionic mechanisms of a hyperpolarizing 5-hydroxytryptmine effect on leech neuropil glial cells, *Brain Res.* **250**:111–121.

Ward, A. A., 1961, Epilepsy, *Int. Rev. Neurobiol.* **3**:137–186.

Wardell, W. M., 1966, Electrical and pharmacological properties of mammalian neuroglial cells in tissue culture, *Proc. R. Soc. London Ser. B* **165**:326–361.

Watson, W. E., 1974, Physiology of neuroglia, *Physiol. Rev.* **54**:245–271.

Windle, W. F. (ed.), 1958, *Biology of Neuroglia*, Thomas Springfield, Ill.

Wood, P., and Bunge, R. P., 1984, The biology of the oligodendrocyte, *Adv. Neurochem.* **5**:1–46.

2

Monoamine Innervation of Cerebral Cortex and a Theory of the Role of Monoamines in Cerebral Cortex and Basal Ganglia

JAMES H. FALLON and SANDRA E. LOUGHLIN

1. Introduction

The historical development of interest in the monoamine innervation of cerebral cortex is highlighted by several key discoveries that have changed our perspectives on cortical function specifically, and brain function in general. The dogma until the early 1960s was that the cortex receives input directly from the thalamus but not from the brain stem. Thus, ascending sensory and nonspecific "activating" neural activity generated in the brain stem was thought to have an obligatory synaptic relay in the thalamus before being sent on to cerebral cortex (Moruzzi and Magoun, 1949; Lorente de Nó, 1949, Scheibel and Scheibel, 1958; Nauta and Kuypers, 1958). In the early 1960s the fluorescence technique for the visualization of monoamines (Falck *et al.*, 1962) led to the discovery that monoamine

JAMES H. FALLON and SANDRA E. LOUGHLIN • Department of Anatomy and Neurobiology, University of California, Irvine, California 92717.

cell bodies are present in the brain-stem reticular formation and monoamine fibers are present in cerebral cortex (Dahlstrom and Fuxe, 1964; Fuxe, 1965). Anden *et al.* (1965), therefore, postulated that these brain-stem norepinephrine- and serotonin-containing neurons in the reticular formation give rise to a direct innervation of cerebral cortex. Moore and Heller (1967) were later able to show biochemically that lesions of the medial forebrain bundle, which contains the ascending monoamine fibers, led to a decrease of serotonin and norepinephrine in cortex. However, because such lesions failed to produce visibly degenerating axons in cortex with silver degeneration methods, it was not clear if the decrease of cortical monoamines was merely a result of a transsynaptic effect induced by the lesions. It was not until significant methodological improvements in the fluorescence technique (Lindvall and Björklund, 1974a) and the use of more sensitive tracing techniques such as horseradish peroxidase retrograde tracing and anterograde autoradiography (Pickel *et al.*, 1974; Segal and Landis, 1974; Moore *et al.*, 1978; Fallon and Moore, 1978a,b) that direct reticulocortical nor- adrenergic and serotonergic projections were convincingly demonstrated. It was then determined that dopamine is also present in cortex (Thierry *et al.*, 1973) and that direct projections from midbrain dopaminergic cells to cerebral cortex formed the basis of a third, independent monoamine projection from brain stem to cortex (Berger *et al.*, 1974; Hökfelt *et al.*, 1974a; Lindvall *et al.*, 1974; Tassin *et al.*, 1975).

In the subsequent sections we will focus on some of the more salient features of the functional anatomy of the monoamine innervation of cerebral cortex. Although we have attempted to separate the relevant from the interesting aspects of this voluminous literature, a more complete appreciation of this subject can be obtained by also reading some recent reviews [Molliver *et al.*, 1982; Lindvall and Björklund, 1983; and earlier contributions to Volume 2 in this series (Krnjević, 1984; Wamsley, 1984a)]. The sections on the dopamine, norepinephrine, and serotonin innervation of cerebral cortex are followed by a theoretical section that attempts to integrate some of the anatomy into a new functional scheme.

2. Synthesis of Monoamines

The monoamine neurotransmitters in cerebral cortex include dopamine, norepinephrine, and serotonin. Dopamine and norepinephrine are catechol- amines, and serotonin is an indoleamine, based on the presence of the catechol or indole nucleus, respectively, in their structure. The catecholamines are de- rived from the amino acid tyrosine (Fig. 1). The synthetic pathway (Fig. 1) begins with the conversion of tyrosine to dopa by the rate-limiting enzyme tyrosine hydroxylase (TH). Dopa is converted to dopamine by an aromatic L-amino acid decarboxylase (AAD); in this case it is referred to as dopa decarboxylase. Do- pamine is oxidized by dopamine β-hydroxylase (DBH), and the resultant nor- epinephrine is converted to epinephrine by phenylethanolamine-*N*-methyl trans- ferase (PNMT). The synthesis of serotonin begins with the conversion of the amino acid tryptophan to 5-hydroxytryptophan by tryptophan hydroxylase (TrH). 5-Hydroxytryptophan is converted to serotonin (5-hydroxytryptamine) by aro- matic L-amino acid decarboxylase (AAD).

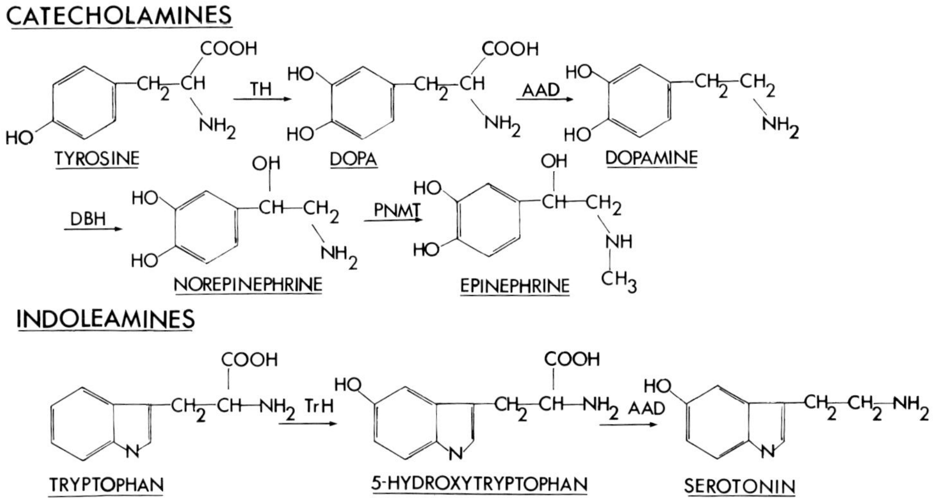

Figure 1. Synthetic pathways of the major catecholamines and indoleamines in neurons. Enzyme abbreviations: TH, tyrosine hydroxylase; AAD, amino acid decarboxylase; DBH, dopamine-β-hydroxylase; PNMT, phenylethanolamine-*N*-methyl transferase; TrH, tryptophan hydroxylase.

3. Techniques of Study

The monoamines have been localized neuroanatomically by histofluorescence and immunohistochemical techniques. These include: (1) the histofluorescence technique based on the condensation of the primary monoamines with gaseous formaldehyde (Falck–Hillarp technique) or glyoxylic acid (glyoxylic acid technique) in a Pictet–Spengler cyclization condensation reaction. The weakly fluorescent fluorophor formed, thus, undergoes an autooxidation or second aldehyde condensation to form strongly fluorescent dihydroisoquinoline compounds (for details see Björklund *et al.*, 1975). The fluorophors are then visible under fluorescent light (excitation of 390–410 nm, emission at 475 nm, green, for catecholamine and 525 nm, yellow, for serotonin). Even with the less sensitive formaldehyde techniques, as little as 5×10^{-4} pg (or 5×10^{-6} pmole) of dopamine or norepinephrine can be visualized in a single terminal or varicosity (Björklund *et al.*, 1975). (2) Another approach to the study of the neuroanatomical visualization of monoamines utilizes immunohistochemical techniques. Antisera raised either against the synthesizing enzymes (e.g., TH, DBH, PNMT, TrH, 1-AADC) or alternatively against the primary monoamines bound to a larger protein such as bovine serum albumin or keyhole limpet hemocyanin have been used to localize monoamine-containing neurons with the indirect immunohistochemical techniques. Other neuroanatomical techniques that have been used to study the localization of monoamines in cortex include: (3) high-resolution autoradiography with ³H-labeled monoamines in light microscopy (Aghajanian and Bloom, 1966; Descarries and Droz, 1968) and electron microscopy (Descarries and Lapierre, 1973); (4) ultrastructural cytochemistry with various fixation techniques and preloading with false neurotransmitters such as 5-hydroxydopamine; (5) standard anterograde and retrograde tracing techniques combined with destruction of catecholamine pathways with neurotoxins such as 6-hydroxydopamine and destruction of indoleamine pathways with 5,6- and 5,7-hydroxytryptamine (Björklund *et al.*, 1973); (6) numerous methodological improvements of the original techniques are detailed in a recent 20-year commemoration of monoamine transmitter histochemistry (Sladek and Björklund, 1982).

In addition to these neuroanatomical techniques, the monoamine systems are commonly studied by biochemical techniques (enzymatic assays, radioimmunoassays, HPLC, amine uptake and turnover techniques, voltammetry, and genomic DNA cloning techniques), pharmacological techniques (receptor binding, receptor autoradiography, drug actions), physiological techniques (physiological recordings, iontophoresis), and behavioral assays. The results of studies using these techniques will be detailed in the following sections.

4. Dopamine

4.1. Introduction

It is initially tempting to consider the monoamine innervation of cortex as a single, global neurochemical system. It is clear that this is far from being the case. The dopamine innervation of cortex is quite different from the norepinephrine and serotonin innervations.

The dopamine innervation was the last to be identified as an independent monoamine system in cortex. Thierry and co-workers initially made this discovery (1973, 1974), and Tassin *et al.* (1974) were able to overcome several obstacles by showing the biochemical independence of the dopamine innervation from the norepinephrine innervation. They used neurotoxic (6-hydroxydopamine) and electrolytic lesions of the norepinephrine systems originating in the locus coeruleus and ascending in the dorsal bundle to show that the dopamine levels were not affected by these lesions (although dopamine levels 5–10% of the norepinephrine content have been considered to be precursor levels of dopamine in norepinephrine terminals). They were then able to show that dopamine fibers, but not cell bodies, are present in cortex (Thierry *et al.*, 1974) and that a specific dopamine uptake system exists in these terminals (Tassin *et al.*, 1974). Studies demonstrating the presence of a dopamine-sensitive adenylate cyclase in cortex and dopaminergic receptors (Mishra *et al.*, 1975; Kuhar *et al.*, 1978; Murrin and Kuhar, 1979) were paralleled by histochemical, lesion, and hodological tract tracing studies (Lindvall *et al.*, 1974, 1978; Fuxe *et al.*, 1974; Fallon *et al.*, 1978a,b; Fallon and Moore, 1978a,b) to prove convincingly the existence of a dopaminergic innervation of specific areas of cortex arising from cell bodies located in the substantia nigra–ventral tegmental area (SN–VTA) of the midbrain tegmentum.

Despite this proof, however, the dopamine system in cortex has been persistently difficult to study. For example, the receptor pharmacology of dopamine is difficult, the physiology is very controversial, and the subcellular binding of dopamine within neurons is weak, rendering electron microscopic analysis of [3H]-dopamine autoradiography relatively ineffective.

4.2. Anatomical Studies

4.2.1. The Mesocortical System

4.2.1a. Origins of the Mesocortical Dopamine Projection. The dopamine neurons innervating the telencephalon, including cerebral cortex, are located in the SN–VTA of the midbrain. The SN–VTA is comprised of a continuum of about 11,000 neurons on each side of the rat brain (Anden *et al.,* 1966). Dopaminergic and nondopaminergic neurons in the SN–VTA that project to cortex are found in the dorsal and ventral "sheet" of cells in the pars compacta of the SN, in the subnuclei paranigralis, parabrachialis pigmentosus, rostral linearis, caudal linearis, and interfascicularis of the VTA, and in the A8 retrorubral field (Fig. 2) (for review see Moore and Bloom, 1978; Lindvall and Björklund, 1983,

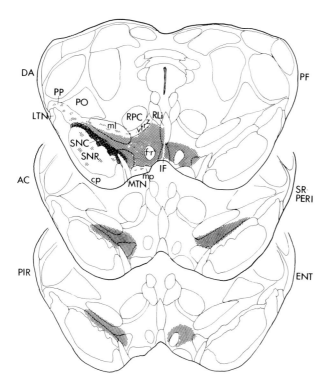

Figure 2. Illustration of the dopamine cells (stippling) that give rise to the mesocortical pathways. The coronal sections of the rat brain are taken at a midrostral level of the SN–VTA. The total dopamine cell distribution at this level is shown at the upper left (DA). The areas giving rise to the anterior cingulate (AC), piriform (PIR), prefrontal (PF), suprarhinal/perirhinal (SR-PERI), and entorhinal (ENT) cortices are illustrated. Other abbreviations are: LTN, lateral terminal nucleus; PP, peripeduncular region; PO, posterior thalamic nucleus; SNC, pars compacta of the substantia nigra; SNR, pars reticulata of the substantia nigra; RPC, parvocellular red nucleus; PP, peripeduncular region; PO, posterior thalamic nucleus; SNC, pars compacta of the substantia nigra; SNR, pars reticulata of the substantia nigra; RPC, parvocellular red nucleus; RLi, rostral linear nucleus; IF, interfascicular nucleus; MTN, medial terminal nucleus; Vtrz, visual tegmental relay zone of Giolli *et al.* (1984); fr, fasciculus retroflexus; cp, cerebral peduncle; ml, medial lemniscus; mp, mammillary peduncle.

1984; Fallon and Loughlin, 1985). This system is referred to as the mesocortical system and is a subset of the mesotelencephalic system. The mesotelencephalic system includes all dopaminergic and nondopaminergic projections to neo- and allo-cortices (mesotelencephalic), striatal structures (mesostriatal) such as the caudate–putamen, nucleus accumbens, and striatal portions of olfactory tubercle (layers I, II, and ventral striatal bridges), amygdala (portions of the central nucleus and analogous portions of the bed nucleus of the stria terminalis), and, possibly, septum. The third portion of the mesotelencephalic system is the so-called mesolimbic system, which frequently changes its membership in the literature. It has included the nucleus accumbens, olfactory tubercle, amygdala, bed nucleus of the stria terminalis, and septum. Since our concept of what constitutes striatal and limbic structures is in flux (Heimer, 1978; Fallon *et al.*, 1983), it is perhaps advisable to drop the term *mesolimbic* unless true "limbic" neurons can be identified. Whereas the mesostriatal projections arise topographically from the SN–VTA, mesocortical projections are more loosely organized (Fallon and Moore, 1976, 1978a; Fallon *et al.*, 1978b; Loughlin and Fallon, 1984; Fallon and Loughlin, 1985).

The data based on these studies indicate that the mesostriatal projection is organized in three planes, with medially placed SN–VTA neurons projecting to the medial (and somewhat anterior) portions of forebrain nuclei and laterally placed SN–VTA neurons projecting to the lateral (and somewhat caudal) portions of these same nuclei. There is also a crude anterior–posterior topography. The third plane of organization is reversed in the dorsal–ventral axis, such that neurons (many with a fusiform shape) in the dorsal "sheet" of the SN–VTA continuum project ventrally in the forebrain, for example, to the olfactory tubercle and amygdala, whereas the ventral "sheet" of SN–VTA neurons (primarily the traditional nigrostriatal neurons in the ventrally located pars compacta of the SN plus the paranigralis VTA neurons located medial to the medial terminal nucleus and just dorsal and anterior to the interpeduncular nucleus) and fewer dorsal "sheet" neurons project more dorsally in the forebrain, for example, to the caudate–putamen and septum. The mesocortical projection, on the other hand, arises from nearly all regions of the dorsal and ventral sheets of SN–VTA neurons but tends to avoid the most ventral mesostriatal neurons of the middle and lateral pars compacta (Fig. 2). As diagrammed in Fig. 2, the projections to prefrontal cortex arise from the VTA, projections to the anterior cingulate cortex arise from the lateral VTA and medial half of the SN, projections to the suprarhinal and perirhinal cortices arise from throughout the SN and most lateral VTA, projections to the piriform cortex arise from the medial two-thirds of the SN and lateral wedge of the VTA, and projections to the entorhinal cortex arise from the VTA and scattered cells in the A8 retrorubral field (not shown). A small percentage (1–5%) of the projections are contralateral.

4.2.1b. Collateralization Patterns. Because there is extensive overlap of the origins of projections to the various cortical and subcortical sites (Fig. 3) it is not surprising that individual SN–VTA neurons send axon collaterals to separate targets in the forebrain (Fig. 4). The zone of the SN–VTA containing the highest percentage (50–70%) of collateralized neurons in the medial SN, with medial VTA having virtually no collateralized projections (Fallon, 1981b; Fallon and Loughlin, 1982; Loughlin and Fallon, 1984). There is some question as to the exact percentage of collateralized neurons in the VTA (cf. only nine double-labeled cells per brain in Swanson, 1982), but it is interesting that this small number of cells gives rise to physiologically identified collateralized projections to frontal cortex, septum, and nucleus accumbens (Deniau *et al.*, 1980).

Anatomical studies have shown that medial SN neurons collateralize to frontal cortex, nucleus accumbens, septum, and medial caudate–putamen (Fallon and Loughlin, 1982). Within cortex (Fig. 4), neurons in the lateral VTA and medial SN send collaterals to pregenual, supragenual, and more posterior por-

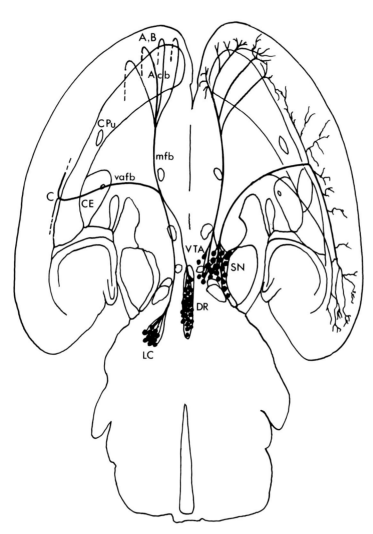

Figure 3. Highly diagrammatic illustration of the monoaminergic pathways from the locus coeruleus (LC), dorsal raphe (DR), and substantia nigra–ventral tegmental area (SN–VTA) to cortex. The major pathways in the forebrain are the medial forebrain bundle and medial internal capsule (mfb) and the ansa peduncularis–ventral amygdalofugal pathway (vafb), also known as the "lateral pathway" to temporal cortices (C). Also shown in this horizontal view of the rat brain are the nucleus accumbens (Acb), caudate–putamen (CPu), and central nucleus of the amygdala (CE).

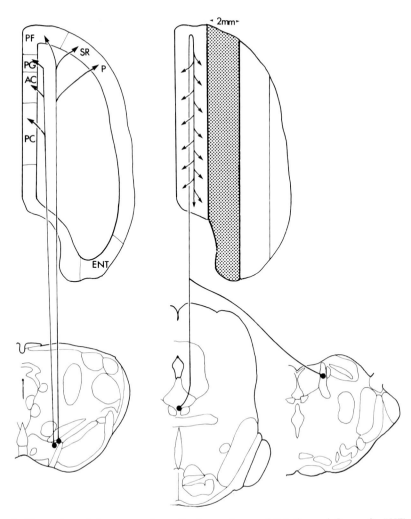

Figure 4. Illustration of the axon collateralization patterns of DA (lower left panel), 5HT (lower middle panel), and NE (lower right panel) neurons to cerebral cortex, shown at top from a horizontal perspective. Note that lateral VTA and medial SN neurons collateralize to pregenual (PG), anterior cingulate (AC), and, to a much lesser extent, posterior cingulate (PC) cortices, whereas other lateral VTA and medial SN neurons collateralize to prefrontal (PF), suprarhinal (SR), and piriform (P) cortices. The entorhinal (ENT) projection is not collateralized. In the case of the 5HT and NE projections, it appears that single neurons collateralize to a longitudinal strip of cortex (stippled) approximately 1.5–2.5 mm in width (Loughlin and Fallon, unpublished).

tions of cingulate cortex, whereas other VTA and SN neurons collateralize to prefrontal and suprarhinal/perirhinal/piriform cortices (Loughlin and Fallon, 1984). Projections to entorhinal cortex are from neurons that have no other identified projections.

4.2.1c. Neurotransmitters in the Mesocortical Projections. It is assumed that dopamine is the predominant neurotransmitter utilized in the SN–VTA projections and while this is generally the case, there are areal differences. The percentage (no. of double labeled per total projection population) of dopaminergic efferents varies from greater than 95% in the mesostriatal (nigrostriatal portion) projection (van der Kooy *et al.*, 1981) to 1–2% in the descending VTA–locus coeruleus pathway (Swanson, 1982; Deutch *et al.*, 1986). Dopaminergic and nondopaminergic neurons projecting to "anterior limbic" cortex form an intermixed matrix in the VTA, and reports of relative percentages of dopaminergic projections range from 0% (Swanson, 1982) to 90% (Albanese and Bentivoglio, 1982). The percentage of dopaminergic projection to the pregenual and supragenual portions of the anterior cingulate cortex (anterior limbic cortex) are similar (27% to VTA, 40% in medial SN), while others include entorhinal cortex (50%) and hippocampus (6%)(Swanson, 1982).

The immunohistochemical studies of Hökfelt and colleagues have shown that some dopamine cells in the SN–VTA also contain the peptides cholecystokinin (CCK) (Hökfelt *et al.*, 1980) or neurotensin (NT) (Hökfelt *et al.*, 1983). We have also recently demonstrated the colocalization and forebrain projections of CCK–NT neurons (Seroogy *et al.*, 1987b). Therefore, we must consider the possibility of dopamine/CCK, dopamine/NT, CCK/NT, and dopamine/CCK/NT mesocortical systems. A dopamine/CCK pathway has been established for the projection to posterior nucleus accumbens, but these experiments indicated that the dopamine and CCK innervation of frontal cortex arises from separate VTA neurons (Studler *et al.*, 1981). Recently in this laboratory, however, we have found that following injections of retrograde fluorescent tracers such as Fluoro-Gold, Stilbene Gold, True Blue, Fast Blue, or Propidium Iodide into frontal cortex, many retrogradely labeled cells in the SN–VTA also contained CCK and tyrosine hydroxylase-like immunoreactivities (Seroogy *et al.*, 1987a). Triple-labeled cells were also found in the SN–VTA after injections of tracer into the anterior caudate–putamen, nucleus accumbens, suprarhinal cortex, and amygdala (Seroogy *et al.*, 1987a), suggesting a commonality of dopamine/CCK input into forebrain structures related to the "prefrontal systems."

4.2.1d. The Retino-mesotelencephalic System. One rather peculiar throughput system of the SN–VTA related to prefrontal and anterior cingulate cortices is the retino-mesotelencephalic system. In recent double-labeling experiments we have found that [^{3}H]adenosine is transported from the retina to neurons of the medial terminal nucleus and some neurons of the SN–VTA that probably send their dendrites into the medial terminal nucleus. Some of these putative retinorecipient neurons of the SN–VTA were found, in the same animals, to be retrogradely labeled by injections of the retrograde fluorescent tracer SITS into prefrontal cortex, anterior cingulate cortex, or anteromedial caudate–putamen (Fallon *et al.*, 1984; Giolli *et al.*, 1985). Such a disynaptic pathway may provide short-latency visual information (perhaps not "consciously" perceived) to the high-order association cortex of the prefrontal system. The neurotransmitter utilized in this potential pathway is unknown.

4.2.2. Pathways of the Mesocortical Dopamine Projection

The axons of the mesocortical pathway collect medially in the rostral–lateral VTA and medial SN (Fig. 14A) and ascend in the medial forebrain bundle (Fig.

3). As the fibers ascend through the lateral hypothalamus, some fibers turn laterally over the supraoptic commissures to enter the ventral amygdalofugal bundle (Fig. 13A*). The fibers pass through the central nucleus of the amygdala and caudal portion of the fundus striata (ventral caudate–putamen), and fan out in the amygdala to innervate the perirhinal and piriform cortices (Fig. 13A) as well as deep layers of dorsal and lateral (somatosensory) neocortex. Some fibers pass caudally in deep layers of the perirhinal cortex and external capsule to innervate the entorhinal cortex and temporal pole of the hippocampal formation (Fig. 14A). Mesocortical fibers continuing their ascent in the medial forebrain bundle and medial edge of the internal capsule may pass ventral and lateral to the nucleus accumbens (rostromedial fundus striata) to reach anterior suprarhinal (lateral prefrontal cortices) and posterior suprahinal cortices (Fig. 12A), or ascend through the medial and ventromedial nucleus accumbens to reach the deep layers of prefrontal cortex, or sweep around the genu of the corpus callosum (Fig. 11A) to innervate superficial and deep layers of supragenual cortex and deep layers of more posterior cingulate cortex (Fig. 13A).

4.2.3. Terminal Projections of the Mesocortical Dopamine System

The terminal projections of the mesocortical dopamine system have been studied in detail in a number of laboratories (Albanese and Bentivoglio, 1982; Beckstead, 1976, 19878; Beckstead *et al.*, 1979; Berger *et al.*, 1974, 1976, 1985; Björklund *et al.*, 1978; Brown and Goldman, 1977; Carter and Fibiger, 1977; Collier and Routtenberg, 1977; Divac *et al.*, 1975, 1978; Emson and Koob, 1978; Fallon, 1981a; Fallon *et al.*, 1978a,b, 1983; Fallon and Moore, 1978a,b; Fallon and Loughlin, 1982; Fuxe *et al.*, 1974; Gerfen and Clavier, 1979; Gessa *et al.*, 1974; Hökfelt *et al.*, 1974a,b; Lewis *et al.*, 1979; Lindvall *et al.*, 1974, 1978, 1984; Markowitsch and Irle, 1981; Reader *et al.*, 1979a,b; Scheibner, 1986; Schmidt *et al.*, 1982; Simon *et al.*, 1976, 1979; Swanson, 1982; Tassin *et al.*, 1977; Thierry *et al.*, 1973; Tork and Turner, 1981; van der Kooy and Kuypers, 1979; for reviews see Lindvall and Björklund, 1983, 1984; Moore and Bloom, 1978; Thierry *et al.*, 1984; Fallon and Loughlin, 1985) and the results of these studies have been used to generate the schematic diagrams of areal terminations (Figs. 10A, 11A, 12A, 13A, 14A, and 15A) and laminar distribution of dopamine fibers (Figs. 16, 17, and 18) in coronal sections of the albino rat brain.

4.2.3a. Prefrontal Cortex. Prefrontal cortex in mammals can be defined as those cortical areas receiving input from the mediodorsal thalamic nucleus (Divac *et al.*, 1975, 1978). These regions also receive a moderately dense dopaminergic input. In the rat these include area 32 of anteromedial prefrontal cortex and agranular insular suprarhinal cortex (Figs. 10A, 11B, and 12A). The fibers are smooth and are distributed densely in layers V and VI with sparsely scattered fibers in more superficial layers. The fibers arise from cell bodies in the VTA (Fig. 2). In primates, recent evidence (Brown and Goldman, 1977; Brown *et al.*, 1979; Levitt *et al.*, 1981, 1984a,b) has shown that a dense dopamine innervation is present in orbital and dorsolateral prefrontal cortices as well as

*Figures 10–19 on pages 77–86.

moderate amounts in premotor and motor cortices. In the rat, the dorsal neo-cortices are sparsely innervated by dopamine fibers. Such species differences in the monoamine innervation of cerebral cortex are commonly found, as will be further seen in subsequent sections.

4.2.3b. Cingulate Cortex. The dopaminergic innervation of cingulate cortex is primarily to the most anterior regions (pregenual) and supragenual regions of anterior cingulate cortex (areas 24a and 24b). In the pregenual region, the fibers are present in the deep cortical layers (Fig. 11A). An abrupt transition takes place in the supragenual portion of anterior cingulate cortex, where a denser innervation of layers III, II, and, to a lesser extent, Ia appears (Fig. 12A and 16). This more superficial innervation, which contains varicose fibers, arises from cell bodies in the medial SN and lateral VTA (Fig. 2). The sparser inner-vation of deeper layers continues caudally into more caudal areas of anterior cingulate cortex (Fig. 13A). Posterior cingulate retrosplenial cortex contains a very sparse innervation in deeper layers (Figs. 14A and 16). Some dopaminergic innervation of layers I–III of retrosplenial granular areas 29c,b and agranular area 29d may also be present (Berger *et al.*, 1985).

4.2.3c. Perirhinal Cortex. Perirhinal cortex includes the strip of agranular insular cortex that begins at the caudal border of suprarhinal ("lateral prefron-tal") cortex and runs caudally with the rhinal sulcus. Dopaminergic fibers are present in all cortical layers, but especially in deep laminae along this strip (Figs. 11A, 12A, 13A, 14A, and 17). The densest fiber concentration runs closely along the lateral border of the claustrum and dorsal endopiriform nucleus (Figs. 11A, 12A, and 13A). These deep figures, running in a loosely organized "extreme capsule" in the rat, originate in the lateral VTA, medial SN (Fig. 2), and A8 cell groups.

4.2.3d. Piriform Cortex. The dopaminergic innervation of piriform cortex is modest, with the medial half (area 51A) receiving a more dense innervation than the lateral half (area 51b) (Figs. 11A, 12A, and 13A). Most medially, the cortex–amygdala transition zone (Cxa) receives the densest innervation (Fig. 13A). Fibers are primarily found in layers II and III, with some occasional clustering of terminal plexuses being present in layer II (Fig. 17). Like perirhinal cortex, dopaminergic fibers in piriform cortex originate in cell bodies located in the lateral VTA, SN, and A8 (A. Deutch, personal communication) (Fig. 2). The fibers reach these cortices by the rostral–lateral route and through the ven-tral–lateral route of the ansa peduncularis–ventral amygdalofugal bundle (Fig. 3). The lateral route becomes more dominant in primates, where an extensive dopaminergic innervation of temporal cortices is present (Levitt *et al.*, 1984b).

4.2.3e. Entorhinal Cortex. The anterior portion of lateral entorhinal cor-tex receives a unique type of dopaminergic innervation (Fig. 14A). The fibers form dense clusters in layers II and III around islands of cells (Fig. 17). Cell bodies in the VTA (Fig. 2) and retrorubral field (A8; not shown in Fig. 2) give rise to these fibers, which reach the entorhinal cortex through the posterior lateral route (Fig. 3).

4.2.3f. Other Cortices. Other areas of neo- and allocortices have been reported to contain a sparse to moderate dopaminergic innervation. After injections of horseradish peroxidase into numerous neocortical regions of the cat, retrogradely labeled cells are present in the VTA (Markowitsch and Irle, 1981). Widespread dopaminergic projections to sensory and motor neocortices in the rat can also be demonstrated with the anterograde autoradiographic technique (Fig. 5 of Fallon and Moore, 1978b) and histochemical techniques (Berger *et al.,* 1985; Berger and Verney, 1984). Although it is thought that projections of the VTA to neocortices as well as to the hippocampus (Cragg, 1961; Wyss *et al.,* 1979; Scatton *et al.,* 1980), may represent some nondopaminergic projections of neurons in the VTA, recent studies support the idea that there are dopaminergic projections to the hippocampus from the VTA (Swanson, 1982) and dorsal raphe (Reymann *et al.,* 1983), and to visual cortex from the VTA (Swanson, 1982) and dorsal raphe (Reymann *et al.,* 1983), and to visual cortex from the VTA in the rat (Tork and Turner, 1981). Berger and colleagues (Berger *et al.,* 1985) have recently reported a widespread dopaminergic projection to virtually all neocortices in the rat.

In the monkey it had been thought that prefrontal and premotor cortices were the only neocortices innervated by DA fibers, suggesting that there is an anterior-to-posterior gradient of DA innervation in the primate cortex. This concept is challenged in a study by Lewis *et al.* (1987) who found that the DA innervation of Old World and New World monkey cortices is more widespread than previously thought. Lewis and colleagues found TH-immunoreactive (and on the basis of NE fiber lesions, DA specific) axons in all cortices, with a preferential innervation of motor versus sensory cortices, agranular versus granular cortices, association versus primary sensory regions, and auditory association versus visual association cortices. Thus, the DA innervation favors association and motor cortices over sensory cortices. Correlated with this area-to-area specialization is the general finding that layer IV is always poorly innervated. These patterns of innervation suggest that DA regulates the activity of cortical output, rather than thalamocortical input projections.

4.2.4. Ontogenetic Development

DA neurons in the SN–VTA are the earliest monoamine cells (both ontogenetically and phylogenetically) to differentiate. In the rat, these neurons derive from a common cell complex (Seiger and Olson, 1973) and are born on days E11–E13 (Lauder and Bloom, 1974). Using TH immunoreactivity as a marker, Berger and Verney (1984) have found DA fibers first reach the cortex on day E16 in the intermediate zone of anteromedial prefrontal cortex. This corresponds to the day of arrival of thalamocortical fibers. At E17, scattered fibers are seen to pierce the striatum and reach lateral frontal cortex. At E18, two prominent bundles are present. One pathway passes ventral to the striatum to innervate the intermediate zone of frontal cortex and the second follows a more medial course to enter the intermediate zone of the medial wall of frontal–cingulate cortices. These pathways pass caudally along the rhinal fissure, suprarhinal cortex, and deep supragenual cortex until birth. The fibers appear to remain in the intermediate zone for several days before penetrating the cortical plate. The postnatal development proceeds for 2 weeks, with more posterior cortices (entorhinal cortex) developing last. Interestingly, Berger and Verney (1984) also found that the superficial plexus of supragenual cortex develops about a week later than the fibers in the deeper layers of supragenual cortex. The superficial plexus appears one day P3 and, like the developing and adult DA fibers of the deep layers of frontal and cingulate cortices, contains fine fibers. During the next 2–3 weeks the superficial plexus acquires the appearance of NE fibers, i.e., they are fine and varicose. The fibers of the deeper layers, on the other hand, arrive on day E20 and remain smooth until adulthood. These findings suggest that the fibers in the superficial layers arise from different cell bodies (SN) than those of the deeper layers (VTA). If this is so, then the superficial plexus would resemble more the terminal DA plexuses in the caudate–putamen than other DA fibers in cerebral cortex, because both the fibers innervating the superficial plexus and caudate–putamen share: (1) a parallel development, (2) a set time of arrival in the terminal areas, (3) a similar origin in the SN, and (4) a similar terminal morphology. The analogy should be taken cautiously, however, since the DA fibers in prefrontal and anterior cingulate cortices are similar in that they both lack autoreceptors (Bannon *et al.*, 1981).

4.3. Functional Studies

Paralleling anatomical studies on the DA innervation of cerebral cortex were numerous biochemical studies (Thierry *et al.*, 1973; Brownstein *et al.*, 1974; Tassin *et al.*, 1975; Kehr *et al.*, 1976; Versteeg *et al.*, 1976; Emson and Koob, 1978; Fallon and Moore, 1978a, Fallon *et al.*, 1978a; Brown *et al.*, 1979 Palkovits *et al.*, 1979; Reader *et al.*, 1979b; Pycock *et al.*, 1980; Slopsema *et al.*, 1982) that confirmed the regional localization of DA in cerebral cortex. [^{3}H]-DA uptake studies (Tassin *et al.*, 1979) and DA turnover studies (Thierry *et al.*, 1976; Lavielle *et al.*, 1979; Agnati *et al.*, 1980) have demonstrated that, despite the confirmation of DA regionalization in cortex by biochemical studies, many biochemical differences exist between cortical regions. Some of these differences can be explained by studies on DA receptors in cerebral cortex.

4.3.1. Receptors

In a previous chapter in this series, Wamsley (1984a) discussed the distribution and characterization of receptors in cortex and emphasized the difficulties in localizing DA receptors in cortex. D_1 receptors, coupled to a DA-sensitive adenylate cyclase, were detected in cerebral cortex over a decade ago (Von Hungen *et al.*, 1974; Mishra *et al.*, 1975). The location of the cyclase activity, biochemically measured DA, and DA histofluorescence overlaps well in cortex. The D_1 receptor appears to be localized postsynaptically on cortical neurons (Tassin *et al.*, 1982, 1986) and may be regulated, in part, by NE input (Tassin *et al.*, 1982). In contrast to these D_1 receptors, cortical D_2 receptors are present presynaptically as autoreceptors in piriform cortex, entorhinal cortex (Bannon *et al.*, 1982, 1983), and subcortical sites, such as the caudate–putamen, olfactory tubercle, and nucleus accumbens (Farnebo and Hamberger, 1971; Bannon *et al.*, 1983; Altar *et al.*, 1985). These autoreceptors are absent in prefrontal and anterior cingulate cortices (Bannon *et al.*, 1982), which helps to explain why there is a higher ratio of DA turnover in these cortices as opposed to DA-rich subcortical sites. However, recent studies suggest that in prefrontal/lateral cingulate cortex, synthesis-modulating autoreceptors are absent but release-modulating autoreceptors may be present; thus, long-term (synthesis) regulation of DA may be lacking, but short-term (release) regulation of DA may exist (Wolf *et al.*, 1986; Galloway *et al.*, 1986). The presence of DA receptors in cerebral cortex is still disputed (cf. Martres *et al.*, 1985; Palacios *et al.*, 1981; Murrin and Kuhar, 1979) since the ligands used (spiroperidol: spiperone) to label D_2 receptors also bind to serotonin receptors (Creese and Snyder, 1978; Palacios *et al.*, 1981). Subtraction techniques following pharmacological manipulations with DA receptor blockers (pimozide), DA agonists (ADTN), or serotonin agonists (pimpamerone) are necessary to localize the D_2 receptors (Murrin and Kuhar, 1979; Marchais *et al.*, 1980). Murrin and Kuhar (1979) have also found that D_2 receptors are present in other DA-rich areas such as the deep (but not superficial) layers of anterior cingulate cortex and suprarhinal cortex. Thus, it is likely that the plexus of DA fibers in layers II and III of anterior cingulate cortex and the deep layers of prefrontal cortex share the characteristic of lacking autoreceptors, and DA fibers in areas such as the deeper laminae of anterior cingulate cortex, piriform cortex, and entorhinal cortex are similar in that they probably possess receptors that inhibit the release of DA. This finding is curious since some DA neurons that innervate prefrontal cortex (no autoreceptors) also innervate piriform cortex (autoreceptors). In addition, neurons that innervate anterior cingulate cortex (no autoreceptors) do not innervate prefrontal cortex or piriform cortex (Loughlin and Fallon, 1984). A recent study (Martres *et al.*, 1985) using iodosulpride as the ligand, however, found that D_2 receptors are present in superficial cingulate and deep frontal cortices. Cortical D_2 receptors may be involved in DA's excitatory influence in cortex (Bradshaw *et al.*, 1985). Adding to this apparent contradiction are numerous controversies regarding the physiology of DA inputs.

4.3.2. Physiology

The electrophysiological effect of DA on postsynaptic cells is still controversial (for reviews see Moore and Bloom, 1978; Groves, 1983; Rolls, 1987). The most common effect reported is inhibition, but in these studies extracellular recordings were made so that direct observation of postsynaptic potentials is, of course, not possible. In intracellular recording situations where postsynaptic potentials have been recorded (Kitai *et al.*, 1976), the initial effect of iontophoretically applied DA is depolarization (EPSP).

In cerebral cortex of the cat, Krnjević and Phillis (1963a,b) initially reported depressant effects of DA on cortical neurons. Subsequent studies (Yarbrough and Lake, 1973; Yarbrough *et al.*, 1974; Bevan *et al.*, 1975; Mora *et al.*, 1976; Bunney and Aghajanian, 1976; Sharma, 1977; Hicks and McLennan, 1978; Reader, 1978; Reader *et al.*, 1979a,b; Ferron *et al.*, 1982; Bannon *et al.*, 1982; Bernardi *et al.*, 1982; Grace and Bunney, 1983; Chiodo *et al.*, 1984; Mercuri *et al.*, 1985) have reported both excitatory and inhibitory effects of DA on cortical neurons. In frontal cortex and caudate–putamen, DA may act to increase the signal-to-noise ratio (Rolls, 1987) and signal detectability of postsynaptic neurons, thus increasing throughput of the frontal striatal system. A recent electrophysiological study using intracellular techniques (Bernardi *et al.*, 1982) supports both concepts. DA was found to produce an initial slow depolarization (excitation) and a decrease in firing rates (inhibition) without any salient changes in membrane resistance. Following stimulation of the cell bodies of origin in the VTA, EPSP–IPSP sequences were induced in frontal cortical neurons.

Other investigators (Guyenet and Aghajanian, 1978; Deniau *et al.*, 1980; Thierry *et al.*, 1980, 1984; Wang, 1981; Grace and Bunney, 1983; Bunney and Chiodi, 1984; Shepard and Gorman, 1984) have demonstrated that two populations of neurons in the VTA project to prefrontal cortex. The axons are probably unmyelinated (Hökfelt and Ungerstedt, 1973) and this finding is supported by the physiological data. One group of axons have a long latency and slow conduction velocity (0.55 m/sec), with a long spike duration (2.2 msec), and are probably dopaminergic, whereas the second group has a faster conduction velocity (3.2 m/sec), shorter spike duration (1.7 msec), and are probably nondopaminergic (Deniau *et al.*, 1980; Thierry *et al.*, 1980). The fact that the neurons projecting to prefrontal cortex have faster firing rates (9.3 spikes/sec) and are more rapid bursters than neurons projecting to other cortical areas (Bunney and Chiodo, 1984) may reflect their lack of self-inhibiting autoreceptors (Bannon *et al.*, 1982).

4.3.3. Interactions

How do DA inputs interact with other inputs to cerebral cortex? It has been discussed how DA is most interactive within its own system of release, i.e., self-inhibition through the actions of autoreceptors. There is little evidence for interactions with other monoamines in cerebral cortex. This is easily explained by the relative isolation of DA terminal receptors from other monoamine inputs to specific cortical laminae. There are examples of interactions between ACh and DA in cortex, with inhibitory actions on release of neurotransmitters either presynaptically (ACh's effect at muscarinic receptors on DA terminals) or postsynaptically (DA's suppression of ACh's excitatory effect) (for review see Reader and Jasper, 1984). DA appears to potentiate the inhibitory effect of GABA on cortical cells, and reduce the excitatory effects of glutamic acid in cortical cells (Reader and Jasper, 1984), thereby having generally inhibiting actions on cerebral cortical output. Because the postsynaptic effects of DA are long-lasting but subtle, and because DA changes the response of cortical cells to "classical" (GABA, glutamate) neurotransmitters, it can be thought of as a neuromodulator in cortical function (Bunney and Chiodi, 1984). Thus, extrinsically derived modulators (DA) and intrinsic local circuit modulators (peptides) may interact to alter cortical neuronal output (Fig. 8). In addition, the presence of coexistent DA, CCK, and NT projections to prefrontal and piriform cortices (Seroogy *et al.*, 1987b) may add another level of complex interactions of peptide modulators (cholecystokinin and neurotensin) and a monoamine inhibitory modulator (DA) within the same terminal in cortex.

4.3.4. Behavioral Studies

The function of DA in cerebral cortex is not well understood. There are, however, a number of findings that suggest DA is involved with higher integrative cortical functions: (1) DA neurons projecting to frontal cortex are activated by low-intensity foot-shocking-induced stress (Thierry *et al.*, 1976; Lavielle *et al.*, 1979; Deutch *et al.*, 1985b). (2) DA neurons projecting to cortex are independently regulated, in that those projecting to cortex have been shown by one group to be influenced by habenular efferents (Lisoprowski *et al.*, 1980), whereas those projecting to subcortical sites are most affected by raphe inputs (Herve *et al.*, 1979, 1981). (3) Changes in DA function in cortex may underlie the etiology of schizophrenia (Hökfelt *et al.*, 1974b) and the antischizophrenic drug, sulpiride, was shown to affect DA turnover in entorhinal cortex (Tagliamonti *et al.*, 1975). (4) Delayed alteration response behavior, long thought to be a prefrontal and/or anterior striatal function, can be interrupted by 6-hydroxydopamine lesions of the VTA (Carter and Pycock, 1978; Simon *et al.*, 1979), and by DA depletion in the principalis sector of prefrontal cortex in the rhesus monkey (Brozoski *et al.*, 1979). (5) In some cases of advanced Parkinson's disease, cognitive defects, intellectual impairment, depression, and schizophrenic thought disorders are present (for review see Javoy-Agid and Agid, 1980). These "frontal" cortical signs are ameliorated by treatment with L-dopa (Loranger *et al.*, 1972). In some cases, such replacement therapy induces hallucinations and mania (Morel-Maroger, 1977), perhaps due to supersensitivity to denervated DA receptors in cortex that normally are innervated by DA from the VTA (Javoy-Agid and Agid, 1980). (6) A permanent behavioral syndrome in the rat, induced by lesions of the VTA (hyperactivity, inability to learn a passive avoidance task, difficulty in suppressing previously learned responses, disappearance of alternation behavior), may be correlated with loss of DA in frontal cortex and nucleus accumbens (Tassin *et al.*, 1977). In addition, damage to orbital frontal cortex, but not anteromedial frontal cortex, appears to be the site affected in locomotor hyperactivity (Kolb, 1974; Tassin *et al.*, 1977). (7) The DA innervation of cerebral cortex (and cortical innervation of midbrain) may play a role in self-stimulation behavior (German and Bowden, 1974; Routtenberg and Sloan, 1972). (8) Normal exploratory behavior depends on the functional integrity of the mesocortical DA system (Fink and Smith, 1980). It should be stressed that many of these data were derived from studies using lesions that were nonselective (e.g., lesioning dopaminergic plus nondopaminergic inputs), or lesions that involved other systems (e.g., destruction of thalamocortical inputs). In addition, it is sometimes presumed that, by lesioning the VTA and SN, mesocortical and mesolimbic projections are selectively affected. In fact, the VTA also projects to the striatum, and the SN projects to some cortical areas (Fallon and Moore, 1978b).

With these caveats in mind, it can be seen from the anatomical, physiological, and behavioral data that the DA input to cerebral cortex affects predominantly agranular "limbic type" of cortex. Isocortex, which can be thought of as acting to organize sensory information and sensory-motor association information in a columnar manner that is then passed back to subcortical structures, is generally less innervated by DA fibers. Very-high-order association, allocortex, and juxta-allocortex of the frontal and temporal regions are richly innervated by DA fibers. The DA-rich cortical regions are generally believed to be involved in inhibition of subcortical sites; when the DA input or cortical output of these cortical areas is damaged, subcortical loops and outputs are released from inhibition and locomotor hyperactivity ensues (Iversen, 1984). However, if the postsynaptic action of DA on cortical neurons is to reduce depolarization and reduce action potentials, and if DA's modulatory interactions on GABA output are facilitatory, and DA's effect on glutamate output is inhibitory, then the net effect of DA on cortical output is inhibitory. Thus, if there is a simple correspondence between neurophysiology and behavior, then the effects of lesions of the DA input to cortex should be opposite to the effects of cortical lesions, which does not appear to be the case (Scatton *et al.*, 1982). This contradiction between the neurophysiological and behavioral manifestations of these lesions is difficult to reconcile. Since Brozoski *et al.*, (1979) found that the behavioral effect of DA depletion in monkey prefrontal cortex could be reversed by apomorphine of L-dopa, some DA receptor effect is implicated. Perhaps there are interactions of DA with other (non-D_1 or D_2) receptor systems in frontal cortex. Additionally, since the DA projection to anterior cingulate cortex probably influences a different type of cortical output neuron (layer II and III pyramidal cells with corticocortical outputs) than those in prefrontal cortex (pyramidal cells of layers V and VI with corticostriatal, corticothalamic, and corticomesencephalic outputs), then separate output systems would be affected by a DA depletion in prefrontal versus anterior cingulate cortices. Likewise, different corticostriatopallidal systems may be impacted by such a DA depletion. In one case, a net excitatory output system would be disrupted [corticostriatopallidal projection involving glutamate and aspartate (+) and substance P and K (+)], and in the other case, a net inhibitory output system might be disrupted [a corticostriatopallidal projection involving glutamate (+) and GABA (−)]. Many other complex cortico-subcortico-loop systems could be called upon to explain the powerful, but perplexing effects of DA depletion in cortex (see Section 7 for theoretical treatment). A different approach could be to view the ascending mesocortical projection as being primarily one that contains CCK (excitatory), rather than DA (inhibitory). Such a view could also reconcile the neurophysiological and behavioral data. The paucity of DA receptors (cf. Martres *et al.*, 1985) in frontal and cingulate cortices, thus, would not be surprising if CCK were the dominant mesocortical neuromodulator. The very high density of CCK receptors in the outer portion of layer I, and layers II and III of anterior cingulate cortex, and the high density in deep layers of frontal cortex (see Wamsley, 1984a,b) overlaps the "dopamine" mesocortical inputs (Fig. 16). Therefore, our ignorance of the function of DA in cerebral cortex may, in part, be due to an epiphenomenal artifact, i.e., DA just happens to be contained in some CCK neurons projecting to cortex.

5. Norepinephrine

5.1. Introduction

The sole source of NE terminals in cerebral cortex in the rat is the nucleus locus coeruleus (LC). As has been discussed, the development of sensitive methods for the demonstration of catecholamine fibers in cortex (Falck *et al.*, 1962; Fuxe *et al.*, 1968) combined with lesions of the pontine cell bodies and/or ascending pathways allowed the demonstration of this system. Many more studies have followed on its pathways, terminal arborization, collateralization, ultrastructure, pharmacology, physiology, and behavior. This monosynaptic monoamine input to cortex parallels the serotonin system in many ways, but shows marked differences in terminal arborization and regional heterogeneity. For many years it was believed that the cells of LC were homogeneous with respect to efferent projection such that the axons of all LC cells collateralized to innervate all terminal fields. Recent work challenges this concept and suggests that LC cells are more restricted in their efferent projections. More recently, the existence of a number of peptidergic neurotransmitters in noradrenergic (NE-containing) LC cells has been demonstrated. As with many other brain systems, our concept of the complexity of LC function must thus be revised.

5.2. Anatomical Studies

5.2.1. The Coeruleocortical System

5.2.1a. Cell Bodies of Origin. The approximately 1600 cells of the LC are located in the pontine tegmentum (See Figs. 3 and 4). All or most of these cells contain NE (Swanson, 1976) and they are most often subdivided into two major groups, the dorsal, compact LC containing pseudofusiform and multipolar "core" cells and the ventral LC containing large multipolar cells. While further subdivisions can be defined (Loughlin and Fallon, 1985; Loughlin *et al.*, 1986a,b), cortical projections arise from core cells and a few fusiform cells scattered across all sections of dorsal compact LC (Mason and Fibiger, 1979; Waterhouse *et al.*, 1983; Loughlin *et al.*, 1986a). A crude topography exists in cortical projections, such that the more anterior cells project to anterior cortical regions, and more posterior cells project posteriorly. Additionally, there is a slight tendency for the innervation (Waterhouse *et al.*, 1983) of lateral cortical regions, such as suprarhinal cortex, to arise from more ventral cells, but largely coextensive distributions of cells are derived after widely separated cortical injections of retrograde tracer (Loughlin *et al.*, 1982). The hippocampally projecting cells are located within the dorsal one-third of LC (Mason and Fibiger, 1979; Loughlin *et al.*, 1986a) and are largely fusiform cells (Loughlin *et al.*, 1986b). Approximately 5–10% of LC projections to cortex arise contralaterally (Ader *et al.*, 1980; Room *et al.*, 1981). In the primate, the LC is bisected by the superior cerebellar peduncle. Cortically projecting cells are located in both divisions (Freedman *et al.*, 1975) and do not appear to be topographically organized.

5.2.1b. Collateralization Patterns. While individual LC cells may not innervate all terminal fields, they do exhibit markedly collateralized axons. Studies utilizing the simultaneous injection of multiple retrograde tracers have shown that one cortically projecting LC cell may also innervate widely disparate brain regions such as hippocampus, thalamus, and/or cerebellum (Nagai *et al.*, 1981; Room *et al.*, 1981; Steindler, 1981). LC cells also collateralize within cortex. Some axons bifurcate to simultaneously innervate bilateral cortices (Ader *et al.*, 1980; Room *et al.*, 1981). Axons of individual LC cells collateralize extensively within

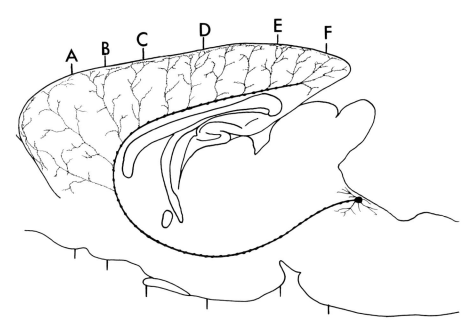

Figure 5. Schematic drawing of a single NE axon arising from the locus coeruleus and innervating cortical regions. Note the anterior-to-posterior course of the axons in cortex and the rich arborization patterns (cf. Fig. 4). It has not been resolved if, alternatively, the plexus in superficial layers forms a separate bundle that first collateralizes from the parent axons in prefrontal cortex. Letters A–F in this parasagittal view show where coronal sections in Figs. 10–15 are taken from in the rat brain. These correspond as follows: Fig. 10A,B is level A in this figure, Fig. 11A,B is level B, Fig. 12A,B is level C, Fig. 13A,B is level D, Fig. 14A,B is level E, Fig. 15A,B is level F.

the anterior-to-posterior dimensions of cortex (see Figs. 4 and 5) but only to a limited extent in the medial-to-lateral dimension (Loughlin *et al.*, 1982). This is consistent with the lesion studies of Morrison *et al.* (1981) and suggests that LC cells innervate longitudinal wedges of cortex of approximately 2 mm in width (see Fig. 4). Most cells that exhibit collateralized axons are the "core cells" in the central region of the compact dorsal division of LC (Fallon and Loughlin, 1982).

5.2.1c. Neurotransmitters. The major neurotransmitter in LC neurons is NE. It is thought that all, or nearly all, cells within LC contain NE and its associated synthetic enzyme, DBH (Swanson, 1976). Only one class of cells, small round cells, have not been conclusively shown to contain NE (Loughlin *et al.*, 1986b). Recent studies have also shown that LC cells in the rat contain one or more peptides. These include vasopressin, neurophysin (Caffee and van Leeuwen, 1983), neurotensin (Uhl *et al.*, 1979), and corticotropin-releasing factor (Swanson *et al.*, 1983). In the cat, in which LC is more diffuse, some LC cells may also contain serotonin (Leger *et al.*, 1979) and enkephalin (Charney *et al.*, 1982). The peptide content of primate LC cells remains unknown. Three recent studies have examined the projections of peptide-containing cells in rat LC directly by a double-labeling technique. Neuropeptide Y- and galanin-containing cells exhibit differential projections to cortex (Gustafson and Moore, 1985; Holets *et al.*, 1985; Skofitsch and Jacobowitz, 1985).

5.2.2. Pathways of the LC Projection to Cortex

The axons of the LC collect into five major efferent bundles, but only one of these contains all or nearly all of the projections to cortex (Ungerstedt, 1971). This major efferent, known as the "dorsal bundle," traverses the midbrain tegmentum ventrolaterally to the periaqueductal gray and then turns laterally at the level of the fasciculus retroflexus, to join the medial forebrain bundle. Here the monoaminergic cells traverse the lateral hypothalamic area predominantly in the medial forebrain bundle. At the level of the caudal septum, the medial forebrain bundle divides into several major branches. Some fibers continue medially along the diagonal band to the septum, continue on into the fornix and contribute to the innervation of the hippocampus (Loy *et al.*, 1980). Some axons traverse the diagonal band and Zuckerkandl's bundle to turn caudally around the corpus callosum. These run in a compact band along the cingulum contributing to the innervation of medial cortex, but probably not dorsal neocortex (Morrison *et al.*, 1978). This bundle continues through the subiculum to hippocampus. Another group of fibers continues in the medial forebrain bundle, ascends in the external capsule, and may contribute to neocortical innervation. The majority of neocortical innervation derives from fibers that ascend in the frontal pole and direct themselves longitudinally in layer VI throughout neocortex (Morrison *et al.*, 1981). The trajectory of these fibers is indicated in Fig. 6. Collaterals then ascend through the cortical layers in complex patterns described in Section 5.2.3a–g (see also Figs. 5, 10–18). In primates, a portion of the neocortical innervations may derive from a lateral pathway (Levitt *et al.*, 1984b).

5.2.3. Terminal Projections of the Locus Coeruleus

The terminations of coeruleocortical axons have been examined by a number of techniques in many laboratories (Beaudet and Descarries, 1978; Brown *et al.*, 1979; Fallon and Loughlin, 1982; Gatter and Powell, 1977 Levitt and Moore, 1978; Levitt *et al.*, 1984a; Lindvall and Björklund, 1984; Loughlin *et al.*, 1982; Morrison *et al.*, 1978a, 1981, 1984). Based on these and other studies, schematic diagrams have been constructed of the terminal arborizations of LC axons on coronal sections through cortex (Figs. 11B, 12B, 13B, 14B, and 15B) and the laminar distribution of NE terminals in each major cortical region (Figs. 16–19).

While regional heterogeneity does exist in the LC terminal patterns, a basic pattern of arborization can be described, especially in rat cortex (see Fig. 17) (Levitt and Moore, 1978a; Morrison *et al.*, 1978). Layer I contains a dense, gridlike plexus of fibers. Layers II and III contain sparse, radially oriented fibers. Layers IV and V have moderately dense, short, oblique fibers, and layer VI exhibits long fibers that are oriented from anterior to posterior within the cortex. NE-containing fibers are rarely observed in white matter in general. The primate cortex exhibits greater regional heterogeneity than the rat. The following sections describe the LC innervation of selected cortical regions.

5.2.3a. Prefrontal Cortex and Anterior Cingulate Cortex. The innervation of rat cortex both in front of and dorsal to the genu of the corpus callosum

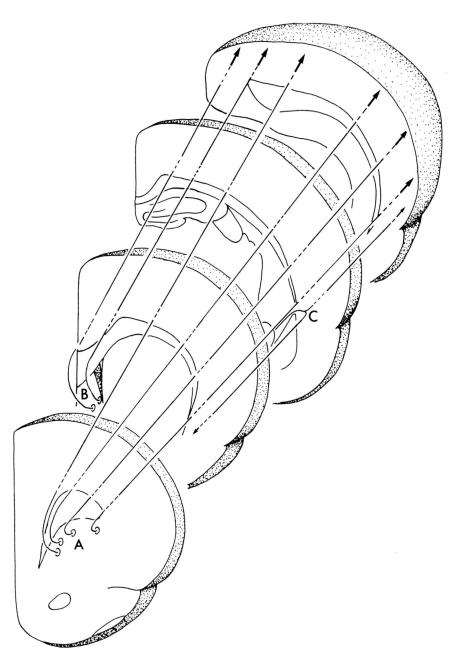

Figure 6. Schematic representation of the three major routes (A, B, C; cf. Fig. 3) whereby NE and 5HT fibers innervate rat cortex. They include the most anterior pathway through the frontal cortex (A), the Zuckerkandl's fasciculus/septal route (B), and the lateral route (C).

(including areas 24 and 32) is quite similar on sections stained with antisera to the NE synthetic enzyme DBH (see Figs. 10B, 11B, 12B, 13B, and 16) (Morrison *et al.*, 1978). Long axons oriented parallel to the pial surface lie in the deep half of layer I, while short fibers of various orientations lie in the superficial half. Radial axons can often be followed from the top of layer V to layer II. Layer V has the lowest density of fibers. The laminar densities of NE innervation in this region are complementary to those of the DA system described above (see Fig. 11 and Section 4.2.3 a,b; Lindvall, *et al.*, 1978; Lewis *et al.*, 1979). Layer VI contains fibers oriented from anterior to posterior and, in contrast to other cortical regions, also in the coronal plane. Unlike other regions of subcortical white matter, the cingulum bundle contains many DBH-positive fibers, especially caudal to the genu of the corpus callosum.

Investigators have only begun to examine the complex prefrontal cortex in primates. In squirrel monkey cortex, while the pattern of innervation is similar to the "typical" pattern described above, the density of innervation is lower in frontal cortex, especially in the frontal association areas (Morrison *et al.*, 1984). In rhesus prefrontal orbital cortex, layers II and V are heavily innervated, and layers III–V contain fibers oriented in all directions.

5.2.3b. Neocortex.   The "typical" pattern of innervation described above (Section 5.2.3) is observed in the majority of neocortical areas in the rat (see Figs. 10B, 11B, 12B, 13B, 14B, and 15B). Primary somatosensory cortex is perhaps most "typical" (see Fig. 18) (Morrison *et al.*, 1978). Layer V is particularly dense. Interestingly, the innervation of the barrel fields in the mouse is specialized such that the density of NE innervation within the barrels is greater than that in the surround (Lidov *et al.*, 1978). In rat motor cortex, as in somatosensory cortex, layers I and VI exhibit predominantly gential DBH-positive fibers, layers II and III have radial fibers, and oblique fibers are observed in layers IV and V. However, the NE innervation of layer V in motor cortex is more dense than in layer V of any other area of cortex (Morrison *et al.*, 1978). It has been proposed that these axons are in close apposition to the basal dendrites of pyramidal cells (Morrison *et al.*, 1978). In visual cortex, the typical pattern is also observed, although the innervation of layer IV is more prominent in contrast to the low density of innervation in layers V and VI (see Fig. 18).

In primate neocortex, NE afferents display a far greater degree of regional variation (Lindvall and Björklund, 1984). As Morrison and co-workers have suggested, it appears that the greater differentiation of primate cortex is paralleled by a specialization of the LC innervation (Morrison *et al.*, 1982a). The pattern of innervation in somatosensory cortex is similar to that in the rat, peaking in density in the regions surrounding the central fissure, and decreasing in density in a graded fashion rostrally and caudally (Morrison *et al.*, 1984). Visual cortex thus exhibits a relatively low density of NE (see Fig. 19). Interestingly, in squirrel monkey the NE innervation is complementary to the 5HT innervation (Morrison *et al.*, 1982b). Layers V and VI receive a moderately dense NE innervation and a sparse 5HT, while layers IVa and IVc receive a dense 5HT projection and virtually no NE fibers. Layer III is also relatively dense. Thus, the NE projection is denser in layers that contain cells projecting out of cortex. Unlike the 5HT innervation, which exhibits species differences, the NE innervation of visual cortex is similar in Old and New World monkeys (Kosofsky *et al.*, 1984).

5.2.3c. Suprarhinal Cortex. The LC innervation of suprarhinal cortex is sparse to moderate and fibers are observed in all layers (see Figs. 10B, 11B, and 12B; Fallon *et al.*, 1978a). Many fibers appear to ascend from deeper layers, bifurcate in layer I, then descend to innervate layer II (see Fig. 17).

5.2.3d. Piriform Cortex. NE axons in piriform cortex are scattered from the deep plexiform layer, through the upper cortical layers (see Figs. 10B, 11B, 12B, 13B, and 17). Collaterals branch off in layers II and III, then branch in layer I to form varicose axons running parallel to the surface (Jones and Moore, 1977; Fallon and Moore, 1978b).

5.2.3e. Posterior Cingulate Cortex. An extensive arborization of NE axons is present throughout layers I–V, unlike the neocortical pattern of largely radial axons on layers II and III (see Figs. 14B, 15B, and 16) (Lindvall and Björklund, 1984).

5.2.3f. Insular Cortex. In primate insular cortex a novel termination pattern is observed (Levitt *et al.*, 1984b). Axons are oriented in the anterior–posterior direction in the deep layers, with very few fibers in superficial layers.

5.2.3g. Entorhinal Cortex. All layers of entorhinal cortex are innervated moderately densely by NE axons (Fallon *et al.*, 1978a). They are especially dense in layer I, forming a gridlike plexus.

5.2.3h. Hippocampus. LC axons travel via three major routes to the hippocampus (Loy *et al.*, 1980; Haring and Davis, 1985). Fibers entering via the fornix innervate the septal pole of the dentate gyrus, and those from the cingulum innervate mainly the ventral dentate gyrus. The fibers traveling in the ventral amygdalofugal bundle innervate the entire hippocampal gyrus as well as the mid-septotemporal and ventral regions of the dentate gyrus (Haring and Davis, 1985). The plasticity of the NE innervation of the hippocampus is striking. Lesions of the fornix and cingulum induce proliferation of remaining NE fibers (Gage *et al.*, 1983). In general, the density of LC innervation (and of [^{3}H]-NE uptake) is greater in the area dentata than Ammon's horn, and is further greater in the temporal hippocampus than the septal (Storm-Mathisen and Guldberg, 1974; Loy *et al.*, 1980). The pattern of innervation is similar throughout the hippocampus with dense plexuses in the infragranular hilus of the dentate gyrus, the stratum lucidum of CA3, and the molecular layer of the subiculum (see Figs. 13B, 14B, 15B, and 18). Terminals appear to innervate the dendrites of granule and pyramidal cells (Loy *et al.*, 1980).

5.2.3i. Other Aspects of the NE Innervation: Do NE Terminals Make Synaptic Contacts? A controversy exists in the literature as to whether LC terminals in cortex exhibit the ultrastructural elements typically associated with synaptic junctions. Investigators who have utilized autoradiographic visualization of [³H]-NE uptake have observed a low incidence (5–20%) of labeled terminals that exhibit synaptic specializations (Beaudet and Descarries, 1978, 1984), suggesting that many LC boutons in cortex do not form conventional synapses. Similar conclusions have been reached by investigators who have utilized permanganate-fixation to label NE-containing varicosities (Maeda *et al.*, 1975). These findings have led to considerable speculation as to the possibility of extrajunctional release of NE or plasticity of LC terminals. In hippocampus, however, a recent study demonstrated synaptic specializations in 50% of [³H]-NE-labeled profiles (Parnavelas *et al.*, 1985). Furthermore, cortical varicosities identified by immunocytochemical localization of DBH exhibit synaptic junctions with a frequency of 40–50% (Olschowka *et al.*, 1981; Molliver *et al.*, 1982). These discrepancies may be due to methodological differences and must be resolved by further study.

5.2.4. Ontogenetic Development

LC neurons are born on gestational days 10–13, with a peak on day 12 (Lauder and Bloom, 1974). Catecholamine-fluorescent cell bodies are observed on day 14 from which axons emerge anteriorly (Loizou, 1972). By embryonic day 16, catecholamine-containing processes penetrate the outer superficial layers of neocortex (Schlumpf *et al.*, 1980). The early fibers arrive via three to four small fiber bundles entering at the ventrorostral aspect of the developing cortex. These bundles appear to bifurcate into the deep and superficial layers. The innervation progresses from ventral to dorsal and rostral to caudal through E21. During this time fibers are observed in the superficial layer and the intermediate zone below the cortical plate, but rarely cross the cortical plate (see Fig. 7). Although catecholamine-fluorescent terminal are sparse in neonatal cortex, there is apparently a population of terminals that take up and store 5-hydroxydopamine or L-dopa in a reserpine-sensitive storage compartment (Coyle and Molliver, 1977). Within the first postnatal week the adult pattern and density is evident (Levitt and Moore, 1979) although the superficial and deep plexuses are still evident (Lidov and Zecevic, 1978; Berger and Verney, 1984). NE content continues to rise through at least P31 (Loizou, 1972). Developmental studies utilizing mouse mutants suggest that NE-containing axons seek out particular cell classes regardless of their positions in cortex (Caviness and Korde, 1981).

In the hippocampus, fibers first appear on E18 in the septal pole of CA3 at the boundary of the marginal zone and cortical plate, the future stratum lucidum. Innervation throughout the dentate and Ammon's horn is fairly complete by P10 (Loy and Moore, 1979).

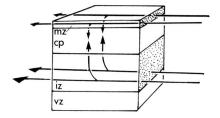

Figure 7. Representation of a small slab of cerebral cortex and the trajectory of NE and 5HT fibers during development. The plexus in the marginal zone (mz) and intermediate zones (iz) of cortex are present first. Later, the cortical plate (cp) is innervated. See text for details. vz, ventricular zone.

In primates, LC neurons are also generated early (Levitt and Rakic, 1982). Little is known of the prenatal development of the cortical innervation (for review see Foote and Morrison, 1985). In visual cortex of *Macaca fascicularis,* there is a low density of NA fibers in all layers at birth (Foote and Morrison, 1985). These fibers increase in density and arborize to the adult pattern by 60 days of age. As in the rat, however, NE storage capacity and rate of synthesis increase long after morphological maturity is achieved (Goldman-Rakic and Brown, 1982).

5.3. Functional Studies

While the intriguing anatomy of the NE system has led to much speculation as to its function, the literature regarding its role is fraught with disagreement. NE in cortex may be involved in memory consolidation (Zornetzer *et al.,* 1978), anxiety (Redmond andHuang, 1979), sleep (Aston-Jones and Bloom, 1981a), plasticity (Kasamatsu *et al.,* 1984), and control of cerebral circulation (Magistretti and Morrison, 1985). Little is known of the subcortical and/or cortical neuronal networks that might underlie these putative functions.

5.3.1. Receptors

Cortical NE receptors have been localized by receptor autoradiography. Three types of NE receptors are found in cortex: α_1, α_2, and β. These receptors also bind epinephrine and they exhibit a complex pharmacology (for review see Wamsley, 1984a,b). α_1 receptors, as labeled by WB-4101, are found fairly uniformly distributed across all cortical layers and regions (Wamsley *et al.,* 1981). Greater regional heterogeneity is observed when prazosin is used as an α_1 ligand in human brain tissue (see Wamsley, 1984b). α_2 receptors can be labeled by clonidine. A relatively low concentration of binding is observed over all layers with a slightly greater density in superficial layers than deeper layers (Young and Kuhar, 1980a; Wamsley *et al.,* 1981). The use of newly developed ligands has led to the proposal that α_2 receptors may be heterogeneous (Boyajian *et al.,* 1985). The localization of these receptor subtypes remains to be determined. β receptors can also be differentiated into β_1 and β_2 receptors. β_1 receptors are localized by dihydroalprenolol and those dihydroalprenolol sites displaced by zinterol are defined as β_2 (Palacios and Kuhar, 1980). β receptors are concentrated in the superficial layers of parietal cortex and in lamina I of cingulate cortex. These are mainly β_1 receptors (Palacios and Kuhar, 1982; Palacios and Wamsley, 1983, 1984). As in many other systems, there is not a direct correspondence between any one NE receptor subtype and NE terminal fields. Many hypotheses have been offered to explain such discrepancies (Wamsley, 1984b). Biochemical characterization of the adrenergic receptors is currently in progress (Caron *et al.,* 1984). The complexity of the receptor interactions with the endogenous ligand NE precludes any conclusions as to their functions.

5.3.2. Physiology

The physiological effects of NE on postsynaptic cells are still the subject of controversy (for review see Foote, 1985; Foote *et al.,* 1983; Van Dengen, 1981).

Early investigators describe inhibitory actions of NE on cortical cells (Morruzzi and Hart, 1955). Later studies reported inhibitory and excitatory effects (Krnjević and Phillis, 1963a,b; Johnson *et al.*, 1969). Some of the discrepancies in the literature may reflect the choice of anesthetic (Johnson *et al.*, 1969; Bunney and Aghajanian, 1976), the pH of the solution in microintophoretic studies (Gruol *et al.*, 1980), and the actual concentration of NE at the synapse (Armstrong-James and Fox, 1983). The complexity of the postsynaptic response to NE is further illustrated by studies addressing the modulation of responses to other inputs. NE has been reported to enhance the "signal-to-noise" ("enabling") ratio of neuronal response to stimuli in rat somatosensory cortex (Waterhouse and Woodward, 1980), cat visual cortex (Kasamatsu and Heggelund, 1982), rat hippocampus (Segal and Bloom, 1976a,b), and monkey auditory cortex (Foote *et al.*, 1975). The molecular basis of these effects is unclear. In hippocampus, evidence suggests that NE effects are mediated by a cyclic AMP system (Segal and Bloom, 1974). Topical application of NE results in a 3- to 4-mV hyperpolarization associated with a decrease in input resistance (Segal, 1980). This is thought to be mediated by a stimulation of the membrane sodium pump (Segal, 1980; Phillis *et al.*, 1982).

LC terminals in cortex are also auto-inhibited by NE, via α_2 receptor-mediated hyperpolarization (Nakamura *et al.*, 1981). In contrast, the inhibition of postsynaptic cells is thought to be mediated by β receptors (Olpe *et al.*, 1980).

5.3.3. Interactions

The suggestion that NE should be termed a neuromodulator rather than a neurotransmitter is dependent on the demonstration of interactions with other transmitters (for review see Reader and Jasper, 1984). However, no clear examples have been defined. NE inhibits the excitatory effects of ACh on cortical neurons. It is possible that this is mediated by an interaction of the two transmitters in modulation of intracellular cyclic AMP and GMP pools (Reader *et al.*, 1979a). In addition, it has been shown that NE and vasoactive intestinal polypeptide (VIP) act synergistically to increase cyclic AMP in mouse cortical slices and thus create "metabolic hot-spots" in their regions of overlap (Magistretti *et al.*, 1981, 1983; Magistretti and Morrison, 1985). The tangentially oriented NE system in cortex is orthogonal to the radially oriented VIP neurons. These systems, thus, might interactively modulate cerebral metabolism in discrete cortical regions (see Fig. 8).

5.3.4. Plasticity

An intriguing, though controversial, line of work has suggested that NE may be an important regulator of neuronal plasticity (for review see Kasamatsu *et al.*, 1984). Briefly, removal of the NE terminals in kitten visual cortex results in a failure of the ocular dominance shift normally associated with monocular deprivation (Kasamatsu *et al.*, 1981). Local perfusion of NE not only restores the ocular dominance shift but also induces plasticity in older animals (Kasamatsu *et al.*, 1979). In addition, stimulation of the LC in monocularly deprived adult cats restored plasticity in mature visual cortex (Kasamatsu *et al.*, 1983). It is

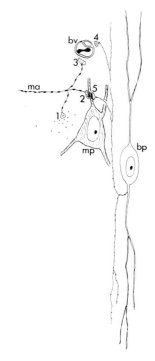

Figure 8. Illustration of some suggested interactions of a mono-amine axon (ma) in cortex. These include "nonsynaptic" release into the extracellular space (1). This neurohumoral or paracrine action would be expected to influence a more widespread area of cortical NE receptors than more classical synaptic effects on neurons (2). In addition, an effect on cerebral vasculature and permeability has been proposed (3). These effects could be enhanced or suppressed by actions of peptidergic bipolar (local circuit) neurons (bp) in cortex. Thus, the combined action of peptides (5, 4) and monoamines (1–3) on multipolar cells (mp) and the vasculature could produce metabolic "hot spots" and "cold spots" in cortex. See text for details. bv, blood vessel.

thought that the β receptor–cyclic AMP system may mediate such effects (Kasamatsu *et al.,* 1984).

5.3.5. Behavior

As mentioned above, the LC system in cortex has been implicated in many behavioral functions including, among others, learning, stress, memory, reinforcement, and attention. Its precise role in any of these remains elusive (for review see Iversen, 1984; Mason, 1980; McNaughton and Mason, 1980; Redmond and Huang, 1979; Stein, 1978; Zornetzer *et al.,* 1978). In general, however, the anatomical organization, physiological effects on postsynaptic cells, and activity of LC cells in various situations suggest that the LC system may be responsible for a subtle, global process. In awake, behaving monkeys, LC neurons respond to a range of complex sensory stimuli (Foote *et al.,* 1980). LC neurons fire less during sleep and instinctive behaviors such as grooming or feeding (Aston-Jones and Bloom, 1981a,b). It has been previously noted that NE application (and LC stimulation) increases the signal-to-noise ratio of the responses of postsynaptic cells, especially to relevant stimuli (Segal and Bloom, 1976a,b). NE also affects cortical metabolism (Magistretti and Morrison, 1985). Based on these and other data, it has been suggested that the LC system in forebrain is important in the switching of "attention" (an admittedly complex term) between internal and external sensory cues (Iverson, 1984). In primates, the NE system in frontal cortex may be important in the form of selective attention important in delayed alternation tasks (Arnsten and Goldman-Rakic, 1985). Such basic functions might underlie many behaviors. The most intriguing aspect of the literature on the LC in behavior is that LC/NE lesions produce few documentable effects (Roberts *et al.*, 1976; Zornetzer *et al.*, 1978). As will be discussed in Section 7, however, analysis of the spatiotemporal integration of this system with other systems may lead to a clarification of its role.

6. Serotonin

6.1. Introduction

Serotonin or 5-hydroxytryptamine (5HT) fibers in cerebral cortex are derived from the dorsal raphe (B7 cell group of Dahlstrom and Fuxe, 1964) and, to a lesser extent, the median raphe (B8) of the mesencephalon (Conrad *et al.*, 1974; Moore and Halaris, 1975; Bobillier *et al.*, 1976; Halaris *et al.*, 1976; Geyer *et al.*, 1976; Jacobs *et al.*, 1978; Azmitia and Segal, 1978; Moore *et al.*, 1978; Fallon and Moore, 1979b; Lidov *et al.*, 1980; Steinbusch, 1981; Azmitia, 1981; Lidov and Molliver, 1982; Kohler and Steinbusch, 1982; Fallon and Loughlin, 1982; Porrino and Goldman-Rakic, 1982). The study of the distribution of 5HT has lagged significantly behind studies of DA and NE in cerebral cortex, primarily for methodological reasons. Thus, there have been significant hiatuses from the time of the initial discoveries of 5HT in the CNS (Twarog and Page, 1953; Amin *et al.*, 1954; Bogdanski *et al.*, 1957), to the determination of 5HT-containing tracts in the CNS (Heller *et al.*, 1962; Dahlstrom and Fuxe, 1964). While laboratories were quite successful in studying the catecholamine systems with the fluorescence techniques (Falck *et al.*, 1962; Dahlstrom and Fuxe, 1964; Fuxe, 1965; Ungerstedt, 1971), the lability and instability of the 5HT-derived fluorophor, β-carboline, impeded progress in the study of 5HT systems, especially in cerebral cortex. Some headway had been made using other techniques such as EM autoradiography (Aghajanian and Bloom, 1967; Descarries *et al.*, 1975), light-level autoradiography, (Conrad *et al.*, 1974; Bobillier *et al.*, 1976, 1979; Moore *et al.*, 1978; Azmitia and Segal, 1978), biochemistry combined with lesions (Geyer *et al.*, 1976), silver degeneration methods (Taber *et al.*, 1960; Brodal *et al.*, 1960), and with improved existing techniques (see Azmitia, 1982). However, it was not until the development of antisera raised against 5HT coupled to bovine albumin or bovine thyroglobulin (Steinbusch *et al.*, 1978; Lidov *et al.*, 1980; Takeuchi and Sano, 1983; Steinbusch and Nieuwenhuys, 1983; Kosofsky *et al.*, 1984) that the study of the precise anatomical distribution of 5HT in the CNS became possible. This technique has shown that, contrary to the findings of many previous studies, the 5HT innervation of cerebral cortex is very rich, indeed.

6.2. Anatomical Studies

6.2.1. The Raphecortical System

6.2.1a. Origins of the Mesocortical 5HT Projection. The 5HT innervation of cerebral cortex originates in cell bodies of the dorsal raphe (B7) and median raphe (B8) of the mesencephalon (Fig. 9). Dahlstrom and Fuxe (1964) used the "B" terminology instead of classical neuroanatomical nomenclature to delineate the 5HT cell groups because not all cells of the raphe nuclei contain 5HT, and many 5HT cells can be found outside of the borders of raphe nuclei. Fortunately, the dorsal raphe nucleus is compact and contains most of the 5HT cells innervating cerebral cortex. In addition, a large majority (70%) of the cells in the dorsal raphe are serotonergic (Descarries *et al.*, 1979; Wiklund *et al.*, 1980). The median raphe or nucleus centralis superior (B8), which gives rise to a smaller component of the mesocortical 5HT pathway, is less compact but still contains a relatively large percentage (35%) of 5HT cells (Wiklund *et al.*, 1980).

The dorsal raphe is the most extensive of the raphe groups, with a length of 3.4 mm. It has a *fleur-de-lis* shape in coronal sections throughout part of its length, and consists of several subregions with a high cell density. These include dorsomedial, ventromedial, and lateral outlying groups. The ventral region located between the paired medial longitudinal fasciculus bundles is also called the Fountain of Sheehan. Of the three types of cells seen in Nissl material (small spherical, 14 μm; medium fusiform, 24 × 20 μm; large multipolar, 35 μm), the medium fusiform and large multipolar cells make up the majority of 5HT cells.

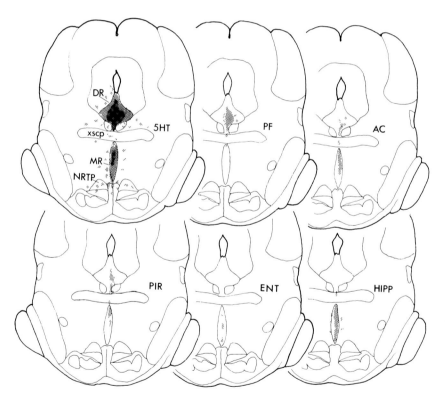

Figure 9. Illustration of serotonin (5HT) cells that give rise to the cortical projection from the dorsal raphe (DR) and median raphe (MR). The coronal sections of the rat brain are taken at a midsection of this DR. The total 5HT cell distribution at this level is shown at the top left. The 5HT projections to prefrontal (PF), anterior cingulate (AC), piriform (PIR), entorhinal (ENT), and hippocampal (HIPP) cortices are shown as stippling. MR, median raphe (B8); NRTP, nucleus reticularis tegmenti pontis of Bechterew (B9); XSCP, decussation of the superior cerebellar peduncle.

The cortical projections from the 5HT cells in the dorsal raphe are predominantly to frontal anterior cingulate, piriform, and neocortices (Fig. 9), although there are also varying proportions of median raphe projections to these cortices (Bobillier *et al.*, 1976; Azmitia, 1978; Fallon and Moore, 1979b). The projections are predominantly ipsilateral, partially contralateral, but not bilateral (van der Kooy and Hattori, 1980; Loughlin and Fallon, 1982).

The median raphe (B8) lies ventral to the dorsal raphe and is approximately 2.2 mm in length in the rat (Fig. 9), with cells scattered from the midline to the tectospinal tracts on each side. This raphe nucleus is more diffuse than the dorsal raphe. It contains small-sized ellipsoid cells (12 × 13 mm), medium-sized ellipsoid cells (18 × 13 μm), and medium-sized fusiform cells (19 × 16 μm) that are spread homogeneously throughout the nucleus (Steinbusch and Nieuwenhuys, 1983). The 5HT cells, which compromise 35% of the nucleus (Wiklund *et al.*, 1980), are of the small ellipsoid (medially) and medium fusiform (laterally) type (Steinbusch and Nieuwenhuys, 1983). The cortical projections of the 5HT cells of the median raphe are predominantly to the hippocampus, entorhinal, piriform, anterior cingulate, and, to a much lesser extent, frontal cortex (Fig. 9) (Bobillier *et al.*, 1976; Azmitia, 1978; Fallon and Moore, 1979b). As in the case of the doral raphe, the median raphe projection is ipsilateral or contralateral, but not bilateral.

In comparing the projections of the dorsal and median raphe, note that dorsal neocortex and frontal cortices are primarily innervated by the dorsal raphe, whereas hippocampus and entorhinal cortex are primarily innervated by the median raphe. The region of the raphe that appears to project to nearly all areas is the ventral portion of the dorsal raphe, in the sector known as the Fountain of Sheehan. This finding suggests that these neurons may have highly colateralized projections, as discussed in the next section.

6.2.1b. Collateralization Patterns. As mentioned above, the ventralmost strip of the dorsal raphe appears to give rise to projections to many regions of cortex (Fig. 9) and subcortical areas (Fallon and Moore, 1979b). In fact, when several fluorescent retrograde tracers are injected into different forebrain areas, multiple-labeled cells (50–80%) are found in this same ventral portion of dorsal raphe (Fallon and Loughlin, 1982). Thus, individual cells in this region may project not only to subcortical sites such as caudate–putamen, septum, amygdala, and olfactory tubercle, but also to prefrontal, supragenual, dorsal parietal, posterior cingulate, and/or entorhinal cortices. On the other hand, the same combination of injections leads to very few multiple-labeled cells in the peripheral regions of the dorsal raphe (5–10%) and median raphe (1%) (Fallon and Loughlin, 1982). The cells in the raphe nuclei project ipsilaterally, contralaterally, but, with the exception of the hippocampal projection (Azmitia, 1981), not bilaterally (van der Kooy and Hattori, 1980; Loughlin and Fallon, 1982). During development these neurons have a double migration pattern, with an initial ventral migration from the ventricular zone and a second migration medially, with fusion of the paired nuclei and overmigration of some cells to the contralateral side (Levitt and Moore, 1978b). These developmental findings help explain why raphe neurons have only unilateral projections (including contralateral projections from neurons that may have originally been derived from the ipsilateral side, but later overmigrated to the contralateral side during development within neocortex. Axons of raphe cells collateralize more extensively from anterior to posterior than in the medial to lateral dimension (Loughlin and Fallon, unpublished results).

6.2.1c. Neurotransmitters in the Mesocortical Projection. In addition to 5HT projections to cerebral cortex from the dorsal and median raphe, there are also non-5HT projections. For example, DA neurons in the median raphe may project to hippocampus (Reymann *et al.*, 1983). Other studies have shown extensive non-5HT raphe inputs to hippocampus and entorhinal cortex (Kohler and Steinbusch, 1982).

The dorsal raphe is known to have not only 5HT but also DA, NE, GABA, CCK, Leu-enkephalin, Met-enkephalin, substance P, and VIP neurons, with 5HT and Leu-enkephalin as well as 5HT and GABA known to be colocalized (for review see Steinbusch and Nieuwenhuys, 1983). It would be interesting to know if these and other peptides are colocalized with 5HT in the raphe projections to cerebral cortex; however, data are still lacking.

6.2.2. Pathways of the Mesocortical 5HT Projections

Some of the same pathways that are used for NE fiber traffic to cerebral cortex are also used by 5HT fibers (Figs. 3, 5, and 6). As determined with several techniques (Björklund *et al.*, 173; Conrad *et al.*, 1974; Bobillier *et al.*, 1976; Moore *et al.*, 1978; Lidov *et al.*, 1980; Parent *et al.*, 1981; Steinbusch, 1981; Lidov and Molliver, 1982) the fibers from the dorsal and median raphe ascend in paramedian bundles that first course through the dorsal VTA to enter the medial forebrain bundle in the lateral hypothalamic area. Some fibers turn laterally toward the amygdala, perirhinal cortex, piriform cortex, and entorhinal cortex via the ansa peduncularis–ventral amygdalofugal bundle (Figs. 3 and 6), the so-called "lateral" pathway that is probably more well-developed in primates. Other fibers continue in the medial forebrain bundle and enter the telencephalon. Medially, some fibers radiate through the diagonal band and septum in Zuckerkandl's fascicles. The fibers then curve around the genu of the corpus callosum to enter cingulate cortex and hippocampus. More laterally, some fibers wrap under the forceps minor and proceed caudally to innervate dorsal neocortex (Figs. 3 and 6). Some laterally directed fibers innervate suprarhinal, perirhinal, and piriform cortices.

6.2.3. Terminal Projections of the 5HT Mesocortical Projections

The pattern of the 5HT innervation of cerebral cortex is similar to the NE projection in that it is generally homogeneous throughout cortical layers and cortical regions, especially in the rat. Exceptions to this will be discussed below. As shown by Lidov, Molliver, and co-workers (Lidov *et al.*, 1980; Kosofsky *et al.*, 1984) and Takeuchi and Sano (1983), *en passage* axons are thicker and straighter than preterminal and terminal fibers, which are thinner and more tortuous. The fibers in layers I and VI run tangentially, whereas those in layers II–IV run radially and irregularly (Figs. 16–19). In general, the 5HT innervation of cortex is more dense than the NE innervation of cortex (Figs. 10B, 11B, 12B, 13B, 14B, and 15B).

6.2.3a. Prefrontal Cortex and Neocortex.

In the rat, prefrontal cortex and dorsal neocortices have very similar patterns of 5HT innervation. Moderately dense numbers of fibers are found in all layers, with fibers running tangentially in layers I and VI. The superficial and deep plexuses of 5HT fibers are reminiscent of the early developing plexuses (see below) in that they appear to run anterior to posterior in cortex (Lidov *et al.*, 1980; Lidov and Molliver, 1982). The widespread distribution of 5HT fibers in cerebral cortex led Lidov *et al.* (1980) to speculate that nearly every cortical neuron could be innervated by a 5HT terminal. 5HT-containing boutons are present as 0.7-μm varicosities along 5HT fibers (0.1–0.5 μm). The boutons contain mitochondria, as well as small, round, agranular vesicles, and large granular vesicles (Descarries *et al.*, 1975).

In contrast to the relative homogeneity of the 5HT innervation of rat neocortex, the 5HT innervation in the primate is more laminated and complex. For example, 5HT fibers are densest in visual cortex and least dense in primary motor cortex of the macaque (*Macaca fuscata*) (Takeuchi and Sano, 1983). In this species, area 17 has an extremely dense 5HT innervation in upper layer IVc. In area 17 of another macaque (*Macaca fascicularis*), Kosofsky *et al.* (1984) found that layer IVc is densely innervated by 5HT fibers with other layers receiving a less robust innervation. Layer IVcβ is poorly innervated (Fig. 19). Although the pattern of 5HT fiber innervation of area 17 in the Old World monkeys is similar (and also appears to partially complement the NE pattern—see Fig. 19), the 5HT innervation of cortex in New World monkeys (e.g., squirrel monkey) is quite different. As discussed by Morrison, Foote, and co-workers (Kosofsky *et al.*, 1984; Morrison *et al.*, 1984), the 5HT innervation of area 17 in the squirrel monkey is less dense than in macaque monkeys. A dense fiber plexus is present throughout the entire thickness of layer IVc in the squirrel monkey. Other differences are also apparent (Fig. 19). Thus, during advancing phylogenetic development from rodent to New World monkeys to Old World monkeys, both the geniculocortical and 5HT projections to layer IV specialize in their sublaminar distribution (Morrison *et al.*, 1984).

6.2.3b. Cingulate Cortex.

As detailed by Lidov *et al.* (1980), cingulate cortex contains a heterogeneous 5HT innervation. The innervation in anterior cingulate cortex is generally uniform, with a somewhat more dense band of fibers in layers I and VI (Figs. 11B and 16). Radial fibers are obvious in layers II and III, especially in the ventral division. In comparing DA, NE, and 5HT in this region, there is an interesting complementary association (Fig. 11).

In posterior cingulate granular retrosplenial cortex, on the other hand, DA fibers are virtually nonexistent and NE fibers are uniformly distributed. 5HT fibers, however, are well laminated, with high fiber densities in layers I, III, and VI (Figs. 13B, 14B, and 16).

6.2.3c. Perirhinal and Suprarhinal Cortex.

The perirhinal and suprarhinal strip contains a moderately dense innervation in layers I and III, with a somewhat less dense innervation in other layers (Figs. 10B, 11B, 12b, 13B, 14B, and 17). This has some complementary features to the DA and NE innervation (Fig. 17).

6.2.3d. Piriform Cortex. Steinbusch and Nieuwenhuys (Steinbusch, 1981; Steinbusch and Nieuwenhuys, 1983) have noted a relatively uniform, moderately dense innervation of piriform cortex (Figs. 10B, 11B, 12B, 13B, and 17), but a precise analysis has not yet been carried out. It appears that piriform cortex receives a modest input from all three of the major monoamines, with all layers being potentially under their influence (Fig. 17).

6.2.3e. Entorhinal Cortex. Kohler and colleagues (Kohler *et al.*, 1980, 1981; Kohler, 1982) have studied the 5HT innervation of entorhinal (and hippocampal) cortex in detail. This cortical region appears to receive a dual 5HT innervation. Thin, varicose fibers are distributed throughout all layers, especially in layer I. This innervation is supplemented by thicker, convoluted fibers in layer III of a 1-mm strip of lateral entorhinal cortex (Figs. 14B and 17). Thus, the DA and 5HT innervations of this region are somewhat similar (overlapping?), whereas the NE innervation is more uniformly distributed in this region (Fig. 17). Therefore, DA and 5HT may have synergistic or antagonistic effects on hippocampal circuitry, since monoamine inputs to layers II and III of entorhinal cortex may directly impact on perforant path inputs to the hippocampus.

6.2.3f. Hippocampus. Lidov and colleagues (Lidov *et al.*, 1980) and Kohler (1982) have described the 5HT innervation of the hippocampus. The hilus of the dentate gyrus of the dorsal hippocampus contains a dense, thin (30 μm wide) band of 5HT fibers just subjacent to the dentate granule cells (Figs. 13B, 14B, and 18). These fibers appear to form pericellular baskets around cells. Some fibers are also present in the molecular layer (Fig. 18). The stratum lacunosum moleculare of CA1 also contains a dense band (140 μm wide) just adjacent to the hippocampal fissure (Fig. 18). The basal portion of the pyramidal cell layer of the stratum oriens in CA1 contains a modest band of 5HT fiber innervation. This region in CA3 and CA4, which contains mossy fibers, is devoid of 5HT input. Scattered 5HT fibers are also present in the other layers. The ventral hippocampal formation appears to contain a greater density of 5HT terminals (but a lower K_m for 5HT uptake) than the dorsal hippocampus (Gage and Thompson, 1980). These results agree with immunohistochemical findings that, although the 5HT innervation of the dorsal and ventral hippocampus has the same laminar distribution, the ventral hippocampus is more richly innervated (Kohler, 1982).

6.2.3g. Other Factors of the 5HT Innervation: Asymmetry and Blood Vessels. Rosen *et al.* (1984) have reported that there is a greater 5HT content in the left striatum and right accumbens of the rat, and that there is a higher concentration of 5HT metabolites (5-HIAA) in the left cortex. This is in contrast to DA an NE asymmetries, where more DA is present in the right cortex and nucleus accumbens and more NE is present in the left striatum. Such findings may be important in our understanding of functional asymmetries in the forebrain.

The 5HT innervation of blood vessels in rat cerebral cortex has recently been studied (Itakura *et al.*, 1985). 5HT terminal boutons were found to make contact directly on the basement membrane of capillaries. Furthermore, the 5HT fibers may regulate carbon dioxide reactivity of the capillaries. Thus, like the NE innervation, extrinsically derived 5HT inputs (3 in Fig. 8) may complement intrinsic peptidergic inputs (4 in Fig. 8) to regulate cerebral vasculature and metabolism. Therefore, the monoaminergic innervation of cerebral cortex appears to contain classical synaptic (2 in Fig. 8), nonsynaptic (1 in Fig. 8), and metabolic vascular (3 in Fig. 8) components.

6.2.4. Ontogenetic Development

Lidov and Molliver (1982) have studied the details of the development of the 5HT innervation of rat forebrain. 5HT cell bodies in the raphe nuclei are born on day 12 of gestation (E12). Ascending fibers are seen arising from the dorsal raphe/median raphe complex on E14. By E16, some fibers have reached the forebrain, and by E17 a few early fibers enter the lateral and medial neocortical primordium. By E19, all major pathways are established and the fibers are clearly present in frontal cortex. The fibers course tangentially in the marginal and intermediate zones, avoiding the cortical plate itself (see four tangential arrows in mz and iz in Fig. 7). The density and areal extent of this bilaminar innervation increase for the next week, until at P6 there is finally an innervation of parietal cortex, which is the last to develop. From P7 to P10 the 5HT axons begin to penetrate the thickness of the cortical plate (see curved arrows in Fig. 7). By P21 the entire neocortical mantle is innervated throughout all cortical layers. Several interesting issues have arisen out of our knowledge of the development of the 5HT innervation of cerebral cortex. These include: (1) Do the superficial (marginal zone) and deep (intermediate zone) fiber plexuses arise independently from different raphe neurons? (2) What is the significance of the tangential 5HT fiber system in cortex, which contrasts so sharply with the radial fiber system originating in thalamus and other cortical areas? (3) Do the monoamine fibers, which develop so early, guide or significantly affect the development of other fiber systems? (4) What is the significance of the very prolonged development of the 5HT innervation of cortex? These questions, although intriguing, are still difficult to answer.

6.3. Functional Studies

Like the NE system, the 5HT system has been implicated in many neural functions. These include control of sensory systems, neuroendocrine systems, induction of slow-wave sleep, inhibition of REM sleep, inhibition of arousal, vasoconstriction, and migraine headache, and regulation of a host of behavioral states (Jouvet, 1972; Azmitia, 1978; Reader *et al.*, 1979b; Steinbusch and Nieuwenhuys, 1983). While many of these functions may be primarily under the control of subcortical structures, the very dense 5HT innervation of cerebral cortex, itself, implies a major role for 5HT serotonin in cortical function.

6.3.1. Receptors

There are two types of 5HT receptors in cerebral cortex, including S_1 (5HT) and S_2 ($5HT_2$) subtypes. The ligands for the S_1 receptor include LSD (lysergic acid diethylamide) (Meibach *et al.*, 1980) and 5HT itself (Young and Kuhar, 1980b). The most widely used ligands for the S_2 receptor include spiperone (spiroperidol) (Palacios *et al.*, 1981) and ketanserin (Leysen *et al.*, 1982). Spiperone is a ligand for both D_2 and S_2 receptors (Peroutka and Snyder, 1979; Palacios *et al.*, 1981) so appropriate preincubation of the tissue with a D_2 competitor such as sulpiride must be used to reveal the S2 receptor alone. Using such techniques combined with computer image analysis, Altar and colleagues (Altar *et al.*, 1985) have been able to produce a quantitative visualization of cortical and subcortical S_2 (and D_2) binding sites.

The results of studies on the localization of 5HT receptors in cerebral cortex (Seeman *et al.*, 1980; Meibach *et al.*, 1980; Palacios *et al.*, 1981; Palacios and Wamsley, 1982; Kohler, 1984; Altar *et al.*, 1985) have shown that the distribution of 5HT receptors does not always closely match the distribution of 5HT itself. S_1 receptors are present in layers V and, especially, VI of cerebral cortex. Some S_1 receptors are found on cholinergic terminals in cortex (Cross and Deakin, 1985). Layers II and III contain lower densities of these receptors. S_1 receptors in the hippocampal region are concentrated in stratum radiatum of subfield CA1 and subiculum, the molecular layer of the dentate gyrus, and all layers of the entorhinal cortex, except layer III where dense 5HT terminal plexuses are found (Fig. 17). S_2 receptors are present in layer IV of parietal cortex. Layer Va also contains high levels of S_2 receptors, as does the claustrum. This lamination of 5HT receptors does not closely match that of 5HT terminals; however, imipramine binding sites do overlap well with 5HT terminals in layers I and IV of neocortex (Grabowsky *et al.*, 1983). Thus, this tricyclic antidepressant may serve as a good marker for locating cells postsynaptic to 5HT terminals (Sette *et al.*, 1981; Wamsley, 1984a,b; Kohler, 1984).

6.3.2. Physiology

As with the other monoamines, the neurophysiological effects of 5HT on postsynaptic cells are still controversial. Much of the available literature focuses on the effects of 5HT as studied with extracellular recording techniques. Such studies (Krnjević and Phillis, 1963a,b; Jordan *et al.*, 1972; Sastry and Phillis, 1977; Sharma, 1977; Reader, 1978; Olpe, 1981) support the contention that 5HT is an inhibitory neurotransmitter in that it depresses the firing rate of cerebral cortical neurons. Some intracellular studies (Phillis *et al.*, 1968; Segal, 1980; Jahnsen, 1980; Phillis, 1984) also suggest that 5HT does, indeed, hyperpolarize postsynaptic cells. Apparently, there is no concurrent increase of membrane conductance to potassium or chloride ions. On the other hand, intracellular analysis of the effect of 5HT in the facial nucleus suggests that 5HT depolarizes these neurons with a concomitant decrease in membrane conductance (Van der Maelen and Aghajanian, 1980). These combined actions of 5HT may result in an "enabling" type of modulatory function that would facilitate the response of these neurons to other excitatory inputs (Cooper *et al.*, 1982). Although there are numerous region-specific differences in the postsynaptic effects of 5HT, it is generally believed that the effects of 5HT in cerebral cortex are suppressive.

6.3.3. Interactions

There are no well-known interactions of 5HT with other monoamines or 5HT autoreceptors in cortex. Interactions of 5HT with GABA (Collinge *et al.*, 1983), ovarian hormones (Dumbrille-Ross and Tang, 983), and β-adrenergic receptors (Stockmeier *et al.*, 1985) have recently been reported.

6.3.4. Behavior

As stated in the Introduction and in a recent review (Cooper *et al.*, 1982), 5HT received attention in the 1950s and 1960s mainly for its suspected role in the regulation of several behavioral states, sensory systems, sleep, arousal, and neuroendocrine functions. It is not known, however, if any of these functions of 5HT are dependent upon its actions in cerebral cortex. For example, the state of general arousal is inhibited by 5HT, and 5HT induces slow-wave sleep and inhibits REM sleep. These actions may be imparted at the cortical level, but it is more likely that they occur between monoaminergic systems at subcortical sites such as the LC. 5HT has long been implicated as the neuronal system most profoundly affected by LSD. LSD may ultimately induce hallucinations by interfering with 5HT transmission at the cerebral cortical level, but it is currently believed that the primary effect of LSD is on the raphe 5HT cell bodies. This is loosely derived from a number of related, but often contradictory findings (for review see Cooper *et al.*, 1982): (1) LSD antagonizes the 5HT system, decreases 5HT turnover and inhibits electrical activity in the 5HT cell bodies, and inhibits raphe output; (2) lesioning the raphe does not cause the same behavioral effects as LSD; (3) the LSD effect is seen in raphe-lesioned animals later treated with LSD; (4) stimulation of the raphe nuclei mimics some of the effects of LSD; (5) LSD administration quiets 5HT neuronal activity, but hallucinations still occur; (6) 5HT neurons are silent during REM sleep when hallucinogenic-like experiences (dreams) occur; and (7) 5HT neurons contain autoreceptors, and are also known to give off local circuit axon collaterals that innervate nearby 5HT neurons. Thus, LSD may act on autoreceptors to presynaptically inhibit 5HT neurons and their output to the forebrain. The presence of LSD receptors in the raphe suggests that the primary inhibitory effect of the hallucinogen is not in cortex. The presence of LSD receptors (S_1) in cerebral cortex and the extensive 5HT innervation of cerebral cortex further suggest that the profound hallucinogenic and behavioral effects of LSD are due, in part, to alterations in cortical function.

In conclusion, the rich and heterogeneous monoamine innervation of cerebral cortex has compelled neuroscientists to propose that they play a significant role in cortical function. When compared with thalamocortical and corticocortical inputs, their developmental patterns and routes of entry into cortex appear unorthodox. The axons of the three monoamine systems often stream tangentially through cortical layers, crossing over cytoarchitectonically and functionally delineated cortical regions. Their physiological effects are not well understood.

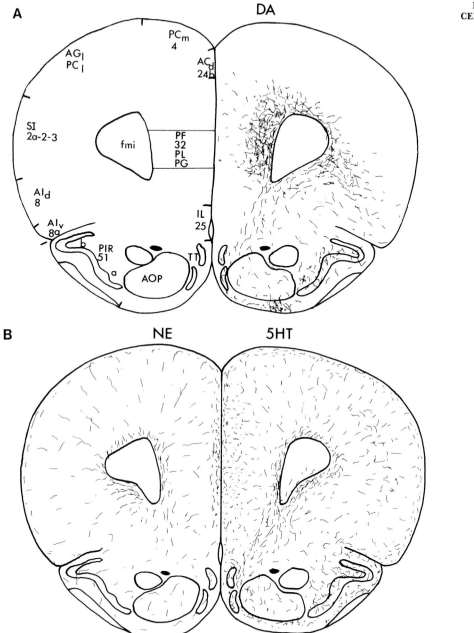

Figure 10. (A) Drawing of coronal section of rat brain showing the DA innervation (at right) of cortex at this level. The cortical regions are identified at the left. The section was taken at the level shown by "A" in Fig. 5. Abbreviations taken from Paxinos and Watson (1982) atlas and several other sources (see text). (B) Same as (A), except the NE (left) and 5HT (right) innervations are shown.

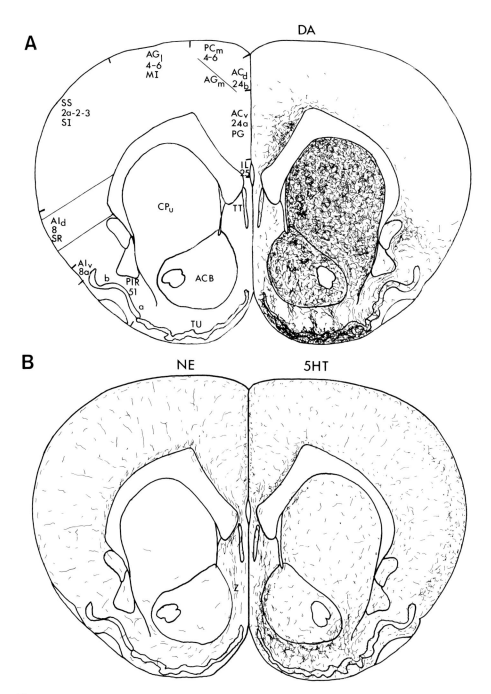

Figure 11. (A) DA innervation. Same as Fig. 10A, except at a more caudal level ("B" in Fig. 5) of the rat brain. (B) Same as (A), except the NE (left) and 5HT (right) innervations are shown.

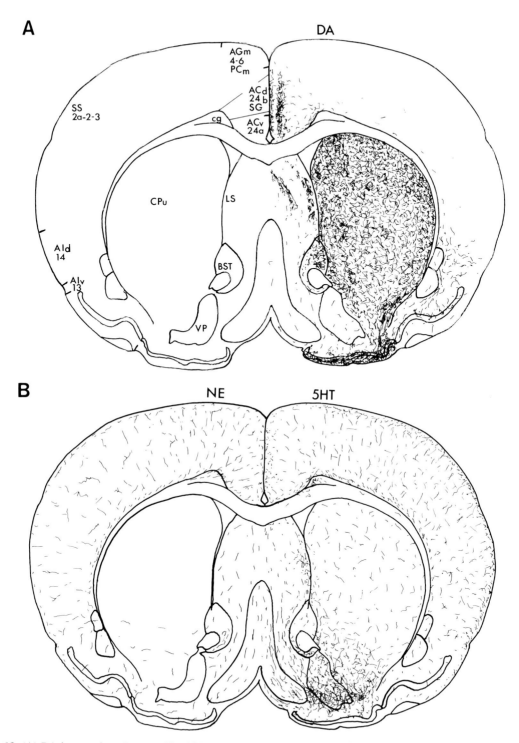

Figure 12. (A) DA innervation. Same as Fig. 10A, except at a more caudal level ("C" in Fig. 5). (B) Same as (A), except the NE (left) and 5HT (right) innervations are shown.

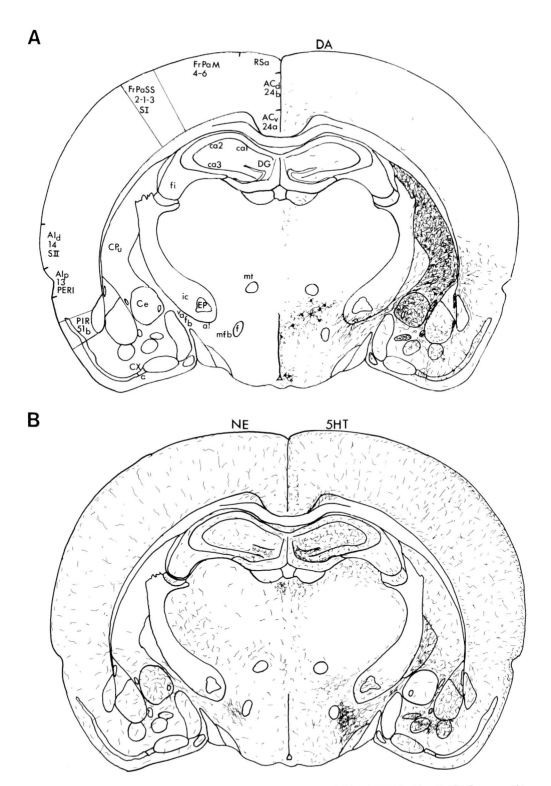

Figure 13. (A) DA innervation. Same as Fig. 10A, except at a more caudal level ("D" in Fig. 5). (B) Same as (A), except the NE (left) and 5HT (right) innervations are shown.

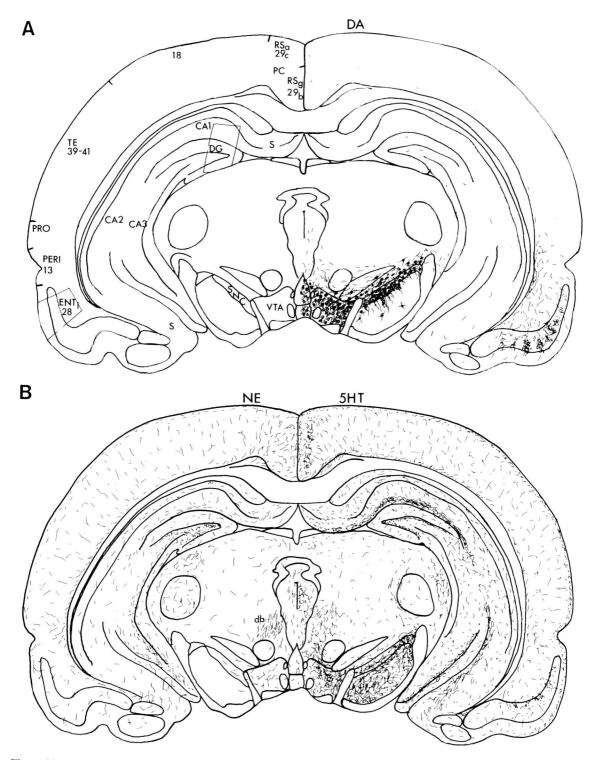

Figure 14. (A) DA innervation. Same as Fig. 10A, except at a more caudal level ("E" in Fig. 5). (B) Same as (A), except the NE (left) and 5HT (right) innervations are shown.

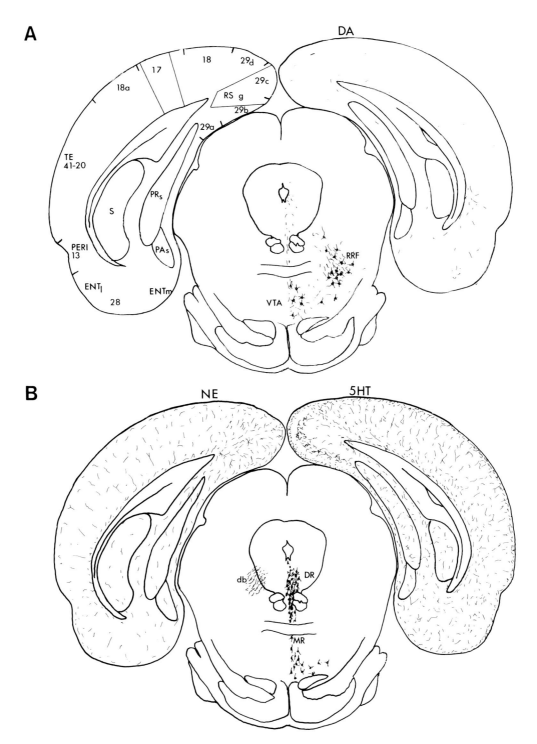

Figure 15. (A) DA innervation. Same as Fig. 10A, except at a more caudal level ("F" in Fig. 5). (B) Same as (A), except the NE (left) and 5HT (right) innervations are shown.

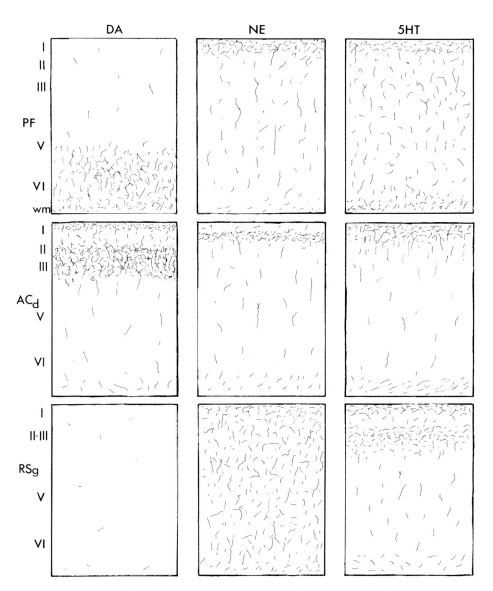

Figure 16. Nine panels illustrating the laminar pattern of DA (left column), NE (center column), and 5HT (right column) innervation of prefrontal (PF), dorsal anterior cingulate (ACd), and granular retrosplenial (RSg) cortices. The areas of cortex shown are indicated by boxes in the left sides of the sections illustrated in Fig. 10A, (PF), Fig. 12A (ACd), and Fig. 15A (region in RSg above RSAg).

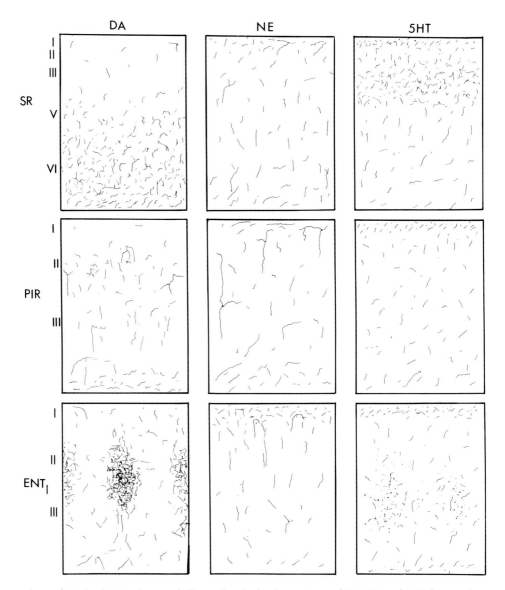

Figure 17. As in Fig. 16, nine panels illustrating the laminar pattern of DA, NE, and 5HT innervation of suprarhinal (SR), piriform (PIR), and lateral entorhinal (ENT$_1$) cortices. The areas of cortex shown are indicated by boxes in Fig. 11A (Al$_d$/8/SR), Fig. 13A (PIR/51$_b$), and Fig. 14A (ENT$_1$/28).

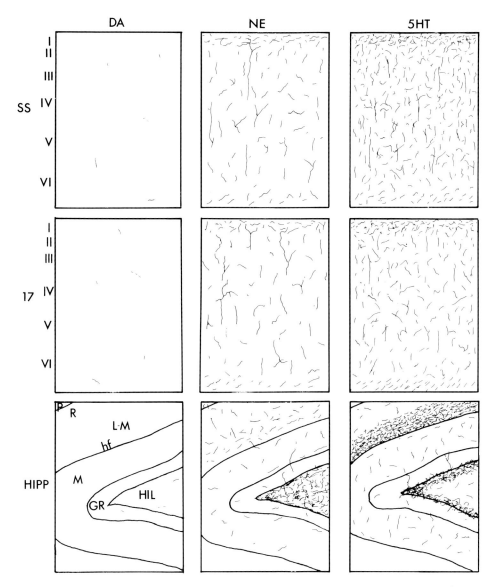

Figure 18. As in Figs. 16 and 17, nine panels illustrating the laminar pattern of DA, NE, and 5HT innervation of somatosensory cortex (SS), area 17 of visual cortex (17), and hippocampus (HIPP). The areas of cortex shown are indicated by boxes in Fig. 13A (FrPaSS/2-1-3/SI), Fig. 15A (17), and Fig. 14A (DG).

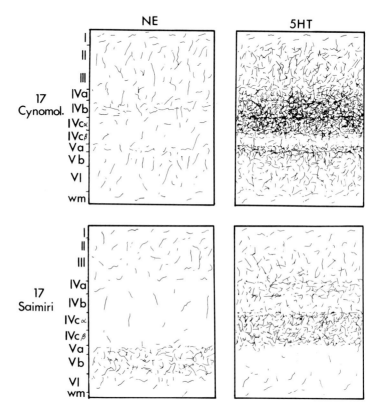

Figure 19. Schematic representation of NE and 5HT innervation of area 17 of visual cortex in the rhesus cynomolgus monkey (Cynomol.) and the squirrel monkey (Saimiri). (Modified from Morrison *et al.*, 1984, and Kosofsky *et al.*, 1984.)

They sometimes behave like classical amino acid neurotransmitters and, on the same cell, behave like long-acting peptidergic modulators. They act at multiple receptors that are often not present where the monoamines are released from terminals. They may make few classical synapses, may interact with local peptidergic neurons to produce metabolic "hot spots," and alter the blood flow through, and permeability of, the cerebral vasculature. Finally, their behavioral functions in cerebral cortex are, unfortunately, very poorly understood but vigorously debated. It is clear that the three major monoamines in cerebral cortex are quite separate systems that may each contain numerous subsystems with many functions.

7. Theoretical Note on the Functions of Monoamines in Cortex and Basal Ganglia

7.1. Introduction

What are the functions of monoamines in cortex and related areas of the basal ganglia? The answer to this question is not obvious.

Investigators from the physiological, biochemical, pharmacological, and behavioral neurosciences have approached this question and have provided fascinating insights (Butcher, 1978; DiChiara and Gessa, 1981; Divac and Oberg, 1979; Fuster, 1980; Garattini *et al.*, 1978; Glowinski *et al.*, 1984; Groves, 1983; Horn *et al.*, 1979; Iversen, 1984; Marsden, 1980; Messiha and Kenny, 1977; Muldrum and Marsden, 1975; Poirier *et al.*, 1979; Roberts *et al.*, 1978; Rolls, 1987; Yahr, 1976). In this section, we will approach this functional question with a bias toward a chemical neuroanatomical and connectional viewpoint of functional relationships. *The general thesis that will be developed is that the monoamine innervation and the corticosubcortical connections involved in the prefrontal system are substantially different from the monoamine innervation and corticosubcortical connections of the other (lateral or dorsal) cortical and basal ganglia systems.* The key differences between the systems are, in many respects, subtle. These subtle differences can be easily overlooked because of the otherwise great similarities in the two systems.

Much of the background literature for this section has been discussed in detail in Sections 4–6. In addition, more detailed reviews of the connections, chemical neuroanatomy, and functions of the systems described below can be found in our previous reports (Fallon, 1981b; Fallon *et al.*, 1983; Fallon and Loughlin, 1985; Loughlin *et al.*, 1986a,b; Loughlin and Fallon, 1982, 1985) and excellent reviews and studies from other laboratories (Graybiel and Ragsdale, 1983; Evarts *et al.*, 1984; Goldman-Rakic, 1984; Wise and Strick, 1984; Milner and Petrides, 1984; Fuster, 1980, 1984; Pickel *et al.*, 1977; Vincent *et al.*, 1983; Groves, 1983; Rolls, 1987; Kolb, 1984; Yahr, 1976; Carpenter, 1976; Dray, 1980; Evarts and Wise, 1984; Fink and Smith, 1980; Horn *et al.*, 1979; Divac and Oberg, 1979; Denny-Brown and Yanagisawa, 1976; DiChiara and Gessa, 1981; DeLong *et al.*, 1983; Fallon, 1981b; Garattini *et al.*, 1978; Kelly *et al.*, 1982; Glowinski *et al.*, 1984; Heimer and Wilson, 1975; Heimer *et al.*, 1982; Hornykiewicz, 1973; Iversen, 1984; Marshall *et al.*, 1974; Matthyse, 1981; Nauta, 1979;

Nauta and Domesick, 1978, 1979, 1984; Newman and Winans, 1980; Stevens, 1979; Ungerstedt, 1974; DiFiglia *et al.*, 1976; Grofova, 1975; Hassler, 1979; Kanazawa *et al.*, 1977, 1984; Lindvall and Björklund, 1984; McGeer *et al.*, 1977; Palkovits *et al.*, 1978; McDonald, 1982, 1983; Swanson and Cowan, 1975; Switzer *et al.*, 1982; Pickel *et al.*, 1977; van der Kooy *et al.*, 1981; Kuypers, 1962; Kuypers and Lawrence, 1967; Leichnetz and Astruc, 1975; Haber *et al.*, 1985; Gerfen, 1985, 1987; Williams and Faull, 1985; Lidsky *et al.*, 1985; Butcher, 1978; Marsden, 1980; Messiha and Kenny, 1977; Muldrum and Marsden, 1975; Versteeg *et al.*, 1976; Sandell *et al.* 1987).

The discussions of the functional anatomy of the monoamine systems in cortex and basal ganglia have been derived from data generated in studies on the rat, cat, Old World monkeys, and humans. It may not seem prudent to interchange data and theory derived from such presumably widely divergent species, but we will follow the concept that frontal cortical (and basal ganglia) functions may be more similar than dissimilar, in the rat, monkey, and humans (for review see Kolb, 1984). Because the rat provides a reasonably good model for many (but not all) frontal cortical and basal ganglia connections and functions, the present discussion will highlight illustrations of connections in the rat brain.

The connections of interest in this section include (1) the ascending mono-amine projections from the SN–VTA (DA), LC (NE), and raphe (5HT) to cortex and basal ganglia, and (2) the descending corticostriatopallidal projections that effect motor behavior. The connectivity of the ascending monoamine inputs to cerebral cortex was discussed in Sections 1–6. Additional details concerning the relevant inputs to basal ganglia structures will be included below. The connectivity of the descending corticostriatopallidal systems will be discussed first.

7.2. Corticostriatopallidal Systems: Overview

Of the many brain systems that may directly control behavior, none seem as extensive as corticostriatopallidal (CSP) systems. This three-tiered system (Nauta, 1979) originates in all regions of cerebral cortex and forms a descending extra-pyramidal, basal ganglia system that parallels the more direct corticospinal motor systems. The CSP systems originate in cortex where topographically organized cortical efferents innervate a mosaic of longitudinal strips of dorsal and ventral striatal structures (Goldman and Nauta, 1977; Yeterian and Van Hoesen, 1978; Kemp and Powell, 1971; Jones *et al.*, 1977; Heimer and Wilson, 1975; Fallon *et al.*, 1978b, 1983; Goldman-Rakic, 1982). These topographically organized cor-ticostriatal projections gain access to pallidal structures that then output to nu-merous brain-stem and diencephalic sites (Nauta, 1979; Fallon *et al.*, 1983) as shown in more detail in Fig. 21. A second nontopographically organized system (not illustrated) appears to originate predominantly in associational cortices (Yet-erian and Van Hoesen, 1978) and project to interdigitating strips in cau-date–putamen (Selemon and Goldman-Rakic, 1985). Subsequently, the nonto-pographical system in the striatum probably arises from neurons in patches or striosomes (see below) in the striatum (Gerfen, 1985, 1987) that project to central globus pallidus (Wilson and Phelan, 1982), and ventral pars compacta of the SN

(Gerfen, 1985, 1987). This secondary nontopographical CSP system probably allows for widespread integration of sensory-motor information in nigral neurons, as suggested by neurophysiological studies (Schwarz *et al.*, 1984; Bunney and Aghajanian, 1976; Hikosaka and Wurtz, 1983a–d).

What are the key features of the primary, topographically organized CSP systems? Following the initial suggestions by Heimer and colleagues (Heimer and Wilson, 1975; Heimer, 1978), we have argued that there are a large number of parallel, topographical, descending CSP systems that originate in classical, and nonclassical (e.g., basolateral amygdaloid nucleus), cortical regions (Fallon *et al.*, 1983; Fallon and Loughlin, 1982; Fallon, 1981b). Three major types of topographical CSP systems are illustrated in Fig. 20. The classical CSP system originates in neocortex (cortex) and descends through caudate–putamen (CP), globus pallidus (GP), entopeduncular nucleus, and substantia nigra (SN). Although many return loops to diencephalon and cortex exist (Fig. 20), brain-stem and spinal cord motor centers are innervated by pallidal (globus pallidus, entopeduncular nucleus, substantia nigra, pars reticulata) outputs to the superior colliculus (SUP COL) and pedunculopontine nucleus (PPN and nearby sectors of the mesencephalic locomotor region). These regions, in turn, form tectospinal and reticulospinal pathways that control motor neurons in the medulla and spinal cord. This classical CSP system parallels direct corticospinal projections that, together with cerebellar efferents, form major control systems for somatic muscles of the body.

A second group of descending CSP systems arise from allocortices such as hippocampus and piriform cortex (Fig. 21). These project to ventral striatal structures (VS) that, in turn, project to ventral pallidum (VP). Thus, a hippocampal–nucleus accumbens–ventral pallidal circuit and a piriform cortex–ventral striatal–ventral pallidal circuit are thought to exist (Heimer, 1978). We have also proposed (Fallon *et al.*, 1983; Fallon, 1981b; Fallon and Loughlin, 1982) other CSP circuits in this system. One is a piriform cortex–islands of Calleja complex (striatum + pallidum) circuit. Another CSP circuit appears to originate in the basolateral nucleus of the amygdala (Fig. 22). Here, pyramidal neurons (cortical-like) project to frontal cortices (the corticocortical connection) as well as several striatal-like regions. These are the nucleus accumbens–ventral caudate–putamen and lateral (striatal-like) subdivisions of the central nucleus of the amygdala and bed nucleus of the stria terminalis (see also McDonald, 1982, 1983; Smith and Millhouse, 1985). These striatal-like structures then project to pallidal-like zones in the medial portions of the ventral pallidum, central nucleus of the amygdala, and bed nucleus of the stria terminalis (Figs. 21 and 22).

It now appears that medial and lateral sectors of each of these CSP regions are distinct from each other in that there is a denser concentration of releasing hormone-containing fibers and steroid (estradiol, dihydrotestosterone, corticosterone)-receptive neurons in the medial sectors (Fallon, 1981b; Fallon *et al.*, 1983; Warembourg, 1981). Thus, these allocortically derived CSP systems originating in amygdala, hippocampus, piriform cortex, and olfactory cortex, contain a medially placed zone that is under the control of releasing hormones and circulating steroids and amines. These observations, combined with known outputs to certain hypothalamic targets, have prompted us (Fallon, 1981b; Fallon *et al.*, 1983) to predict that a third, endocrine-related group of CSP systems is present.

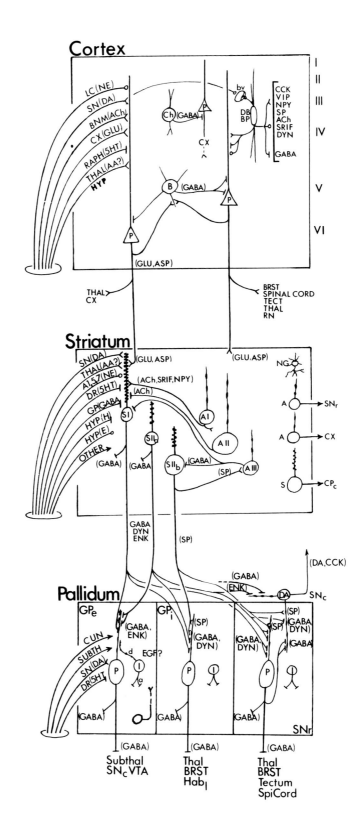

The endocrine-related group of CSP systems in the medial olfactory tubercle, cortico-medial amygdala, medial hippocampal–accumbens circuit, and, perhaps, septum are positioned to receive not only limbic neuronal inputs, but also bloodborne steroid hormonal inputs. Thus, their afferents are derived from the body's internal environment (autonomics, hormones) in a way parallel to the exteroceptive-derived afferents of the neocortical CSP systems. The inputs (e.g., bloodborne hormones) and outputs (pituitary-derived hormones and autonomics) of the endocrine CSP have a much longer time constant than the classical CSP systems, counterparts that utilize fast inputs (visual, auditory, and somatosensory) and relatively fast outputs (muscle contractions).

How do the allocortical and endocrine CSP systems fit into the scheme of motor systems? Two examples would be as follows: Neurons in the amygdala and septum (predicted here to be pallidal-like) project to the perifornical region of the hypothalamus (the so-called "hypothalamic area controlling emotional responses" or HACER—see Smith and DeVito, 1984). The perifornical region projects to the intermediolateral cell column of the spinal cord (IML in Fig. 21),

←
_____

Figure 20. Some features of the neurochemical anatomy of the cortex, striatum, and pallidum are shown. Some *cortical inputs* and their associated neurotransmitters/neuromodulators include: (1) locus coeruleus (LC)—norepinephrine (NE); (2) substantia nigra–ventral tegmental area (SN)–dopamine (DA) (plus cholecystokinin and neurotensin); (3) basal nucleus of Meynert–pallidum (BNM)–acetylcholine (ACh); (4) other cortical areas (CX)–glutamate (GLU); (5) raphe (RAPH)–serotonin (5HT); (6) thalamic (THAL)–amino acids? (AA?); (7) hypothalamus (HYP)–GABA input. *Cortical neurons* and some of their associated neurotransmitters/neuromodulators include (1) pyramidal output neurons (P)–glutamate, aspartate (GLU, ASP); (2) basket cells (B)–GABA; (3) chandelier cells (Ch)–GABA; and (4) double bouquet/bipolar cells (DB/BP)–cholecystokinin (CCK), vasoactive intestinal polypeptide (VIP), neuropeptide Y (NPY), substance P (SP), acetylcholine (ACh), somatostatin (SRIF), dynorphin (DYN), GABA. *Cortical outputs* using GLU and ASP as neurotransmitters are shown projecting to medium-sized spiny cells (SI) of the striatum, as well as thalamus (THAL), other cortical regions (CX), brain-stem locomotor regions, reticular formation, and pons (BRST), spinal cord (SPINAL CORD), tectum (TECT), and red nucleus (RN). Other projections, e.g., to SN–VTA, hypothalamus are not shown. *Striatal inputs* and their associated neurotransmitters/neuromodulators include: (1) substantia nigra–ventral tegmental area (SN)–dopamine (DA); (2) thalamus (THAL)–amino acids? (AA?); (3) lateral tegmental catecholamine cell groups (A1,5,7)–norepinephrine (NE); (4) dorsal raphe (DR)–serotonin (5HT); (5) globus pallidus (GP)–GABA; (6) hypothalamus (HYP)–histamine (H), (7) hypothalamus (HYP)–epinephrine (E); and others (OTHER). *Striatal neurons* and some of their associated neurotransmitters/neuromodulators include: (1) medium spiny (SI)–GABA, DYN, enkephalin (ENK); (3) spiny type IIb (SIIb)–SP; (4) aspiny I (AI)–ACh, SRIF, NPY; (5) aspiny II (AII)–ACh; (5) aspiny III (AIII)–GABA; (6) long projecting aspiny (A) and other large spiny (S) neurons; and (7) neurogliaform/granule cells (NG). *Striatal outputs* using GABA, DYN, ENK, SP, SK, and TGF are shown to project to external globus pallidus (GPe), internal globus pallidus or entopeduncular nucleus (GPi), substantia nigra pars reticulata (SNr), substantia nigra pars compacta (SNc), cortex (CX), and caudal caudate putamin (CPc). Some *pallidal inputs* and their associated neurotransmitters/neuromodulators include: (1) cuneiform nucleus (CUN); (2) subthalamus (SUBTH); (3) substantia nigra pars compacta (SN)–DA; and (4) dorsal raphe (DR)–5HT. *Pallidal neurons* and the associated neurotransmitters/neuromodulators include: (1) medium large, aspiny, varicose principal neuron (P)–GABA; (2) interneurons (I); and basal nucleus/pallidal neurons containing ACh and/or GABA. *Pallidal outputs* containing GABA include subthalamus (Subthal) and SN–VTA, ventral thalamus (Thal), brain-stem pedunculopontine nucleus (BRST), lateral habenula (HAB1), tectum (Tectum), and spinal cord (SpiCord). The symbols at the synaptic terminals indicate that an input is thought to be primarily excitatory (—<), inhibiting (—|), enabling (—○), or disenabling (—●). Inputs with unknown physiology are indicated by an arrow (→).

as well as many regions, such as the nucleus of the solitary tract and parabrachial complex, that also project to the IML. The perifornical-to-IML projection system, which ultimately controls sympathetic outflow to smooth musculature of the body (AUTONOMIC in Fig. 21), is the allocortical CSP system homologue to the neocortically derived CSP projection to α motor neurons that innervate voluntary muscles (VOLUNTARY in Fig. 21). What are the parallel homologous circuits in the endocrine CSP system? One example could be a ventral pallidal output from the bed nucleus of the stria terminalis, which innervates the paraventricular nucleus in the hypothalamus (Schmued and Fallon, unpublished observation) (HYP in Fig. 21). The paraventricular nucleus contains three major zones, which project to either the IML, posterior pituitary, or median eminence (Swanson and Sawchenko, 1983). The two latter projections control endocrine output of the posterior and anterior pituitary (AP), respectively. Thus, this endocrine CSP can be thought of as having a HORMONAL motor output

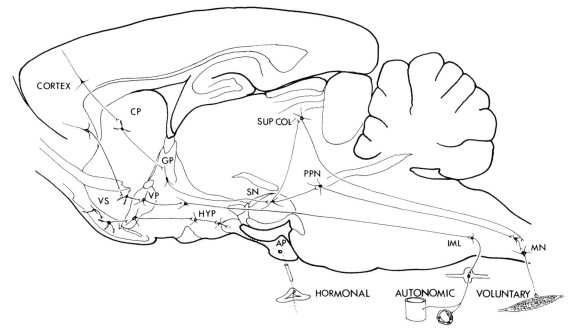

Figure 21. Sagittal view of the rat brain illustrating the three proposed parallel corticostriatopallidal (CSP) motor systems. The *classical CSP systems* originate in neocortex (CORTEX), innervate caudate–putamen (CP), which innervates globus pallidus (GP). GP neurons innervate SN and pedunculopontine nucleus/mesencephalic locomotor area (PPN). SN also innervates PPN and tectum (SUP COL). PPN and SUP COL innervate ventral horn neurons. PPN may also directly innervate hypophysiotrophic zones of the hypothalamus. Ultimately, motor neurons (MN) innervate voluntary muscles (VOLUNTARY). In the second *allocortical (limbic-type)* CSP system, allocortices (CORTEX) innervate ventral striatum (VS), which innervates ventral pallidum (VP). VP neurons also project to SN and PPN (not shown) as well as hypothalamic neurons such as the perifornical region (also called the hypothalamic area controlling emotional responses). These hypothalamic neurons innervate the intermediolateral cell column (IML), which controls the sympathetic autonomics (AUTONOMIC) controlling the smooth muscles of the gut and vasculature, as well as glands. A third parallel CSP system is proposed. It is called the *endocrine CSP system* and originates in medial limbic allocortices rich in releasing hormone and/or steroid hormone receptors and innervates medial regions of VS, which then innervate VP regions such as those found in the islands of Calleja complex and bed nucleus of the stria terminalis. These regions project to the proposed hypothalamic equivalents of the upper motor neuron complex, such as the paraventricular hypothalamic nucleus (HYP). Paraventricular neurons innervate the median eminence, posterior pituitary, or IML. The pituitary hormones, for example, trophic hormones of the anterior pituitary (AP), can be thought of as the endocrine hormonal equivalent of a motor output in the voluntary or autonomic motor system.

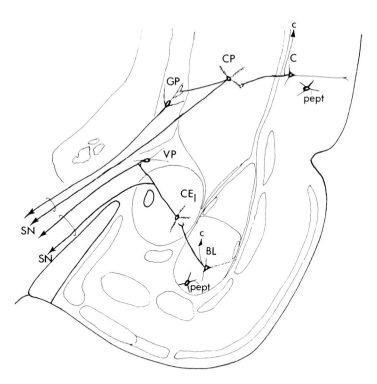

Figure 22. This illustration of the right amygdaloid complex of the rat suggests how amygdaloid structures can be viewed as novel corticostriatopallidal (CSP) systems. The neocortically derived classical CSP system is shown at the top of the figure for comparison, i.e., neocortex (C) contains local circuit peptidergic neurons (pept) such as a CCK neuron. The pyramidal neuron has corticostriatal projections to caudate–putamen (CP). CP projects to globus pallidus (GP) and substantia nigra pars reticulata (SN). GP also projects to SN. In the model of *amygdaloid CSP circuitry,* local circuit peptidergic neurons (pept) and pyramidal-like neurons (*but* with their apical dendrite pointed anterolaterally) are present in the basolateral nucleus (BL). The BL projection to prefrontal cortex (arrow to C) can be considered a corticocortical projection, whereas the BL projection to ventral striatum and lateral central nucleus (CE$_l$) can be considered the corticostriatal projections. Ventral striatal and amygdaloid ventral striatal (CE$_l$) projections to ventral pallidum, including pallidal-like neurons in the medial central nucleus and ansa lenticularis region (VP), could represent the amygdaloid equivalent of the striatopallidal projection of the dorsal (classical) system. Amygdaloid projections to SN are likewise analogous. This example further highlights the concept that the CSP systems comprise a large, finite constellation of similar systems throughout the forebrain. That is anatomically and functionally related CSP systems may be the dominant organizational feature of the entire forebrain.

that parallels AUTONOMIC motor output and VOLUNTARY motor output of the other CSP systems (Fig. 21). When the three great extrapyramidal motor systems are reviewed in this way, it is likely that CSP systems form many parallel longitudinal columns originating in cortex and progressing through several convergent synaptic stations *en route* to their final common "motor" cells, whether they be α motor neurons (classical CSP) or releasing hormone-producing neurons controlling the anterior pituitary (endocrine CSP). In this way, the columnar organization of cortex could be maintained throughout the entire neuraxis. The afferent arcs of sensory input that impinge back on these systems also appear to be parallel, but distinct. That is, the classical CSP systems are dominated by "fast" sensory input to cortex (vision, audition, somatosensation) whereas the allocortical CSP systems are determined by "slower" sensory systems (olfaction, taste, autonomics) and endocrine CSP systems are dominated by "very slow" sensory input (hormones, immunomessengers and other chemical signals in the blood such as osmolarity, pH, O_2/CO_2). In the context of CSP systems, then, cortex can be viewed as the internal CNS sensory organ that reorders peripheral sensory input to give more equipotential access and interaction of all known inputs to CSP systems.

It would appear that if all of the extrapyramidal systems were active at once, a maladaptive motor state would be present. How would individual "preferred channels" of CSP activity dominate other "channels" to maximize survival? As discussed in detail previously (Fallon *et al.*, 1983), there are GABAergic neurons present at all levels of the CSP systems. Thus, GABAergic neurons would exert lateral inhibiting influences at the cortical, striatal, and pallidal levels to inhibit adjacent CSP channels. DA input may also function to focus CSP activity at the subcortical sites. Coordinated activity of several CSP units could be brought about at the cortical level, since cortical regions that are reciprocally connected have projections to the same areas of caudate–putamen (Yeterian and van Hoesen, 1978).

In summary, the general organization of extrapyramidal motor systems can be viewed as consisting of many parallel CSP systems belonging to the classical neocortical, allocortical, and/or endocrine-originating forebrain regions. Each CSP probably originates as a cortical column or small group of cortical columns and maintains a complex but topographical group of descending projections to specific motor neurons. Each CSP system may inhibit its neighbor at the cortical, striatal, and pallidal levels, thus forming "preferred channels" of CSP activity to carry out specific motor tasks. The extrapyramidal pathways are, likewise, paralleled by pyramidal pathways that project directly from cortex to motor neuronal areas in the spinal cord (classical system), lateral hypothalamus (allocortical system), or medial hypothalamus (endocrine, immune systems). Functionally related, but widely separated, CSP systems could be coactivated at the cortical level by well-established corticocortical connections.

Although the foregoing discussion stresses the common, unifying principles of organization of CSP systems, it is also the purpose of this section to discuss how key differences in the organization of CSP systems help to maintain why the prefrontal system is unique. It is also the purpose of this section to demonstrate how the ascending monoamine inputs to the three levels of different CSP systems may differentially regulate behavior. In order to differentiate the CSP organization of the prefrontal systems from other forebrain systems, it is necessary to look more closely at the connectional organization, especially at the striatal level.

7.3. Unique Organization of the Prefrontal System with Regard to Monoamine Input and Corticostriatopallidal Circuitry

The prefrontal system is composed of prefrontal cortex and a set of anatomically and functionally associated cortical and subcortical areas (Rosvold and Szwarcbart, 1964; Divac *et al.*, 1978; Divac, 1979; Divac and Diemer, 1980).

These include prefrontal cortex, supragenual cortex, perirhinal cortex, mediodorsal thalamic nucleus, amygdala, intermediodorsal globus pallidus, anteromedial caudate–putamen, claustrum, entopeduncular nucleus, and SN–VTA. In terms of CSP systems, the prefrontal system includes several associated, interconnected neocortical (prefrontal cortex, supragenual cortex)- and allocortical (perirhinal cortex, claustrum, basolateral nucleus of the amygdala)-originating CSP systems. Functionally and behaviorally, the prefrontal system includes those CSP systems related to both high-order and limbic functions of prefrontal cortex and amygdala (Kolb, 1984; Goldman-Rakic, 1984; Fuster, 1980).

The prefrontal system is a special type of CSP system for a number of reasons. First, this system can be differentiated from most of the other CSP systems on the basis of its dense DA input at the cortical level since most neocortices in the rat are only sparsely to moderately innervated by DA fibers. This differentiation was discussed in detail in Section 4 (and cf. DA innervation of rat and monkey premotor cortex). Second, the organization of cortical and DA inputs at the striatal level appears to be different than other CSP systems. This observation deserves further comment.

The subnuclear organization of striatal structures can be subdivided at the cellular level (DiFiglia *et al.*, 1976), and at the cellular island level (Mensah, 1977; Fallon *et al.*, 1983; Fallon, 1983; Ribak and Fallon, 1982). Our previous work on the islands of Calleja complex demonstrated the organization of striatal and pallidal structures as microunits in each island of Calleja region of ventral striatopallidum (Fallon *et al.*, 1983; Ribak and Fallon, 1982; Fallon, 1981b, 1983). Recent studies by Graybiel, Gerfen, Goldman-Rakic, and others (Graybiel and Chesselet, 1984a,b; Graybiel *et al.*, 1981; Ragsdale and Graybiel, 1981, 1984; Graybiel and Ragsdale, 1978; Nastuk and Graybiel, 1983, 1985; Jimenez-Castellanos and Graybiel, 1985; Sandell *et al.*, 1986; Chesselet and Graybiel, 1987; Gerfen, 1984, 1985, 1987; Gerfen *et al.*, 1985; Vincent *et al.*, 1983; Goedert *et al.*, 1983; Herkenham and Pert, 1981; Moon and Herkenham, 1984; Donoghue and Herkenham, 1983; van der Kooy, 1983; Goldman-Rakic, 1982) have uncovered what may be the predominant modular input–output organizational scheme of the striatum. Although there are some species differences, and despite the fact that some of the modules are obvious only in the developing animal, certain basic patterns of histochemical staining and input–output relationships appear to be present in adult animals.

The modular scheme of the "generalized" mammalian striatum (particularly in the developing animal) can be defined according to the relationship of striatal markers to striosomes or patchy areas of low acetylcholinesterase (AChE) staining. The striosomes are 0.25–5 mm wide in coronal sections and are surrounded by an AChE-rich matrix. As summarized in Fig. 23, striosomes are populated by dynorphin-, enkephalin-, substance P-, substance K-, ACh-, GABA-, and some somatostatin-containing cell bodies, as well as opiate receptor binding ("opiate patches"), muscarinic ACh receptors, neurotensin-containing terminals, D_2 receptors, and DA fibers originating in the "ventral sheet" of the SN (Fig. 25). Other inputs to the striosome patches (where topographically appropriate—see below) arise from cortex and amygdala. In the extrastriasomal matrix, D_2 receptors, calcium-binding protein, as well as somatostatin-, neuropeptide Y-, avian polypeptide-, enkephalin-, and AChE-containing cell bodies are present. DA fibers to this zone arise from the "intermediate" sheet of SN and paranigralis nucleus of the VTA (Fig. 25). This zone is dominated by GABA, ACh, and somatostatin interneurons that project locally, as well as neurons projecting to globus pallidus, entopeduncular nucleus, and SN.

There are also differential outputs of patch and matrix zones to the SN such that neurons in the patch or striosomal zones of dorsal caudate–putamen are thought to project to the cell bodies and proximal dendrites of lateral VTA and SN pars compacta neurons (the nontopographic system) whereas the matrix neurons of the caudate–putamen and ventral striatum project to SN pars reticulata (the topographical system) where they contact distal DA dendrites and GABA neurons (Gerfen, 1984, 1985, 1987; Wassef *et al.*, 1981; Domesick, 1981; Somogyi *et al.*, 1981). Inputs to the matrix (where topographically appropriate—see below) arrive from thalamus, cortex, amygdala, VTA, dorsal sheet of the SN pars compacta and A8 cell group. It should be pointed out that some local circuit neurons tend to be distributed near the matrix–striosome border (AChE-containing: excitatory; and GABA- and somatostatin-containing: inhibitory interneurons). In addition, enkephalin-containing neurons may lie in, or outside, the striosomes, depending on the fixation and immunohistochemical protocol used (Graybiel and Chesselet, 1984b).

What differentiates the prefrontal CSP system from other CSP systems in the context of striosomal organization in the striatum? As illustrated in Fig. 24, there appear to be some basic differences between the input–output organization of striatal striosomes with respect to the prefrontal limbic (PF/LIMBIC in Fig. 24) CSP systems and other CSP systems. First, the VTA DA input to anteromedial caudate–putamen (of the prefrontal system) predominantly innervates the matrix zone, whereas in more lateral–posterior caudate–putamen the SN DA input is denser to the striosomal patches, although in all striatal regions there is matrix and patch innervation. Second, the cortical input from rat prefrontal cortex and basolateral amygdala to anteromedial caudate–putamen of the prefrontal (area 32) system is to the striosomal patches, whereas cingulate and dorsal–lateral

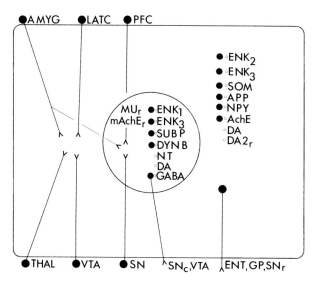

Figure 23. Highly schematic representation of a striosome/matrix unit in striatum. The center circle forms the striosomal patch zone ("in") and the surround forms in matrix zone ("out"). See text for details.

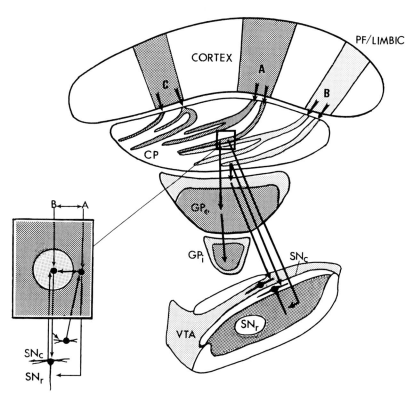

Figure 24. Schematic comparison of the prefrontal/limbic (PF/LIMBIC at "B") CSP systems with dorsal/lateral mesocortical ("A," "B") CSP systems. Cortex (CORTEX), caudate–putamen (CP), globus pallidus (GPe), and entopeduncular nucleus (GP$_i$) are represented in the sagittal plane to illustrate how the corticostriatal projections originate in cortical columns (and slabs) to innervate interdigitating, longitudinally oriented strips in the caudate–putamen. The "limbic" related outputs originating in area 32 of prefrontal cortex are shown in light stippling whereas other neocortical outputs more related to "motor" control are shown in dense stippling. Note that the PF/LIMBIC cortical projections are to patch neurons and other cortical projections are predominantly to matrix neurons (see insert at left). The limbic (light stippling) and motor (dense stippling) zones in the GP$_e$, GP$_i$, and SN/VTA are also shown. The prefrontal system inputs are positioned to control patches in the striatum, peripallidal zones, and interestingly, the proximal dendrites and somata of ventral sheet (SN$_c$), intermediate sheet, and dorsal sheet DA neurons. The dorsal/lateral neocortical system inputs are best positioned to influence matrix neurons in the striatum, central pallidal zones, and distal dendrites (in SN$_c$) of ventral sheet DA neurons.

cortical and amygdala input to more lateral caudate–putamen is to the matrix zone (Donoghue and Herkenham, 1986). [The projection from area 8 of prefrontal cortex to striatum in the monkey is to the matrix zone (Goldman-Rakic, 1982), unlike the area 32 projection in the rat.] Thus, although in both systems the cortical and DA inputs do not overlap extensively, in one CSP system (prefrontal system) the DA projection from the VTA and A8 is primarily to the matrix zone and in the other CSP systems (lateral or dorsal system), the DA projection is to both striosomal patches and matrix. Since striosomal patch neurons project somewhat nontopographically to SN pars compacta neurons and matrix neurons project topographically to SN pars reticulata (and dendrites of pars compacta) neurons, prefrontal cortex has more direct control over the synaptology of SN pars compacta cell bodies and proximal dendrites, whereas the lateral/dorsal neocortices have a more direct control over the synaptology of SN pars compacta distal dendrites and GABA neurons in SN pars reticulata (Fig. 24). There is also an interesting reversal or "switch" in the system, since prefrontal/limbic cortex receives DA input from VTA/SN dorsal sheet neurons that seem to be under descending control from patch neurons in the striatum. These patch neurons themselves receive their DA input predominantly from SNc/ventral sheet neurons. Therefore, this reversal of connections in the CSP system may form part of the basis whereby the prefrontal/limbic CSP system and lateral/dorsal neocortical CSP systems interact. They also interact by local circuit neurons connecting striatal patches and matrix, as well as by corticocortical connections (see arrows in insert in Fig. 24).

In summary, the prefrontal CSP system is unique in the DA and cortical innervation of striosomal patches and matrix regions of striatum. The patch/matrix organization gives a clue as to the differentiation of the prefrontal/limbic CSP from the lateral/dorsal CSP systems. The former dominates the patches, the latter dominates the matrix. Within one striatal region, the matrix may receive input from layer V pyramidal neurons of, for example, a column of somatic sensory cortex and the enclosed patch receives input from prefrontal cortex. This interdigitated, but largely nonoverlapping, system may extend throughout pallidal and nigral zones, such that at one localized nigral zone (specified by its medial–lateral and dorsal–ventral topographical connections with the striatal zone in question) the ventralmost DA neuron projects to the patch, whereas its more dorsal neighbor in the intermediate sheet of SNc projects to the matrix. These findings, together with other unique features of the DA, NE, and 5HT innervation of prefrontal cortices (see Sections 4–6), further suggest that the prefrontal CSP system has a unique functional organization. Other features of the system will be discussed in the next section.

7.4. Unique Organization of the Prefrontal System with Regard to Body Representation in the SN–VTA

The organization of SN–VTA projections to cerebral cortex is described in detail in Section 4. The SN–VTA projections to the entire telencephalon are also well characterized with respect to topography, laterality, collateralization, and neurochemistry (Fallon and Loughlin, 1985). The SN–VTA, surrounding ventral tegmentum, and related fiber pathways can also be viewed with respect to body representation as illustrated in Fig. 25. The topographical somatotopic representation of the medial lemniscus and the somatomotor representation of the cerebral peduncle can be seen to be in register with respect to head, arm, trunk, and leg representation. In a similar way, the accessory optic tract and associated medial terminal nucleus of the accessory optic system located medially in this region, may represent visual space (EYE), whereas lateral SN and A8 regions are bordered by the brachium of the inferior colliculus and appear to partially represent auditory space (EAR). Sandwiched between these lemniscal systems are the subnuclei of the SN–VTA. A dorsally located sheet of DA/CCK neurons in the SN–VTA projects to cortical and limbic structures (CORTI-CAL–LIMBIC ZONE). Just ventral to this zone lie the two sheets of SN–VTA including the intermediate sheet of DA/CCK (light stippling) neurons projecting to the striatum. This sheet may correspond to the MPP-sensitive neurons. They also appear to correspond to the pars compacta neurons that form the DA innervation of striatal matrix regions (see below). Below this intermediate sheet is a "ventral sheet" of DA neurons that forms the classical nigrostriatal pathway. Fewer of these DA neurons are colocalized with CCK. This sheet may be the major source of the DA innervation of striatal patches or striosomes (see below). Thus, DA neurons in adjacent intermediate and ventral sheets could provide adjacent matrix and patch innervation in striatal zones, although data on this proposal are scanty. More ventrally, and just dorsal to the cerebral peduncle, lies the pallidal-like pars reticulata of the SN (MOTOR ZONE). It projects to thalamus, superior colliculus, and pedunculopontine region. Figure 25 is presented not only to draw attention to the organization of body space in this region, but also to point out that neurons in this region probably receive sensory/motor inputs from axon collaterals of the four major lemniscal systems resident in this region. These collaterals may have been missed with conventional neuroanatomical techniques. In an example we have studied in some detail, lateral VTA and medial SN neurons that are located in the region just medial, dorsal, and lateral to the medial terminal nucleus ("EYE" region in Fig. 25) project to frontal and cingulate cortices [including Hall and Lindholm's (1974) "eye fields" in the rat] and anteromedial caudate–putamen. We have recently shown that these SN–VTA neurons, many of which have dendrites extending into the medial terminal nucleus, may also receive direct visual input from the retina (Fallon *et al.*, 1984; Giolli *et al.*, 1985), thus providing the prefrontal system with short-latency (but perhaps "nonconscious") visual input. It is also possible that other SN–VTA neurons, with cell bodies or dendrites lying within the medial-lying accessory optic tracts or brachium of the inferior colliculus, may receive topographically relevant sensory stimuli that may then be relayed to other cortical and limbic forebrain sites via mesotelencephalic projections. We have found

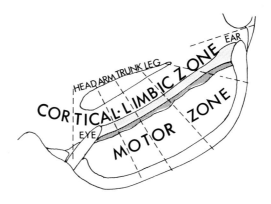

Figure 25. Schematic illustration of the ventral mesencephalon of the right side of the rat brain demonstrating the correspondence of the various body space regions in the medial lemniscus, cortical limbic zone of the SN–VTA, motor zone of the SN pars reticulata, cerebral peduncle, accessory optic systems, and auditory system. Ventral to the cortical limbic "dorsal sheet" of the SN are the "intermediate" sheet of DA/CCK neurons projecting to the caudate–putamen (light stippling). These neurons are probably "ventral" in the MPP-sensitive zone (A. Deutch, personal communication). Ventral to this sheet is the sheet of DA neurons projecting only to caudate–putamen (heavy stippling). See text for discussion.

similar lemniscal projections to hypothalamic neurons whose dendrites invade the optic tract (Fallon and Moore, 1979a).

In summary, the input–output relationships of the SN–VTA can be viewed in several ways, including topographical representations of sensory and motor body space. In this regard, it is interesting to note that SN–VTA neurons projecting to the prefrontal system are located primarily in the regions representing the head and visual space. This observation further demonstrates another unique aspect of the prefrontal system, i.e., its dominant head and visual space representation in the SN–VTA. This topographical organization is likely to be paralleled by the secondary nontopographical CSP system that provides an additional nonsomatotopic organization to SN neurons (see discussion in Section 7.2).

7.5. Unique Organization of the Prefrontal System with Regard to Corticosubcortical Loops in the SN–VTA

In this section, the prefrontal system will be discussed in terms of the connections and neurotransmitter/neuromodular relationships in the SN–VTA. Although much of the data to be presented here were discussed in Sections 4–6 as well as in this section, the information will be viewed in a somewhat different context in order to propose how corticosubcortical loops and motor outputs of the prefrontal CSP systems are different from those of the more lateral and dorsal neocortical CSP systems. These differences will form the basis of a novel set of hypotheses on the functions of monoamines in cortex and basal ganglia. The basic plan of the discussion is shown in Fig. 26. The prefrontal and lateral CSP systems will be analyzed and compared for "LOOP" circuits and motor "OUTPUT" pathways to tectum, motor thalamus, midbrain, and spinal cord. We will argue that the LOOP and OUTPUT circuits are different for the prefrontal and lateral CSP systems.

Two different types of topographic corticosubcortical loops can be envisaged in the SN–VTA. These parallel the "nontopographically" organized CSP systems (see above and Schwarz *et al.*, 1984; Bunney and Aghajanian, 1976; Yeterian and van Hoesen, 1978; Gerfen, 1984, 1985, 1987; Gerfen *et al.*, 1985; Wilson and Phelan, 1982). As shown schematically in Fig. 27, two broad medial–lateral groups of SN–VTA neurons can be identified. The medially placed group I neurons (neurons 1–3) are associated with the prefrontal CSP system and the more laterally placed group II neurons (neurons 4–6) are related to the other

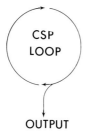

Figure 26. Simple control diagram upon which Figs. 27 and 28 are based. Extrapyramidal motor pathways in the CSP circuits are considered to be loop (LOOP) pathways between cortex and subcortex, or motor output pathways to motor neurons (OUTPUT) from cortex and subcortex.

neocortical CSP systems originating in dorsal and lateral sensory and motor neocortex. This is based on the principle of medial–lateral topography of the mesotelencephalic and telomesencephalic projections. Within each group there are further distinctions such that group I neurons (prefrontal CSP system) have VTA neurons (neuron 1) projecting to either prefrontal cortex (neuron 11) or medial nucleus accumbens (neuron 12—the mesolimbic projections), SN pars compacta neurons (neuron 2) projecting to many striatal and cortical sites in the prefrontal system (nigrostriatal, mesolimbic, and mesocortical projections), and an SN pars reticulata neuron (neuron 3) projecting to thalamus (neuron 8), tectum (neuron 7), or pedunculopontine nucleus (neuron 7). Group II neurons (lateral or dorsal neocortical CSP systems) have similar types of projections, i.e., a dorsal SN pars compacta neuron (neuron 4) projecting to cortical sites (neuron 11), a ventral SN pars compacta neuron (neuron 5) projecting strongly to patches in striatal sites (neuron 12) and, to a lesser extent, cortical/limbic sites (neuron 11), and an SN pars reticulata neuron (neuron 6), projecting to thalamus (neuron 8), tectum (neuron 7), or pedunculopontine nucleus (neuron 7). The return loops from the telencephalon include cortical projections to striatum (neuron

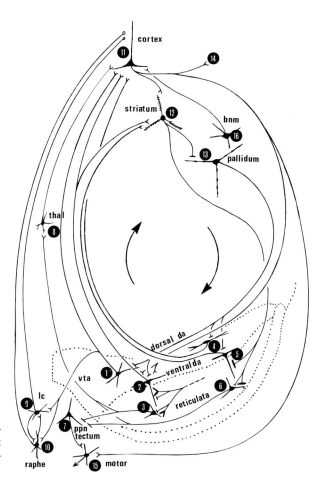

Figure 27. Anatomy and connections of the CSP system. See text for details, abbreviations, and discussion of pathways.

12), striatal projections SN–VTA, and striatal patch and pallidal projections back to the region near the somata and dendrites of the VTA and SN pars compacta neurons (neurons 1–4). In addition, cortical neurons project directly back to SN–VTA, with prefrontal cortex projecting to the regions medially (neurons 1 and 2) and other cortical neurons projecting laterally. Other cortical projections include axon collaterals to the spinal cord (neuron 15: corticospinal projections) and other cortices such as premotor cortex and hippocampal formation (neuron 14). The striatal neurons not only project to pallidum, but also project directly to the SN pars reticulata neurons (neurons 3 and 6) as well as the dendrites of some SN pars compacta neurons (neuron 3). Neuron 16 is the ACh basal nucleus of Meynert neuron that resides in peripallidal regions and projects to cortex. Some other connections have not been included (e.g., pallidotegmental connections, subthalamic area interconnections) (see Fig. 20) because they are not considered here to have as much of an impact in differentiating corticosubcortical loops and outputs in the prefrontal and lateral/dorsal CSP systems. The potential role of other mesencephalic regions such as the superior colliculus and midbrain reticular formation in differentiating medial and lateral nigral outputs is discussed in detail by Vaccarino and Prupas (1985; Vaccarino *et al.*, 1985).

Another facet to consider are the neurotransmitters and neuromodulators in the pathways illustrated in Fig. 27. The neurons are assumed to contain (in descending order) one or more of the following neuroactive compounds: Neuron 1, DA, CCK, NT; 2, DA, some have CCK; 3, GABA; 4, DA, NT, CCK; 5, DA, some have CCK; 6, GABA; 7, ACh, other excitatory transmitters; 8, excitatory transmitters; 9, NE, some NPY, galanin, CRF; 10, 5HT; 11, glutamate, aspartate; 12, GABA, substance P, substance K, dynorphin, epidermal growth factor, transforming growth factor, enkephalin, taurine; 13, GABA, enkephalin; 14, glutamate, aspartate, GABA, enkephalin; 15, ACh; 16, ACh. Some of the neurotransmitters and neuromodulators are colocalized in the same neurons (e.g., neuron 1 may contain DA, CCK, and NT). In contrast, some neurons in these regions do not have identified neurotransmitters in the projections (especially in VTA, thalamus, pedunculopontine nucleus, and tectum).

For this discussion, some assumptions will be made concerning the postsynaptic effects of neurotransmitters and neuromodulators in these pathways (see Sections 4–6 for details). However, we acknowledge that the true synaptic effects of inputs are complex, and have diverse interactions with other inputs. Additionally, it is an understatement to add that the synaptic effects are poorly known and highly controversial. Nonetheless, we shall attempt to crudely reconstruct the synaptology of this system with the same assumptions concerning the synaptic effect of each transmitter or modulator. Using consistent assumptions, it is still apparent that the prefrontal CSP system is unique. The assumptions are as follows:

Neuron 1 has a nonclassical type of facilitatory effect on cortical (11) and striatal neurons (12). DA is assumed to exert an initial depolarizing effect (EPSP) on postsynaptic neurons, and a subsequent suppression of action potentials. DA may increase signal-to-noise ratio of other afferent inputs and, therefore, may increase excitatory or inhibitory throughput of postsynaptic neurons. Because of the complex synaptic relationships within target regions of the striatum, i.e., the striosome/matrix modules, DA may have various effects. First, most DA input is to spines and dendritic shafts of medium spiny type I neurons, which are the major input and output neurons of the striatum. Thus, DA's facilitating effect on these neurons would increase the total throughput in the module receiving DA input. If, however, DA were to project to inhibitory interneurons (e.g., containing somatostatin) that projected to a second neuron (e.g., containing ACh), a net inhibition would result. Thus, until the details of the synaptic relationships within modules are worked out, many ambiguities may result. It should be emphasized, though, that the synaptic relationships within these striatal modules appear to be different for the prefrontal system and more lateral systems (see above). Regardless of DA's effect, many of the VTA neurons (neuron 1) also contain CCK, which is a powerfully excitatory neuron messenger that may be released by the same or different neuronal mechanisms that release DA. Therefore, when neuron 1 is viewed as a CCK-containing neuron that projects to prefrontal cortex and other prefrontal system sites in striatal areas, its effect would also be considered facilitatory. Some of these neurons also contain NT, which increases DA turnover by blocking presynaptic DA receptors or by upregulating tyrosine hydroxylase (Reches *et al.*, 1983). However, any simplistic view of DA, CCK, and NT interactions is unwarranted, for it should be kept in mind that electrophysical, pharmacological, and behavioral effects of such interactions are complex, site dependent (VTA cell bodies versus terminal sites), and highly controversial (Nemeroff *et al.*, 1982; Widerlov and Bresse, 1982; Kalivas *et al.*, 1982; Glimcher *et al.*, 1982; Vaccarino and Koob, 1984; White and Wang, 1984; Skirboll *et al.*, 1981; Schneider *et al.*, 1983; Studler *et al.*, 1982). It would be most helpful if anteromedial caudate–putamen (prefrontal CSP system target) and nucleus accumbens (hippocampal CSP system target) were compared in such interaction studies on "limbic" and "motor" types of behavior (e.g., self-stimulation, stereotypy, hyperlocomotion). Such comparison studies would be critical in differentiating the functions and interactions of DA, CCK, and NT in the different CSP systems. Neuron 1 is also assumed to have few axonal collaterals to different forebrain sites (prefrontal cortex, nucleus accumbens, anteromedial caudate–putamen, septum, amygdala, olfactory tubercle). These neurons also appear to be independently regulated by habenular, raphe, and LC inputs, depending on where these VTA neurons project (see Section 4 for details). They have few autoreceptors and have higher spontaneous firing rates than other SN–VTA neurons. Using double-labeling retrograde tracer injections, we have recently found that some VTA neurons (about 5%) project to both prefrontal cortex and LC in the rat with numerous other VTA neurons projecting to either site (unpublished observations). Thus, activation of some VTA neurons (neuron 1) projecting to prefrontal cortex would also coactivate LC (and possibly dorsal raphe) neurons (Fig. 27, neurons 9 and 10) that also project to prefrontal cortex. Our double-labeling experiments suggest that most, but not all, of the VTA neurons projecting to LC do not also project to cortex; therefore, coactivation may be indirect through VTA interneuronal connections. LC and raphe neurons have additional reciprocal projections with each other and the VTA (not illustrated). Neuron 1 is also well positioned to receive an excitatory aspartatergic input returning from prefrontal cortex (Christie *et al.*, 1985), descending projections from hypothalamus and nucleus accumbens (Nauta *et al.*, 1978), excitatory and inhibiting serotonergic inputs from the raphe, and excitatory substance P, and especially substance K inputs (Quirion *et al.*, 1985; Kanazawa *et al.*, 1984; Kalivas *et al.*, 1985; Kalivas, 1985a; Elliot *et al.*, 1986).

Neuron 2 lies in the most lateral VTA and medial SN pars compacta and contains DA and CCK and many of the assumptions concerning its facilitatory effects will be the same as with neuron 1. Although this type of neuron projects to many of the same areas as neuron 1, its axons collateralize to many prefrontal system regions. Some of these SN neurons form "island" or "patchy" type terminals in striatal regions. This neuron has dendrites extending into pars reticulata in a region where very dense substance K and substance P inputs terminate (Kalivas *et al.*, 1985; Deutch *et al.*, 1985a). The substance K input is powerfully excitatory on both DA and non-DA SN neurons (Innis *et al.*, 1985). Substance P input to this region arising from anterior striatal regions predominantly activates the prefrontal mesocortical system whereas the substance K input, arising from more caudal striatal regions, activates the mesolimbic system (Deutch *et al.*, 1985a; Elliot *et al.*, 1986). The striatal projection to the dendrites of neuron 2 extending into pars reticulata can be considered topographical, whereas the striatal and pallidal projections to the somata and proximal dendrites of neuron 2 in pars compacta are probably nontopographical. Inputs to the somata, proximal dendrites and distal dendrites of these DA neurons may have different and unusual effects on the excitability and neuronal discharge of these cells, since K^+, Na^+-dependent conductances are differentially activated at somal and dendritic sites (Llinas *et al.*, 1984). This nontopographical innervation may be more related to motivationally related behavioral state than are the topographical inputs, which may be more related to motor function *per se*.

Neuron 4, like neurons 1 and 2, contains DA and CCK. It projects to cingulate cortex, some parts of amygdala, lateral olfactory tubercle, and matrix regions of ventral striatum. Like VTA neuron 1, the axons are not highly collateralized. Some direct projections from cortex, hypothalamus, and nucleus accumbens are also present, but to a lesser extent than neuron 1.

Neuron 5 lies in the ventral sheet of SN pars compacta and forms the classical nigrostriatal DA pathway. Some of the neurons also contain CCK, but to a lesser extent than neurons 1, 2, or 4. This neuronal somata, like neuron 4, is positioned to receive direct inhibitory (GABA) and "disenabling" (enkephalin) input from patch neurons of caudate–putamen as well as pallidal inputs. The pallidonigral inputs are predominantly GABAergic whereas the striatonigral inputs are only partially GABAergic (Araki *et al.*, 1985). Some of its distal dendrites (analogous to distal parts of apical dendrites of cortex) extend into pars reticulata where they may receive inhibitory input (GABA) from the striatal matrix neurons, local projections (van den Pol *et al.*, 1985), or nonsynaptic dendrodendritic inputs from the adjacent DA dendrites (Cuello and Iversen, 1978). When compared to neuron 2, this neuron is in a region of less dense substance P and K fibers and terminals; thus, the returning striatonigral terminals are less likely to be excitatory. [We have observed that substance P is concentrated in the medial SN, rostrally, and the ventral and lateral SN, caudally in the rat and the middle of the SN pars reticulata near group II neurons (Fig. 27) contains the least concentration of substance P. However, Inagaki and Parent (1984) observed gradients of tachykinin innervation in the SN in the cat and monkey, but not in the rat.]

Neurons 3 and 6 are GABA SN pars reticulata cells with inhibitory projections to local DA dendrites (not illustrated), thalamus, tectum, and pedunculopontine nuclei. When activated, they probably would inhibit postsynaptic neurons and motor behavior. When inhibited, the effect on postsynaptic neurons and motor behavior would be disinhibition. Because of the relatively high densities of excitatory substance K and P inputs medially (near neuron 3), and inhibitory GABA inputs to these neurons laterally (near neuron 6), different effects on motor behavior would be expected. Descending striatonigral inputs are biased toward topographically selective activation of neuron 3 (thus decreasing motor output) and inhibition of neuron 6 (thus increasing motor output).

Another key difference between the prefrontal system SN–VTA neurons (group I—neurons 1–3) and more lateral system of SN–VTA neurons (group II—neurons 4–6) is that electrical stimulation of the medial group supports very high rates of self-stimulation when compared to other brain structures (Corbett and Wise, 1980; Vaccarino and Franklin, 1982; L. Stein and J. Beluzzi, personal communication).

Based on the connections and neurochemical synaptology of the medial (group I) and lateral (group II) SN–VTA neurons, it is likely that simulation of the prefrontal CSP system, especially in the medial (group I) SN–VTA, would lead to *increased* activity of corticosubcortical loops and *inhibition* of general motor behavior. The effect of stimulation of the lateral and dorsal CSP systems and associated lateral (group II) SN–VTA would lead to the opposite effects, i.e., *inhibition* of the loop circuit and *enhancement* of motor output.

Where can the prefrontal CSP system be initiated and what starts the positive feedback loop? In Fig. 28, the loop and motor outputs of group I neurons have been isolated to illustrate additional features of the loop circuit and corticocortical connections. According to the hypothesis, the loop could be initiated at any level of the CSP system. However, the region where the probability that initiation of the loop would be the greatest is where the greatest convergence and divergence intersect, i.e., the group I neurons and 1 and 2 in the SN–VTA. For other parts of the loop system, a broader (mass action) or more intense stimulation would be necessary. Specific drive states or spontaneous activity could activate many of the CSP systems. Internally driven drives would be mediated by autonomic and hormonal signals activating (or inhibiting) endocrine systems at the CSP or hypothalamic (HYP) levels (Fig. 28). Thus, the hypothalamus would monitor neocortical, allocortical, and endocrine CSP input, circulating hormones and chemical signals in the blood, and internally driven circadian rhythms would further integrate this activity. Projections from the hypothalamus to the SN–VTA and cortex would ultimately mediate the activation or inhibition of the CSP loop circuit depending on the presence of a particular drive or drive-reduction state (e.g., hunger, thirst, electrical stimulation, cocaine addiction).

How do other chemically defined inputs, such as the opioid peptide pathways, affect these systems? Enkephalin and dynorphin projections from the caudate–putamen and pallidum terminate in different SN–VTA zones with enkephalin ending around SN pars compacta and dynorphin ending around SN pars reticulata (Fallon and Leslie, 1986). Although both these systems are thought to be inhibiting or disenabling, some evidence suggests that enkephalin and dynorphin effects are antagonistic and may oppose each other's action in

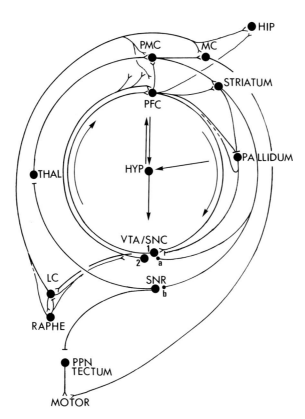

Figure 28. This figure is a redrawing of the CSP loops and outputs introduced in Fig. 26 and developed in detail in Fig. 27. See text for discussion.

SN-mediated motor behavior. The facilitating effect of enkephalin on motor behavior is also substantiated by pharmacological data (Kalivas, 1985b). In the loops described, enkephalin would activate specific motor balance (e.g., for acquiring food or water by a bar press) by inhibiting both SN pars compacta and pars reticulata neurons. The net effect of the opioid peptides may depend on their ability to inhibit GABAergic neurotransmission (Agmo and Avila, 1985; Starr, 1985).

How are specific sets of motor activities, (e.g., bar pressing for a reward) reinforced if the prefrontal CSP system loop is activated and general motor behavior is inhibited by descending CSP activity? In order to approach this question in the present theoretical context, corticocortical and monoamine (especially LC) inputs will not be considered as depicted in an illustration of a dorsal view of the right hemisphere (Fig. 29). For this example, a rat is in a behavioral box where pressing a bar delivers a reward. Many motor acts, such as pressing with a paw or sitting on the bar, will activate the reward stimulus, as long as the bar is pressed. Two premotor or motor cortical regions, labeled 1 and 2, are shown. These are two groupings of cortical columns that have recently (e.g., within 1–5 sec of each other) been active, through either volitional or spontaneous activity. Cortical region 1 was recently active, leading to a bar press with the left paw, which led to a reward. The motor cortical region 2 was also recently active 2 sec prior to the bar press with the left paw, but in this case, activity in region 2 resulted in the animal activating the bar with its nose, which also led to a reward. It is assumed at this point that these two cortical regions will have

an altered excitability for a finite time period by one or more synaptic mechanisms. Several possible mechanisms may explain this altered excitability, including local increase in extracellular K^+ concentration following activation of the
cortical columnar neurons, associative or homosynaptic long-term potentiation
(Johnston and Brown, 1984), reciprocal excitatory synaptic effects, disinhibiting
synaptic mechanisms (Ben-Ari *et al.*, 1981), desensitization of GABA receptors
in recently active cortical columns, or by long-lasting changes in specific ionic
(e.g., calcium influx) currents controlled by phosphorylation of proteins regulating ion channels (Alkon, 1984). In this model, if rewards follow these two
motor acts, the limbic/hypothalamic, and/or corticocortical inputs would signal
activation (or disinhibition) of the prefrontal CSP system loop. Stimulation of
the prefrontal system would lead to transsynaptic activation of LC, raphe, and
prefrontal cortex (Fig. 28). Prefrontal cortical projections to premotor cortex
(Fig. 29) could activate a region that encompasses the recently active sites 1 and
2 in premotor cortex. This posterolaterally directed flow of excitation would
then be supplemented by a concomitant input from LC and raphe fibers. Following state-dependent (e.g., stress, reward) act and/or prefrontal system activation of LC, the "enabling" input from noradrenergic LC fibers (small arrows
in Fig. 29) would increase or "enable" the excitatory synaptic effects of prefrontal
input to regions 1 and 2 in premotor cortex. Thus, the three combined excitatory
effects would increase the probability of those recently rewarded motor acts
occurring again. This model (Fig. 29) predicts that any recently reinforced motor
act (bar pressing with paw, nose, tail, and so on) leading to a reward would have
an increased probability of reactivation. The model also helps explain why there
is the puzzling anterior-to-posterior noradrenergic fiber trajectory in cortex; it
provides for a better timing and synchronizing of enabling input to parallel
posteriorly directed prefrontal-to-premotor projections to "reinforce" specific
motor acts. The combined anterior-to-posterior wave of this dual excitation could
also form the basis of the contingent negative variation wave (CNV), which is a
slow current that can be recorded over the frontal lobe in the interval between

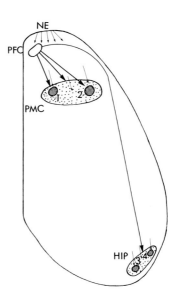

Figure 29. Horizontal view of the right side of the mammalian cerebral cortex illustrating the proposed role of
monoamines in cerebral cortical function. The functions discussed include motor output, reinforcement, learning, and
memory. See text for discussion of this cortical level representation of the CSP model.

successive motor acts. It is also called the "expectancy" wave (see Fuster, 1984). The premotor and motor cortices, once reactivated, would provide corticospinal and descending CSP activity that would lead to motor output. If descending hypothalamic/limbic inputs to the SN–VTA regions involved in the prefrontal CSP loop system signaled that the drive state (e.g., hunger) was reduced sufficiently by the reward (e.g., food pellet), the prefrontal loop system would be inhibited, thus inhibiting subsequent goal-directed (especially orofacial) behavior.

What is the relationship of these pathways to short-term memory acquisition and learning? In this model, some memory and learning systems could be accessed by topographically organized prefrontal connections to hippocampal formation (HIP in Fig. 29). Again, recently active hippocampal zones related to specific sensory/motor activity (3 and 4 in Fig. 29) would be reactivated by combined prefrontal cortical input (arrow from PFC to HIP in Fig. 29) and enabling input from noradrenergic LC fibers (small arrows in Fig. 29). Access to the hippocampal circuitry related to learning and acquisition of short-term memory would depend, in part, either on the repetition of these projections or on the presence of more potent, singly occurring prefrontal inputs.

The roles of 5HT and ACh (nucleus basalis) inputs to cortex in this scheme are less clear. 5HT raphe input, paralleling noradrenergic input to cortex, might also affect these circuits by inhibiting fine tuning or modulation of other inputs to cortex. ACh input from nucleus basalis is unlike that of the other monoamine inputs to cortex. The ACh-containing cell bodies are present in specific pallidal and peripallidal zones (neuron 16 in Fig. 27) and project topographically to defined cortical regions. Such input, presumably excitatory, could be activated or inactivated by specific CSP input (e.g., from striatal inputs to peripallidal regions containing nucleus basalis neurons) related to a specific subregion of cortex (e.g., somatosensory). Thus, nucleus basalis cholinergic neurons could monitor descending CSP activity. Based on this monitoring by peripallidal nucleus basalis neurons, input would be looped back to cortical regions where such input originated. Thus, ACh input to cortical regions (e.g., premotor cortex or hippocampal formation) could provide an additional excitatory input (an ascending pallidocortical component of CSP systems) that would parallel prefrontal input to these cortical regions (Fig. 29). Such input would also effect activation of specific motor acts, as well as memory and learning aspects of the task.

Does the current hypothesis of prefrontal CSP systems fit behavioral/clinical data? Prefrontal (systems)-lesioned animals have an inability to inhibit behavioral reactions when they need to be suppressed; they are hyperactive, and drives, internal impulses, and irrelevant stimuli are disinhibited; they are incapable of changing motor set, especially when a delay is present; they are unable to benefit from errors and have problems with immediate or provisional memory; they are unable to benefit from rule changes and have proactive interference in behavioral testing; they have maladaptive motor responses and a general inability to temporally organize behavior (for review see Fuster, 1980; Milner and Petrides, 1984). These deficits are consistent with the proposed CSP model of prefrontal system function and the functional roles of monoamine inputs to cerebral cortex and striatum.

The purpose of this section was to demonstrate how the prefrontal CSP system is unique when compared to other, more lateral CSP systems. This uniqueness is based on morphological, connectional, neurochemical, and functional features of the system. Although this model is highly simplistic and based on some controversial assumptions, it does help to reorganize cortical and subcortical function in a unified, interactive way that emphasizes the unorthodox, subtle, yet profound ways that monoamines can affect cerebral function.

ACKNOWLEDGMENTS. We wish to thank A. Deutch and F. Leslie for their invaluable comments on the manuscript. We also thank N. Sepion who typed the manuscript. Supported by NIH Grant NS 15321 and a grant from the United Parkinson Foundation.

8. References

Ader, J.-P., Room, P., Postema, F., and Korf, J., 1980, Bilaterally diverging axon collaterals and contralateral projections from rat locus coeruleus neurons, demonstrated by fluorescent retrograde double labeling and norepinephrine metabolism, *J. Neural Transm.* **49:**207–218.

Aghajanian, G. K., and Bloom, F. E., 1966, Electron-microscopic autoradiography of rat hypothalamus after intraventricular H³-norepinephrine, *Science* **153:**308–310.

Aghajanian, G. K., and Bloom, F. E., 1967, The formation of synaptic junctions in developing brain: A quantitative electron microscopic study, *Brain Res.* **6:**716–727.

Agmo, A., and Avila, N. D., 1985, Interactions between enkephalin and dopamine in the control of locomotor activity in the rat: A new hypothesis, *Pharmacol. Biochem. Behav.* **22:**599–603.

Agnati, L. F., Fuxe, K., Benfenati, F., Cortelli, P., and D'Alessandro, R., 1980, The mesolimbic dopamine system: Evidence for a high amine turnover and for a heterogeneity of the dopamine neuron population, *Neurosci. Lett.* **18:**45–51.

Albanese, A., and Bentivoglio, M., 1982, The organization of dopaminergic and nondopaminergic mesencephalo-cortical neurons in the rat, *Brain Res.* **238:**421–425.

Alkon, K. D., 1984, Calcium-mediated reduction of ionic currents: A biophysical memory trace, *Science* **226:**1037–1045.

Altar, C. A., O'Neil, S., Water, R. J., and Marshall, J. F., 1985, Widespread distribution of brain dopamine receptors evidenced with ^{125}I iodosulpride, a highly selective ligand, *Science* **228:**597–600.

Amin, A. H., Crawford, T. B., and Gaddum, J. N., 1954, The distribution of substance P and 5-hydroxytryptamine in the central nervous system of the dog, *J. Physiol. (London)* **126:**596–618.

Anden, N. E., Dahlstrom, A., Fuxe, K., and Larsson, K., 1965, Mapping out of catecholamine and 5-hydroxytryptamine neurons innervating the telencephalon and diencephalon, *Life Sci.* **4:**1275–1279.

Anden, N. E., Dahlstrom, A., Fuxe, K., Larsson, K., Olson, L., and Ungerstedt, U., 1966, Ascending monoamine neurons to the telencephalon and diencephalon, *Acta Physiol. Scand.* **67:**313–326.

Araki, M., McGeer, P. L., and McGeer, E. G., 1985, Striatonigral and pallidonigral pathways studied by a combination of retrograde horseradish peroxidase tracing and a pharmacohistochemical method for gamma-amino butyric acid transaminase, *Brain Res.* **331:**17–24.

Armstrong-James, M., and Fox, K., 1983, Effects of iontophoresed noradrenaline on the spontaneous activity of neurons in rat primary somatosensory cortex, *J. Physiol. (London)* **355:**427–447.

Arnsten, A., and Goldman-Rakic, P., 1985, Alpha-2 adrenergic mechanisms in prefrontal cortex associated with cognitive decline in aged non-human primates, *Science* **230:**1273–1277.

Aston-Jones, G., and Bloom, F., 1981a, Activity of norepinephrine-containing locus coeruleus rats anticipates fluctuations in the sleep walking cycle, *J. Neurosci.* **1:**876–886.

Aston-Jones, G., and Bloom, F., 1981b, Norepinephrine containing locus coeruleus neurons in behaving rats exhibit pronounced responses to non-noxious environmental stimuli, *J. Neurosci.* **1:**887–900.

Azmitia, E. C., 1978, The serotonin-producing neurons of the midbrain median and dorsal raphe nuclei, in: *Handbook of Psychopharmacology* (L. L. Ivesen, S. D. Iversen, and S. H. Snyder, eds.), Plenum Press, New York, pp. 232–314.

Azmitia, E. C., 1981, Bilateral serotonergic projections to the dorsal hippocampus of the rat; simultaneous localization of retrogradely transported ³H-5HT and HRP, *J. Comp. Neurol.* **203:**737–750.

Azmitia, E. C., 1982, Recent advances in serotonin methods, *J. Histochem. Cytochem.* **30:**739–743.

Azmitia, E. C., and Segal, M., 1978, An autoradiographic analysis of the differential ascending projections of the dorsal and median raphe nuclei in the rat, *J. Comp. Neurol.* **179:**641–668.

Bannon, M. J., Michaud, R. L., and Roth, R. H., 1981, Mesocortical dopamine neurons: Lack of autoreceptors modulating dopamine synthesis, *Mol. Pharmacol.* **1981**(2):270–275.

Bannon, M. J., Reinhard, J. F., Bunney, B., and Roth, R. H., 1982, Unique response to antipsychotic drugs is due to absence of terminal autoreceptors in mesocortical dopamine neurons, *Nature* **296:**444–445.

Bannon, M. J., Wolf, M. E., and Roth, R. H., 1983, Pharmacology of dopamine neurons innervating the prefrontal cingulate and piriform cortices, *Eur. J. Pharmacol.* **92:**119–125.

Beaudet, A., and Descarries, L., 1978, The monoamine innervation of rat cerebral cortex: Synaptic and nonsynaptic axon terminals, *Neuroscience* **3:**851–860.

Beaudet, A., and Descarries, L., 1984, Fine structure of monoamine axon terminals in cerebral cortex, in: *Monoamine Innervation of Cerebral Cortex* (L. Descarries, T. Reader, and H. Jasper, eds.), Liss, New York, pp. 77–93.

Beckstead, R. M., 1976, Convergent thalamic and mesencephalic projections to the anterior medial cortex in the rat, *J. Comp. Neurol.* **166:**403–416.

Beckstead, R. M., 1978, Afferent connections of the entorhinal area in the rat as demonstrated by retrograde cell-labeling with horseradish peroxidase, *Brain Res.* **152:**249–264.

Beckstead, R. M., Domesick, V. B., and Nauta, W. J. H., 1979, Efferent connections of the substantia nigra and ventral tegmental area in the rat, *Brain Res.* **175:**191–217.

Ben-Ari, Y., Krnjević, K., Reiffenstein, R. J., and Reinhardt, W., 1981, Inhibitory conductance changes and action of gamma-amino-butyrate in rat hippocampus, *Neuroscience* **6:**2442–2463.

Berger, B., and Verney, C., 1984, Development of the catecholamine innervation in rat neocortex: Morphological features, in: *Monoamine Innervation of Cerebral Cortex* (L. Descarries, T. Reader, and H. Jasper, eds.), Liss, New York, pp. 95–121.

Berger, B., Tassin, J. P., Blanc, G., Moyne, M. A., and Thierry, A. M., 1974, Histochemical confirmation for dopaminergic innervation of the rat cerebral cortex after destruction of the noradrenergic ascending pathways, *Brain Res.* **81:**332–337.

Berger, B., Thierry, A. M., Tassin, J. P., and Moyne, M. A., 1976, Dopaminergic innervation of the rat prefrontal cortex: A fluorescence histochemical study, *Brain Res.* **106:**133–145.

Berger, B., Verney, C., Alvarez, C., Veginy, A., and Helle, K. B., 1985, New dopaminergic terminal fields in the motor, visual (area 18b) and retrospenial cortex in the young and adult rat: Immunocytochemical and catecholamine histochemical analyses, *Neuroscience* **15:**983–998.

Bernardi, G., Cherubini, E., Marciani, M. G., Mercuri, N., and Stanzione, P., 1982, Responses of intracellularly recorded cortical neurons to the iontophoretic application of dopamine, *Brain Res.* **245:**267–274.

Bevan, P., Bradshaw, C. M., and Szabadi, E., 1975, Proceedings: Comparison of the effects of DOPA and noradrenaline on single cortical neurones, *Br. J. Pharmacol.* **55:**301P–302P.

Björklund, A., Nobin, A., and Stenevi, U., 1973, The use of neurotoxic dihydroxytryptamines as tools for morphological studies and localized lesioning of central indolamine neurons, *Z. Zellforsch.* **145:**479–501.

Björklund, A., Baumgarten, H. G., Lachenmayer, L., and Rosengren, E., 1975, Recovery of brain noradrenaline after 5,7-dihydroxytryptamine-induced axonal lesions in the rat, *Cell Tissue Res.* **161:**145–155.

Björklund, A., Divac, I., and Lindvall, O., 1978, Regional distribution of catecholamines in monkey cerebral cortex, evidence for a dopaminergic innervation of the primate prefrontal cortex, *Neurosci. Lett.* **7:**115–119.

Bobillier, P., Seguin, S., Petitjean, F., Salvert, D., Touret, M., and Jouvet, M., 1976, The raphe nuclei of the cat brain stem: A topographical atlas of their efferent projections as revealed by autoradiography, *Brain Res.* **113:**449–486.

Bobillier, P., Seguin, S., DeGueurce, A., Lewis, B. D., and Pujol, J. F., 1979, The efferent connections of the nucleus raphe centralis superior in the rat as revealed by radioautography, *Brain Res.* **166:**1–8.

Bogdanski, D. F., Weissbach, H., and Underfriend, S., 1957, The distribution of serotonin, 5-hydroxytryptophan decarboxylase and monoamine oxidase in brain, *J. Neurochem.* **1:**272–278.

Boyajian, C., Loughlin, S., and Leslie, F., 1985, Differential binding properties of two alpha-2 adrenoceptor agonists in rat brain, *Soc. Neurosci. Abstr.* **11:**104.3.

Bradshaw, C. M., Sheridan, R. D., and Szabadi, E., 1985, Excitatory neuronal responses to dopamine in the cerebral cortex: Involvement of D2 but not D1 dopamine receptors, *Br. J. Pharmacol.* **86:**483–490.

Brodal, D., Taber, E., and Walberg, F., 1960, The raphe nuclei of the brainstem in the cat. II. Efferent connections, *J. Comp. Neurol.* **114:**239–260.

Brown, R., and Goldman, P. S., 1977, Catecholamines in neocortex of rhesus monkeys: Regional distribution and ontogenetic development, *Brain Res.* **124:**576–580.

Brown, R. M., Crane, A. M., and Goldman, P. S., 1979, Regional distribution of monoamines in the cerebral cortex and subcortical structures of the rhesus monkey: Concentrations and *in vivo* synthesis rates, *Brain Res.* **168:**133–150.

Brownstein, M., Saavedra, J M., and Palkovits, M., 1974, Norepinephrine and dopamine in the limbic system of the rat, *Brain Res.* **79:**431–436.

Brozoski, T. J., Brown, R. M., Rosvold, H. E., and Goldman, P. S., 1979, Cognitive deficit caused by regional depletion of dopamine in prefrontal cortex of rhesus monkey, *Science* **205:**929–932.

Bunney, B. S., and Aghajanian, G. K., 1976, Dopamine and norepinephrine innervated cells in rat prefrontal cortex: Pharmacological differentiation using microiontophoretic techniques, *Life Sci.* **19:**1783–1792.

Bunney, B. S., and Chiodo, L. A., 1984, Mesocortical dopamine systems: Further electrophysiological and pharmacological characteristics, in: *Monoamine Innervation of Cerebral Cortex* (L. Descarries, T. Reader, and H. Jasper, eds.), Liss, New York, pp. 263–277.

Butcher, L. L. (ed.), 1978, *Cholinergic Monoaminergic Interactions in the Brain*, Academic Press, New York.

Caffee, A. R., and van Leeuwen, F. W., 1983, Vasopressin-immunoreactive cells in dorsomedial hypothalamic region, medial amygdaloid nucleus and locus coeruleus of the rat, *Cell Tissue Res.* **233:**23–33.

Caron, M., Leeb-Lundberg, L., Strader, C., Dickinson, K., Pickel, V., Joh, T., and Lefkowitz, R., 1984, Biochemical characterization of adrenergic receptors: Photo affinity labelling and immunocytochemical localization in brain, in: *Monoamine Innervation of Cerebral Cortex* (L. Descarries, T. Reader, and H. Jasper, eds.), Liss, New York, pp. 135–151.

Carpenter, M. B., 1976, Anatomical organization of the corpus striatum and related nuclei, *Res. Publ. Assoc. Res. Nerv. Ment. Dis.* **55:**1–35.

Carter, C. J., and Pycock, C. J., 1978, Lesions of the frontal cortex of the rat: Changes in neurotransmitter systems in subcortical regions, *Br. J. Pharmacol.* **64:**430P.

Carter, D. A., and Fibiger, H. C., 1977, Ascending projections of presumed dopamine-containing neurons in the ventral tegmentum of the rat as demonstrated by horseradish peroxidase, *Neuroscience* **2:**569–576.

Caviness, V., and Korde, M., 1981, Monoaminergic afferents to the neocortex: A developmental histofluorescence study in normal and reeler mouse embryos, *Brain Res.* **209:**1–9.

Charney, Y., Leger, L., Berod, A., Jouvet, M., Pujol, J., and Dubois, P., 1982, Evidence for the presence of enkephalin in catecholaminergic neurons of cat locus coeruleus, *Neurosci. Lett.* **30:**147–151.

Chesselet, M.-F., and Graybiel, A. M., 1987, Striatal neurons expressing somatostatin-like immunoreactivity: Evidence for a peptidergic interneuronal system in the cat, *Neuroscience* in press.

Chiodo, L. A., Bannon, M. J., Grace, A. A., Roth, R. H., and Bunney, B. S., 1984, Evidence for the absence of impulse-regulating somatodendritic and synthesis-modulating nerve terminal autoreceptors and subpopulations of mesocortical dopamine neurons, *Neuroscience* **12:**1–16.

Christie, M, J., Bridge, S., James, L. B., and Beart, P. M., 1985, Excitation lesions suggest an aspartatergic projection from rat medial prefrontal cortex to ventral tegmental area, *Brain Res.* **333:**169–172.

Collier, T. J., and Routtenberg, A., 1977, Entorhinal cortex: Catecholamine fluorescence and Nissl staining of identical Vibratome sections, *Brain Res.* **128:**354–360.

Collinge, J., Pycock, C. J., and Taberna, P. V., 1983, Studies on the interaction between cerebral 5-hydroxytryptamine and gamma-aminobutyric acid in the mode of actions of diazepam in the rat, *Br. J. Pharmacol.* **79:**637–643.

Conrad, L. C., Leonard, C. M., and Pfaff, D. W., 1974, Connections of the median and dorsal raphe nuclei in the rat: An autoradiographic and degeneration study, *J. Comp. Neurol.* **156:**179–206.

Cooper, J. R., Bloom, F. E., and Roth, R. H. (eds.), 1982, *The Biochemical Basis of Neuropharmacology*, Oxford University Press, London, pp. 223–248.

Corbett, D., and Wise, R. A., 1980, Intracranial self-stimulation in relation to the ascending dopaminergic systems of the midbrain: A moveable electrode mapping study, *Brain Res.* **185**:1–15.

Coyle, J. T., and Molliver, M. E., 1977, Major innervation of newborn rat cortex by monoaminergic neurons, *Science* **196**:444–447.

Cragg, B. G., 1961, Olfactory and other afferent connections of the hippocampus in the rabbit, rat, and cat, *Exp. Neurol.* **3**:588–600.

Creese, I., and Snyder, S. H., 1978, ^{3}H-spiroperidol labels serotonin receptors in rat cerebral cortex and hippocampus, *Eur. J. Pharmacol.* **49**:201–202.

Cross, A. J., and Deakin, J. F., 1985, Cortical serotonin receptor subtypes after lesion of ascending cholinergic neurones in rat, *Neurosci. Lett.* **60**:261–265.

Cuello, A. C., and Iverson, L. L., 1978, Interactions of dopamine with other neurotransmitters in the rat substantia nigra: A possible functional role of dendritic dopamine, in: *Interactions between Putative Neurotransmitters in the Brain* (S. Garattini, ed.), Raven Press, New York, pp. 127–149.

Dahlstrom A., and Fuxe, K., 1964, Evidence for the existence of monoamine-containing neurons in the central nervous system. I. Demonstration of monoamines in the cell bodies of brain stem neurones, *Acta Physiol. Scand. Suppl.* **232**:1–55.

DeLong, M. R., Georgopoulos, A. P., and Crutcher, M. D., 1983, Cortical-basal ganglia loops and coding of motor performance, *Exp. Brain Res. Suppl.* **7**:30–40.

Deniau, J. M., Thierry, A. M., and Feger, J., 1980, Electrophysiological identification of mesencephalic ventromedial tegmental (VMT) neurons projecting to the frontal cortex, septum, and nucleus accumbens, *Brain Res.* **189**:315–326.

Denny-Brown, D., and Yanagisawa, N., 1976, The role of the basal ganglia in the initiation of movement, *Res. Publ. Assoc. Res. Nerv. Ment. Dis.* **55**:115–148.

Descarries, L., and Droz, B., 1968, Incorporation de noradrenaline-^{3}H (NA-^{3}H) dans le systeme nerveux central du rat adulte: Etude radioautographique en microscopie electronique, *C.R. Acad. Sci.* **266**:2480–2482.

Descarries, L., and Lapierre, Y., 1973, Noradrenergic axon terminals in the cerebral cortex of the rat. I. Radioautographic visualization after topical application of DI-^{3}H norepinephrine, *Brain Res.* **51**:141–160.

Descarries, L., Beaudet, A., and De Champlain, J., 1975, Selective deafferentation of rat neocortex by destruction of catecholamine neurons with intraventricular 6-hydroxydopamine, in: *Chemical Tools in Catecholamine Research I* (G. Jonsson, ed.), North-Holland, Amsterdam, pp. 101–106.

Descarries, L., Beaudet, A., Watkins, K. C., and Garcia, S., 1979, The serotonin neurons in nucleus raphe dorsalis of adult rat, *Anat. Rec.* **193**:520.

Deutch, A. Y., Maggio, J. E., Bannon, M. J., Kalivas, P. W., Tam, S.-Y., Goldstein, M., and Roth, R. H., 1985a, Substance K and substance P differentially modulate mesolimbic and mesocortical systems, *Peptides* **6**:113–122.

Deutch, A. Y., Tam, S.-Y., and Roth, R. H., 1985b, Footshock and conditioned stress increase 3,4-dihydroxyphenyl acetic acid (DOPAC) in the ventral tegmental area but not substantia nigra, *Brain Res.* **333**:143–146.

Deutch, A. Y., Goldstein, M., and Roth, R. H., 1986, Activation of the locus coeruleus induced by secretive stimulation of ventral tegmental area, *Brain Res.* **363**:307–314.

DiChiara, G., and Gessa, G. L. (eds.), 1981, *GABA and the Basal Ganglia, Adv. Biochem. Psychopharmacol.* **30**.

DiFiglia, M., Pasik, P., and Pasik, T., 1976, A Golgi study of neuronal types in the neostriatum of monkeys, *Brain Res.* **114**:245–256.

Divac, I., 1979, Patterns of subcortical–cortical projections as revealed by somatopetal HRP tracings, *Neuroscience* **4**:455–461.

Divac, I., and Diemer, N. H., 1980, Prefrontal systems in the rat visualized by means of labeled deoxyglucose: Further evidence for functional heterogeneity of the neostriatum, *J. Comp. Neurol.* **190**:1–13.

Divac, I., and Oberg, R. G. E., 1979, Current concepts of neostriatal functions, in: *The Neostriatum* (I. Divac and R. G. E. Oberg, eds.), Pergamon Press, Elmsford, N.Y., pp. 215–230.

Divac, I., Lindvall, O., Björklund, A., and Passingham, R. E., 1975, Converging projections from the mediodorsal thalamic nucleus and mesencephalic dopaminergic neurons to the neocortex in three species, *Exp. Brain Res.* **23**:58 (abstr.).

Divac, I., Björklund, A., Lindvall, O., and Passingham, R. E., 1978, Converging projections from the mediodorsal thalamic nucleus and mesencephalic dopaminergic neurons to the neocortex in three species, *J. Comp. Neurol.* **180**:59–71.

Domesick, V. B., 1981, The anatomical basis for feedback and feedforward in the striatonigral system, in: *Apomorphine and other Diaminomimetics, Basic Pharmacology* (G. L. Class and G. U. Corsini, eds.), Raven Press, New York, pp. 302–322.

Donoghue, J. P., and Herkenham, M., 1983, Multiple patterns of corticostriatal projections and their relationship to opiate receptor patches in rats, *Neurosci. Abstr.* **9:**15.

Donoghue, J. P., and Herkenham, M., 1986, Neostriatal projections from individual cortical fields conform to histochemically distinct striatal compartments in the rat, *Brain Res.* **365:**397–403.

Dray, A., 1980, The physiology and pharmacology of the mammalian basal ganglia, *Prog. Neurobiol.* **14:**221–335.

Dumbrille-Ross, A., and Tang, S. W., 1983, Manipulations of synaptic serotonin: Discrepancy of effects on serotonin S1 and S2 sites, *Life Sci.* **32:**2677–2684.

Elliot, P. J., Alpert, J. E., Bannon, M. J., and Iversen, S. D., 1986, Selective activation of mesolimbic and mesocortical dopamine metabolism in rat brain by infusion of a stable substance P analogue into the ventral tegmental area, *Brain Res.* **363:**145–147.

Emson, P. C., and Koob, G. F., 1978, The origin and distribution of dopamine-containing afferents to the rat frontal cortex, *Brain Res.* **142:**249–267.

Evarts, E. V., and Wise, S. P., 1984, Basal ganglia outputs and motor control, *Ciba Found. Symp.* **107:**83–96.

Evarts, E. V., Kimura, M., Wurtz, R. H., and Hikosaka, O., 1984, Behavioral correlates of activity in basal ganglia neurons, *Trends Neurosci.* **447:**453.

Falck, B., Hillarp, N. A., Thieme, G., and Torp, A., 1962, Fluorescence of catecholamines and related compounds condensed with formaldehyde, *J. Histochem. Cytochem.* **10:**348–354.

Fallon, J. H., 1981a, Collateralization of monoamine neurons: Mesotelencephalic dopamine projections to caudate, septum and frontal cortex, *J. Neurosci.* **4:**1361–1368.

Fallon, J. H., 1981b, Comment on Chairman's Report, in: *The Amygdala Revisited.* Plenum Press, New York, pp. 11–12.

Fallon, J. H., 1983, The islands of Calleja complex or rat basal forebrain. II. Connection of medium and large cells, *Brain Res. Bull.* **10:**775–793.

Fallon, J. H., and Leslie, F. M., 1986, Distribution of dynorphin and enkephalin peptides in the rat brain, *J. Comp. Neurol.* **249:**293–336.

Fallon, J. H., and Loughlin, S. E., 1982, Monoamine innervation of the forebrain: Collateralization, *Brain Res. Bull.* **9:**295–307.

Fallon, J. H., and Loughlin, S. E., 1985, The substantia nigra, in: *The Rat Central Nervous System: A Handbook for Neuroscientists* (G. Paxinos and J. Watson, eds.), Academic Press, New York, pp. 353–374.

Fallon, J. H., and Moore, R. Y., 1976, Topography of dopamine cell projection to the telencephalon, *Anat. Rec.* **185:**485.

Fallon, J. H., and Moore, R. Y., 1978a, Catecholamine innervation of the basal forebrain. IV. Topography of dopamine cell projections to the basal forebrain and neostriatum, *J. Comp. Neurol.* **180:**545–580.

Fallon, J. H., and Moore, R. Y., 1978b, Catecholamine innervation of the basal ganglia. III. Olfactory bulb, olfactory tubercle and piriform cortex, *J. Comp. Neurol.* **180:**495–508.

Fallon, J. H., and Moore, R. Y., 1979a, Superior colliculus efferents to the hypothalamus, *Neurosci. Lett.* **14:**265–270.

Fallon, J. H., and Moore, R. Y., 1979b, Raphe nuclei in the rat: Efferent projections to forebrain studied using the HRP-retrograde transport method, *Soc. Neurosci. Abstr.* **4:**272.

Fallon, J. H., Koziell, D. A., and Moore, R. Y., 1978a, Catecholamine innervation of the basal forebrain. II. Amygdala, suprarhinal cortex and entorhinal cortex, *J. Comp. Neurol.* **180:**509–532.

Fallon, J. H., Riley, J., and Moore, R. Y., 1978b, Substantia nigra dopamine neurons: Separate populations project to neostriatum and allocrotex, *Neurosci. Lett.* **7:**157–162.

Fallon, J. H., Loughlin, S. E., and Ribak, C. E., 1983, The islands of Calleja complex of rat basal forebrain. III. Histochemical evidence for a striato-pallidal system, *J. Comp. Neurol.* **16:**91–120.

Fallon, J. H., Schmued, L., Wang, C., Miller, R., and Banales, G., 1984, Neurons in the ventral tegmentum have separate populations projecting to telencephalon and inferior olive, are histochemically different and may receive direct visual input, *Brain Res.* **321:**332–336.

Farnebo, L. O., and Hamberger, B., 1971, Drug-induced changes in the release of ^{3}H-monoamines from field stimulated rat brain slices, *Acta Physiol. Scand. Suppl.* **371:**35–44.

Ferron, A., Descarries, L., and Reader, T. A., 1982, Altered neuronal responsiveness to biogenic amines in rat cerebral cortex after serotonin denervation or depletion, *Brain Res.* **231**:93–108.

Fink, J. S., and Smith, G. P., 1980, Mesolimbic and mesocortical dopaminergic neurons are necessary for normal exploratory behavior in rats, *Neurosci. Lett.* **17**:61–65.

Foote, S. L., 1985, Anatomy and physiology of brain monoamine systems, *Psychiatry* **3**:1–14.

Foote, S., and Morrison, J., 1985, Postnatal development of laminar innervation patterns by monoaminergic fibers in monkey primary visual cortex, *J. Neurosci.* **4**:2667–2680.

Foote, S., Freedman, R., and Oliver, R., 1975, Effects of putative neurotransmitters on neuronal activity in monkey auditory cortex, *Brain Res.* **86**:229–242.

Foote, S., Aston-Jones, G., and Bloom, F., 1980, Impulse activity of locus coeruleus neurons in awake rats and monkeys is a function of sensory stimulation and arousal, *Proc. Natl. Acad. Sci. USA* **77**:3033–3037.

Foote, S., Bloom, F., and Aston-Jones, G., 1983, Nucleus locus coeruleus: New evidence of anatomical and physiological specificity, *Physiol. Rev.* **63**:844–914.

Freedman, R., Foote, S. L., and Bloom, F. E., 1975, Histochemical characterization of a neocortical projection of the nucleus locus coeruleus in the squirrel monkey, *J. Comp. Neurol.* **164**:209–231.

Fuster, J. M., 1980, *The Prefrontal Cortex*, Raven Press, New York.

Fuster, J. M., 1984, Behavioral electrophysiology of the prefrontal cortex, *Trends Neurosci.* **7**:408–414.

Fuxe, K., 1965, Evidence for the existence of monoamine neurons in the central nervous system. IV. Distribution of monoamine nerve terminals in the central nervous system, *Acta Physiol. Scand. Suppl.* **247**:39–85.

Fuxe, K., Hamberger, B., and Hökfelt, T., 1968, Distribution of noradrenaline nerve terminals in cortical areas of the rat, *Brain Res.* **8**:125–131.

Fuxe, K., Hökfelt, T., Johansson O., Jonsson, G., Lidbrink, P., and Ljungdahl, A., 1974, The origin of the dopamine nerve terminals in limbic and frontal cortex: Evidence for mesocortico dopamine neurons, *Brain Res.* **82**:349–355.

Gage, F. W., and Thompson, R. G., 1980, Differential distribution of norepinephrine and serotonin along the dorsal–ventral areas of the hippocampal formation, *Brain Res. Bull.* **5**:771–773.

Gage, F., Björklund, A., and Stenevi, U., 1983, Local regulation of compensatory noradrenergic hyperactivity in the partially denervated hippocampus, *Nature* **303**:819–821.

Galloway, M. P., Wolf, M. E., and Roth, R. H., 1986, Regulation of dopamine synthesis in the medial prefrontal cortex is mediated by release modulating autoreceptors: Studies *in vivo*, *J. Pharmacol. Exp. Ther.* **236**:689–698.

Garattini, S., Pujal, J. F., and Samanin, R. (eds.), 1978, *Interaction between Putative Neurotransmitters in the Brain*, Raven Press, New York.

Gatter, K., and Powell, T., 1977, The projection of the locus coeruleus upon the neocortex in the macaque monkey, *Neuroscience* **2**:441–445.

Gerfen, C. R., 1984, The neostriatal mosaic: Compartmentalization of corticostriatal input and striatonigral output systems, *Nature* **311**:461–464.

Gerfen, C. R., 1985, The neostriatal mosaic. I. Compartmental organization of projections from the striatum to the substantia nigra in the rat, *J. Comp. Neurol.* **236**:454–476.

Gerfen, C. R., 1987, The neostriatal mosaic: The reiterated processing unit, in: *Neurotransmitter Interactions in the Basal Ganglia* (C. Feurstein, B. Scatton, and M. Sandler, eds.), Raven Press, New York, in press.

Gerfen, C. R., and Clavier, R. M., 1979, Neural inputs to the prefrontal agranular insular cortex in the rat: Horseradish peroxidase study, *Brain Res. Bull.* **4**:347–353.

Gerfen, C. R., Baimbridge, K. G., and Miller, J. J., 1985, The neostriatal mosaic: Compartmental distribution of calcium binding protein and paralbumin in the basal ganglia of the rat and monkey, *Proc. Natl. Acad. Sci. USA* **82**:8780–8784.

German, D., and Bowden, D. M., 1974, Catecholamine systems as the neural substrate for intracranial self stimulation: A hypothesis, *Brain Res.* **73**:381–419.

Gessa, G. L., Biggio, G., Vergiu, L., Napoleone, F., and Tagliamonte, A., 1974, Norepinephrine and dopamine concentrations in the cerebral cortex of man, monkeys and other mammals, *Experientia* **30**:1295–1296.

Geyer, M. A., Puerto, A., Dawsey, W. J., Knapp, S., Bullard, W. P., and Mandell, A. J., 1976, Histological and enzymatic studies of the mesolimbic and mesostriatal serotonergic pathways, *Brain Res.* **106**:241–256.

Giolli, R. A., Blanks, R. H. I., and Torigoe, Y., 1984, Pretectal and brain stem projections of the medial terminal nucleus of the accessory optic system of the rabbit and rat as studied by anterograde and retrograde neuronal trading methods, *J. Comp. Neurol.* **227**:228–251.

Giolli, R. A., Schmued, L. C., and Fallon, J. H., 1985, A retino-mesotelencephalic pathway in the albino rat, *Neurosci. Lett.* **53**:1–7.

Glimcher, P., Margalin, D., and Haebel, D. G., 1982, Rewarding effects of neurotensin in the brain, *Proc. N.Y. Acad. Sci.* **77**:422–424.

Glowinski, J., Tassin, J. P., and Thierry, A. M., 1984, The mesocortico-prefrontal dopaminergic neurons, *Trends Neurosci.* **7**:415–418.

Goedert, M., Mantyh, P. W., Hunt, S. P., and Emson, P. C., 1983, Mosaic distribution of neurotensin-like immunoreactivity in cat striatum, *Nature* **307**:543–546.

Goldman, P. S., and Nauta, W. J. H., 1977, An intricately patterned prefronto-caudate projection in the rhesus monkey, *J. Comp. Neurol.* **171**:369–385.

Goldman-Rakic, P. S., 1982, Cytoarchitectonic heterogeneity of the primates neostriatum: Subdivision into island and matrix cellular compartments, *J. Comp. Neurol.* **205**:398–413.

Goldman-Rakic, P. S., 1984, Modular organization of prefrontal cortex, *Trends Neurosci.* **7**:419–424.

Goldman-Rakic, P. S., and Brown, R. M., 1982, Postnatal development of monoamine content and synthesis in the cerebral cortex of rhesus monkeys, *Dev. Brain Res.* **4**:339–349.

Grabowsky, K., McCabe, R. T., and Wamsley, J. K., 1983, Localization of ^{3}H imipramine binding sites in rat brain, *Life Sci.* **32**:2355–2361.

Grace, A. A., and Bunney, B. S., 1983, Intracellular and extracellular electrophysiology of nigral dopaminergic neurons. I. Identification and characterization, *Neuroscience* **10**:301–315.

Graybiel, A. M., and Chesselet, M.-F., 1984a, Distribution of cell bodies expressing substance P, enkephalin and dynorphin B in kitten and cat striatum, *Anat. Rec.* **208**:64A

Graybiel, A. M., and Chesselet, M.-F., 1984b, Compartmental distribution of striatal cell bodies expressing met-enkephalin-like immunoreactivity, *Proc. Natl. Acad. Sci. USA* **81**:7980–7984.

Graybiel, A. M., and Ragsdale, C. W., 1978, Histochemically distinct compartments in the striatum of human, monkey, and cat demonstrated by acetylcholinesterase staining, *Proc. Natl. Acad. Sci. USA* **75**:5723–5727.

Graybiel, A. M., and Ragsdale, C. W., 1983, Biochemical anatomy of the striatum, in: *Chemical Neuroanatomy* (P. C. Emson, ed.), Raven Press, New York, pp. 427–504.

Graybiel, A. M., Ragsdale, C. W., Yoneoka, E. S., and Elde, R. P., 1981, An immunohistochemical study of enkephalins and other neuropeptides in the striatum of the cat with evidence that the opiate peptides are arranged to form mosaic patterns in register with the striosomal compartments visible by acetylcholinesterase staining, *Neuroscience* **6**:377–387.

Grofova, I., 1975, The identification of striatal and pallidal neurons projecting to substantia nigra: An experimental study by means of retrograde axonal transport of horseradish peroxidase, *Brain Res.* **31**:286–291.

Groves, P. M., 1983, A theory of the functional organization of the neostriatum and the neostriatal control of voluntary movement, *Brain Res. Rev.* **5**:109–139.

Gruol, D. L., Barker, J. L., Huang, L. Y. M., MacDonald, J. F., and Smith, T. G., 1980, Hydrogen ions have multiple effects on the excitability of cultured mammalian neurons, *Brain Res.* **183**:247–252.

Gustafson, E. L., and Moore, R. Y., 1985, Differential projections of neuropeptide Y containing neurons in the locus coeruleus of the rat, *Soc. Neurosci. Abstr.* **11**:27.10.

Guyenet, P. C., and Aghajanian, G. K., 1978, Antidromic identification of dopaminergic and other output neurons of the rat substantia nigra, *Brain Res.* **150**:69–84.

Haber, S. N., Groeneinegar, H. J., Grove, E. A., and Nauta, W. J. H., 1985, Efferent connections of the ventral pallidum: Evidence of a dual striato pallidofugal pathway, *J. Comp. Neurol.* **235**:322–335.

Halaris, A. E., Jones, B. E., and Moore, R. Y., 1976, Axonal transport in serotonin neurons of the midbrain raphe, *Brain Res.* **107**:555–574.

Hall, R. D., and Lindholm, E. P., 1974, Organization of motor and somatosensory neocortex in the albino rat, *Brain Res.* **66**:23–38.

Haring, J., and Davis, J., 1985, Differential distribution of locus coeruleus projections to the hippocampal formation: Anatomical and biochemical evidence, *Brain Res.* **325**:366–369.

Hassler, R., 1979, Electron microscopic differentiation of the extrinsic and intrinsic types of nerve cells and synapses in the striatum and their putative transmitters, *Adv. Neurol.* **24**:93–108.

Heimer, L., 1978, The olfactory cortex and the ventral striatum, in: *The Continuing Evolution of the Limbic System Concept* (K. E. Livingston and O. Hornykiewicz, eds.), Plenum Press, New York, pp. 95–187.

Heimer, L., and Wilson, R. D., 1975, The subcortical projections of the allo-cortex: Similarities in the neural associations of the hippocampus, the piriform cortex and the neocortex, *Golgi Centennial Symposium, Perspectives in Neurobiology* (M. Santini, ed.), Raven Press, New York, pp. 177–193.

Heimer, L., Switzer, R. D., and Van Hoesen, G. W., 1982, Ventral striatum and ventral pallidum: Components of the motor system?, *Trends Neurosci.* **5**:83–87.

Heller, A., Harvey, J. A., and Moore, R. Y., 1962, A demonstration of a fall in brain serotonin following central nervous system lesions in the rat, *Biochem. Pharmacol. Exp. Ther.* **150**:1–9.

Herkenham, M., and Pert, C. B., 1981, Mosaic distribution of opiate receptors, parafascicular projections and acetylcholinesterase in the rat striatum, *Nature* **291**:415–418.

Herve, D., Simon, H., Blanc, G., Lisoprawski, A., LeMoal, M., Glowinski, J., and Tassin, J. P., 1979, Increased utilization of dopamine in the nucleus accumbens but not in the cerebral cortex after dorsal raphe lesion in the rat, *Neurosci. Lett.* **15**:127–133.

Herve, D., Simon, H., Blanc, G., LeMoal, M., Glowinski, J., and Tassin, J. P., 1981, Opposite changes in dopamine utilization in the nucleus accumbens and the frontal cortex after electrolytic lesion of the median raphe in the rat, *Brain Res.* **216**:422–428.

Hicks, T. P., and McLennan, H., 1978, Comparison of the actions of octopamine and catecholamines on single neurons of the rat cerebral cortex, *Br. J. Pharmacol.* **64**:485–491.

Hikosaka, H., and Wurtz, R. H., 1983a, Visual and oculomotor functions of monkey substantia nigra pars reticulata. I. Relation of visual and auditory responses to saccades, *J. Neurophysiol.* **49**:1230–1253.

Hikosaka, H., and Wurtz, R. H., 1983b, Visual and oculomotor functions of monkey substantia nigra pars reticulata. II. Visual responses related to fixation of gaze, *J. Neurophysiol.* **49**:1254–1267.

Hikosaka, H., and Wurtz, R. H., 1983c, Visual and oculomotor functions of monkey substantia nigra pars reticulata. III. Memory-contingent visual and saccade responses, *J. Neurophysiol.* **49**:1268–1284.

Hikosaka, H., and Wurtz, R. H., 1983d, Visual and oculomotor functions of monkey substantia nigra pars reticulata. IV. Relation of substantia nigra to superior colliculus, *J. Neurophysiol.* **49**:1285–1301.

Hökfelt, T., and Ungerstedt, U., 1973, Specificity of 6-hydroxydopamine induced degeneration of central monoamine neurons: An electron and light microscopic study with special reference to intra-cerebral injection on the nigro-striatal dopamine system, *Brain Res.* **60**:269–297.

Hökfelt, T., Fuxe, K., Johansson, O., and Ljungdahl, A., 1974a, Pharmacohistochemical evidence of the existence of dopamine nerve terminals in the limbic cortex, *Eur. J. Pharmacol.* **25**:108–112.

Hökfelt, T., and Ljungdahl, A., Fuxe, K., and Johansson, O., 1974b, Dopamine nerve terminals in the rat limbic cortex: Aspects of the dopamine hypothesis of schizophrenia, *Science* **184**:177–179.

Hökfelt, T., Skirboll, L., Rehfeld, J. F., Goldstein, M., Markey, K., and Dann, O., 1980, A subpopulation of mesencephalic dopamine neurons projecting to limbic areas contains a cholecystokinin-like peptide: Evidence from immunochemistry combined with retrograde tracing, *Neuroscience* **5**:2093–2124.

Hökfelt, T., Everitt, B. J., Norheim, E., Rosell, S., and Goldstein, M., 1983, Neurotensin-like immunoreactivity in dopamine neurons in the arcuate nucleus and the ventral mesencephalon, 5th CA Symposium. Suppl. to *Progress in Neuro-Psychopharmacology and Biological Psychiatry*, Pergamon Press, Elmsford, N.Y., p. 171.

Holets, V., Hökfelt, T., Terenius, L., and Goldstein, M., 1985, Differential projections of locus coeruleus neurons containing tyrosine hydroxylase and neuropeptide Y and/or galanin, *Soc. Neurosci. Abstr.* **11**:47.5.

Horn, A. S., Korf, J., and Westernak, B. H. C. (eds.), 1979, *The Neurobiology of Dopamine*, Academic Press, New York.

Hornykiewicz, O., 1973, Dopamine in the basal ganglia: Its role and therapeutic implications, *Br. Med. Bull.* **29**:172–178.

Inagaki, S., and Parent, A., 1984, Distribution of substance P and enkephalin-like immunoreactivity in the substantia nigra of rat, cat and monkey, *Brain Res. Bull.* **13**:319–329.

Innis, R. B., Andrade, R., and Aghajanian, G. K., 1985, Substance K excites dopaminergic and non-dopaminergic neurons in rat substantia nigra, *Brain Res.* **335**:381–383.

Itakura, T., Yakate, H., Kimura, H., Kamei, I., Nakakita, K., Naka, Y., Nakai, K., Imai, H., and Komai, N., 1985, 5-Hydroxytryptamine innervation of vessels in the rat cerebral cortex: Immunohistochemical finding and hydrogen clearance studies, *J. Neurosurg.* **62**:42–47.

Iversen, S. D., 1984, Cortical monoamines and behavior, in: *Monoamine Innervation of Cerebral Cortex* (L. Descarries, T. Reader, and H. Jasper, eds.), Liss, New York, pp. 321–349.

Jacobs, B. L., Foote, S. L., and Bloom, F. E., 1978, Differential projections of neurons within the dorsal raphe nucleus of the rat: A horseradish peroxidase (HRP) study, *Brain Res.* **147**:149–153.

Jahnsen, H., 1980, The action of 5-hydroxytryptamine on neuronal membranes and synaptic transmission in area CA1 of the hippocampus in vitro, *Brain Res.* **197**:83–94.

Javoy-Agid, F., and Agid, Y., 1980, Is the mesocortical dopaminergic system involved in Parkinson disease?, *Neurology* **30**:1326–1330.

Jimenez-Castellanos, J., and Graybiel, A. M., 1985, The dopamine-containing innvervation of striosomes: Nigral subsystems and their striatal correspondents, *Soc. Neurosci. Abstr.* **11**:365.10.

Johnson, E. S., Roberts, M. H. T., and Straughan, D. W., 1969, The responses of cortical neurones to monoamines under differing anesthetic conditions, *J. Physiol. (London)* **203**:261–280.

Johnston, D., and Brown, T. H., 1984, The synaptic nature of the paroxysmal depolarizing shift in hippocampal neurons, *Ann. Neurol.* **16**:565–571.

Jones, B. E., and Moore, R. Y., 1977, Ascending projections of the locus coeruleus in the rat. II. Autoradiographic study, *Brain Res.* **127**:23–53.

Jones, E. G., Coulter, J. D., Burton, H., and Porter, R., 1977, Cells of origin and terminal distribution of corticostriatal fibres arising in sensory motor cortex of monkeys, *J. Comp. Neurol.* **181**:53–80.

Jordan, L. M., Frederickson, R. C. A., Phillis, J. W., and Lake, N., 1972, Microelectrophoresis of 5-hydroxytryptamine: A clarification of its action on cerebral cortical neurones, *Brain Res.* **40**:552–558.

Jouvet, M., 1972, The role of monoamine and acetylcholine containing neurons in the regulation of the sleep–walking cycle, *Orgeb. Physiol.* **64**:166–307.

Kalivas, P. W., 1985a, Interactions between neuropeptides and dopamine neurons in the ventromedial mesencephalon, *Neurosci. Biobehav. Rev.* **9**:573–587.

Kalivas, P. W., 1985b, Sensitization to repeated enkephalin administration in the ventral tegmental area of the rat. II. Involvement of the mesolimbic dopamine system, *J. Pharmacol. Exp. Ther.* **235**:544–550.

Kalivas, P. W., Nemeroff, C. B., and Prange, A. J., Jr., 1982, Neuroanatomical sites of action of neurotensin, *Proc. N.Y. Acad. Sci.* **77**:307–318.

Kalivas, P. W., Deutch, A. Y., Maggio, J. F., Mantyh, P. W., and Roth, R. H., 1985, Substance K and substance P in the ventral tegmental area, *Brain Res.* **57**:241–246.

Kanazawa, I., Emson, C. P., and Cuello, C. A., 1977, Evidence for the existence of substance P containing fibers in striato-nigral and pallido-nigral pathways in rat brain, *Brain Res.* **119**:445–467.

Kanazawa, I., Ogawa, T., Kimura, S., and Munekata, E., 1984, Regional distribution of substance P, neurokinin alpha and neurokinin beta in rat central nervous system, *Neurosci. Res.* **2**:111–120.

Kasamatsu, T., and Heggelund, P., 1982, Single cell responses in cat visual cortex to visual stimulation during iontophoresis of noradrenaline, *Exp. Brain Res.* **45**:317–327.

Kasamatsu, T., Pettigrew, J. D., and Ary, M., 1979, Restoration of visual cortical plasticity by local microperfusion of norepinephrine, *J. Comp. Neurol.* **185**:163–182.

Kasamatsu, T., Pettigrew, J. D., and Ary, M., 1981, Cortical recovery from effects of monocular deprivation: Acceleration with norepinephrine and suppression with 6-hydroxydopamine, *J. Neurophysiol.* **45**:254–266.

Kasamatsu, T., Watabe, K., Scholler, E., and Heggelund, P., 1983, Restoration of neuronal plasticity in cat visual cortex by electrical stimulation of the locus coeruleus, *Soc. Neurosci. Abstr.* **9**:911.

Kasamatsu, T., Hakura, T., Jonnson, G., Heggelund, P., Pettigrew, J., Nakai, K., Watabe, K., Kupperman, B., and Ary, M., 1984, Neuronal plasticity in cat visual cortex: A proposed role for the central noradrenaline system, in: *Monoamine Innervation of Cerebral Cortex* (L. Descarries, T. Reader, and H. Jasper, eds.), Liss, New York, pp. 301–319.

Kehr, W., Lindquist, M., and Carlsson, A., 1976, Distribution of dopamine in the rat cerebral cortex, *J. Neural Transm.* **38**:173–180.

Kelley, A. E., Domesick, V. B., and Nauta, W. J. H., 1982, The amygdalostriatal projection in the rat—An anatomical study by anterograde and retrograde tracing methods, *Neuroscience* **7**:615–630.

Kemp, J. M., and Powell, T. P. S., 1971, The structure of the caudate nucleus of the cat: Light and electron microscopy, *Philos. Trans. R. Soc. London* **262**:383–401.

Kitai, S. T., Sugimori, M., and Kocsis, J D., 1976, Excitatory nature of dopamine in the nigrocaudate pathway, *Exp. Brain Res.* **24**:351–363.

Kohler, C., 1982, On the serotonergic innervation of the hippocampal region: An analysis employing immunohistochemistry and retrograde fluorescent tracing in the rat brain, in: *Cytochemical Methods in Neuroanatomy* (S. Palay and V. Chan-Palay, eds.), Liss, New York, pp. 387–407.

Kohler, C., 1984, The distribution of serotonin binding sites in the hippocampal region of the rat brain: An autoradiographic study, *Neuroscience* **13**:667–680.

Kohler, C., and Steinbusch, H., 1982, Identification of serotonin and nonserotonin-containing neurons of the midbrain raphe projecting to the entorhinal area and the hippocampal formation: A combined immunohistochemical fluorescent retrograde tracing study in the rat brain, *Neuroscience* **7**:951–975.

Kohler, C., Chan-Palay, V., Haglund, L., and Steinbusch, H., 1980, Immunohistochemical localization of serotonin nerve terminals in the lateral entorhinal cortex of the rat: Demonstration of two separate patterns of innervation from the midbrain raphe, *Anat. Embryol.* **160**:121–129.

Kohler, C., Chan-Palay, V., and Steinbusch, H., 1981, The distribution and orientation of serotonin fibers in the entorhinal and other retrohippocampal areas: An immunohistochemical study with anti-serotonin antibodies in the rat's brain, *Anat. Embryol.* **161**:237–264.

Kolb, B., 1974, Dissociation of the effect of lesions of the orbital or medial aspect of the prefrontal cortex of the rat with respect to activity, *Behav. Biol.* **10**:329–343.

Kolb, B., 1984, Functions of the frontal cortex of the rat: A comparative review, *Brain Res. Rev.* **8**:65–98.

Kosofsky, B., Molliver, M., Morrison, J., and Foote, S., 1984, The serotonin and norepinephrine innervation of primary visual cortex in cynomolgous monkey, *J. Comp. Neurol.* **230**:168–178.

Krnjević, K., 1984, Neurotransmitters in cerebral cortex: A general account, in *Cerebral Cortex*, Vol. 2 (E. G. Jones and A. Peters, eds.), Plenum Press, New York, pp. 39–62.

Krnjević, K., and Phillis, J. W., 1963a, Actions of certain amines on cerebral cortical neurons, *Br. J. Pharmacol. Chemother.* **20**:471–490.

Krnjević, K., and Phillis, J. W., 1963b, Iontophoretic studies of neurons in the mammalian cerebral cortex, *J. Physiol. (London)* **165**:274–304.

Kuhar, M. J., Murrin, L. C., Malouf, A., and Klemn, N., 1978, Dopamine receptor binding *in vivo*: The feasibility of autoradiography studies, *Life Sci.* **22**:203–210.

Kuypers, H. G. J. M., 1962, Corticospinal connections: Postnatal development in the rhesus monkey, *Science* **138**:678–680.

Kuypers, H. G. J. M., and Lawrence, D. G., 1967, Cortical projections to the red nucleus and the brain stem in the rhesus monkey, *Brain Res.* **4**:487–492.

Lauder, J., and Bloom, F., 1974, Ontogeny of monoaminergic neurons in the locus coeruleus, raphe nuclei and substantia nigra of the rat, *J. Comp. Neurol.* **155**:469–482.

Lavielle, S., Tassin, J. P., Thierry, A. M., Blanc, G., Herve, D., Barthelemy, C., and Glowinski, J., 1979, Blockade by benzodiazepines of the selective high increase in dopamine turnover induced by stress im mesocortical dopaminergic neurons of the rat, *Brain Res.* **168**:585–594.

Leger, L., Wiklund, L., Descarries, L., and Persson, M., 1979, Description of an indole aminergic cell component in the cat locus coeruleus, *Brain Res.* **168**:43–56.

Leichnetz, G. R., and Astruc, J., 1975, Preliminary evidence for a direct projection of the prefrontal cortex to the hippocampus in the squirrel monkey, *Brain Behav. Evol.* **11**:355–364.

Levitt, P., and Moore, R. Y., 1978a, Noradrenaline neuron innervation of the neocortex in the rat, *Brain Res.* **139**:219–231.

Levitt, P., and Moore, R. Y., 1978b, Developmental organization of raphe serotonin neuron groups in the cat, *Anat. Embryol.* **154**:241–251.

Levitt, P., and Moore, R. Y., 1979, Development of the noradrenergic innervation of neocortex, *Brain Res.* **162**:243–259.

Levitt, P., and Rakic, P., 1982, The time of genesis, embryonic origin and differentiation of the brainstem monoamine neurons in the rhesus monkey, *Dev. Brain Res.* **4**:35–57.

Levitt, P., Rakic, P., and Goldman-Rakic, P. S., 1981, Region-specific catecholamine innervation of primate cerebral cortex, *Soc. Neurosci. Abstr.* **7**:801.

Levitt, P., Rakic, P., and Goldman-Rakic, P.S., 1984a, Comparative assessment of monoamine afferents in mammalian cerebral cortex, in: *Monoamine Innervation of Cerebral Cortex* (L. Descarries, T. Reader, and H. Jasper, eds.), Liss, New York, pp. 41–60.

Levitt, P., Rakic, P., and Goldman-Rakic, P. S., 1984b, Region-specific distribution of catecholamine afferents in primate cerebral cortex: A fluorescence histochemical analysis, *J. Comp. Neurol.* **227**:23–36.

Lewis, D. A., Campbell, M. J., Foote, S. L., Goldstein, M., and Morrison, J. H., 1987, The dopaminergic innervation of primate neocortex: Widespread yet regionally specific, *Proc. Natl. Acad. Sci. USA* in press.

Lewis, M. S., Molliver, M. E., Morrison, J. H., and Lidov, H. G. W., 1979, Complementarity of dopaminergic and noradrenergic innervation of anterior cingulate cortex of the rat, *Brain Res.* **164**:328–333.

Leysen, J. E., Geerts, R., Gommeren, W., Verwimp, M., and Van Gompel, P., 1982, Regional distribution of serotonin-2 receptor binding sites in the brain and effects of neuronal lesions, *Arch. Int. Pharmacodyn. Ther.* **256**:301–305.

Lidov, H. G. W., and Molliver, M. E., 1982, An immunohistochemical study of serotonin neuron development in the rat: Ascending pathway and terminal fields, *Brain Res. Bull.* **8**:389–430.

Lidov, H. G. W., and Zecevic, N. R., 1978, Characterization of the monoaminergic innervation of immature rat neocortex: A histofluorescence analysis, *J. Comp. Neurol.* **181**:663–680.

Lidov, H. G. W., Rice, F. L., and Molliver, M. E., 1978, The organization of the catecholamine innervation of somatosensory cortex: The barrel field of the mouse, *Brain Res.* **153**:577–584.

Lidov, H. G. W., Grzanna, R., and Molliver, M. E., 1980, The serotonin innervation of the cerebral cortex in the rat—An immunohistochemical analysis, *Neuroscience* **5**:207–227.

Lidsky, T. T., Manetto, C., and Schneider, J. S., 1985, Consideration of sensory factors involved in motor functions of the basal ganglia, *Brain Res. Rev.* **9**:133–141.

Lindvall, O., and Björklund, A., 1974a, The glyoxylic acid fluorescence histochemical method: A detailed account of the methodology for the visualization of central catecholamine neurons, *Histochemistry* **39**:97–127.

Lindvall, O., and Björklund, A., 1983, Dopamine and noradrenaline-containing neuron systems: Their anatomy in the rat brain, in: *Chemical Neuroanatomy* (P. C. Emson, ed.), Raven Press, New York, pp. 229–255.

Lindvall, O., and Björklund, A., 1984, General organization of cortical monoamine systems, in: *Monoamine Innervation of Cerebral Cortex* (L. Descarries, T. Reader, and H. Jasper, eds.), Liss, New York, pp. 9–40.

Lindvall, O., Björklund, A., Moore, R. Y., and Stenevi, U., 1974, Mesencephalic dopamine neurons projecting to neocortex, *Brain Res.* **81**:325–331.

Lindvall, O., Björklund, A., and Divac, I., 1978, Organization of catecholamine neurons projecting to the frontal cortex of the rat, *Brain Res.* **142**:1–24.

Lindvall, O., Björklund, A., and Skagerberg, G., 1984, Selective histochemical demonstration of dopamine terminal systems in rat di- and telencephalon: New evidence for a dopaminergic innervation of hypothalamic neurosecretory nuclei, *Brain Res.* **306**:19–30.

Lisoprawski, A., Herve, D., Blanc, G., Glowinski, J., and Tassin, J. P., 1980, Selective activation of the mesocortico-frontal dopaminergic neurons induced by lesion of the habenula in the rat, *Brain Res.* **183**:229–234.

Llinas, R., Greenfield, S. A., and Jahnsen, H., 1984, Electrophysiology of pars compacta cells with *in vitro* substantia nigra—A possible mechanism for dendrite release, *Brain Res.* **294**:127–132.

Loizou, L. A., 1972, The postnatal ontogeny of monoamine containing neurons in the central nervous system of the albino rat, *Brain Res.* **40**:395–418.

Loranger, A. W., Goodell, H., and McDowell, F. H., 1972, Intellectual impairment in Parkinson's syndrome, *Brain* **95**:405–412.

Lorente de Nó, R., 1949, Cerebral cortex: Architecture, intracortical connections, motor projections, in: *Physiology of the Nervous System* (J. F. Fulton, ed.), Oxford University Press, London, pp. 288–312.

Loughlin, S. E., and Fallon, J. H., 1982, Mesostriatal projections from ventral tegmentum and dorsal raphe: Individual cells project ipsilaterally and contralaterally but not bilaterally, *Neurosci. Lett.* **32**:11–16.

Loughlin, S.E., and Fallon, J. H., 1984, Substantia nigra and ventral tegmental area projections to cortex: Topography and collateralization, *Neuroscience* **11**:425–436.

Loughlin, S. E., and Fallon, J. H., 1985, The locus coeruleus, in: *The Rat Central Nervous System* (G. Paxinos, ed.), Academic Press, New York, pp. 79–94.

Loughlin, S. E., Foote, S. L., and Fallon, J. H., 1982, Locus coeruleus projections to cortex: Topography, morphology and collateralization, *Brain Res. Bull.* **9**:287–294.

Loughlin, S. E., Foote, S. L., and Bloom, F., 1986a, Efferent projections of nucleus locus coeruleus: Topographic organization of cells of origin demonstrated by three-dimensional reconstruction, *Neuroscience* **18**:291–306.

Loughlin, S. E., Foote, S., and Grzanna, R., 1986b, Efferent projections of nucleus locus coeruleus: Morphologic subpopulations have different efferent targets, *Neuroscience* **18**:307–320.

Loy, R., and Moore, R., 1979, Ontogeny of the noradrenergic innervation of the rat hippocampal formation, *Anat. Embryol.* **157:**243–253.

Loy, R., Koziell, D., Lindsey, J., and Moore, R., 1980, Noradrenergic innervation of the adult rat hippocampal formation, *J. Comp. Neurol.* **189:**699–710.

McDonald, A., 1982, Cytoarchitecture of the central amygdaloid nucleus of the rat, *J. Comp. Neurol.* **208:**401–418.

McDonald, A., 1983, Neurons of the bed nucleus of the stria terminalis: A Golgi study in the rat, *Brain Res. Bull.* **10:**111–120.

McGeer, P. L., McGeer, E. G., Scherer, U., and Singh, K., 1977, A glutamatergic corticostriatal pathway, *Brain Res.* **128:**369–373.

McNaughton, N., and Mason, S., 1980, The neuropsychology and neuropharmacology of the dorsal ascending bundle—A review, *Prog. Neurobiol.* **14:**157–219.

Maeda, T., Kashiba, A., Tohyama, M., Hori, M., Itakura, T., and Shimizu, N., 1975, Demonstration of aminergic terminals and their contacts in rat brain by perfusion fixation with potassium permanganate, *Abstr. 10th Int. Congr. Anat.* p. 142.

Magistretti, P., and Morrison, J., 1985, VIP neurons in the neocortex, *Trends Neurosci.* **8:**7–8.

Magistretti, P. J., Morrison, J. H., Shoemaker, W. J., Sapin, V., and Bloom, F. E., 1981, Vasoactive intestinal polypeptide induces glycogenolysis in mouse cortical slices: A possible regulatory mechanism for the local control of energy metabolism, *Proc. Natl. Acad. Sci. USA* **78:**6535–6539.

Magistretti, P. J., Morrison, J. H., Shoemaker, W. J., and Bloom, F. E., 1983, Effect of 6-hydroxydopamine lesions on norepinephrine-induced (^{3}H) glycogen hydrolysis in mouse cortical slices, *Brain Res.* **26:**159–162.

Marchais, D., Tassin, J. P., and Bockaert, J., 1980, Dopaminergic component of (^{3}H) spiroperidol binding in the rat anterior cerebral cortex, *Brain Res.* **183:**235–240.

Markowitsch, H. J., and Irle, E., 1981, Widespread cortical projections of the ventral tegmental area and of other brain stem structures in the cat, *Exp. Brain Res.* **41:**233–246.

Marsden, C. D., 1980, The enigma of the basal ganglia and movement, *Trends Neurosurg.* **3:**284–287.

Marshall, J. P., Richardson, J. S., and Teitelbaum, P., 1974, Nigrostriatal bundle damage and the lateral hypothalamic syndrome, *J. Comp. Physiol. Psychol.* **87:**808–830.

Martres, M. P., Bouthenet, M. L., Sales, N., Sokoloff, P., and Schwartz, J. C., 1985, Widespread distribution of brain dopamine receptors evidenced with ^{125}I iodosulpride, a highly selective ligand, *Science* **228:**752–755.

Mason, S., 1980, Noradrenaline and selective attention: A review of the model and the evidence, *Life Sci.* **27:**617–631.

Mason, S. T., and Fibiger, H. C., 1979, Regional topography within noradrenergic locus coeruleus as revealed by retrograde transport of horseradish peroxidase, *J. Comp. Neurol.* **187:**703–724.

Matthyse, S., 1981, Nucleus accumbens and schizophrenia, in: *The Neurobiology of the Nucleus Accumbens* (R. B. Chronister and J. F. DeFrance, eds.), Haer, Brunswick, N.J., pp. 351–359.

Meilbach, R. C., Maayani, S., and Green, J. P., 1980, Characterization and radioautography of ^{3}H LSD binding by rat brain slices *in vitro:* The effect of 5-hydroxytryptamine, *Eur. J. Pharmacol.* **67:**371–382.

Mensah, P. L., 1977, The internal organization of the mouse caudate nucleus: Evidence for cell clustering and regional variation, *Brain Res.* **137:**53–66.

Mercuri, N., Calabresi, P., Stanzione, P., and Bernardi, G., 1985, Electrical stimulation of mesencephalic cell groups (A9–A10) produces monosynaptic excitatory potentials in rat frontal cortex, *Brain Res.* **338:**192–195.

Messiha, F. S., and Kenny, A. D. (eds.), 1977, *Parkinson's Disease: Neurophysiological, Clinical and Related Aspects, Adv. Exp. Med. Biol.* **90.**

Milner, B., and Petrides, M., 1984, Behavioral effects of frontal lobe lesions in man, *Trends Neurosci.* **7:**403–407.

Mishra, R. K., Demirjian, C., Katzman, R., and Makman, M. H., 1975, A dopamine-sensitive adenylate cyclase in anterior limbic cortex and mesolimbic region of primate brain, *Brain Res.* **96:**395–399.

Molliver, M E., Grzanna, R., Lidov, H. G. W., Morrison, J. H., and Olschowka, J. A., 1982, Monoamine systems in the cerebral cortex, in: *Cytochemical Methods in Neuroanatomy* (V. Chan-Palay and S. L. Palay, eds.), Liss, New York, pp. 255–277.

Moon, S., and Herkenham, M., 1984, Heterogeneous dopaminergic projections to the neostriatum of the rat: Nuclei of origin dictate discrete relationship to opiate receptor patches, *Soc. Neurosci. Abstr.* **14:**120.

Moore, R. Y., and Bloom, F. E., 1978, Central catecholamine neuron systems: Anatomy and physiology of the dopamine systems, *Annu. Rev. Neurosci.* **1:**129–169.

Moore, R. Y., and Halaris, A. E., 1975, Hippocampal innervation by serotonin neurons of the midbrain raphe in the cat, *J. Comp. Neurol.* **164:**161–184.

Moore, R. Y., and Heller, A., 1967, Monoamine levels and neuronal degeneration in rat brain following lateral hypothalamic lesions, *J. Pharmacol. Exp. Ther.* **156:**12–23.

Moore, R. Y., Halaris, A. E., and Jones, B. E., 1978, Serotonin neurons of the midbrain raphe: Ascending projections, *J. Comp. Neurol.* **180:**417–438.

Mora, F., Sweeney, K. F., Rools, E. T., and Sanguinetti, A. M., 1976, Spontaneous firing rate of neurons in the prefrontal cortex of the rat: Evidence for a dopaminergic inhibition, *Brain Res.* **116:**516–522.

Morel-Maroger, A., 1977, Effects of levodopa on frontal signs in parkinsonism, *Br. Med. J.* **2:**1543.

Morrison, J. H., Grzanna, R., Molliver, M. E., and Coyle, J. T., 1978, The distribution and orientation of noradrenergic fibers in neocortex of the rat: An immunofluorescence study, *J. Comp. Neurol.* **181:**17–40.

Morrison, J. H., Molliver, M. E., Grzanna, R., and Coyle, J. T., 1981, The intracortical trajectory of the coeruleo-cortical projection in the rat: A tangentially organized cortical afferent, *Neuroscience* **6:**139–158.

Morrison, J. H., Foote, S. L., O'Connor, D., and Bloom, F. E., 1982a, A laminar, tangential and regional organization of the noradrenergic innervation of monkey cortex: Dopamine-β-hydroxylase immunohistochemistry, *Brain Res. Bull.* **9:**309–319.

Morrison, J. H., Foote, S. L., Molliver, M. E., Bloom, F. E., and Lidov, G. W., 1982b, Noradrenergic and serotonergic fibers innervate complementary layers in monkey primary visual cortex: An immunohistochemical study, *Proc. Natl. Acad. Sci. USA* **79:**2401–2405.

Morrison, J., Foote, S., and Bloom, F., 1984, Regional, laminar, developmental and functional characteristics of noradrenaline and serotonin innervation patterns in monkey cortex, in: *Monoamine Innervation of Cerebral Cortex* (L. Descarries, T. Reader, and H. Jasper, eds.), Liss, New York, pp. 61–75.

Morruzzi, A. S., and Hart, E. R., 1955, Evoked cortical responses under the influence of hallucinogens and related drugs, *Electroencephalogr. Clin. Neurophysiol.* **7:**146.

Moruzzi, G., and Magoun, H. W., 1949, Brain stem reticular formation and activation of the cortex, *Electroencephalogr. Clin. Neurophysiol.* **1:**455–473.

Muldrum, B. S., and Marsden, C. D. (eds.), *Primate Models of Neurological Disorders, Adv. Neurol.* **10**.

Murrin, K. C., and Kuhar, M. J., 1979, Dopamine receptors in rat frontal cortex: An autoradiographic study, *Brain Res.* **177:**279–285.

Nagai, T., Satoh, K., Imamoto, K., and Maeda, T., 1981, Divergent projections of catecholamine neurons of the locus coeruleus as revealed by fluorescent retrograde double labeling technique, *Neurosci. Lett.* **23:**117–123.

Nakamura, S., Tepper, J. M., Young, S. J., and Groves, P. M., 1981, Neurophysiological consequences of presynaptic receptor activation: Changes in noradrenergic terminal excitability, *Brain Res.* **226:**155–170.

Nastuk, M. A., and Graybiel, A. M., 1983, The distribution of muscarinic binding sites in the feline striatum and its relationship to other histochemical staining patterns, *Soc. Neurosci. Abstr.* **9:**15.

Nastuk, M. A., and Graybiel, A. M., 1985, Patterns of muscarinic cholinergic binding in the striatum and their relation to dopamine islands and striosomes, *J. Comp. Neurol.* **237:**176–194.

Nauta, W. J. H., 1979, A proposed conceptual reorganization of the basal ganglia and telencephalon, *Neuroscience* **4:**1875–1881.

Nauta, W. J. H., and Domesick, V. B., 1978, Crossroads of limbic and striatal circuitry: Hypothalamonigral connections, in: *Limbic Mechanisms* (K. E. Livingstone and O. Hornykiewicz, eds.), Plenum Press, New York, pp. 75–93.

Nauta, W. J. H., and Domesick, V. B., 1979, The anatomy of the extrapyramidal system, in: *Dopaminergic Ergot Derivatives and Motor Function* (K. Fuxe and D. B. Calne, eds.), Pergamon Press, Elmsford, N.Y., pp. 3–22.

Nauta, W. J. H., and Domesick, V. B., 1984, Afferent and efferent relationships of the basal ganglia, *Ciba Found. Symp.* **107:**3–29.

Nauta, W. J. H., and Kuypers, H. G. J. M., 1958, Some ascending pathways in the brain stem reticular formation, in: *Reticular Formation of the Brain* (H. H. Jasper, L. D. Proctor, R. S. Knighton, W. C. Noshay, and R. T. Costello, eds.), Little, Brown, Boston, pp. 3–30.

Nauta, W. J. H., Smith, G. P., Faull, R. L. N., and Domesick, V. B., 1978, Efferent connections and nigral afferents of the nucleus accumbens septi in the rat, *Neuroscience* **3:**345–401.

Nemeroff, C. B., Hernandez, D. E., Luttinger, D., Kalivas, P. W., and Prange, A. J., 1982, Sites of neurotensin action in the brain, *Proc. N.Y. Acad. Sci.* **77:**330–344.

Newman, R., and Winans, S. S., 1980, An experimental study of the ventral striatum of the golden hamster. I. Neuronal connections of the nucleus accumbens, *J. Comp. Neurol.* **191:**167–192.

Olpe, H. R., 1981, Differential effects of clomipramine and clorgyline on the sensitivity of cortical neurons to serotonin: Effect of chronic treatment, *Eur. J. Pharmacol.* **69:**375–377.

Olpe, H. R., Glatt, A., Laszlo, J., and Schellenberg, A., 1980, Some electrophysiological and pharmacological properties of the cortical, noradrenergic projection of the locus coeruleus in the rat, *Brain Res.* **186:**9–19.

Olschowka, J. A., Molliver, M. E, Grzanna, R., Rice, F. L., and Coyle, J. T., 1981, Ultrastructural demonstration of noradrenergic synapses in the rat central nervous system by dopamine-β-hydroxylase immunocytochemistry, *J. Histochem. Cytochem.* **29:**271–280.

Palacios, J. M., and Kuhar, M. J., 1980, Beta-adrenergic-receptor localization by light microscopic autoradiography, *Science* **208:**1378–1380.

Palacios, J. M., and Kuhar, M. J., 1982, Beta-adrenergic receptor localization in rat brain by light microscopic autoradiography, *Neurochem. Int.* **4:**473–490.

Palacios, J. M., and Wamsley, J. K., 1982, Receptor for amines, amino acids and peptides. *Prog. Brain Res.* **55:**265–278.

Palacios, J. M., and Wamsley, J. K., 1983, Microscopic localization of adrenoreceptors, in: *Adrenoreceptors and Catecholamine Action*, Part B, Vol. 2 (G. Kinos, ed.), Wiley, New York, pp. 295–313.

Palacios, J. M., and Wamsley, J. K., 1984, Autoradiographic distribution of receptor ligand binding—Catecholamine receptors, in: *Handbook of Chemical Neuroanatomy* (A. Björklund, T. Hökfelt, and M. J. Kuhar, eds.), Vol. 3, Elsevier/North-Holland, Amsterdam, pp. 325–351.

Palacios, J. M., Niehoff, D. L., and Kuhar, M. J., 1981, [3H] spiperone binding sites in brain: Autoradiographic localization of multiple receptors, *Brain Res.* **213:**277–289.

Palkovits, M., Mroz, E. A., Brownstein, M. J., and Leeman, S. E., 1978, Descending substance P-containing pathway: A component of the ansa lenticularis, *Brain Res.* **156:**124–128.

Palkovits, M., Zaborsky, L. Brownstein, M. J., Fekete, M. I., Herman, J. P., and Kanyicska, B., 1979, Distribution of norepinephrine and dopamine in cerebral cortical areas of the rat, *Brain Res. Bull.* **4:**593–601.

Parent, A., Descarries, L., and Beaudet, A., 1981, Organization of ascending serotonin systems in the adult rat brain: A radioautographic study after intraventricular administration of ([3H])-hydroxytryptamine, *Neuroscience* **6:**115–138.

Parnavelas, J., Moises, H., and Speciale, S., 1985, The monoaminergic innervation of the rat visual cortex, *Proc. R. Soc. London Ser. B* **223:**319–329.

Paxinos, G., and Watson, C., 1982, *The Rat Brain in Stereotaxic Coordinates.* Academic Press, New York.

Peroutka, S. J., and Snyder, S. H., 1979, Multiple serotonin receptors: Differential binding of ([3H])-hydroxytryptamine, ([3H]) lysergic acid diethylamide and ([3H]) spiroperidol, *Mol. Pharmacol.* **16:**687–699.

Phillis, J. W., 1984, Micro-iontophoretic studies of cortical biogenic amines, in: *Monoamine Innervation of Cerebral Cortex* (L. Descarries, T. Reader, and H. Jasper, eds.), Liss, New York, pp. 175–194.

Phillis, J. W., Tebecis, A. K., and York, D. H ., 1968, Depression of spinal motoneurons by noradrenaline, 5-hydroxytryptamine and histamine, *Eur. J. Pharmacol.* **7:**471–475.

Phillis, J. W., Wu, P. H., and Thierry, D. L., 1982, The effect of β-adrenergic receptor agonists and antagonists on the efflux on ^{22}Na and uptake of ^{42}K by rat brain cortical slices, *Brain Res.* **236:**133–142.

Pickel, V. M., Segal, M., and Bloom, F. E., 1974, A radioautographic study of the efferent pathways of the nucleus locus coeruleus, *J. Comp. Neurol.* **155:**15–42.

Pickel, V. M., Joh, T. H., and Reis, D. J., 1977, A serotonergic innervation of noradrenergic neurons in nucleus locus coeruleus: Demonstration by immunocytochemical localization of the transmitter specific enzymes tyrosine and tryptophan hydroxylase, *Brain Res.* **131:**197–214.

Poirier, L. J., Sourkes, T. L., and Bedard, P. J. (eds.)., 1979, *The Extrapyramidal System and Its Disorders, Adv. Neurol.* **24.**

Porrino, L. J., and Goldman-Rakic, P. S., 1982, Brainstem innervation of prefrontal and anterior cingulate cortex in the rhesus monkey revealed by retrograde transport of HRP, *J. Comp. Neurol.* **205:**63–76.

Pycock, C. J., Kerwin, R. W., and Carter, C. J., 1980, Effect of lesion of cortical dopamine terminals on subcortical dopamine receptors in rats, *Nature* **286**:74–77.

Quirion, R., Chiueh, C., Evenist, H., and Pert, A., 1985, Comparative localization of neurotensin receptors on nigrostriatal and mesolimbic dopaminergic terminals, *Brain Res.* **327**: 385–389.

Ragsdale, C. W., and Graybiel, A., 1981, The fronto-striatal projection in the cat and monkey and its relationship to inhomogeneities established by acetylcholinesterase histochemistry, *Brain Res.* **208**:259–266.

Ragsdale, C. W., and Graybiel, A. M., 1984, Further observations on the striosomal organization of frontostriatal projections in cats and monkeys, *Soc. Neurosci. Abstr.* **10**:514.

Reader, T. A., 1978, Effects of dopamine, noradrenaline and serotonin in visual cortex of cat, *Experientia* **34**:1586–1588.

Reader, T. A., and Jasper, H. H., 1984, Interactions between monoamines and other transmitters in cerebral cortex, in: *Monoamine Innervation of Cerebral Cortex* (L. Descarries, T. Reader, and H. Jasper, eds.), Liss, New York, pp. 195–225.

Reader, T. A., De Champlain, J., and Jasper, H. H., 1979a, Interactions between biogenic amines and acetylcholine, in: *Catecholamines: Basic and Clinical Frontiers* (E. Usdin, I. J. Kopin, and J. Barchas, eds.), Pergamon Press, Elmsford, N.Y., pp. 1074–1076.

Reader, T. A., Ferron, A., Descarries, L., and Jasper, H. H., 1979b, Modulatory role for biogenic amines in the cerebral cortex: Microiontophoretic studies, *Brain Res.* **160**:217–229.

Reches, A., Burke, R. E., Jiang, D., Wagner, H. R., and Fahn, S., 1983, Neurotensin interacts with dopaminergic neurons in rat brain, *Peptides* **4**:43–48.

Redmond, D. E., and Huang, Y. H., 1979, New evidence for a locus coeruleus norepinephrine connection with anxiety, *Life Sci.* **25**:2149–2162.

Reymann, K., Pohle, W., Muller-Welde, P., and Ott, T., 1983, Dopaminergic innervation of the hippocampus: Evidence for midbrain raphe neurons as the site of origin, *Biomed. Biochem. Acta.* **42**:1247–1255.

Ribak, C. E., and Fallon, J. H., 1982, The islands of Calleja complex of the basal forebrain of the rat. I. Light and electron microscopic observations, *J. Comp. Neurol.* **205**:207–218.

Roberts, D., Price, M., and Fibiger, H., 1976, The dorsal tegmental noradrenergic projection: An analysis of its role in maze learning, *J. Comp. Physiol. Psychol.* **90**:363–372.

Rolls, E. T., 1987, Investigations of the functions of different regions of the basal ganglia, in: *Parkinson's Disease* (G. Stern, ed.), Chapman & Hall, London, in press.

Room, P., Postema, F., and Korf, J., 1981, Divergent axon collaterals of rat locus coeruleus neurons: Demonstration by a fluorescent double labeling technique, *Brain Res.* **221**:219–230.

Rosen, G. D., Finklestein, S., Stall, A. K., Yutzey, D. A., and Denenberg, V. N., 1984, Neurochemical asymmetries in the albino rat's cortex, striatum, and nucleus accumbens, *Life Sci.* **34**:1143–1148.

Rosvold, H. E., and Szwarcbart, M. K., 1964, Neural structures involved in delayed response performance, in: *The Frontal Granular Cortex and Behavior* (J. M. Warren and K. Akert, eds.), McGraw–Hill, New York, pp. 1–15.

Routtenberg, A., and Sloan, M., 1972, Self stimulation in the frontal cortex of Rattus norwegiens, *Behav. Biol.* **7**:567–572.

Sandell, J. H., Graybiel, A. M., and Chesselet, M.-F., 1987, A new enzyme marker for striatal compartmentalization: NADPH diaphorase activity in the caudate nucleus and putamen of the cat, *J. Comp. Neurol.* in press.

Sastry, B. S., and Phillis, J. W., 1977, Metergoline as a selective 5-hydroxytryptamine antagonist in the cerebral cortex, *Can. J. Physiol. Pharmacol.* **55**:130–133.

Scatton, B., Simon, H., LeMoal, M., and Bischoof, S., 1980, Origin of dopaminergic innervation of the rat hippocampal formation, *Neurosci. Lett.* **18**:125–133.

Scatton, B., Rouquier, L., Javoy-Agid, F., and Agid, Y., 1982, Dopamine deficiency in the cerebral cortex in Parkinson's disease, *Neurology* **32**:1039–1040.

Scheibel, M. E., and Scheibel, A. B., 1958, Structural substrates for integrative patterns in the brain stem reticular core, in: *Reticular Formation of the Brain* (H. H . Jasper, L. D. Proctor, R. S. Knighton, W. C. Noshay, and R. T. Costello, eds.), Little, Brown, Boston, pp. 31–55.

Scheibner, T., 1986, The morphology and distribution of the mesocortical and mesostriatal projections in the cat, Ph.D. thesis, University of New South Wales.

Schlumpf, M., Shoemaker, W. J., and Bloom, F. E., 1980, Innervation of embryonic rat cerebral cortex by catecholamine-containing fibers, *J. Comp. Neurol.* **192**:361–377.

Schmidt, R. H., Björklund, A., Lindvall, O., and Loren, I., 1982, Prefrontal cortex: Dense dopaminergic input in the newborn rat, *Dev. Brain Res.* **5:**222–228.

Schneider, L. H., Alpert, J. E., and Iversen, S. D., 1983, CCK-8 modulation of mesolimbic dopamine: Antagonism of amphetamine-stimulated behavior, *Peptides* **4:**749–753.

Schwarz, M., Sontag, K.-H., and Wand, P., 1984, Sensory-motor processing in substantia nigra pars reticulata in conscious cats, *J. Physiol. (London)* **347:**129–147.

Seeman, P., Westman, K., Coscina, D., and Marsh, J. J., 1980, Serotonin receptors in hippocampus and frontal cortex, *Eur. J. Pharmacol.* **66:**179–191.

Segal, M., 1980, The action of serotonin in the rat hippocampal slice preparation, *J. Physiol. (London)* **303:**423–439.

Segal, M., and Bloom, F., 1974, The action of norepinephrine in the rat hippocampus, I. Iontophoretic studies, *Brain Res.* **72:**79–97.

Segal, M., and Bloom, F., 1987a, The action of norepinephrine in the rat hippocampus. III. Hippocampal cellular responses to locus coeruleus stimulation in the awake rat, *Brain Res.* **107:**499–511.

Segal, M., and Bloom, F., 1976b, The action of norepinephrine in the rat hippocampus. IV. The effects of locus coeruleus stimulation on evoked hippocampal unit activity, *Brain Res.* **107:**513–525.

Segal, M., and Landis, S. C., 1974, Afferents to the hippocampus of the rat studied with the method of retrograde transport of horseradish peroxidase, *Brain Res.* **78:**1–15.

Seiger, A., and Olson, L., 1973, Late prenatal ontogeny of central monoamine neurons in the rat: Fluorescence histochemical observations, *Z. Anat. Entwicklungsgesch.* **140:**281–318.

Selemon, L. D., and Goldman-Rakic, P. S., 1985, Longitudinal topography and interdigitation of corticostriatal projections in the rhesus monkey, *J. Neurosci.* **5:**776–794.

Seroogy, K. B., Dangaran, K., Lin, S., Haycock, J., and Fallon, J. H., 1987a, Innervation of forebrain structures by ventral mesencephalic neurons containing both CCK and TH-like immunoreactivity, *Brain Res.* in press.

Seroogy, K. B., Mehta, A., and Fallon, J. H., 1987b, Neurotensin and cholecystokinin coexist within neurons of the ventral mesencephalon and project to forebrain regions, *J. Neurosci.* in press.

Sette, M., Raisman, R., Briley, M., and Langer, S. Z., 1981, Localization of tricyclic antidepressant binding sites on serotonin nerve terminals, *J. Neurochem.* **37:**40–42.

Sharma, J. N., 1977, Microiontophoretic application of some monoamines and their antagonists to cortical neurons of the rat, *Neuropharmacology* **16:**83–88.

Shepard, P. D., and Gorman, D. C., 1984, A subpopulation of mesocortical dopamine neurons possesses autoreceptors, *Eur. J. Pharmacol.* **98:**555–566.

Simon, H., Le Moal, M., Galey, D., and Carbo, B., 1976, Silver impregnation of dopaminergic systems after radio frequency and 6-OHDA lesions of the rat ventral tegmentum, *Brain Res.* **115:**215–231.

Simon, H., Le Moal, M., and Calas, A., 1979, Efferents and afferents of the ventral tegmental–A10 region studied after local injection of (^{3}H) leucine and horseradish peroxidase, *Brain Res.* **178:**17–40.

Skirboll, L. R., Grace, A. A., Hommer, J., Rehfeld, J., Goldstein, M., Hökfelt, T., and Bunney, B. S., 1981, Peptide–monoamine co-existence: Studies of the actions of cholecystokinin-like peptide on the electrical activity of midbrain dopamine neurons, *Neuroscience* **6:**2111–2124.

Skofitsch, G., and Jacobowitz, D. M., 1985, Immunohistochemical mapping of galanin-like neurons in the rat central nervous system, *Peptides* **6:**509–546.

Sladek, J. R., and Björklund, A., 1982, Monoamine transmitter histochemistry: A twenty year commemoratum, *Brain Res. Bull.* **9.**

Slopsema, J. S., Van der Guten, J., and De Bruin, J., 1982, Regional concentration of noradrenaline and dopamine in the frontal cortex of the rat: Dopaminergic innervation of the prefrontal subareas and lateralization of prefrontal dopamine, *Brain Res.* **250:**197–200.

Smith, B. S., and Millhouse, O. E., 1985, The connections between the basolateral and central amygdaloid nuclei, *Neurosci. Lett.* **56:**307–309.

Smith, O. A., and DeVito, J. L., 1984, Central neural integration for the control of autonomic responses associated with emotion, *Annu. Rev. Neurosci.* **7:**43–65.

Somogyi, P., Bolan, J. P., and Smith, A. D., 1981, Monosynaptic cortical input and local axon collaterals of identified striatonigral neurons: A light and electron microscopic study using the Golgi–peroxidase transport degeneration procedure, *J. Comp. Neurol.* **195:**567–584.

Starr, M. S., 1985, Multiple opiate receptors may be involved in suppressing gamma-aminobutyrate release in substantia nigra, *Life Sci.* **37:**2249–2255.

Stein, L., 1978, Reward transmitters: Catecholamines and opioid peptides, in: *Psychopharmacology: A Generation of Progress* (M. Lipton, A. DiMascio, and K. Killam, eds.), Raven Press, New York, pp. 569–581.

Steinbusch, H. W. M., 1981, Distribution of serotonin-immunoreactivity in the central nervous system of the rat—cell bodies and terminals, *Neuroscience* **6:**557–618.

Steinbusch, H. W. M., and Nieuwenhuys, R., 1983, The raphe nuclei of the rat brainstem: A cytoarchitectonic and immunohistochemical study, in: *Chemical Neuroanatomy* (P. C. Emson, ed.), Raven Press, New York, pp. 131–207.

Steinbusch, H. W. M., Verhofstad, A. A. J., and Joosten, H. W. J., 1978, Localization of serotonin in central nervous system by immunohistochemistry: Description of a specific and sensitive technique and some applications, *Neuroscience* **3:**811–819.

Steindler, D. A., 1981, Locus coeruleus neurons have axons that branch to the forebrain and cerebellum, *Brain Res.* **223:**367–373.

Stevens, J. R., 1979, Schizophrenia and dopamine regulation in the mesolimbic system, *Trends Neurosci.* **2:**103–105.

Stockmeier, C. A., Martin, A. M., and Kellar, K. J., 1985, A strong influence of serotonin axons on β-adrenergic receptors in rat brain, *Science* **230:**323–325.

Storm-Mathisen, J., and Guldberg, H., 1974, 5-Hydroxytryptamine and noradrenaline in the hippocampal region, *J. Neurochem.* **22:**793–803.

Studler, J. M., Simon, H., Cesselin, F., Legrand, J. C., Glowinski, J., and Tassin, J. P., 1981, Biochemical investigation in the localization of the cholecystokinin octapeptide in dopaminergic neurons originating from the ventral tegmental area of the rat, *Neuropeptides* **2:**131–139.

Swanson, L. W., 1976, The locus coeruleus: A cytoarchitectonic Golgi and immunohistochemical study in the albino rat, *Brain Res.* **110:**39–56.

Swanson, L. W., 1982, The projections of the ventral tegmental area and adjacent regions: A combined fluorescent retrograde tracer and immunofluorescence study in the rat, *Brain Res. Bull.* **9:**321–353.

Swanson, L. W., and Cowan, W. M., 1975, A note on the connections and development of the nucleus accumbens, *Brain Res.* **92:**324–330.

Swanson, L. W., and Sawchenko, P. E., 1983, Hypothalamic integration: Organization of the paraventricular and supraoptic nuclei, *Annu. Rev. Neurosci.* **6:**269–324.

Swanson, L. W., Sawchenko, P. E., Rivier, J., and Vale, W. W., 1983, Organization of ovine corticotropin releasing factor immunoreactive cells and fibers in the rat brain: An immunohistochemical study, *Neuroendocrinology* **36:**165–186.

Switzer, R. C., Hill, J., and Heimer, L., 1982, The globus pallidus and its rostroventral extension into the olfactory tubercle of the rat: A cyto- and chemoarchitectural study, *Neuroscience* **7:**1891–1904.

Taber, E., Brodal, A., and Walberg, F., 1960, The raphe nuclei of the brain stem in the cat. I. Normal topography and cytoarchitecture and general discussion, *J. Comp. Neurol.* **114:**161–187.

Tagliamonte, A., DeMontis, G., and Olianas, M., 1975, Selective increase of brain dopamine synthesis by sulpiride, *J. Neurochem.* **24:**707–710.

Takeuchi, Y., and Sano, Y., 1983, Immunohistochemical demonstration of serotonin nerve fibers in the neocortex of the monkey (Macaca fuscata), *Anat. Embryol.* **166:**155–168.

Tassin, J. P., Thierry, A. M., Blanc, G., and Glowinski, J., 1974, Evidence for a specific uptake of dopamine by dopaminergic terminals of the rat cerebral cortex, *Naunyn Schmiedebergs Arch. Pharmacol.* **282:**239–244.

Tassin, J. P., Velley, L., Stinus, L., Blanc, G., Glowinski, J., and Thierry, A. M., 1975, Development of cortical and nigro-neostriatal dopaminergic systems after destruction of central noradrenergic neurons in fetal or neonatal rats, *Brain Res.* **83:**93–106.

Tassin, J. P., Stinus, L., Simon, H., Blanc, G., Thierry, A. M., Le Moral, M., Cardo, B., and Glowinski, J., 1977, Distribution of dopaminergic terminals in rat cerebral cortex: Role of dopaminergic mesocortical system in ventral tegmental area syndrome, *Adv. Biochem. Psychopharmacol.* **16:**21–28.

Tassin, J. P., Lavielle, S., Herve, D., Blanc, G., Thierry, A. M., Alvarez, C., Berger, B., and Glowinski, J., 1979, Collateral sprouting and reduced activity of the rat mesocortical dopaminergic neurons after selective destruction of the ascending noradrenergic bundles, *Neuroscience* **4:**1569–1582.

Tassin, J. P., Simon, H., Herve, D., Blanc, G., Le Moal, M., Glowinski, J., and Bockaert, J., 1982, Non-dopaminergic fibers may regulate dopamine-sensitive adenylate cyclase in the prefrontal cortex and nucleus accumbens, *Nature* **295:**696–698.

Tassin, J. P., Studler, J. M., Herve, D., Blanc, G., and Glowinski, J., 1986, Contribution of norad-renergic neurons to the regulation of dopaminergic (DI) receptor denervation supersensitivity in rat prefrontal cortex, *J. Neurochem.* **46:**243–248.

Thierry, A. M., Stinus, L., Blanc, G., and Glowinski, J., 1973, Some evidence for the existence of dopaminergic neurons in the rat cortex, *Brain Res.* **50:**230–234.

Thierry, A. M., Hirsch, J. C., Tassin, J. P., Blanc, G., and Glowinski, J., 1974, Presence of dopa-minergic terminals and absence of dopaminergic cell bodies in the cerebral cortex of the cat, *Brain Res.* **79:**77–88.

Thierry, A. M., Tassin, J. P., Blanc, G., and Glowinski, J., 1976, Selective activation of the mesocortical DA system by stress, *Nature* **263:**242–244.

Thierry, A. M., Deniau, J. M., Herve, D., and Chevalier, G., 1980, Electrophysiological evidence for non-dopaminergic mesocortical and mesolimbic neurons in the rat, *Brain Res.* **201:**210–214.

Thierry, A. M., Tassin, J. P., and Glowinski, J., 1984, Biochemical and electrophysiological studies of the mesocortical dopamine system, in: *Monoamine Innervation of Central Cortex* (L. Descarries, T. Reader, and H. Jasper, eds.), Liss, New York, pp. 233–261.

Tork, I., and Turner, S., 1981, Histochemical evidence for a catecholaminergic (presumably do-paminergic) projection from the ventral mesencephalic tegmentum to visual cortex in the cat, *Neurosci. Lett.* **24:**215–219.

Twarog, B. M., and Page, I. H., 1953, Serotonin content of some mammalian tissues and urine, *Am. J. Physiol.* **175:**157–161.

Uhl, G. R., Goodman, R. R., and Snyder, S., 1979, Neurotensin-containing cell bodies, fibers and nerve terminals in the brainstem of the rat: Immunohistochemical mapping, *Brain Res.* **167:**77–91.

Ungerstedt U., 1971, Stereotaxic mapping of the monoamine pathways of the rat brain, *Acta Physiol. Scand. Suppl.* **367:**1–49.

Ungerstedt, U., 1974, Brain dopamine neurones and behavior, in: *The Neurosciences: Third Study Program* (F. O. Schmitt and F. G. Worden, eds.), MIT Press, Cambridge, Mass. pp. 695–705.

Vaccarino, F. J., and Franklin, K. B. J., 1982, Self-stimulation and circling reveal functional differ-ences between medial and lateral substantia nigra, *Behav. Brain Res.* **5:**281–295.

Vaccarino, F. J., and Koob, G. F., 1984, Microinjections of nanogram amounts of sulfated CCK-8 into the rat nucleus accumbens attenuates brain stimulation reward, *Neurosci. Lett.* **52:**61–66.

Vaccarino, F. J., and Prupas, D., 1985, The role of the midbrain reticular formation in the expression of two opposing nigral denervation syndromes, *Physiol. Behav.* **35:**749–752.

Vaccarino, F. J., Franklin, K. B., and Prupas, D., 1985, Opposite locomotor asymmetries elicited from the medial and lateral substantia nigra: Role of the superior colliculus, *Physiol. Behav.* **35:**741–747.

van den Pol, A. N., Smith, A. D., and Powell, J. F., 1985, GABA axons in synaptic contact with dopamine neurons in the substantia nigra: Double immunochemistry with biotin–peroxidase and protein A–colloidal gold, *Brain Res.* **348:**146–154.

van der Kooy, D., 1983, Developmental relationships between opiate receptors and dopamine in-formation of caudate–putamen patches, *Soc. Neurosci. Abstr.* **9:**659.

van der Kooy, D., and Hattori, T., 1980, Bilaterally situated dorsal raphe cell bodies have only unilateral forebrain projections in rat, *Brain Res.* **192:**550–554.

van der Kooy, D., and Kuypers, H. G. J. M., 1979, Fluorescent retrograde double labeling: Axonal branching in the ascending raphe and nigral projections, *Science* **204:**873–875.

van der Kooy, D., Coscina, D. V., and Hattori, T., 1981, Is there a non-dopaminergic nigrostriatal pathway?, *Neuroscience* **6:**345–357.

Van der Maelen, C P., and Aghajanian, G. K., 1980, Intracellular studies showing modulation of facial motorneurons excitability by serotonin, *Nature* **287:**346–347.

Van Dengen, P., 1981, The central norepinephrine transmission and the locus coeruleus: A review of the data, *Prog. Neurobiol.* **16:**117–143.

Versteeg, D., Van der Gugten, J., De Jong, W., and Palkovits, M., 1976, Regional concentrations of noradrenaline and dopamine in the rat brain, *Brain Res.* **113:**563–574.

Vincent, S. R., Johansson, O., Hökfelt, T., Skirboll, L., Elde, R. P., Terenius, L., Kimmel, J., and Goldstein, M., 1983, NADPH diaphorase: A histochemical selective marker for striatal neurons containing both somatostatin and avian pancreatic polypeptide (AP) like immunoreactivities, *J. Comp. Neurol.* **217:**252–263.

Von Hungen, K., Roberts, S., and Hill, D. F., 1974, LSD as an agonist and antagonist at central dopamine receptors, *Nature* **252:**588–589.

Wamsley, J. K., 1984a, Autoradiographic localization of receptor sites in the cerebral cortex, in: *Cerebral Cortex*, Vol. 2 (E. G. Jones and A. Peters, eds.), Plenum Press, New York, pp. 173–202.

Wamsley J., 1984b, Autoradiographic localization of cortical biogenic amine receptors, in: *Monoamine Innervation of Cerebral Cortex* (L. Descarries, T. Reader, and H. Jasper, eds.), Liss, New York, pp. 153–174.

Wamsley, J. K., Palacios, J. M., Young, W. S., and Kuhar, M. J., 1981, Autoradiographic determination of neurotransmitter receptor distributions in the cerebral and cerebellar cortices, *J. Histochem. Cytochem.* **29:**125–135.

Wang, R., 1981, Dopaminergic neurons in the rat ventral tegmental area. III. Effects of *d* and *l*-amphetamine, *Brain Res. Rev.* **3:**153–165.

Warembourg, M., 1981, Localization of steroid receptors in the amygdaloid complex, in: *The Amygdaloid Complex* (Y. Ben-Ari, ed.), Elsevier, Amsterdam, pp. 203–208.

Wassef, M., Berod, A., and Sotelo, C., 1981, Dopaminergic dendrites in the pars reticulata of the rat substantia nigra and their striatal input: Combined immunocytochemical localization of tyrosine hydroxylase and anterograde degeneration, *Neuroscience* **6:**2125–2139.

Waterhouse, B. D., and Woodward, D. J., 1980, Interaction of norepinephrine with cerebrocortical activity evoked by stimulation of somatosensory afferent pathways in the rat, *Exp. Neurol.* **67:**11–34.

Waterhouse, B. D., Lin, C. S., Burne, R. A., and Woodward, D. J., 1983, The distribution of neocortical projection neurons in the locus coeruleus, *J. Comp. Neurol.* **217:**418–431.

White, F. J., and Wang, R. Y., 1984, Interactions of cholecystokinin octapeptide and dopamine on nucleus accumbens neurons, *Brain Res.* **300:**161–166.

Widerlov, E., and Breese, G. R., 1982, Actions of neurotensin on dopaminergic and serotonergic pathways in rat brain, *Proc. N.Y. Acad. Sci.* **77:**428–430.

Wiklund, L., Leger, L., and Persson M., 1980, Monoamine cell distribution in the cat brain stem: A fluorescence histochemical study with quantification of indolaminergic and locus coeruleus cell groups, *J. Comp. Neurol.* **203:**613–647.

Williams, M. N., and Faull, R. L., 1985, The striatonigral projection and nigrostriatal neurons in the rat: A correlated light and electron microscopic study demonstrating a monosynaptic striatal input to identified nigrotectal neurons using a combined degeneration and horseradish peroxidase procedure, *Neuroscience* **14:**991–1010.

Wilson, C. J., and Phelan, K. D., 1982, Dual topographic representation of neostriatum in the globus pallidus of rats, *Brain Res.* **243:**354–359.

Wise, S. P., and Strick, P. L., 1984, Anatomical and physiological organization of the nonprimary motor cortex, *Trends Neurosci.* **7:**442–446.

Wolf, M. E., Galloway, M. P., and Roth, R. H., 1986, Regulation of dopamine synthesis in the medial prefrontal cortex: Studies in brain slices, *J. Pharmacol. Exp. Ther.* **236:**699–707.

Wyss, J. M., Swanson, L. W., and Cowan, W. M., 1979, A study of subcortical afferents to the hippocampal formation in the rat, *Neuroscience* **4:**463–476.

Yahr, M. R. (ed.), 1976, *The Basal Ganglia*, Raven Press, New York.

Yarbrough, G., and Lake, N., 1973, The role of calcium in monamine induced depression of cerebral cortical neurones, *Life Sci.* **13:**703–711.

Yarbrough, G. G., Lake, N., and Phillis, J. W., 1974, Calcium antagonism and its effect on the inhibitory actions of biogenic amines on cerebral cortical neurones, *Brain Res.* **67:**77–88.

Yeterian, E. H., and van Hoesen, G. W., 1978, Cortico-striate projections in the rhesus monkey: The organization of certain cortico-caudate connections, *Brain Res.* **139:**43–63.

Young, W. S., and Kuhar, M. J., 1980a, Noradrenergic, alpha$_1$ and alpha$_2$ receptors: Light microscopic autoradiographic localization, *Proc. Natl. Acad. Sci. USA* **77:**1696–1700.

Young, W. S., and Kuhar, M. J., 1980b, Serotonin receptor localization in rat brain by light microscopic autoradiography, *Eur. J. Pharmacol.* **62:**237–239.

Zornetzer, S., Abraham, W., and Appleton, R., 1978, Locus coeruleus and labile memory, *Pharmacol. Biochem. Behav.* **9:**227–234.

3

Cholinergic Innervation in Cerebral Cortex

FELIX ECKENSTEIN and ROBERT W. BAUGHMAN

1. Introduction

This chapter summarizes current knowledge about the anatomical organization of cholinergic innervation in cerebral cortex. Many investigations over the last five decades have contributed to establishing ACh as a neurotransmitter in cerebral cortex. It was realized early that cerebral cortex contains all of the components of cholinergic metabolism in moderately high amounts, including ACh itself, the ACh-synthesizing enzyme choline acetyltransferase (ChAT, EC 2.3.1.6), and the ACh-degrading enzyme acetylcholinesterase (AChE, EC 3.1.1.7). Later, the presence in cortex of both muscarinic and nicotinic binding sites (probably reflecting ACh receptors) was described (for review see Fonnum, 1973, 1975; Kuhar, 1976; Emson and Lindvall, 1979; Fibiger, 1982; Parnavelas and McDonald, 1983). Cortical synaptosomes, subcellular fractions containing mainly isolated synaptic complexes, have been shown to contain ACh, ChAT, AChE, and sodium-dependent high-affinity choline uptake (HACU) (Yamamura and Snyder, 1973; Kuhar and Murrin, 1978), and ACh can be released from cortex *in vivo* (Mitchell, 1963: Collier and Mitchell, 1966) and from synaptosomes in a Ca^{2+}-dependent manner (Kuhar and Murrin, 1978). Many studies have investigated the pharmacological and physiological effects of ACh in cortex (Krnjević

FELIX ECKENSTEIN and ROBERT W. BAUGHMAN • Department of Neurobiology, Harvard Medical School, Boston, Massachusetts 02115. *Present address of F.E.:* Department of Neurology, Oregon Health Sciences University, Portland, Oregon 97201.

and Phillis, 1963a–c; Crawford, 1970; Lamour *et al.*, 1982b). Altogether, the evidence strongly suggests that ACh acts as a neurotransmitter in cerebral cortex, although the complex anatomical organization of this tissue has not permitted experiments as straightforward and conclusive as those that have characterized cholinergic transmission at the neuromuscular junction.

In contrast to this large body of biochemical, pharmacological, and physiological data, our knowledge of the anatomical features underlying cholinergic transmission in cortex until recently was limited, mainly because specific anatomical methods for localizing cholinergic neurons were not available. This review will concentrate on recent immunocytochemical studies that have importantly added to our understanding of cholinergic innervation in cerebral cortex. The focus will be on rat cortex, since studies on this species are particularly advanced.

2. The Specificity of Markers for Cholinergic Neurons

In addition to ACh itself, the mechanisms associated with ACh metabolism (ChAT, AChE, and HACU) provide possible markers for cholinergic neurons, and in fact all of these have been tested. It has become evident, however, that not all of these markers are equally reliable. For example, some of them are not restricted to cholinergic neurons, which of course can lead to erroneous identifications.

ACh is the most obvious marker, and so far no evidence of its presence in noncholinergic neurons has been reported. On the other hand, ACh is synthesized by several types of nonneuronal cells, including Schwann cells at the frog neuromuscular junction following nerve section (Birks *et al.*, 1960), the primate placenta and sperm (Chang and Gaddum, 1933), as well as bacteria and plants (Hebb and Krnjević, 1962). Within neuronal populations, however, ACh appears to be a reliable marker for cholinergic function. Anatomical localization of endogenous ACh could not be achieved, as no fixative is known that retains ACh within tissue [although this recently may have been achieved (Geffard *et al.*, 1984)]. The use of other anatomical markers for localizing cholinergic neurons has therefore received much attention.

AChE is an enzyme that relatively specifically hydrolyzes ACh to choline and acetate. As a result of the pioneering work of Koelle and Friedenwald (1949), AChE can be easily localized by histochemical methods. With the use of specific inhibitors that have become available, it is possible to characterize the type of esterase giving rise to the observed staining (for review see Main, 1976). Further improvements of the original technique, allowing clear visualization of AChE-positive cell bodies, also have been introduced (Nichols and Koelle, 1967; Butcher, 1978). The long availability and ease of use of this technique have led to a vast literature on AChE localization, but there are concerns about its reliability as a cholinergic marker. In two recent studies of forebrain nuclei in the rat (Eckenstein and Sofroniew, 1983; Levey *et al.*, 1983b), most ChAT-positive neurons were found also to contain AChE, but the distribution of AChE through the brain does not completely parallel that of other cholinergic markers. For example, high AChE levels have been found in areas containing little ACh or ChAT, such as the cerebellum (Hoover *et al.*, 1978). In addition, the catecholaminergic neurons of the substantia nigra and the locus coeruleus, and the serotonergic neurons in the brain stem have been shown to stain heavily for AChE (Butcher *et al.*, 1975), as do some ChAT-negative but AChE-positive neurons in the forebrain (Eckenstein and Sofroniew, 1983; Levey *et al.*, 1983b). The physiological significance of AChE not directly associated with cholinergic structures is unknown. It has been hypothesized that some neurons receiving cholinergic input might express AChE (McGeer *et al.*, 1974). The observation that AChE is able to hydrolyze, at a somewhat slow rate, certain neuroactive peptides (Chubb *et al.*, 1980) might imply enzyme functions not associated with cholinergic transmission. In any event, it is obvious that AChE alone cannot be employed as a marker for cholinergic structures, although it might serve as a useful tool if supported by other data.

HACU replenishes choline in cholinergic neurons after release of ACh, and it appears that this system is mainly localized in cholinergic synapses (Yamamura and Snyder, 1973; Kuhar and Murrin, 1978). Localization of HACU requires a sophisticated technique, since, like ACh, choline cannot be fixed within the tissue with normal histological procedures. Dry autoradiography of freeze-dried tissue has been employed to identify the structures accumulating radiolabeled choline by means of HACU (Baughman and Bader, 1977), but the difficulty of this technique has limited the number of studies undertaken. The correlation between ACh, ChAT, and HACU is reasonably good, but the observation that HACU is found in noncholinergic photoreceptors in rabbit retina (Masland and Mills, 1979) and in some nonneuronal cells in tissue culture (Barrald and Berg, 1978), raises concern about the specificity of HACU as a marker for cholinergic neurons.

Reliable, relatively simple methods for biochemical measurement of ACh, ChAT, AChE, and HACU in small quantities of tissue are available, and another approach to studying the distribution of cholinergic markers in the CNS has been to measure the concentration of each marker in microdissected areas (Hoover *et al.*, 1978) When combined with lesions, this approach can provide information about cholinergic projection patterns (Fonnum, 1973; Hoover and Jacobowitz, 1979; Johnston *et al.*, 1979; Lehmann *et al.*, 1980). Although this technique is limited in that it does not identify the precise type of cholinergic structure present, it has provided much basically accurate data that have been confirmed by more precise, recent studies based on immunocytochemistry of ChAT.

ChAT synthesizes ACh from acetyl-*S*-coenzyme A and choline. The mammalian enzyme appears to consist of a single polypeptide chain with a molecular weight around 68,000 (Rossier, 1977; Eckenstein *et al.*, 1981). [The observation of multiple molecular weight forms (Cozzarri and Hartman, 1980; Dietz and Salvaterra, 1980) may be due to limited proteolysis during the purification.] No other mechanism has been reported so far to synthesize ACh efficiently. ChAT appears to have a specificity for cholinergic neurons similar to that of ACh, and the distribution of the two markers throughout the brain is similar (Kuhar, 1976;

Hoover *et al.*, 1978). No evidence so far suggests the presence of ChAT in noncholinergic neurons, but like ACh, ChAT is found in primate placenta (Comline, 1946), sperm, plants, and bacteria (Hebb and Krnjević, 1962).

The first attempts to localize ChAT were based on histochemical procedures (Kasa *et al.*, 1970; Burt, 1970). Although at first the results seemed promising, it became obvious that the methods used were not specific for ChAT (for review see Rossier, 1977). The approach of raising specific antibodies to ChAT, which can be used for immunohistochemical detection of the enzyme, has been more successful. ChAT is present at very low concentrations, and thus very high purification factors are needed to obtain preparations suitable for production of specific antisera (Eckenstein *et al.*, 1981; Eckenstein and Thoenen, 1982). For this reason the results of some early studies, using antisera raised against incompletely purified ChAT (Chao and Wolfgram, 1973; Singh and McGeer, 1974), have been questioned (Rossier, 1977). By using more sophisticated purification protocols or the monoclonal antibody technique (Eckenstein and Thoenen, 1982; Crawford *et al.*, 1982; Levey *et al.*, 1983a), these problems seem to have been overcome.

For the reader's ease, in discussing immunohistochemical staining of ChAT we will use the terms *ChAT-positive* and *ChAT-containing* instead of the more precise but cumbersome term *ChAT-like-immunoreactivity-positive*, and the like. We have also chosen, for the reasons outlined earlier in this section, to consider ChAT-positive neurons as cholinergic and to discuss them accordingly.

3. The Anatomical Characterization of Cholinergic Innervation in Cortex

ACh, ChAT, AChE, and HACU are found at levels high enough to indicate cholinergic activity throughout cerebral cortex (see above). Within a single cortical region, ChAT activity, measured in microdissected horizontal slabs, appears to vary maximally threefold from pia to white matter (Beesley and Emson, 1975; Johnston *et al.*, 1981b; Parnavelas and McDonald, 1983). This diffuse, widespread presence of cholinergic markers has been taken to indicate that ACh might have some very general effect in cortex, such as arousal (Celesia and Jasper, 1966; Phillis, 1968). The anatomical characterization of cholinergic structures is a key element in determining the role of ACh in cerebral cortex.

On the basis of ChAT immunohistochemistry, in some cases combined with retrograde labeling techniques employing fluorescent dyes and horseradish peroxidase, three anatomically different cholinergic systems have been found in rat cerebral cortex. Two of the systems originate in nuclei of the forebrain and midbrain, respectively, while the third is an intrinsic cortical system. So far, only the subcortical projection systems have been conclusively demonstrated in species other than the rat. The experiments demonstrating intrinsic cortical cholinergic neurons are technically difficult, however, and more work is required to establish whether these neurons are present in species other than the rat. We will consider the evidence for the three systems separately, and propose some hypotheses for their function in the Discussion.

3.1. The Cholinergic Projection from Magnocellular Forebrain Nuclei to Cerebral Cortex

The preparation *in vivo* of chronically isolated cortical areas by undercutting of the cortex has been found to reduce ChAT activity in the isolated areas by as much as 90% (Hebb *et al.*, 1968; Green *et al.*, 1970; Johnston *et al.*, 1981a; for review see Emson and Lindvall, 1979; Parnavelas and McDonald, 1983). This suggests that the majority of cholinergic cortical innervation originates in sub-cortical areas. Undercutting, however, did not lead to the total disappearance of ChAT activity, which might be accounted for by incomplete deafferentation, the presence of intrinsic cortical cholinergic neurons, or the presence of cholinergic fibers reaching the cortex from the pia (see below).

Shute and Lewis (1963), in their pioneer work using AChE histochemistry, concluded that the heavily AChE-stained magnocellular neurons found in the globus pallidus, the entopeduncular nucleus, and the lateral preoptic area of the rat project to neocortex. This observation was later confirmed and extended in the rat (Lehman *et al.*, 1980; Bigl *et al.*, 1982) and the monkey (Mesulam and Van Hoesen, 1976) by simultaneous localization of HRP retrogradely transported from cortex, with AChE staining. Double-labeled neurons were most numerous in the nucleus basalis of Meynert (NBM), but some were also observed in the globus pallidus and the nucleus of the diagonal band. These neurons have large, multipolar cell bodies of up to 30- to 40-μm diameter and some of their dendrites can be followed for over 200 μm. In the rat (Fig. 1), these nuclei form a diffuse network throughout the entire basal forebrain; the borders of the individual nuclei are not well defined. In contrast, the corresponding nuclei in primates seem to be more tightly organized and anatomically better defined.

As described above, AChE is not completely reliable as a cholinergic marker, but subsequent studies have confirmed the cholinergic nature of the NBM projection to cortex. There is a high level of ChAT activity in the magnocellular nuclei of the forebrain (Brownstein *et al.*, 1975; Hoover *et al.*,1978) and after electrolytic or chemical lesions of the NBM there is a marked decrease of ChAT and AChE activity and HACU (Johnston *et al.*, 1979, 1981a,b; Lehmann *et al.*, 1980; Wenk *et al.*, 1980; Pedata *et al.*, 1982) in the ipsilateral cortex. Most convincingly, with the advent of ChAT immunohistochemistry, neurons staining for ChAT were found in the magnocellular forebrain nuclei of the rat (Kimura *et al.*, 1980; Sofroniew *et al.*, 1982; Armstrong *et al.*, 1983; Houser *et al.*, 1983), cat (Kimura *et al.*, 1981; Wahle *et al.*, 1984), and monkey (Mesulam *et al.*, 1983a; Hendreen *et al.*, 1983) with a frequency and morphology similar to those of the AChE-positive cells; and with double-labeling techniques at least 80–90% of the AChE-rich neurons also stain for ChAT (Eckenstein and Sofroniew, 1983; Levey *et al.*, 1983b) (Fig. 2). The projection of these cells to cortex has been confirmed by the colocalization of ChAT or AChE with either HRP (Mesulam *et al.*, 1983a,b; Wahle *et al.*, 1984; Fig. 3) or fluorescent dyes (Woolf *et al.*, 1983) in cells retrogradely labeled following cortical injections (Fig. 4). Very recently the presence of the neuropeptide galanin has been observed in some of the cholinergic basal forebrain neurons (Melander *et al.*, 1985).

Many current efforts are centered on achieving a more detailed anatomical analysis of the magnocellular projection to cortex. One question is whether

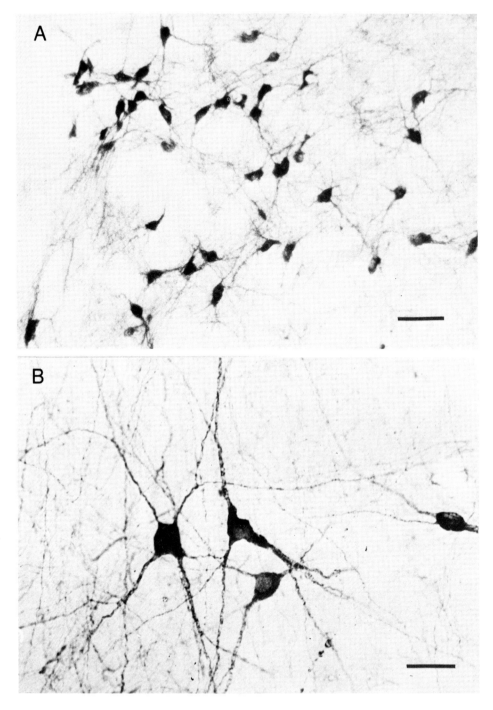

Figure 1. Photomicrographs of rat basal forebrain sections stained for ChAT immunoreactivity. Numerous cells in the basal nucleus of Meynert (A, B) and the diagonal band of Broca (C, D) are heavily stained. These cells have large, fusiform somata (30–40 μm in diameter) and multiple dendrites, which taper off gradually from the cell body. Bars = 80 μm (A, C), 40 μm (B, D).

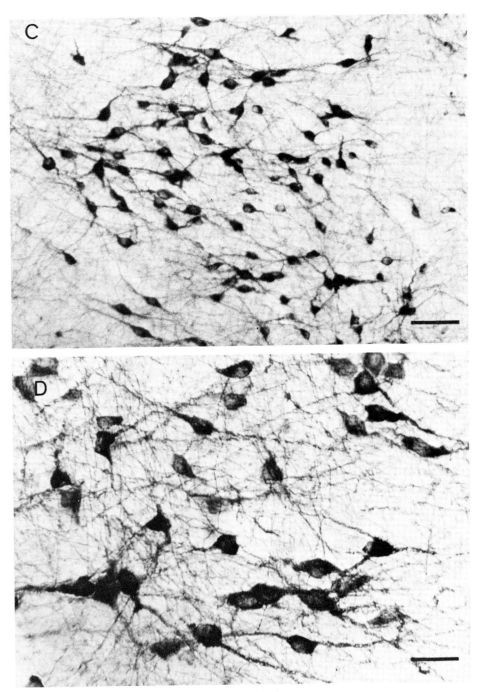

Figure 1. (*continued*)

cholinergic neurons, in particular magnocellular nuclei, project in an ordered manner to restricted cortical areas. Retrograde labeling with fluorescent dyes and HRP (see below) clearly demonstrate topological order in the projections (Bigl *et al.*, 1982; Lamour *et al.*, 1982a; Mesulam *et al.*, 1983a,b; McKinney *et al.*, 1983; Saper, 1984). Anterograde studies based on lesioning the basal forebrain and measuring the decrease in ChAT activity in cortex have cruder resolution,

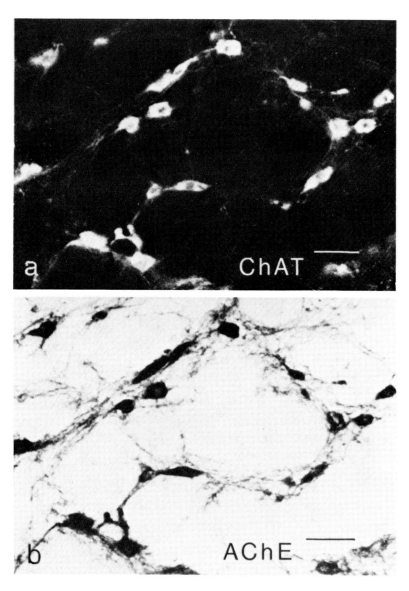

Figure 2. Photomicrographs of the basal nucleus of Meynert of the rat, stained for ChAT immunoreactivity (a) and AChE (b). All ChAT-positive neurons in this area contain AChE as well, and all AChE-positive neurons stain for ChAT. ChAT was localized by immunofluorescence and photographed; the same section was then stained with a histochemical method for AChE and rephotographed. Bars = 50 μm. From Eckenstein and Sofroniew (1983) with permission.

but reach the same conclusion (Hartgraves *et al.*, 1982). Studies using autoradiographic visualization of anterogradely transported [³H]proline (Nauta, 1979) have given some idea of the detailed pattern of the projection, but the most informative results have come from anterograde transport studies with HRP coupled to wheat germ agglutinin (HRP–WGA) (Lamour *et al.*, 1984), which demonstrate that in most cortical areas the majority of the basal forebrain input is concentrated in layers 5 and 6. Studies with agglutinins (lectins) have the advantage that projection fibers are directly visualized, but they have the disadvantage that they are not specific to cholinergic neurons. The HRP–WGA technique may in principle permit the ultrastructural analysis of postsynaptic targets in cortex.

The results of the tracing studies suggest that there is a clear, but not yet completely characterized topological order in the projection from basal forebrain to cortex. Cells labeled retrogradely from cortex usually are found in more than one magnocellular nucleus, but the nuclei appear to have a limited preference as to the extent to which they innervate cortical areas. The most detailed analysis of this topographical organization was performed by Saper (1984) in the rat. In this study, most of the techniques cited above were used. Saper concluded that both the previously proposed rostrocaudal organization (Wenk *et al.*, 1980; Bigl *et al.*, 1982; McKinney *et al.*, 1983; Price and Stern, 1983), and the idea that the basal forebrain nuclei are divided into those innervating neocortex and those innervating allocortex (Lehmann *et al.*, 1980), are not fully compatible with his observations. Instead, he proposed that cholinergic basal forebrain projection neurons innervating specific cortical areas are organized on the basis of a reciprocal, descending corticodiencephalic projection. That is, the ascending basal forebrain projection is topographically mirrored by a descending corticofugal projection. In addition, he concluded that the basal forebrain axons take two different pathways, a diffuse lateral and a more confined medial to reach cortex. We recently have obtained direct evidence for these two pathways by ChAT immunohistochemistry (Eckenstein and Baughman, manuscript submitted, Fig. 5).

More observations are required, however, to confirm Saper's proposal for reciprocal, descending projections from cortex to basal forebrain. This is especially true in view of the observation of Mesulam and Mufson (1984) that the basal forebrain cholinergic neurons of the monkey appear to receive input from only a limited number of cortical areas. In this context a study of the topography of the cholinergic basal forebrain innervation of the hippocampus (Amaral *et al.*, 1984) is relevant. Amaral *et al.* (1984) made a very small HRP injection in the hippocampus and then analyzed the distribution of retrogradely labeled ChAT-positive cells in the basal forebrain. In order to obtain a fine-grained resolution of the projection pattern, over 35 animals were used. It was observed that the septal area could be subdivided into at least four distinct nuclei, all preferentially innervating specific hippocampal areas, and that, in addition, topographical organization was present within each nucleus. These findings suggest that the basal forebrain projections may be much more precise than originally thought. The proposal of a new nomenclature (Mesulam *et al.*, 1983b) for the cholinergic basal forebrain nuclei thus appears to be justified, but additional refinements will likely be required as more precise anatomical data become available. Once the basal forebrain cholinergic cell groups can be defined ac-

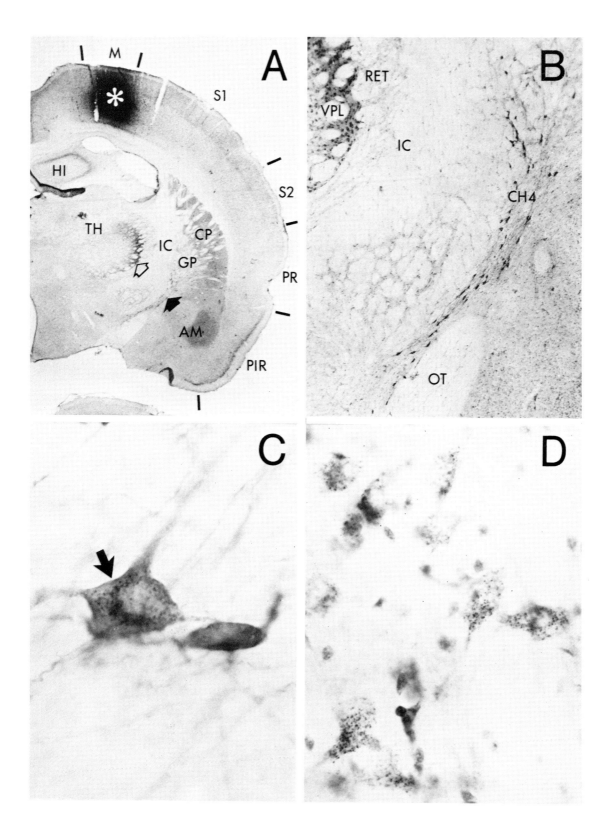

cording to their input and projection patterns, we will be closer to understanding the physiological importance of this system.

In addition to learning about the overall topographical order of projections, it is also of interest to know the size of the cortical area innervated by a single basal forebrain neuron. This question has been addressed directly in several studies (Price and Stern, 1983; McKinney *et al.*, 1983; Saper, 1984) by similar methods. Briefly, two different fluorescent dyes were injected into adjacent cortical areas and the percentage of neurons retrogradely labeled with both dyes was analyzed. Two studies (Price and Stern, 1983; Saper, 1984) concluded that the diameter of the innervated cortical area was small, less than 1.5 mm in diameter, while one study (McKinney *et al.*, 1983) demonstrated evidence for a larger area. In view of the technical difficulties of restricting the size of the marker injection site, and at the same time obtaining adequate retrograde labeling of cell bodies, the available data are most consistent with each basal forebrain neuron having only a small area of innervation in cortex. More work, however, is clearly needed in this area.

3.2. The Cholinergic Projection from Midbrain to Frontal Cerebral Cortex

In addition to the basal forebrain system, two other putative cholinergic projections were discovered by Shute and Lewis (1967). These two projections,

←———————————————————————————————————————

Figure 3. Cholinergic projections to neocortex in the rat: a combination of retrograde tracing and immunocytochemical localization of ChAT. An injection of horseradish peroxidase–wheat germ agglutinin was placed in motor cortex. Following a 48-hr survival period the brain was perfusion fixed, the retrograde tracer was visualized with cobalt intensification of the diaminobenzidine chromogen followed by immunocytochemical localization of ChAT using the peroxidase–antiperoxidase method according to the procedure of Wainer and Rye (B. H. Wainer and D. B. Rye, 1984, Retrograde horseradish peroxidase tracing combined with localization of choline acetyltransferase immunoreactivity, *J. Histochem. Cytochem.* **32**:439–443), and the sections were lightly counterstained with thionin. In (A), a low-power photomicrograph (10×) illustrates the injection site (white asterisk) in motor cortex (M) as well as retrogradely labeled neurons in the ventral posterolateral (VPL) nucleus of the thalamus (TH) (open arrowhead) and retrogradely labeled and immunostained cholinergic neurons of the CH4 group of the basal forebrain (closed arrowhead). At this level the CH4 neurons are ventromedial to the globus pallidus (GP) and ventral to the internal capsule (IC). Other abbreviations are: S1, primary somatosensory cortex; S2, secondary somatosensory cortex; PR, perirhinal cortex; PIR, piriform cortex; AM, amygdala; CP, caudate putamen; HI, hippocampus. In (B), a higher-power photomicrograph (40×) shows retrogradely labeled cells in the VPL and retrogradely labeled/immunostained cells of CH4. Additional abbreviations are: RET, reticular nucleus of the thalamus; and OT, optic tract. In (C), a high-power photomicrograph (750×) shows a retrogradely labeled (dark granular reaction product) and immunostained (diffuse reaction product) cholinergic neuron of CH4 (arrow). This cell is adjacent to another ChAT-positive neuron that does not contain retrograde label. In (D), a high-power photomicrograph (600×) shows VPL neurons that are labeled only for retrograde tracer. The photomicrographs were provided by Bruce H. Wainer and David B. Rye, and material is derived from a recent combination retrograde tracing/ChAT immunocytochemical study of the topography of cholinergic–cortical projections (D. B. Rye, B. H. Wainer, M.-M. Mesulam, E. J. Mufson, and C. B. Saper, 1984, Cortical projections arising from the basal forebrain: A study of cholinergic and non-cholinergic components applying combined retrograde tracing and immunohistochemical localization of choline acetyltransferase, *Neuroscience* **13**:627–643).

originating in the midbrain and innervating more frontal areas including thalamus and basal forebrain, were termed the ventral and dorsal tegmental pathways of the ascending cholinergic reticular system. The evidence was based on AChE histochemistry and the observation that, after lesioning of an AChE-containing fiber tract, the enzyme accumulates on the side of the cut proximal to the origin of the severed fibers, whereas the enzyme activity of the distal side appears to decrease. Thus, by placing cuts at different levels through the medial forebrain bundle (MFB), Shute and Lewis (1967) were able to trace the AChE-containing fiber bundles innervating the forebrain back to their origin in the midbrain. It was clearly demonstrated that the strongly AChE-positive neurons found in such midbrain locations as the substantia nigra, the tegmental area, and the reticular formation projected to various thalamic, hypothalamic, and forebrain areas. No direct innervation of cerebral cortex by this so-called ascending reticular cholinergic system could be demonstrated, largely because of the difficulty in differentiating a minor midbrain contribution to the major AChE-rich projection to cortex from the various magnocellular forebrain nuclei. Nonetheless, the observation that electrical stimulation of the reticular formation leads to an increased release of ACh from cortex (Kanai and Szerb, 1965; Celesia

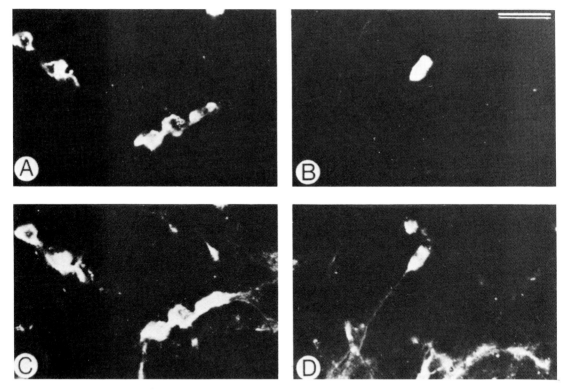

Figure 4. Photomicrographs demonstrating the colocalization of a fluorescent dye (A, B), transported retrogradely from cerebral cortex in ChAT-positive (C, D) neurons in the basal nucleus of Meynert. Propidium iodide was used as retrograde marker and fluorescein-labeled antibodies were used for the immunofluorescent localization of ChAT, permitting simultaneous localization of the two stains in the same structure. Bar = 50 μm. From Woolf *et al.* (1983) with permission.

and Jasper, 1966; Phillis, 1968) was cited as evidence for a cholinergic ascending reticular projection.

Subsequently, however. monoamines were demonstrated to be present in many of the AChE-rich midbrain neurons by the work of Butcher *et al.* (1975). Using a combination of (1) formaldehyde-induced fluorescence to demonstrate monoamines and (2) AChE histochemistry, neurons in the substantia nigra were shown to contain both AChE and dopamine. In addition, lesions of the MFB led to a decrease of tyrosine hydroxylase, a marker for catecholaminergic structures, and not ChAT in frontal cortex (Fonnum *et al.,* 1977). The existence of a direct cholinergic projection from midbrain to cortex was therefore considered to be unlikely (Emson and Lindvall, 1979).

On the other hand, MFB lesions did lead to a decrease of ChAT in subcortical forebrain areas (Hoover and Jacobowitz, 1979), and recently ChAT-positive neurons resembling the AChE-stained neurons (Armstrong *et al.,* 1983; Fig. 6) were found in the mesencephalic tegmental area and the reticular formation. Mesulam *et al.* (1983b), by combining ChAT staining with localization of retrogradely transported HRP, demonstrated that some of these cholinergic neurons project to frontal cortex. Earlier, a projection from these midbrain areas to frontal cortex by neurons staining for the neuropeptide substance P (SP) was described (Sakanaka *et al.,* 1983). This led Vincent *et al.* (1983) to carry out an elegant study to identify the targets of these tegmental cells. A fluorescent dye, True Blue, was used to label retrogradely neurons projecting to medial frontal cortex, followed by immunofluorescent localization of ChAT, using fluorescein-labeled second antibodies. Many unequivocally double-labeled neurons were observed in the reticular formation and tegmentum. In addition, Vincent *et al.* (1983) demonstrated, using rhodamine-labeled second antibodies, that more than 30% of the retrogradely labeled, ChAT-positive neurons also stained for SP. As the three dyes—True Blue, fluorescein, and rhodamine—fluoresce at different wavelength, it was possible to localize them simultaneously (Fig. 7). Colchicine, an axonal transport blocker, was needed to accumulate SP to a detectable level in the tegmental neurons, and it is possible that, despite the treatment, some cells still contained subthreshold levels of SP. The percentage of ChAT and SP coexistence thus might be even higher than 30%. Recently, it has been confirmed that many ChAT-positive midbrain neurons innervate thalamic and basal forebrain areas (McGurk *et al.,* 1984; Sofroniew *et al.,* 1985).

In conclusion, there is convincing evidence of a cholinergic contribution to the AChE-positive system originating in the midbrain, although the system is largely monoaminergic. The cholinergic component is directed largely into the thalamus and basal forebrain, although medial frontal cortex is also innervated. The restriction of the midbrain cholinergic system to one area of cortex, in contrast to the basal forebrain system that diffusely innervates all of cortex suggests that these two pathways have different functions.

3.3. Intrinsic Cholinergic Neurons in Cerebral Cortex

Chronic isolation of cortical tissue by undercutting leads to a marked decrease in ChAT activity, reaching up to 70% in the rat, and up to 90% in the cat (for review see Emson and Lindvall, 1979; Fibiger, 1982; Parnavelas and McDonald, 1983). As described above, this approach has led to the identification of cholinergic projections to cortex. Considering the wealth of data confirming these findings, the result of one study (McGeer *et al.*, 1977), demonstrating no loss of cortical ChAT following undercutting, appears erroneous. In all the studies, however, a small amount of ChAT activity was found to persist in the isolated tissue. It is difficult to achieve complete deafferentation, and therefore the low ChAT levels persisting might result from a few nonsevered cholinergic fibers still reaching the undercut area. Such fibers might even be of peripheral origin, reaching cortex by following blood vessels from the pia, a hypothesis discussed by Fibiger (1982). To our knowledge, no evidence in support of this has so far been presented. The idea that cerebral cortex itself might contain cholinergic neuronal cell bodies was viewed with skepticism (Fibiger, 1982), mainly based on the absence of intensely AChE-positive cortical neurons, al-

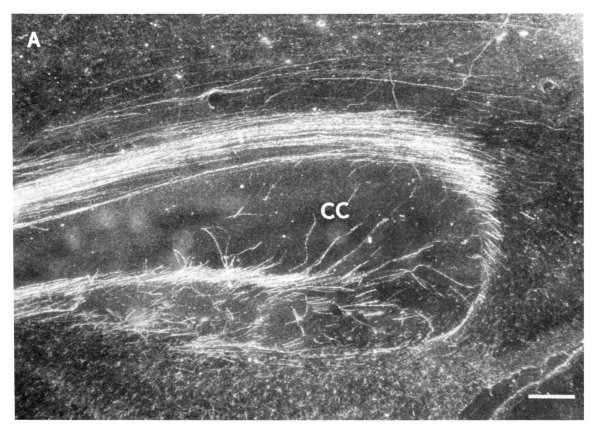

Figure 5. Darkfield photomicrographs showing the two main pathways by which cholinergic, ChAT-positive fibers reach cerebral cortex in the rat. The medial pathway (A), originating in the diagonal band of Broca, extends around the genu of the corpus callosum (CC) and runs caudally in the cingulate bundle. This panel shows the ChAT-positive fibers at the caudal pole of the corpus callosum. The lateral path-way (B) is taken mainly by the cholinergic neurons of the basal nucleus of Meynert. Their axons fan out laterally through the caudate (CD) to the corpus callosum (CC), which they then appear to follow for some distance before turning into cortex (CX). The medial pathway consists of a discrete fiber-bundle, whereas the lateral pathway fans out diffusely through the entire caudate. Bars = 100 μm.

though some lightly stained cell bodies are observed. On the other hand, kainic acid injections into cortex were reported to reduce cortical ChAT by up to 30% (Johnston *et al.*, 1981a), although these data in some cases were not confirmed (Fibiger, 1982). A reduction in ChAT could suggest the presence of intrinsic cholinergic cortical neurons, since kainic acid is thought to lead to degeneration of cell bodies only, in the injected area, and not of fibers and terminals. It is of course possible that ChAT would be reduced in a terminal that innervated a now-degenerated target. An anatomical method for identifying ChAT-containing structures is clearly desirable to resolve such issues.

In early study that used indirect immunofluorescence to localize ChAT in rat cortex, most neurons appeared to be stained (McGeer *et al.*, 1974). This result was questioned by Rossier (Rossier, 1977) on the basis of the apparent lack of specificity of the ChAT antiserum used. More recent experiments (Eckenstein *et al.*, 1981) have demonstrated the validity of Rossier's arguments concerning specificity. In subsequent studies, employing either monoclonal (Armstrong *et al.*, 1983) or specific polyclonal (Sofroniew *et al.*, 1982) antibodies, no ChAT-positive perikarya were found in rat cerebral cortex and only terminals were observed in cat cortex (Kimura *et al.*, 1981). More recently, however, when we (Eckenstein and Thoenen, 1983; Eckenstein and Baughman, 1984) and Houser

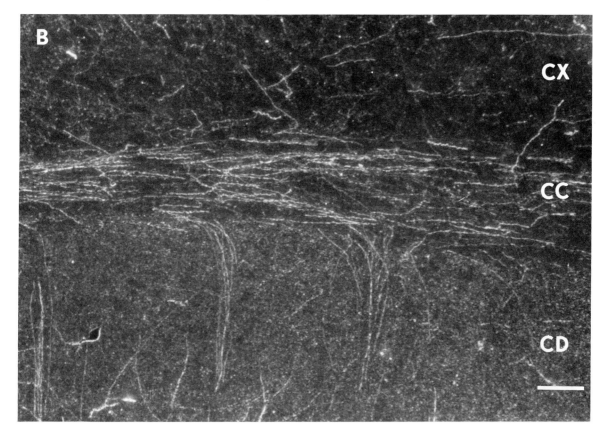

Figure 5. (*continued*)

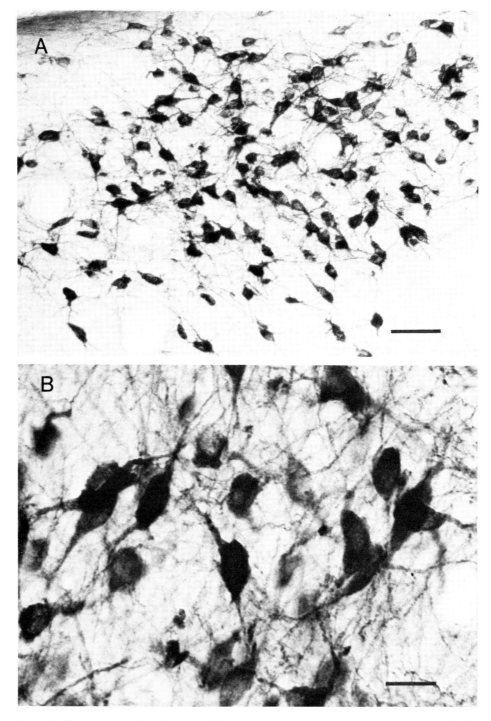

Figure 6. Photomicrographs of the rat midbrain tegmentum, stained immunohistochemically for ChAT. Numerous strongly ChAT-positive, multipolar neurons with large cell bodies (30–40 μm in diameter) are found in this area. The morphology of these cells is similar to that of the cholinergic neurons found in the basal forebrain. Bars = 80 μm (A), 30 μm (B).

et al. (1983) started to use highly sensitive staining methods, ChAT-positive cell bodies were found in rat cerebral cortex.

These cortical neurons are not observed with indirect immunofluorescence techniques (Coons, 1978) and are only faintly labeled by a peroxidase–antiperoxidase (PAP) (Sternberger, 1979) protocol. On the other hand, when the biotin–avidin technique (Hsu *et al.*, 1981) or a PAP-cycling protocol (Vacca *et al.*, 1980; Ordronneau *et al.*, 1981) is employed, strongly labeled cell bodies, fibers, and terminals are observed in cortex (Fig. 8). The stained neurons,

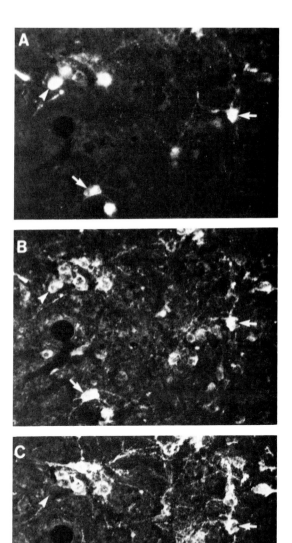

Figure 7. Photomicrographs demonstrating in neurons of the rat midbrain tegmentum, retrogradely labeled from frontal cortex (A), the colocalization of ChAT (B), and the neuropeptide substance P (C). Note that all SP-containing neurons stain also for ChAT, but appear to represent only a subpopulation of all the ChAT-containing neurons. The use of three different molecules fluorescing at different wavelengths made it possible to localize simultaneously SP, ChAT, and the retrograde marker True Blue. Bar = 50 μm. From Vincent *et al.* (1983) with permission.

representing about 1–2% of total cortical neurons, are found in all cortical areas and layers, but are more numerous in layers 2 and 3. The majority of stained neurons are bipolar in shape and have small, radially oriented cell bodies (7-μm diameter in the short axis, 13 μm in the long). They most commonly have two long, vertically running primary fibers (Fig. 9), but up to five fibers can be observed. These fibers, presumably representing dendrites, appear beaded toward their ends and span several layers; in general, the stained cells have direct contact with layers 1–5. In the deeper layers, some of the stained cells have a multipolar appearance. So far, ChAT-positive cortical neurons have only been reported in the rat; although we have made an effort to localize similar neurons in the monkey, we have only observed stained fibers and terminals. Whether this is due to a true species difference or to technical problems is not clear. The

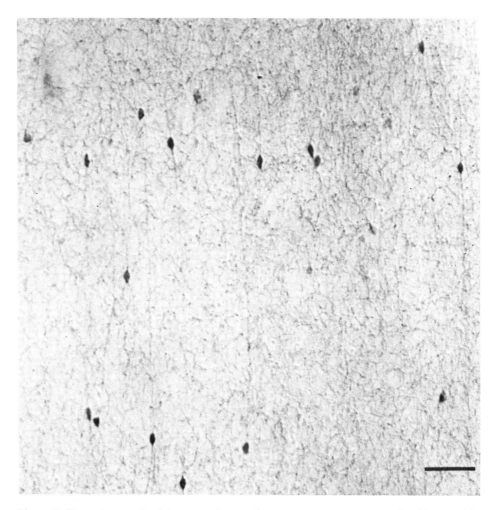

Figure 8. Photomicrograph of the upper layers of rat somatosensory cortex, stained immunohistochemically for ChAT. Small bipolar neurons with cell bodies of 10 to 13-μm diameter in the long axis are stained with moderate intensity. A dense network of stained fibers and terminals is also observed. Bar = 60 μm.

morphology of ChAT neurons in rat cortex is very similar to that of neurons containing vasoactive intestinal polypeptide (VIP) immunoreactivity (Loren *et al.*, 1979; McDonald *et al.*, 1982). We therefore investigated the possible coexistence of ChAT and VIP in these neurons by cutting 6-μm-thick serial sections of cortex and staining them alternately for the two antigens (Eckenstein and Baughman, 1984). Since the cells are larger than the section thickness, a single cell is represented in more than one section, which permits serial double labeling. By camera lucida analysis it was found that more than 80% of the ChAT-containing cells were also VIP-positive in an adjacent section (Fig. 10). The actual percentage of coexistence might be even higher in view of the technical difficulties of the method.

The physiological role of this ChAT–VIP coexistence is clearly of interest. We have observed in the light microscope many ChAT and VIP fibers in close association with cortical blood vessels. This observation was confirmed in the electron microscope, where many labeled structures were seen in close apposition with both capillaries and larger blood vessels (Fig. 11). Synaptic specializations ending on blood vessels, were not observed, however, for either VIP or ChAT, although numerous labeled synapses innervating neuronal profiles were observed. Although these anatomical data do not confirm the existence of functional connections with blood vessels, several observations support the idea that ACh and VIP might be coreleased onto cortical blood vessels to control per-

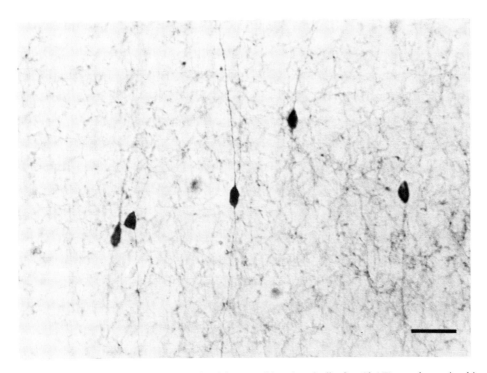

Figure 9. Bipolar cortical neurons stained immunohistochemically for ChAT are shown in this micrograph taken from layer 2 of rat somatosensory cortex. The stained neurons represent a minor fraction, about 1–2%, of all cortical cells. They have long dendrites, which in many cases span through cortical layers 1– 5. Bar = 25 μm.

meability or blood flow. For example, VIP and ACh dilate cerebral arteries (Larsson *et al.*, 1976; Iadecola *et al.*, 1983), and VIP receptors (Huang and Rorstod, 1983) and muscarinic receptors (Grammas *et al.*, 1983) have been demonstrated in preparations of cortical microvessels. Also, it has been shown that VIP is present in some peripheral cholinergic nerves (Lundberg *et al.*, 1982a), and one study (Lundberg *et al.*, 1982b) demonstrated a dramatic increase of muscarinic binding affinity in the presence of VIP. VIP in addition appears to stimulate glycogenolysis in cortical glial cells (Magistretti *et al.*, 1981), giving indirect evidence for involvement of the ChAT–VIP neurons in the control of local catabolic processes.

Cortical ChAT- and VIP-localization were studied in detail at the electron

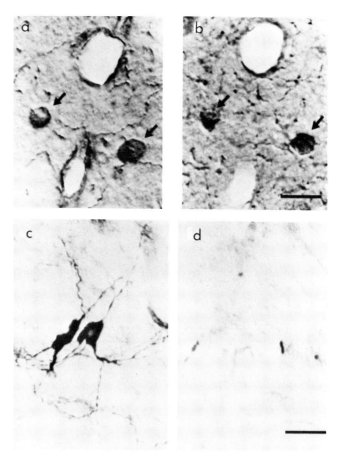

Figure 10. Photomicrographs demonstrating the colocalization of vasoactive intestinal polypeptide VIP(a) in the bipolar, ChAT-positive neurons (b) of rat cortex. Six-micrometer-thick serial sections were alternatively stained for VIP and ChAT. The sections were aligned by using blood vessels as landmarks. The two cells staining for ChAT in (a) (arrows) also contain VIP (b, arrows). Overall, more than 80% of the ChAT-positive cortical neurons contained VIP. In contrast to these neurons, the ChAT-positive cells in the basal nucleus of Meynert (c), which innervate cerebral cortex, do not stain for VIP (d). Bars = 10 μm (a, b), 20 μm (c, d). From Eckenstein and Baughman (1984) with permission.

microscopic level by Houser *et al.* (1985) and by Connor and Peters (1984), respectively. These authors similarly did not observe stained synaptic specializations contacting blood vessels. ChAT-positive synapses were mainly of the symmetric type and were found to contact many dendritic shafts of unidentified origin, pryamidal cell dendrites, and nonprymidal cell bodies. VIP synapses were found to share some characteristics of both symmetric and asymmetric terminals and to end predominantly on dendritic shafts.

In summary, ChAT-positive cholinergic cortical neurons have been observed only in the rat. The neuronal populations containing ChAT and VIP appear to be identical. In addition to acting on neurons, this system might be involved in control of blood flow. More information is clearly needed to ascertain the place of these neurons in cortical microcircuitry. The observation that the

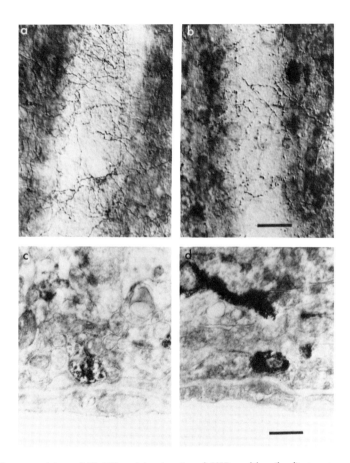

Figure 11. The apposition of ChAT-positive (a, c) and VIP-positive (b, d) structures with blood vessels in rat cerebral cortex. With the light microscope (a, b), many stained fibers are observed close to the lumen of a blood vessel, represented by the light area in the center of the field. No obvious increase, however, in the number of stained structures is observed in the vicinity of blood vessels. Electron microscopic analysis (c, d) indicates that the stained structures are in close apposition with cells of the blood vessel wall. No obvious synaptic specializations, however, are observed in the stained structures. Bars = 30 μm (a, b), 300 nm (c, d). From Eckenstein and Baughman (1984) with permission.

basal forebrain cholinergic projection does not contain VIP (Eckenstein and Baughman, 1984) might prove useful in this respect, as it offers a means to differentiate the two systems.

4. Discussion

The evidence for the existence of three different cholinergic systems in rat cortex has been discussed in detail above. In this section we will compare some features of these systems, propose some testable hypotheses concerning possible functions, and point out some still unanswered questions.

An important question is whether the three different cholinergic systems found in rat cortex are also present in other mammalian species, including primates and man. Thus far, all species examined have extrinsic cholinergic projections to cortex, but it is still unclear whether the intrinsic cholinergic cortical cells are present in species other than the rat.

Some features of the three cholinergic cortical systems of the rat are summarized and compared in Table I. One difference is the location of the cell bodies giving rise to each of the three systems. The intrinsic cortical ChAT–VIP neurons are found throughout the entire cortex, and they appear to innervate a restricted local area (Morrison *et al.*, 1984). The basal forebrain and midbrain cholinergic neurons must project several millimeters to reach their cortical targets. Both projection systems innervate noncortical CNS areas as well: the basal forebrain system projects to the hippocampus (Shute and Lewis, 1967; for review see Fibiger, 1982) and amygdala (Nagai *et al.*, 1982; Woolf and Butcher, 1982), and the midbrain projection innervates several subcortical targets, including basal forebrain and thalamus (Shute and Lewis, 1967; McGurk *et al.*, 1984; Sofroniew *et al.*, 1984). In terms of cortical projections, the cholinergic midbrain neurons appear to project exclusively to medial frontal cortex, whereas the basal forebrain system projects in a topographic manner to the entire cerebral cortex. It is not clear whether single projection neurons may innervate different areas by axon collaterals or whether these systems are composed of different subsystems innervating different areas. The area of cortex innervated by a single afferent neuron remains unknown, but an area 1.5 mm or less in diameter seems likely for the basal forebrain afferents (Price and Stern, 1983; Saper, 1984). An interesting possibility is that the two subcortical cholinergic projection systems may perform similar tasks in a variety of areas, including cortex, analogous to the widespread noradrenergic innervation of various CNS areas by the locus coeruleus (Moore and Bloom, 1979).

The source of innervation of the cholinergic neurons of the three systems is poorly characterized, although some evidence suggests the possibility that basal forebrain neurons receive reciprocal cortical input.

The recent discoveries that VIP, SP, and galanin immunoreactivities are found in cortical (Eckenstein and Baughman, 1984), midbrain (Vincent *et al.*, 1983), and basal forebrain ChAT neurons, respectively, raise some important questions. First, assuming that the peptides and ACh are coreleased, do ACh and the peptides act on identical targets? Although this seems likely at first, it is possible that ACh, which is broken down efficiently close to its site of release,

Table I. Comparison of the Three Known Types of Cholinergic Innervation in Cerebral Cortex

	I	II	III
Area of origin	Basal forebrain (extrinsic)	Midbrain (extrinsic)	Cortex (intrinsic)
Type of system	Projection, axons of several millimeters' length	Projection, axons of several millimeters' length	Local, short axons
Cortical areas innervated	Entire cortex	Medial frontal cortex	Entire cortex
Noncortical areas innervated	Hippocampus, olfactory bulb, amygdala	Thalamus, basal forebrain, spinal cord	None
Neuropeptide coexistence	Galanin	Substance P	Vasoactive intestinal polypeptide
Species differences	Found in all mammalian species studied	Found in all mammalian species studied	Found so far in rat and mouse only

might act locally, whereas the peptides might diffuse longer distances and exert their physiological action on a different target cell. Such an observation has been described for the sympathetic ganglion of the bullfrog (Jan and Jan, 1982). It is also important to know whether the peptides modulate the response to ACh. So far, VIP has been correlated with muscarinic (Lundberg *et al.*, 1982a,b), and SP with nicotinic (Belcher and Ryall, 1977; Krnjević and Lekic, 1977) mechanisms. These observations were made in the periphery and spinal cord, respectively. It will be interesting to see whether analogous physiological actions are found in cortex. The observation that peptides are correlated with some, but not all, cortical cholinergic systems raises the possibility of differentiating these systems anatomically. We have attempted in recent experiments to use VIP as a marker to decide which fractions of the ChAT-positive fibers are of intrinsic origin, by comparing VIP- and ChAT-stained serial sections under darkfield illumination. Preliminary results indicate that throughout cerebral cortex, the intrinsic cholinergic system, visualized by staining the VIP–ChAT bipolar cells for VIP, is relatively evenly distributed through all cortical layers, although it is somewhat less dense in layer 6. On the other hand, ChAT-positive terminals, which include both the intrinsic VIP–ChAT terminals and basal forebrain ter-

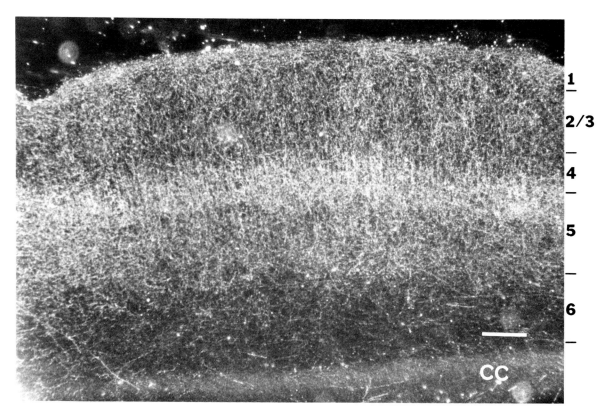

Figure 12. Low-power darkfield photomicrograph showing the distribution of ChAT-positive structures in rat visual cortex. Mainly fibers and terminals are observed, because of the tendency of darkfield illumination to preferentially reveal structures of small diameter. A band containing a high concentration of stained structures is seen at the border of cortical layers 4 and 5, and only few stained structures are observed in cortical layer 6. The number of stained structures in the other layers is of intermediate density. CC, corpus callosum. Bar = 200 μm.

minals, show a varying degree of lamination in different cortical areas. The laminar aspects of the ChAT staining thus appear to be associated with the basal forebrain input. An example of the laminar pattern of ChAT staining is visual cortex is given in Fig. 12. The heaviest concentration of basal forebrain terminals appears to be in upper layer 5, extending somewhat into layer 4.

The observed concentration of labeling in upper layer 5, together with the presence of ChAT-positive terminals on pyramidal cell dendrites (Houser *et al.*, 1985), suggests that a substantial fraction of the basal forebrain projection innervates neurons projecting to subcortical areas. Modulation of cortical efferent activity thus might represent a function for this pathway. The intrinsic cortical cholinergic system, on the other hand, seems to be involved in local cortical functions. It might integrate the activity of a small cortical area and relay this information to other neurons in the vicinity, as well as regulate local blood flow, blood vessel permeability, or other local catabolic functions. The cholinergic midbrain projection differs from the two other systems in innervating only a restricted cortical area. Thus, its function is presumably related to specific tasks performed by medial frontal cortex. Additional ultrastructural and physiological data are needed to evaluate these hypotheses and to characterize more completely the role of these systems.

5. Alzheimer's Disease and Cortical Cholinergic Function

Persons affected with Alzheimer's disease or senile dementia of the Alzheimer's type (both will be abbreviated here as AD) show gross disorientation of mental state and loss of memory functions. The neuroanatomical correlates of the disease are the presence of numerous argyrophilic plaques and neurofibrillary tangles in cerebral cortex and hippocampus. Recently, it was found that AD is accompanied by decreases in cholinergic parameters in these areas and in the NBM (for review see Terry and Davis, 1980; Marchbanks, 1982; Coyle *et al.*, 1983). This degeneration process seems to show some selectivity for the cholinergic system, as indices for GABAergic function appear to be normal (Davies, 1979; Rossor *et al.*, 1984). Some, but not all, peptidergic (Rossor *et al.*, 1980a,b; Davies *et al.*, 1980; Crystal and Davies, 1982) or monoaminergic (Adolfsson *et al.*, 1979) cortical parameters also seem impaired in AD. In the NBM a marked decrease in the number of large ChAT-positive cells has been observed. This could be due either to cell death (Rossor *et al.*, 1982; Nagai *et al.*, 1983) or to shrinkage of the large cholinergic NBM cells (Perry *et al.*, 1982). In one AD case examined by ChAT immunohistochemistry, cell shrinkage without cell death was observed (Pearson *et al.*, 1983). A reduction in cell size without cell death in NBM neurons was also observed in rats following cortical lesions (Sofroniew *et al.*, 1983). From the available data, it is unclear whether two different types of AD exist, one resulting in shrinkage in cell size, the other in cell death; or whether the disease sequentially progresses through cell shrinkage to cell death. In any case, in AD patients the cholinergic projection from NBM to cortex is largely degenerated. Although much attention has been focused on the cholinergic system, it is clear that an explanation of the observed neurological symptoms by an exclusive cholinergic hypothesis might be overly simplistic. This point is noteworthy since attempts to treat AD by increasing cholinergic metabolism in affected patients have not been particularly successful (for review see Marchbanks, 1982).

The primary cause for the lesions associated with AD remains unknown. Evidence for the following, not mutually exclusive, mechanisms has been presented: (1) AD might have a genetic component (Heston *et al.*, 1981); (2) high levels of aluminum in cortex and NBM of patients indicate a possible role for metal intoxication (Terry and Pena, 1965; Crapper *et al.*, 1976); and (3) general metabolic changes (Hagberg and Ingvar, 1976) as well as changes in RNA metabolism have been observed in diseased cortex (Sajdel-Sulkowska and Marotta, 1984).

A different possibility was raised recently, when it was demonstrated that rat basal forebrain cholinergic neurons respond to a well-known neuronal survival and trophic factor, nerve growth factor (NGF) (for review see Thoenen and Barde, 1980), by an increase in specific ChAT activity (Gnahn *et al.*, 1982; Hefti *et al.*, 1985). These neurons also show specific retrograde transport of NGF injected into cortex (Seiler and Schwab, 1984). This suggests the existence in cortex and hippocampus of a trophic substance that is needed to maintain cholinergic innervation; and production of this substance might be affected in AD patients. Additional, circumstantial evidence for such a hypothesis comes from the observation in the rat that cortical cholinergic parameters appear to recover over time following the initial loss induced by lesions of the basal forebrain (Wenk and Olton, 1984). This hypothetical trophic factor might not be identical with NGF, since anti-NGF antibodies produced no effect on cholinergic basal forebrain neurons *in vivo* or in tissue culture (Gnahn *et al.*, 1982; Hefti *et al.*, 1985).

It is obvious that much additional information is needed to understand the relationship of the different neurological, anatomical, and biochemical alterations described above to the behavioral deficits associated with AD.

ACKNOWLEDGMENT. Support by ADRDA (FSA 85–011) is gratefully acknowledged.

6. References

Adolfsson, R., Gottfries, C. G., Roos, B. E., and Winblad, B., 1979, Changes in brain catecholamine in patients with dementia of the Alzheimer type, *Br. J. Psychiatry* **135**:216–223.

Amaral, D. G., Kurz, J., and Eckenstein, F., 1984, An analysis of the origins of the cholingeric and non-cholinergic septal projections to the hippocampal formation of the rat: A double labeling study using WGA-HRP and an antibody to choline acetyltransferase, *Soc. Neurosci. Abstr.* **10**:612.

Armstrong, D. E., Saper, C. B., Levey, A. I., Wainer, B. H., and Terry, R., 1983, Distribution of cholinergic neurons in rat brain: Demonstrated by immunocytochemical localization of choline acetyltransferase, *J. Comp. Neurol.* **216**:53–68.

Barrald, K. F., Berg, D. K., 1978, High affinity choline uptake by spinal cord neurons in dissociated cell culture, *Dev. Biol.* **65**:90–99.

Baughman, R. W., and Bader, C. R., 1977, Biochemical characterization and cellular localization of the cholinergic system in the chicken retina, *Brain Res.* **138**:469–485.

Beesley, P. W., and Emson, P. C., 1975, Distribution of transmitter related enzymes in the rat sensorimotor cortex, *Biochem. Soc. Trans.* **3**:936–939.

Belcher, G., and Ryall, R. W. 1977, Substance P and Renshaw cells: A new concept of inhibitory synaptic interactions, *J. Physiol. (London)* **272**:105–119.

Bigl, V., Woolf, N. J., and Butcher, L. L., 1982, Cholinergic projections from the basal forebrain to frontal parietal, temporal, occipital and cingulate cortices: A combined fluorescent tracer and acetylcholinesterase analysis, *Brain Res. Bull.* **8**:727–749.

Birks, R., Katz, B., and Miledi, R., 1960, Physiological and structural changes at the amphibian myoneural junction in the course of nerve degeneration, *J. Physiol. (London)* **150**:145–168.

Brownstein, M., Kobayashi, R., Palkovits, M., and Saavedra, J. M., 1975, Choline acetyltransferase levels in diencephalic nuclei of the rat, *J. Neurochem.* **24**:35–38.

Burt, A. M., 1970, A histochemical procedure for the localization of choline acetyltransferase activity, *J. Histochem. Cytochem.* **18**:408–415.

Butcher, L. L., 1978, Recent advances in histochemical techniques for the study of central cholinergic mechanisms, in: *Cholinergic Mechanisms and Psychopharmacology* (J. Jenden, ed.), Plenum Press, New York, pp. 93–124.

Butcher, L. L., Talbot, K., and Bilezikjian, L., 1975, Acetylcholinestrase in dopamine-containing regions of the brain, *J. Neural Transm.* **37**:127–153.

Celesia, C. G., and Jasper, H. H., 1966, Acetylcholine released from the cerebral cortex in relation to state of excitation, *Neurology* **16**:1053–1064.

Chang, H. C., and Gaddum, J. H., 1933, Choline esters in tissue extracts, *J. Physiol. (London)* **79**:255–275.

Chao, L. P., and Wolfgram, F., 1973, Purification and some properties of choline acetyltransferase (E.C. 2.3.16) from bovine brain, *J. Neurochem.* **20**:1075–1082.

Chubb, I. W., Hodgson, A. J., and White, G. H., 1980, Acetylcholinesterase hydrolyzes substance P, *Neuroscience* **5**:2065–2072.

Collier, B., and Mitchell, J. F., 1966, The central release of acetylcholine from the cerebral cortex, *J. Physiol. (London)* **184**:239–254.

Comline, R. S., 1946, Synthesis of acetylcholine by non-nervous tissue, *J. Physiol. (London)* **105**:6P.

Connor, J. R., and Peters, A., 1984, Vasoactive intestinal polypeptide-immunoreactive neurons in rat visual cortex, *Neuroscience* **12**:1027–1044.

Coons, A. H., 1978, Fluorescent antibody methods, in: *General Cytochemical Methods* (J. F. Danielli, ed.), Academic Press, New York, pp. 399–422.

Coyle, J. T., Price, D. L., DeLong, M. R., 1983, Alzheimer's disease: A disorder of cortical cholinergic innervation, *Science* **219**:1184–1190.

Cozzarri, C., and Hartman, B. K., 1980, Preparation of antibodies specific to choline acetyltransferase from bovine caudate nucleus and immunohistochemical localization of the enzyme, *Proc. Natl. Acad. Sci. USA* **77**:7453–7457.

Crapper, D. R., Krishnan, S. S., and Quittkat, S., 1976, Aluminum, neurofibrillary degeneration and Alzheimer's disease, *Brain* **99**:67–80.

Crawford, G. D., Correa, L., and Salvaterra, P. M., 1982, Interaction of monoclonal antibodies with mammalian choline acetyltransferase, *Proc. Natl. Acad. Sci. USA* **79**:7031–7035.

Crawford, J. M., 1970, The sensitivity of cortical neurons to acidic amino acids and acetylcholine, *Brain Res.* **17**:287–296.

Crystal, H. A., and Davies, P., 1982, Cortical substance P-Like immunoreactivity in cases of Alzheimer's disease and senile dementia of the Alzheimer type, *J. Neurochem.* **38**:1781–1784.

Davies, P., 1979, Neurotransmitter-related enzymes in senile dementia of the Alzheimer type, *Brain Res.* **171**:319–327.

Davies, P., Katzmann, R., and Terry, R. D., 1980, Reduced somatostatin-like immunoreactivity in cerebral cortex from cases of Alzheimer disease and Alzheimer senile dementia, *Nature* **288**:279–280.

Dietz, G. W., and Salvaterra, P. M., 1980, Purification and peptide mapping of rat brain choline acetyltransferase, *J. Biol. Chem.* **255**:10612–10617.

Eckenstein, F., and Baughman, R. W. 1984, Two types of cholinergic innervation in cortex, one co-localized with vasoactive intestinal polypeptide, *Nature* **309**:153–155.

Eckenstein. F., and Sofroniew, M. V., 1983, Identification of central cholinergic neurons containing both choline acetyltransferase and acetylcholinesterase and of central neurons containing only acetylcholinesterase, *J. Neurosci.* **3**:2286–2291.

Eckenstein, F., and Thoenen, H., 1982, Production of specific antisera and monoclonal antibodies to choline acetyltransferase: Characterization and use for identification of cholinergic neurons, *EMBO J.* **1**:363–368.

Eckenstein, F., and Thoenen, H., 1983, Cholinergic neurons in the rat cerebral cortex demonstrated by immunohistochemical localization of choline acetyltransferase, *Neurosci. Lett.* **36:**211–215.

Eckenstein, F., Barde, Y. A., and Thoenen, H., 1981, Production of specific antibodies to choline acetyltransferase purified from pig brain, *Neuroscience* **6:**993–1000.

Emson, P. C., and Lindvall, O., 1979, Distribution of putative neurotransmitters in cortex, *Neuroscience* **4:**1–30.

Fibiger, H. C., 1982, The organization and some projections of cholinergic neurons of the mammalian forebrain, *Brain Res. Rev.* **4:**327–388.

Fonnum, F., 1973, Recent developments in biochemical investigations of cholinergic transmission, *Brain Res.* **62:**497–507.

Fonnum, F., 1975, Review of recent progress in the synthesis, storage, and release of acetylcholine, in: *Cholinergic Mechanisms* (P. G. Waser, ed.), Raven Press, New York, pp. 145–160.

Fonnum, F., Walaas, I., and Iversen, E., 1977, Localization of GABAergic, cholinergic and aminergic structures in the mesolimbic system, *J. Neurochem.* **29:**221–230.

Geffard, M., Rock, A. M., Souan, M. L., Delluc, J., and LeMoal, M., 1984, Simultaneous detection of dopamine, noradrenaline and acetylcholine in brain using specific antibodies, *Soc. Neurosci, Abstr.* **10:**443.

Gnahn, H., Hefti, F., Heumann, R., Schwab, M. E., and Thoenen, H., 1982, NGF-mediated increase in choline acetyltransferase (ChAT) in the neonatal rat forebrain; evidence for a physiological role of NGF in the brain? *Dev. Brain Res.* **9:**45–52.

Grammas, P., Diglio, C. A., Marks, B. H., Giacomelli, F., and Weiner, J., 1983, Identification of muscarinic receptors in rat cerebral cortical microvessels, *J. Neurochem.* **40:**645–651.

Green, J. R., Halpern, L. M., and Van Niel, S., 1970, Alterations in the activity of selected enzymes in chronic isolated cerebral cortex of the rat, *Brain* **93:**57–64.

Hagberg, B. O., and Ingvar, D. H., 1976, Cognitive reduction in presenile dementia related to regional abnormalities of the cerebral blood flow, *Br. J. Psychiatry* **128:**209–222.

Hartgraves, S. L., Mensah, P. L., and Kelly, P. H., 1982, Regional decreases of cortical choline acetyltransferase after lesions of the septal area and in the area of nucleus basalis cellularis. *Neuroscience* **7:**2369–2376.

Hebb, C. O., and Krnjević, K., 1962, The physiological significance of acetylcholine, in: *Neurochemistry* (K. A. C. Elliot, I. H. Page, and J. H. Quastel, eds.), Thomas, Springfield, Ill., pp. 452–481.

Hebb, C. O., Krnjević, K., and Silver, A., 1968, Effect of undercutting on the acetylcholinesterase and choline acetyltransferase activity in the cat's cerebral cortex, *Nature* **198:**692.

Hedreen, J. C., Bacon, S. J., Cork, L. C., Kitt, C. A., Crawford, G. D., Salvaterra, P. M., and Price, D. L., 1983, Immunocytochemical identification of cholinergic neurons in the monkey central nervous system using monoclonal antibodies against choline acetyltransferase, *Neurosci. Lett.* **43:**173–177.

Hefti, F., Harlikka, J., Eckenstein, F., Gnahn, H., Heumann, R., Schwab, M., and Thoenen, H., 1985, Nerve growth factor (NGF) induces choline acetyltransferase but fails to affect survival or fiber outgrowth of cholinergic neurons in cultures of siddociated septal neurons of fetal rat brains, *Neuroscience* **14:**55–68.

Heston, L. L., Mastri, A. R., and Anderson, E., 1981, Dementia of the Alzheimer type: Clinical genetics, natural history, and association conditions, *Arch. Gen. Psychiatry* **38:**1085–1090.

Hoover, D. B., and Jacobowitz, D. M., 1979, Neurochemical and histochemical studies on the effect of a lesion of the nucleus cuneiformis on the cholinergic innervation of discrete areas of the rat brain, *Brain Res.* **170:**113–122.

Hoover, D. B., Muth, E. A., and Jacobowitz, D. M., 1978, A mapping of the distribution of acetylcholine, choline acetyltransferase and acetylcholinesterase in discrete areas of rat brain, *Brain Res.* **153:**295–306.

Houser, C. R., Crawford, G. D., Barber, R. P., Salvaterra, P. M., and Vaughn, J. E., 1983, Organization and morphological characteristics of cholinergic neurons: An immunocytochemical study with a monoclonal antibody to choline acetyltransferase, *Brain Res.* **266:**97–119.

Houser, C. R., Crawford, G. D., Salvaterra, P. M., and Vaughn, J. E., 1985, Immunocytochemical localization of choline acetyltransferase in rat cerebral cortex: A study of cholinergic neurons and synapses, *J. Comp. Neurol.* **234:**17–34.

Hsu, S. M., Raine, L., and Fanger, H., 1981, Use of avidin–biotin–peroxidase complex (ABC) in immunoperoxidase techniques: A comparison between ABC and unlabeled antibody (PAP) procedures, *J. Histochem. Cytochem* **29:**577–580.

Huang, M., and Rorstad, O. P., 1983, Effects of vasoactive intestinal polypeptide, monoamines, prostaglandins, and 2-chloroadenosine on adenylte cyclase in rat cerebral microvessels, *J. Neurochem* **40:**719–726.

Iadecola, C., Mraovitch, S., Meeley, M. P., and Reis, D. J., 1983, Lesions of the basal forebrain in rat selectively impair the cortical vasodilation elicited from cerebellar fastigial nucleus, *Brain Res.* **279:**41–52.

Jan, L. Y., and Jan, J. N., 1982, Peptidergic transmission in sympathetic ganglia of the frog, *J. Physiol. (London)* **327:**219.

Johnston, M. V., McKinney, M., and Coyle, J. T., 1979, Evidence for a cholinergic projection to neocortex from neurons in the basal forebrain, *Proc. Natl. Acad. Sci. USA* **76:**5392–5396.

Johnston, M. V., McKinney, M., and Coyle, J. T., 1981a, Neocortical cholinergic innervation: A description of extrinsic and intrinsic components in the rat, *Exp. Brain Res.* **43:**159–172.

Johnston, M. V., Young, A. C., and Coyle, J. T., 1981b, Laminar distribution of cholinergic markers in cortex: Effect of lesions, *J. Neurosci. Res.* **6:**597–607.

Kanai, T., and Szerb, J. C., 1965, The mesencephalic reticular activating system and cortical acetylcholine output, *Nature* **205:**81–82.

Kasa, P., Mann, S. P., and Hebb, C., 1970, Localization of choline acetyltransferase, *Nature* **226:**812–816.

Kimura, H., McGeer, P. L., Peng, F., and McGeer, E. G., 1980, Choline acetyltransferase-containing neurons in the rodent brain demonstrated by immunohistochemistry, *Science* **208:** 1057–1059.

Kimura, H., McGeer, P. L., Peng, J. H., and McGeer, E. G., 1981, The central cholinergic system studied by choline acetyltransferase immunohistochemistry in the cat, *J. Comp. Neurol.* **200:**151–201.

Koelle, G. B., and Friedenwald, J. S., 1949, A histochemical method for localizing cholinesterase activity, *Proc. Soc. Exp. Biol. Med.* **70:**617–622.

Krnjević, K., and Lekic, D., 1977, Substance P selectively blocks excitation of Renshaw cells by acetylcholine, *Can. Physiol. Pharmacol.* **55:**958–961.

Krnjević, K., and Phillis, J. W., 1963a, Iontophoretic studies of neurones in the mammalian cerebral cortex, *J. Physiol. (London)* **165:**274–304.

Krnjević, K., and Phillis, J. W., 1963b, Acetylcholine-sensitive cells in the cerebral cortex, *J. Physiol. (London)* **166:**296–327.

Krnjević, K., and Phillis, J. W., 1963c, Pharmacological properties of acetylcholine sensitive cells in the cerebral cortex, *J. Physiol. (London)* **166:**328–350.

Kuhar, M. J., 1976, The anatomy of cholinergic neurons, in: *Biology of Cholinergic Function* (A. H. Goldberg and I. Hanin, eds.), Raven Press, New York, pp. 3–27.

Kuhar, M. J., and Murrin, L. C., 1978, Sodium-dependent, high affinity choline uptake, *J. Neurochem.* **30:**15–21.

Lamour, Y., Dutar, P., and Jobert, A., 1982a, Topographic organization of basal forebrain neurons projecting to the rat cerebral cortex, *Neurosci. Lett.* **34:**117–122.

Lamour, Y. P., Dutar, P., and Jobert, A., 1982b, Excitatory effect of acetylcholine on different types of neurons in the first somatosensory neocortex of the rat: Laminar distribution and pharmacological characteristics, *Neuroscience* **10:107–117.**

Lamour, Y., Dutar, P., and Jobert, A., 1984, Cortical projections of the nucleus of the diagonal band of Broca and of the substantia innominata in the rat: An anatomical study using the anterograde transport of a conjugate of wheat germ agglutinin and horseradish peroxidase, *Neuroscience* **12:**395–408.

Larsson, L. I., Edvinsson, L., Fahrenkrug, J., Hakanson, R., Owman, C., Schaffalitzky de Muckadell, O., and Sundler, F., 1976, Immunohistochemical localization of a vasodilatory polypeptide (VIP) in cerebrovascular nerves, *Brain Res.* **113:**400–404.

Lehmann, J., Nagy, J. I., Atmadja, S., and Fibiger, H. C., 1980, The nucleus basalis magnocellular is: The origin of a cholinergic projection to the neocortex of the rat, *Neuroscience* **5:**1161–1174.

Levey, A. I., Armstrong, D. M., Atweh, S. F., Terry, R. D., and Wainer, B. H., 1983a, Monoclonal antibodies to choline acetyltransferase: Production, specificity, and immunohistochemistry, *J. Neurosci.* **3:**1–9.

Levey, A. I., Wainer, B. H., Mufson, E. J., and Mesulam, M. M., 1983b, Co-localization of acetylcholinesterase and choline acetyltransferase in the rat cerebrum, *Neuroscience* **9:**9–22.

Loren, I., Emson, P. C., Fahrenkrug, J., Björklund, A., Alumeh, J., Hakanson, R., and Sundler, F., 1979, Distribution of vasoactive intestinal polypeptide in the rat and mouse brain, *Neuroscience* **4:**1953–1976.

Lundberg, J. M., Auggard, A., Fahrenkrug, J., Johansson, O., and Hökfelt, T., 1982a, Vasoactive intestinal polypeptide in cholinergic neurons of exocrine gland, in: *Vasoactive Intestinal Polypeptide* (S. I. Said, ed.), Raven Press, New York, 1982b, pp. 373–389.

Lundberg, J. M., Hedlund, B., and Bartfai, T., 1982b, Vasoactive intestinal polypeptide enhances muscarinic ligand binding in cat submandibular salivary gland, *Nature* **295:** 147–149.

McDonald, J. K., Parnavelas, J. G., Karamanlidis, A. N., and Brecha, N., 1982, The morphology and distribution of peptide containing neurons in the adult and developing visual cortex of the rat. II. Vasoactive intestinal polypeptide, *J. Neurocytol.* **11:**825–837.

McGeer, P. L., McGeer, E. G., Singh, V, K., and Chase, W. H., 1974, Choline acetyltransferase localization in the central nervous system by immunohistochemistry, *Brain Res.* **81:**373–379.

McGeer, P. L., McGeer, E. G., Scherer, U., and Singh, V. K., 1977, A glutaminergic cortico-strital pathway, *Brain Res.* **128:**369–373.

McGurk, S. R., Woolf, N. J., Eckenstein, F., and Butcher, L. L., 1984, Cholinergic pathways III: Projections from the cholinergic pontine tegmentum to the thalamus, tectum, basal forebrain and basal ganglia of the rat, *Soc. Neurosci. Abstr.* **10:**1182.

McKinney, M., Coyle, J. T., and Hedreen, J. C., 1983, Topographical analysis of the innervation of the rat neocortex and hippocampus by the basal forebrain cholinergic system, *J. Comp. Neurol.* **217:**103–121.

Magistretti, P. J., Morrison, J. H., Shoemaker, W. J., Sapin, V., and Bloom, F. E., 1981, Vasoactive intestinal polypeptide induces glycogenolysis in mouse cortical slices: A possible regulatory mechanism for the local control of energy metabolism, *Proc. Natl. Acad. Sci. USA* **78:** 6535–6539.

Main, A. R., 1976, Structure and inhibitors of cholinesterase, in: *Biology of Cholinergic Function* (A. Goldberg and I. Hanin, eds.), Raven Press, New York, pp. 269–353.

Marchbanks, R. M., 1982, Biochemistry of Alzheimer's dementia, *J. Neurochem.* **39:**9–15.

Masland, R. H., and Mills, J. W., 1979, Autoradiographic identification of acetylcholine in the rabbit retina, *J. Cell Biol.* **83:**159–178.

Melander, T., Staines, W. A., Hökfelt, T., Rokaeus, A., Eckenstein, F., Salvaterra, P. M., and Wainer, B. H., 1985, Galanin-like immunoreactivity in cholinergic neurons of the septum-basal forebrain complex projecting to the hippocampus of the rat, *Brain Res.* **360:**130–138.

Mesulam, M. M., and Mufson, E. J., 1984, Neural inputs into the nucleus basalis of the substantia innominata (Ch 4) in the rhesus monkey, *Brain* 107:253–274.

Mesulam, M. M., and Van Hoesen, G. W., 1976, Acetylcholinesterase-rich projections from the basal forebrain of the rhesus monkey to neocortex, *Brain Res.* **109:**152–157.

Mesulam, M. M., Mufson, E. J., Levey, A. I., and Wainer, B. H., 1983a, Cholinergic innervation of cortex by the basal forebrain: Cytochemistry and cortical connections of the septal area, diagonal band nuclei, nucleus basalis (substantia innominata), and hypothalamus in the rhesus monkey, *J. Comp. Neurol.* **214:**170–197.

Mesulam, M. M., Mufson, E. J., Wainer, B. H., and Levey, A. I., 1983b, Central cholinergic pathways in the rat: An overview based on an alternative nomenclasure (Ch1–Ch6), *Neuroscience* **10:**1185–1201.

Mitchell, J. F., 1963, The spontaneous and evoked release of acetylcholine from the cerebral cortex, *J. Physiol. (London)* **165:**98–116.

Moore, R. Y., and Bloom, F. E., 1979, Central catecholamine neuron systems: Anatomy and physiology of the norepinephrine and epinephrine systems, *Annu. Rev. Neurosci.* **2:**113–168.

Morrison, J. H., Magistretti, P. J., Benoit, R., and Bloom, F. E., 1984, The distribution and morphological characteristics of the intracortical VIP-positive cell: An immunohistochemical analysis, *Brain Res.* **292:**269–282.

Nagai, T., Kimura, H., Maeda, T., McGeer, P. L., Peng, F., and McGeer, E. G., 1982, Cholinergic projections from the basal forebrain of the rat to the amygdala, *J. Neurosci.* **2:**513–520.

Nagai, T., McGeer, P. L., Peng, J. H., McGeer, E. G., and Dolman, C. E., 1983, Choline acetyltransferase immunohistochemistry in brains of Alzheimer's disease patients and controls, *Neurosci. Lett.* **36:**195–199.

Nauta, H. J. W., 1979, Projections of the pallidal complex: An autoradiographic study in the cat, *Neuroscience* **4:**1853–1873.

Nichols, C. W., and Koelle, G. B., 1967, Acetylcholinesterase: Method for demonstration of amacrine cells of rabbit retina, *Science* **155:**477–478.

Ordronneau, P., Lindstrom, P. B. M., and Petrusz, P., 1981, Four unlabeled antibody bridge techniques: A comparison, *J. Histochem. Cytochem.* **29:**1397–1404.

Parnavelas, J. G., and McDonald, J. K., 1983, The cerebral cortex, in: *Chemical Neuroanatomy* (P. C. Emson, ed.), Raven Press, New York, pp. 505–549.

Pearson, R. C. A., Sofroniew, M. V., Cuello, A. C., Powell, T. P. S., Eckenstein, F., Esin, M. M., and Wilcock, G. K., 1983, Persistence of cholinergic neurons in the basal nucleus in a brain with senile dementia of the Alzheimer's type demonstrated by immunohistochemical staining for choline acetyltransferase, *Brain Res.* **289:**375–379.

Pedata, F., LoConte, G., Sorbi, S., Marcoucini-Pepen, I., and Pepen, G., 1982, Changes in high affinity choline uptake in rat cortex following lesions of the magnocellular forebrain nuclei, *Brain Res.* **233:**359–367.

Perry, R. H., Candy, J. M., Perry, E. K., Irving, D., Blessed, G., Fairbairn, A. F., and Tomlinson, B. E., 1982, Extensive loss of choline acetyltransferase activity is not reflected by neuronal loss in the nucleus of Meynert in Alzheimer's disease, *Neurosci. Lett.* **33:**311–315.

Phillis, J. W., 1968, Acetylcholine release from cerebral cortex: Its role in cortical arousal, *Brain Res.* **7:**378–382.

Price, J. L., and Stern, R., 1983, Individual cells in the nucleus basalis–diagonal band complex have restricted axonal projection patterns to the cerebral cortex in rat, *Brain Res.* **269:**352–356.

Rossier, J., 1977, Choline acetyltransferase: A review with special reference to its cellular and subcellular localization, *In. Rev. Neurobiol.* **20:**284–337.

Rossor, M. N., Emson, P. C., Mountjoy, C. Q., Roth, M., and Iversen, L. L., 1980a, Reduced amounts of immunoreactive somatostatin in the temporal cortex in senile dementia of Alzheimer type, *Neurosci. Lett.* **20:**373–377.

Rossor, M. N., Fahrenkrug, J., Emson, P., Mountjoy, C., Iversen, L. L., and Roth, M., 1980b, Reduced cortical choline acetyltransferase activity in senile dementia of Alzheimer's type is not accompanied by changes in vasoactive intestinal polypeptide, *Brain Res.* **201:**249–253.

Rossor, M. N., Svendsen, C., Hunt, S. P., Mountjoy, C. Q., Roth, M., and Iversen, L. L., 1982, The substantia innominata in Alzheimer's disease: An histochemical and biochemical study of cholinergic marker enzymes, *Neurosci. Lett.* **28:**217–222.

Rossor, M. N., Iversen, L. L., Reynolds, G. P., Mountjoy, C. Q., and Roth, M., 1984, Neurochemical characteristics of early and late onset types of Alzheimer's disease, *Br. Med. J.* **288:**961–964.

Sajdel-Sulkowska, E. M., and Marotta, C. A., 1984, Alzheimer's disease brain: Alterations in RNA-levels and in a ribonuclease–inhibitor complex, *Science* **225:**947–949.

Sakanaka, M., Shiosaka, S., Takatsuki, K., and Tohyama, M., 1983, Evidence for the existence of a substance P-containing pathway from the nucleus laterodorsalis tegmenti (Castaldi) to the medial frontal cortex of the rat, *Brain Res.* **259:**123–126.

Saper, C. B., 1984, Organization of cerebral cortical afferent systems in the rat. I. Magnocellular basal nucleus, *J. Comp. Neurol.* **222:**313–342.

Seiler, M., and Schwab, M. E., 1984, Specific retrograde transport of nerve growth factor (NGF) from neocortex to nucleus basalis in the rat, *Brain Res.* **300:**33–38.

Shute, C. C. D., and Lewis, P. R., 1963, Cholinesterase-containing systems of the brain of the rat, *Nature* **199:**1160–1164.

Shute, C. C. D., and Lewis, P. R., 1967, The ascending cholinergic reticular system: Neocortical, olfactory and subcortical projections, *Brain* **90:**497–520.

Singh, V. K., and McGeer, P. L., 1974, Antibody production to choline acetyltransferase purified from human brain, *Life Sci.* **15:**901–913.

Sofroniew, M. W., Eckenstein, F., Thoenen, H., and Cuello, A. C., 1982, Topography of choline acetyltransferase-containing neurons in the forebrain of the rat, *Neurosci. Lett.* **33:**7–12.

Sofroniew, M. V., Pearson, R. C. A., Eckenstein, F., Cuello, A. C., and Powell, T. P. S., 1983, Retrograde changes in cholinergic neurons in the basal forebrain of the rat following cortical damage, *Brain Res.* **289:**370–374.

Sofroniew, M. V., Priestley, J. V., Consolazione, A., Eckenstein, F., and Cuello, A. C., 1985, Cholinergic projections from the midbrain and pons to the thalamus in the rat, identified by combining retrograde tracing and choline acetyltransferase immunohistochemistry, *Brain Res.* **329:**213–223.

Sternberger, L. A., 1979, *Immunocytochemistry,* Wiley, New York, pp. 104–179.

Terry, R. D., and Davies, P., 1980, Dementia of the Alzheimer type, *Annu. Rev. Neurosci.* **3:**77–95.

Terry, R. D., and Pena, C., 1965, Experimental production of neurofibrillary degeneration: Electron microscopy, phosphatase histochemistry and electron probe analysis, *J.Neuropathol. Exp. Neurol.* **24:**200–210.

Thoenen, H., and Barde, Y. A., 1980, Physiology of nerve growth factor, *Physiol. Re.* **60**:1284–1335.

Vacca, L. L., Abrahams, S. J., and Naftchi, N. E., 1980, A modified peroxidase–antiperoxidase procedure for improved localization of tissue antigens: Localization of substance P in rat spinal cord, *J. Histochem. Cytochem.* **28**:297–307.

Vincent, S. R., Satoh, K., Armstrong, D. M., and Fibiger, H. C., 1983, Substance P in the ascending cholinergic reticular system, *Nature* **306**:688–691.

Wahle, P., Sanides-Buchkolz, C., Eckenstein, F., and Albus, K., 1984, Concurrent visualization of choline acetyltransferase-like immunoreactivity and retrograde transport of neocortically injected markers in basal forebrain neurons of cat and rat, *Neurosci. Lett.* **44**:223–228.

Wenk, G. L., and Olton, D. S., 1984, Recovery of neocortical choline acetyltransferase activity following ibotenic acid injection into the nucleus basalis of Meynert in rats, *Brain Res.* **293**:184–186.

Wenk, H., Bigl, V., and Meyer, U., 1980, Cholinergic projections from magnocellular nuclei of the basal forebrain to cortical areas in rats, *Brain Res. Rev.* **2**:295–316.

Woolf, N. J., and Butcher, L. L., 1982, Cholinergic projections to the basolateral amygdata: A combined Evans blue and acetylcholinesterase analysis, *Brain Res. Bull.* **8**:751–763.

Woolf, N. J., Eckenstein, F., and Butcher, L. L., 1983, Cholinergic projections from the basal forebrain to the frontal cortex: A combined fluorescent tracer and immunohistochemical analysis in the rat, *Neurosci. Lett.* **40**:93–98.

Yamamura, H. I., and Snyder, S. H., 1973, High affinity transport of choline into synaptosomes of rat brain, *J. Neurochem.* **21**:1355–1374.

The Cholinergic Modulation of Cortical Function

ADAM MURDIN SILLITO and PENELOPE CLARE MURPHY

1. Introduction

The cholinergic input to neocortex has long been considered to mediate a nonspecific influence over its function (Hebb, 1957; Shute and Lewis, 1967, Szerb, 1967, Spehlmann, 1971) rather than convey specific thalamic inputs (Spehlmann *et al.*, 1971). The general view has been that it produces the changes in cortical function that are normally associated with arousal (Singer, 1979). However, not only does the situation appear to be more complex than earlier work suggested, but we now have a much greater insight into the mechanisms of action of acetylcholine (ACh) at pre- and postsynaptic levels. In this account I shall attempt to bring together a summary of the various components of our knowledge regarding the cholinergic innervation of neocortex together with its possible function, and then discuss the ways in which the cholinergic system may interact with the other nonspecific inputs to neocortex. Some sections will draw heavily on information available for visual cortex because this is to date one of the best models of cortical function that we have. While there has been a tendency to regard the nonspecific inputs as simply shifting the cortex backwards and for-

ADAM MURDIN SILLITO and PENELOPE CLARE MURPHY • Department of Physiology, University College, Cardiff CF1 1XL, United Kingdom.

wards between the sleeping and waking states, what now emerges is a much more complex picture. The interplay between the nonspecific systems and the cortex appears to be very subtle; it suggests roles in selective attention and interactions that influence the control of cortical blood flow, metabolism, and brain plasticity. Further to this, considerable attention has been given in recent time to the fact that there is a deficit in the cholinergic innervation of neocortex in persons with Alzheimer's disease. This has given rise to the view that cholinergic processes may be involved in memory and the issue will be discussed.

2. The Cholinergic Innervation of Neocortex

Following the discovery that cortex receives an extrinsic cholinergic innervation (Hebb, 1957; Hebb *et al.,* 1963), Shute and Lewis (1967), taking the presence of the enzyme acetylcholinesterase (AChE) as a criterion for identifying cholinergic cells, mapped the course and cells of origin of the cholinergic projection to neocortex. Subsequent investigations utilizing a combination of AChE histochemistry and retrograde transport have largely confirmed these observations (Henderson, 1981; Johnston *et al.,* 1981; Parent *et al.,* 1981; Ribak and Kramer, 1982; Bigl *et al.,* 1982; Bear *et al.,* 1985). However, the interpretation of these data has to be viewed in the context of the fact that AChE is found in neuronal systems that are not associated with ACh (Butcher *et al.,* 1975; Lehmann and Fibiger, 1978). Only recently has the situation been clarified following the development and use of specific monoclonal antibodies to choline acetyltransferase (ChAT), the enzyme involved in the synthesis of ACh (Houser *et al.,* 1983). In the basal forebrain at least, there appears to be a good correlation between ChAT-labeled cells and those that stain intensely for AChE (Mesulam *et al.,* 1983a,b, 1984a; Levey *et al.,* 1983) and the AChE fibers in cortex appear to be associated with the input from these cells rather than from other AChE-rich sources (Bear *et al.,* 1985), although lamina I may be the exception (see below and Kristt *et al.,* 1985).

It is now clear that in the rat, cat, and monkey, the cells of origin of this projection lie in the magnocellular nuclei of the basal forebrain, in a region that in the primate at least can be broadly considered to encompass the nucleus basalis of Meynert (Henderson, 1981; Johnston *et al.,* 1981; Houser *et al.,* 1983; Mesulam *et al.,* 1983a,b; Saper, 1984; Bear *et al.,* 1985). The precise anatomical organization of the region providing the cholinergic innervation of cortex is complex, the exact boundaries of some of the structures are difficult to define (see Mesulam *et al.,* 1983a,b, 1984a) and show species variation (Gorry, 1963). Furthermore, the problems of accurate definition of the structures involved have been compounded by variation in the terms used to describe specific areas within this region. In this account I shall use the term *nucleus basalis magnocellularis* (NBM) as a general name for the cells giving rise to the cholinergic projection to neocortex. In man and monkey this is an extensive group of large, often fusiform, hyperchromic neurons, 90% of which are ChAT-positive. It lies ventral to the globus pallidus (although some cells may cross into this), stretching from the subcommissural region rostrally to a more lateral location at the level of the

LGN. The region is traversed by fiber bundles that include among others the fornix, diagonal band, stria terminalis, medial forebrain bundle, ansa lenticularis, inferior thalamic peduncle, internal capsule, anterior commissure, and the medullary laminae of the globus pallidus (Mesulam *et al.*, 1983a, 1984a; Pearson *et al.*, 1983). The dendrites, and occasionally the somata, of these neurons appear to extend among the associated fiber bundles. Although the "nucleus" is not as clearly defined morphologically in other species, a similar overall pattern seems to apply in the rat (Mesulam *et al.*, 1983b; Saper, 1984) and cat (Parent *et al.*, 1981; Ribak and Kramer, 1982; Wahle *et al.*, 1984; Bear *et al.*, 1985) with the proviso that the magnocellular cell group is more clearly differentiated in man and primates (see also Tigges and Tigges, Volume 3 of this series). Of particular interest is the fact that the evidence supports the view that there is a topographical relationship between cortex and NBM, with particular groups of NBM neurons innervating and receiving innervation from particular areas of cortex (Jones *et al.*, 1976; Lehmann *et al.*, 1980; Wenk *et al.*, 1980; Bigl *et al.*, 1982; Mesulam *et al.*, 1983a; McKinney *et al.*, 1983; Price and Stern, 1983; Saper, 1984). At present, the best evidence for the topographical organization is derived from studies on the rat although the available data for the monkey are not inconsistent with a similar pattern (Mesulam *et al.*, 1983a). In the rat it appears that individual NBM neurons innervate very restricted terminal fields (Bigl *et al.*, 1982; Price and Stern, 1983; Saper, 1984) with little overlap in the distribution of cells projecting to separate cortical areas. Saper (1984) argues that the widespread distribution of the projection neurons in the rat reflects their location along the pathway of descending corticodiencephalic fibers derived from the cortical areas that they innervate, with some modification resulting from the division of the system between medial and lateral outflow pathways. The cells are thus in a position to receive a reciprocal projection from the cortical areas that they innervate, a view that receives some support from recent anatomical evidence (Lemann and Saper, 1985). This raises the possibility of a high degree of specialization in the functional organization of the NBM. It is pertinent to note that neocortex also seems to receive a small cholinergic projection from the mesencephalic reticular formation (Mufson *et al.*, 1982).

The cholinergic innervation of neocortex, although apparently distributed to all layers, shows some variation in density between layers. The precise pattern differs from cortical area to area, and from species to species (Mesulam *et al.*, 1984b; Hedreen *et al.*, 1984; Stichel and Singer, 1985; Houser *et al.*, 1985; Bear *et al.*, 1985). Taking visual cortex as a model, monoclonal antibodies to ChAT have revealed a dense network of branching fibers extending through all the layers of cat area 17, with maximum density in layers I–III decreasing through IV to the deeper layers. The fibers show numerous varicosities, and there is evidence for a predominantly horizontal distribution in layers I and VI although no systematic pattern is found in other laminae (Stichel and Singer, 1985). In contrast, a directly comparable study in cat visual cortex, but using AChE staining, showed the most prominent fiber density in layers I, lower III, the IV/V border, and deep layer VI (Bear *et al.*, 1985). This is very similar to the data obtained by Hedreen *et al.* (1984) in monkey area 17 using immunocytochemical techniques to localize AChE, but obviously rather different from Stichel and Singer's (1985) data. There is, of course, some question as to whether all the fibers stained are truly cholinergic. Certainly some could for example be those bringing serotonergic input from the raphe nuclei or noradrenergic input from the locus coeruleus. Both these groups of afferents may contain AChE. Further to this, some cells in layers V and VI are AChE-positive (Fitzpatrick and Diamond, 1980; Hedreen *et al.*, 1984; Bear *et al.*, 1985) although it seems clear that they are not cholinergic cells. Nevertheless, the fact that a significant depletion of cortical AChE results from lesions in the basal forebrain (Johnston *et al.*, 1981; Bear *et al.*, 1985) suggests that the cortical staining pattern does relate to the cholinergic input. Hence, although data based on the identification of AChE-containing fibers must be regarded with caution, they should at least provide a broad indication of the pattern of cholinergic innervation. Despite the variations in laminar density just described, all these works underline the fact that putative cholinergic fibers are distributed throughout all layers. This latter point is illustrated in Fig. 1, which shows the fiber patterns obtained from Hedreen *et al.* (1984), Bear *et al.* (1985), and Stichel and Singer (1985). It is to be emphasized that an assessment of the full subtlety of the pattern of innervation needs to take note of the precise distribution of the synaptic contacts and not simply the fiber distribution. The fibers seem to make symmetrical type I synapses on dendritic shafts and spines (Wainer *et al.*, 1984) and as discussed below the way

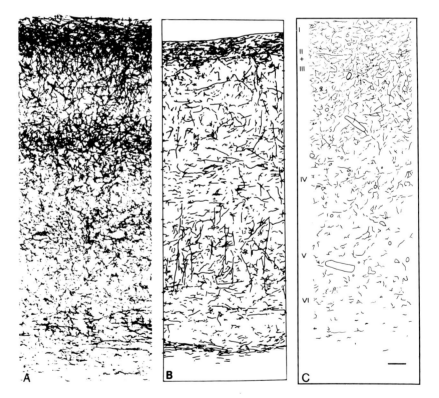

Figure 1. Patterns of acetylcholinesterase (A, B) and choline acetyltransferase (C) staining fibers in the visual cortex of A: cat (from Bear *et al.*, 1985); B: macaque monkey (from Hedreen *et al.*, 1984); C: cat (from Stichel and Singer, 1985). Drawings represent sections through the cortex, from layer I (top) to layer VI. Bar = 50μm.

in which this pattern of innervation is organized could have enormous functional implications. The fact that the synapses appear to be symmetric suggests that they are inhibitory, but it is not clear that the asymmetric/symmetric classification scheme is meaningful for synapses mediating a modulatory influence of the type ACh appears to exert on neocortical cells.

A further complication is the demonstration of ChAT-positive cells in visual cortex of the rat (Eckenstein and Thoenin, 1983; Eckenstein and Baughman, 1984) although not in the cat or ferret (Kimura *et al.*, 1981; Stichel and Singer, 1985; Henderson, 1986). These ChAT-positive cells are bipolar and are found throughout the depth of the cortex, with the greatest concentration being in layers II and III. In addition, it seems that VIP is colocalized with ACh in these cells (Eckenstein and Baughman, 1984) and that they make synaptic contact with blood vessels as well as the dendritic spines, dendritic shafts, and somata of other cortical cells (Morrison *et al.*, 1984). It must be stressed that they are distinct from the AChE-positive pyramidal cells that have been identified in the deeper layers of the cat and monkey visual cortex, but seem not to be cholinergic. Further to this, it seems that the rat cortex contains a population of cells, mainly multipolar, that stain moderately for AChE but do not contain ChAT and are found in all layers (Levey *et al.*, 1984).

3. Mechanisms of Action of ACh at the Cellular Level

ACh has been observed to produce both slow facilitatory and inhibitory effects in neocortex (Krnjević and Phillis, 1963a; Phillis and York, 1967; Spehlmann, 1971; Jordan and Phillis, 1972; Stone, 1972; Lamour *et al.*, 1982; Sillito and Kemp, 1983) but to date there is only clear evidence for the ionic mechanism underlying the facilitatory effects. These appear to be largely muscarinic (Krnjević and Phillis, 1963b; Stone, 1972; Lamour *et al.*, 1982; Cole and Nicoll, 1984) and can be regarded as exerting a modulatory influence over the cell's activity rather than mediating a fast excitatory process. The first clear indication of the possible mechanisms involved came from the work of Krnjević *et al.* (1971), who suggested that ACh produced a reduction in the resting potassium conductance and the delayed potassium current following an action potential. Further work largely carried out in the hippocampus has extended this original observation and indicates that ACh reduces the conductance of two potassium channels. One is a low-threshold voltage-dependent current activated by depolarization, first described in sympathetic neurons by Brown and Adams (1980) and termed the "M" current, the other is the calcium activated potassium conductance (Benardo and Prince, 1982a,b; Halliwell and Adams, 1982). The implication of these actions in terms of the cell firing pattern is that they increase the tendency of the cell to fire repetitively in response to a depolarizing input, without directly producing a strong depolarization (Fig. 2A). In their discussion, Halliwell and Adams (1982) postulate that the cholinergic input to the hippocampus is an enabling device, allowing cells to respond more briskly to conventional excitation. In this sense, this component of the cholinergic input clearly falls into the category of an extrinsic modulatory influence, with the potential to significantly modify the responsiveness of cortical cells. The lack of information on the ionic mechanisms underlying the inhibitory effects of ACh, should not detract from consideration of its potential importance in regulating the pattern of cortical activity. The fact that some cells are facilitated while others are inhibited suggests that various components of the neocortical circuit may be affected differentially by ACh. The inhibitory effect of ACh in neocortex appears to be muscarinic (e.g., Stone, 1972) and there is evidence for a rapid muscarinic hyperpolarization in the hippocampal slice that may involve an increase in potassium conductance (Segal, 1982). Alternatively, it is just possible that some of the inhibitory effects are mediated indirectly via facilitatory effects on GABAergic interneurons (see below for further discussion).

Another facet of the potential mechanism of action of ACh is that in the hippocampus at least, it exerts a rapid muscarinic presynaptic inhibitory effect on both excitatory and inhibitory inputs (Yamamoto and Kawai, 1967; Hounsgaard, 1978; Ben-Ari *et al.*, 1981; Valentino and Dingledine, 1981; Rovira *et al.*, 1983). This raises the potential for both disinhibition and disfacilitation (Fig. 2B). Furthermore, the nature of the effect exerted by the natural cholinergic input is likely to be influenced by the distribution of the cholinergic fibers in

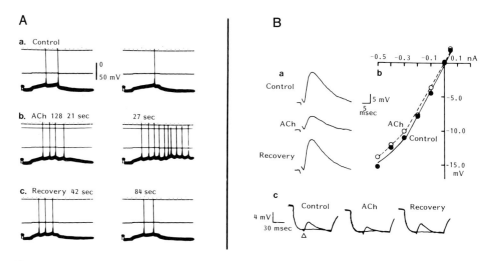

Figure 2. A: Burst firing evoked by ACh in a pyramidal neuron. (a) In control, standard depolarizing current pulses delivered through the microelectrode elicit one or two action potentials at long latency. The current monitor is shown in the middle trace, and a 20-msec timebase in the upper trace. (b) At 21 and 27 sec after starting ACh iontophoresis, the current pulse elicits repetitive firing that lasts beyond the duration of the current pulse. (c) Recovery at 42 and 84 sec after terminating the ACh application.   B: ACh-evoked depression of excitatory and inhibitory synaptic potentials in the hippocampus. (a) An EPSP recorded from a CA1 pyramidal cell before (Control), 2 to 6 sec after (ACh), and following recovery from an iontophoretic dose of ACh (100 nA, 8 sec) into the layer of activated apical dendritic synapses. Each trace is the average of four sweeps. (b) Current–voltage plot of the same cell. Input slope resistance 37MΩ in control and 35MΩ during ACh. (c) A depolarizing recurrent IPSP evoked by alveus stimulation during a hyperpolarizing current pulse prior to (Control), 3 sec after (ACh), and 52 sec after (Recovery) the start of a 15-sec iontophoretic application of ACh (100 nA) into the cell layer. The small open triangle denotes the stimulus artifact. From Dingledine (1984).

relation to the synaptic input on a given cell. In the case of hippocampal pyramidal cells, focal application of ACh in the dendritic field reduces intracellularly recorded EPSPs while focal somatic application reduces somatic IPSPs (Valentino and Dingledine, 1981). There is no clear evidence at present regarding the precise mechanism of the presynaptic inhibitory effect although it seems that it may not involve direct depolarization of terminals (Dingledine, 1984). In addition to the presynaptic and postsynaptic effects discussed so far, ACh may alter the coupling of the synaptic input to the cell output in yet another way. This would be secondary to the rise in membrane resistance following from the action on potassium channels, which has the potential to modulate the electrotonic properties of the cell and the coupling of the dendrites to the cell body. Further to this, the presence of cholinergic synapses on dendritic spines as well as shafts (Wainer *et al.*, 1984; Houser *et al.*, 1985) raises the question of whether the cholinergic synapses may exert a crucial role in regulating the transfer of information from the spine via an action on stem resistance (Miller *et al.*, 1985; Perkel and Perkel, 1985) in those spines so innervated.

4. Mechanisms of Action at the Level of System Function

As suggested at the beginning of this chapter, the evidence has consistently favored the view that ACh exerts a generalized influence over neocortical function associated in most earlier work with the concept of the "ascending reticular activating system" and arousal. However, in addition to the cholinergic input there are at least two other inputs that provide an extrinsic and presumably modulatory influence on cortical function, which are also considered to be most active during arousal. It is not clear which of the changes in cortical function associated with arousal can be reliably taken to follow the influence of the cholinergic input. The additional inputs referred to here include the serotonergic input from the dorsal and medial raphe nuclei (Moore *et al.*, 1978; Trulson and Jacobs, 1979; Lidov *et al.*, 1980) and the noradrenergic input from the locus coeruleus (Ungerstedt, 1971; Levitt and Moore, 1978; Aston-Jones and Bloom, 1981). Aside from the work on the ionic mechanisms, studies of the action of ACh in specific cortical regions have largely been restricted to assessing whether, when iontophoretically applied, it produces an increase or decrease in the background discharge of cells (Krnjević and Phillis, 1963a,b; Stone, 1972; Wallingford *et al.*, 1973; Lamour *et al.*, 1982, 1983). Given the capacity of ACh to modulate the effectiveness of other inputs without necessarily affecting the background firing rate of the cell, it is evident that these experiments cannot provide any realistic demonstration of the way in which the system-related functional properties of neocortical cells may be affected by ACh. The main attempt to date to tackle this issue has come from our own laboratory and is concerned with the cholinergic modulation of the visual response properties of cells in visual cortex (Kemp *et al.*, 1981; Sillito and Kemp, 1983). In many ways, visual cortex is an ideal model for this type of investigation; the response properties of the cells are highly stimulus selective, they can be precisely and quantitatively documented with computer-controlled visual stimuli and moreover seem to reflect the psychophysically determined properties of the intact visual system. Thus, there is a unique opportunity for access to neuronal response variables that can be related to the behaviorally determined system function. These comments should be judged in the further context of our detailed knowledge of the neuronal circuitry and possible mechanisms underlying the response properties, which at present is better formulated for visual cortex than any other neocortical area (see Sillito, 1984, 1985, and chapters in Volume 1 and 2 of the present series). The experiments I shall refer to below involve the determination of the effects of iontophoretically applied ACh on the visually driven responses of cells in primary visual cortex of the lightly anesthetized, paralyzed cat (for further details of methods see Sillito, 1979; Sillito and Kemp, 1983).

One of the first points to make is that, when tested on visual responses, iontophoretically applied ACh can be shown to exert an effect on the majority of cells (92% in Sillito and Kemp, 1983). This contrasts with the 20% reported in most studies where effects were assessed on the cell's resting discharge (Spehl-

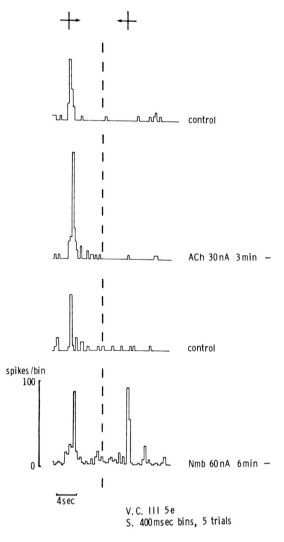

Figure 3. Cholinergic modulation of simple cell properties. Records show effect of iontophoretically applied ACh on a simple cell in area 17 of the cat visual cortex, and compare this with that of an inhibitory blockade elicited by the GABA antagonist N-methyl bicuculline (Nmb). Each peristimulus time histogram (PSTH) shows the response of the cell to an optimally oriented bar of light crossing the receptive field in two directions of motion, averaged for five trials. The sequence is as follows: control response, response during continuous application of ACh at an ejection current of 30 nA that was started 3 min prior to the trial, control for recovery from ACh, response during the continuous application of Nmb at a current of 60 nA started 6 min prior to this trial. Bin size 400 msec; calibration as indicated. Note that ACh provokes a large increase in response magnitude in the preferred direction but has no effect on background discharge. Nmb, on the other hand, raises the background discharge and eliminates the directional selectivity. From Sillito and Kemp (1983).

mann, 1971; Spehlmann *et al.*, 1971; Wallingford *et al.*, 1973), although Krnjević and Phillis (1963a,b) found up to 50% in some of their experiments. Of this 92%, we observed 61% to involve facilitatory effects and 31% inhibitory effects. The facilitatory effects involved an increase in response magnitude without a loss of receptive field selectivity in the majority of cases (90% of cells facilitated) and in just under a third of these (29%) receptive field selectivity was actually enhanced. This is illustrated in Fig. 3, which shows the responses of a directionally specific simple cell to an optimally oriented bar of light passing forwards and backwards over its receptive field. As is clear from the upper record, in the control situation the cell responds only to one direction of motion. During ACh application, there is a marked enhancement of the response to the preferred direction of motion, but still no response to the other and no enhancement of background discharge. In contrast, following recovery from the effect of ACh, application of the GABA antagonist bicuculline (lower record) produces a notable increase in background discharge (as judged from the counts in the regions of the histogram on either side of the visual response zone), a modest increase in response magnitude, and a loss of directional selectivity. The loss of directional selectivity during bicuculline application is the obvious consequence of blockade of the inhibitory input (Sillito, 1977, 1984). It is clear that despite the increase in response magnitude seen during ACh application, ACh does not cause any disinhibition as judged by the directional selectivity. This latter observation taken together with the increase in response magnitude would seem to rule out obvious presynaptic inhibitory effects of ACh in this instance. The results are, however, entirely compatible with what would be expected to occur following the postsynaptic potassium channel effects discussed above. The cell's response to its excitatory input is increased and it shows a higher peak frequency; effects that are the logical consequence following from a reduction in the "M" current and the calcium-activated potassium channel (Brown and Adams, 1980; Halliwell and Adams, 1982). Similar effects are shown in Figs. 4 and 5 for a simple cell

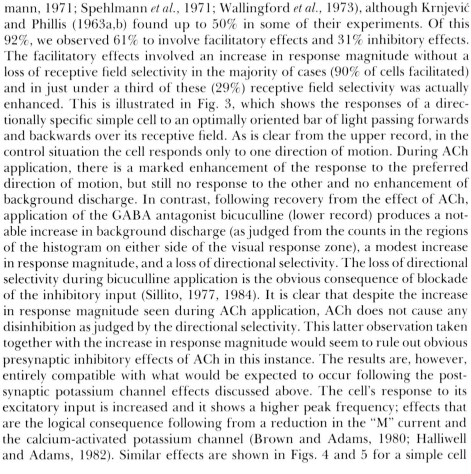

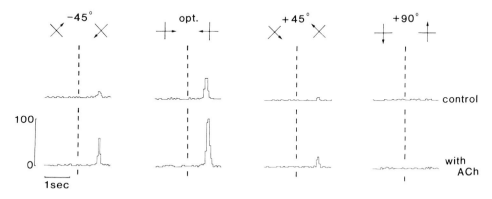

Figure 4. Cholinergic enhancement of stimulus-selective responses shown on the orientation tuning of a simple cell. PSTHs show response of cell to a bar of light moving back and forth over the receptive field at four different test orientations, averaged in each case for 25 trials. "opt." indicates optimal orientation, with others designated in degrees clockwise (+) or anticlockwise (−) from this. Upper records show control responses, lower records responses to the same stimuli during the application of ACh at an ejection current of 60 nA. Bin size 50 msec; calibration as indicated. From Sillito and Kemp (1983).

A **B**

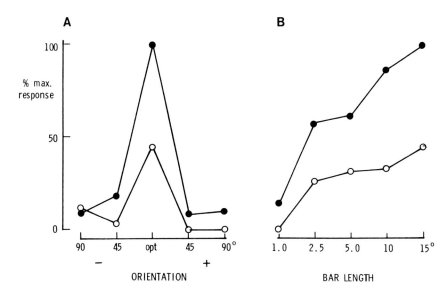

Figure 5. Cholinergic enhancement of stimulus-selective responses shown on the orientation and length tuning of a complex cell. Responses expressed as percentage of maximum response, assessed from peak frequency averaged over ten trials. ○, control responses; ●, responses during the application of ACh at an ejection current of 80 nA. (A) Orientation tuning. Orientation shown as degrees clockwise (+) or anticlockwise (−) of the optimal (opt). (B) Length tuning assessed for response to preferred direction of motion only, at the optimal orientation. From Sillito and Kemp (1983).

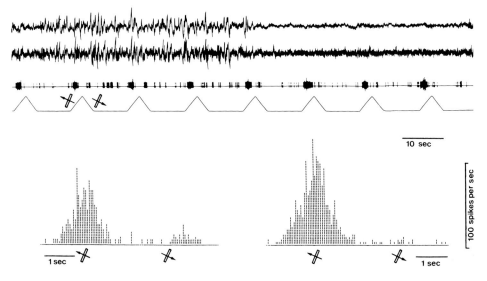

Figure 6. Effects of arousal from slow-wave sleep on response magnitude and response selectivity of a cell in layer II of striate cortex. About halfway through the 2-min record, the cat is aroused by a noise. An optimal slit, $\frac{1}{2}° \times 3°$, oriented 25° clockwise to vertical, evokes a response (third trace) that is much greater to one direction than to the other. Arousal, shown by loss of the EEG slow waves, results in an enhancement of the response to the preferred direction and the virtual elimination of the response to the other. From Livingstone and Hubel (1981).

tested with a range of different orientations and a layer VI complex cell tested at a range of different orientations and stimulus lengths. In each case the stimulus-selective response properties are enhanced. These and the similar observations in our sample all show an enhancement of the signal-to-noise ratio in stimulus-selective neurons. Assuming that the activity of these cells is significant to the perception of the events that precipitate the activity (which is virtually the central tenet of the neuronal doctrine), then it can only be beneficial to the perceptual capabilities of an alert animal to have this type of cholinergic influence operating. In their paper documenting the response properties of cells in cats passing from the sleeping to waking states, Livingstone and Hubel (1981) report some observations that are remarkably similar to those shown here for the facilitatory effects of ACh with, for example, an illustration of a cell showing an increase in response magnitude and an improvement in directional selectivity as reproduced in Fig. 6. They never observed a loss in response selectivity during the arousal from sleep.

While the above observations are compatible with the postsynaptic effects of ACh on potassium channels, the other facets of the action of ACh discussed in Section 3 suggest a capability for a range of different influences. In a small number of cells, we observed more complex patterns of action and two of these are illustrated in Figs. 7 and 8. The first shows the response of a complex cell to an optimally oriented bar of light passing in both directions over its receptive field. The cell shows a background resting discharge and although responding to both directions of motion with almost identical peak frequency, exhibits an asymmetry in the response profile to these. In the presence of ACh the response is remarkably changed, the resting discharge level is almost eliminated, the peak

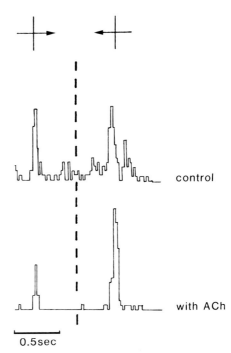

Figure 7. Cholinergic enhancement of response magnitude and directional selectivity in a complex cell. PSTHs show response of cell to an optimally oriented light bar moving back and forth over receptive field, averaged for 25 trials. Upper record is a control, lower record shows response during the application of ACh at an ejection current of 30 nA started 30 sec prior to the trial. Bin size 20 msec; vertical calibration 25 spikes/bin. From Sillito and Kemp (1983).

response to one direction of motion is enhanced, and the response to the other direction of motion is diminished. This type of change seems to require an effect on several mechanisms. First, the responsiveness of the cell to one direction of motion has been facilitated, in a way that would be compatible with the post-synaptic effects of ACh on potassium channels. Second, the reduction in response

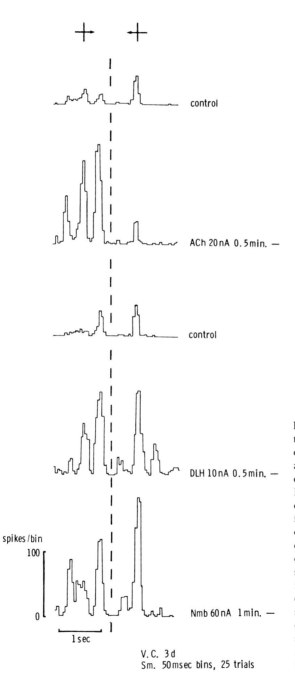

Figure 8. Cholinergic modulation of the responses of a multimodal simple cell, compared with effects secondary to a simple enhancement of excitability and inhibitory blockade. PSTHs show responses to optimally oriented light bar moving back and forth over receptive field, averaged over 25 trials. Sequence is as follows: control, response during application of ACh at ejection current of 20 nA started 30 sec prior to trial, control for recovery from ACh, response during application of DLH at 10 nA started 30 sec prior to trial, response during application of Nmb at 60 nA started 1 min prior to trial. Bin size 50 msec; calibration as indicated. From Sillito and Kemp (1983).

to the other direction of motion and the reduction in background discharge suggest the facilitation of an inhibitory mechanism having both a tonic and to some extent a directionally selective, stimulus-dependent component. Facilitation of an inhibitory interneuron with dendrites within the zone of iontophoretically released ACh would be compatible with these results. Alternatively a background excitatory input generating the resting discharge may have been diminished via a postsynaptic inhibitory action or via a presynaptic action on the excitatory terminals associated with the background discharge. It is also important to note that our electrodes are unlikely to produce a uniform distribution of the drug over the cell's dendritic field, particularly if it is a pyramidal cell with extensive basal and apical dendritic arborizations. Hence, it is quite likely that any pre-synaptic effects will be restricted to certain groups of synapses, presumably those on the cell body and proximal dendrites. In the case of the cell shown in Fig. 8 there appears to have been a selective facilitation of one component of the cell's responsiveness, generating a pattern of selectivity that is distinct from that apparently pertaining under control conditions. This shows a simple cell of the multimodal type with several discharge zones in its receptive field as tested by stationary flashing stimuli. Under control conditions, in response to an optimally oriented moving bar, it shows a clearly resolved single peak to one direction of motion and three smaller peaks to the other direction of motion. Surprisingly, the application of ACh does not enhance the sharply defined single peak response, yet produces a massive increase in the response to the three peaks generated by the other direction of motion. The single peak response is if anything diminished! After recovery from the effects of ACh, testing for the effects of simply increasing excitability by iontophoretically applying an excitatory amino acid (DLH) brings up the response to both directions of motion more or less equally, revealing each response zone. Application of the GABA antagonist N-methyl bicuculline does virtually the same thing as DLH. Both are in sharp contrast to the ACh effect. There is no easy explanation for the observations on this cell. One possibility is that a shift in the pattern of dendritic coupling, secondary to an effect on the electrotonic properties of the cell, could have shifted the influence of a background wave of facilitation received by the cell to favor a stimulus approaching from one direction. Similarly, an asymmetric distribution of the drug may have exerted a presynaptic inhibitory influence on terminals mediating an inhibitory input from one direction of motion but not the other.

While we clearly are not in a position to elucidate exactly what has occurred in the case of the cells just discussed, the central point is that the data for these cells and those discussed earlier illustrate the potential for the type of influence that can be expected to follow from activation of the cholinergic input to visual cortex. The effects seem to be strongly biased toward enhancing response selectivity and in some cases generating it. The effects are not simply reproduced by globally shifting cell excitability or by blockade of inhibitory input. From this viewpoint the precise orientation of cholinergic fibers and patterns of synaptic contact on dendritic shafts and spines could be expected to exert patterns of modulation of cortical function that are not immediately open to deduction following from a knowledge of the "*in vitro*" action of ACh on ionic events and synaptic input. The illustrations in Fig. 1 suggest a variation in the laminar organization of cholinergic fibers and it is logical to assume that this will have functional significance. Although the cells purely inhibited by ACh in our sample showed nothing more than a reduction of responsiveness (Fig. 9), their laminar location was interesting: while cells facilitated by ACh were found through all laminae, those inhibited by it were restricted to laminae III and IV and the III/IV border region (Fig. 10). The dense plexus in this area in the data of Bear *et al.* (1985; see Fig. 1) is most interesting from this viewpoint. The implication is that the cholinergic input may selectively inhibit a group of cells at this laminar location, but not all the cells, and not cells in other laminae. It is possible that these cholinergic inhibitory effects are not direct, but mediated by a muscarinic facilitatory influence on inhibitory interneurons. Were this to be the case, it would imply that locally acting inhibitory interneurons were in a particularly close proximity to some of the cells studied in the III/IV region and that they were rapidly and strongly excited by ACh, possibly because they had a high background discharge. Moreover, it would be necessary to assume that this did not apply in other laminae. In short, this still suggests a facet of the cholinergic influence that is unique to this laminar location and this in turn supports the view that the cholinergic input has the potential to exert selective influence on components of the neocortical circuit.

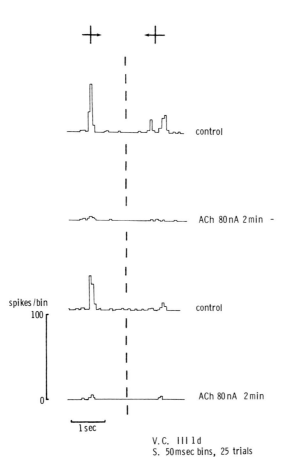

Figure 9. Inhibitory action of ACh on a simple cell. PSTHs show responses to optimally oriented light bar in two directions of motion, averaged for 25 trials. First and third records are controls, second and final records show responses during application of ACh at ejection current of 80 nA started 2 min prior to each trial. Bin size 50 msec; calibration as indicated. From Sillito and Kemp (1983).

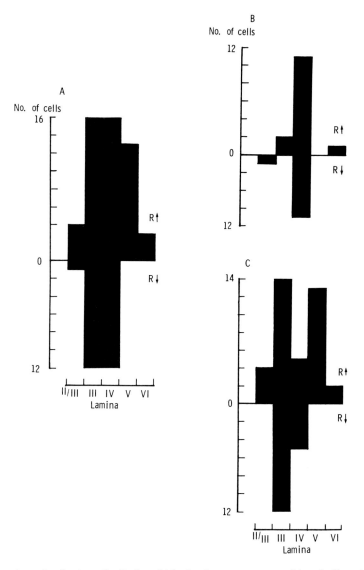

Figure 10. Laminar distribution of cells for which visual responses were either facilitated (R ↑) or depressed (R ↓) by iontophoretically applied ACh. (A) Total sample; (B) simple family cells only; (C) complex family cells only. From Sillito and Kemp (1983).

5. Interactions with VIP and the Other Extrinsic Modulatory Systems

The first insight into the way in which a peptide may interact with another neurotransmitter has come from studies of the action of VIP and ACh in the peripheral nervous system (Lundberg *et al.*, 1982; Kawatani *et al.*, 1985). It is thus of some interest to ascertain whether there is any such interaction in neocortex. The issue is underlined by the fact that at least in the rodent, VIP and

ACh appear to be coexistent in the same neurons. Although this coexistence does not seem to apply in the carnivore (Stichel and Singer, 1986; Henderson, 1986), there is evidence to suggest that ACh and VIP may have complementary actions in cat neocortex. Iontophoretic application of VIP to cat visual cortical cells produces either facilitations or depressions of the visually elicited responses that are directly comparable with those produced by ACh in terms of both the time course, and the nature of the action on stimulus-specific responses (Grieve *et al.*, 1985). Moreover, in the majority of cases the direction of action of VIP and ACh on cortical cells is the same; thus, where ACh facilitates the visual response, so does VIP, and where both substances are applied together, the effects appear to be additive. At present, we cannot determine whether the effects of VIP on its own reflect an interaction with the endogenous ACh; certainly, this would provide a simple explanation of the fact that the effects of VIP appear to follow the polarity of the effects of iontophoretically applied ACh on the various cells studied. If the actions of VIP and ACh are, as they appear, complementary, this raises the question of the functional significance in the carnivore of an interaction between the extrinsic cholinergic input and the intrinsic VIP-containing bipolar cells. The VIP-containing bipolars make type I asymmetric synapses with the spines and shafts of the apical dendrites of pyramidal cells, the dendrites and cell bodies of nonpyramidal cells (Peters and Kimerer, 1981), and blood vessels (Morrison *et al.*, 1984). They are considered to have a role in the control of neocortical blood flow and cyclic AMP-mediated glycogenolysis (Magistretti *et al.*, 1981; Lee *et al.*, 1984; Morrison *et al.*, 1984) and show a relatively uniform spatial dispersion through neocortex suggestive of a mosaic, with each bipolar apparently innervating a 30-μm column of cortex through laminae I–IV (Morrison *et al.*, 1984). This raises the possibility that they may be uniquely placed to regulate blood flow and metabolism on a columnar basis, where their output would reflect the local activity levels in the cortical circuit at that point. Thus, demand, blood flow, and metabolism could be matched at the level of what appears to be the elemental subunit of cortical function. The influence of the extrinsic cholinergic system would not appear to be this discrete, but the topological organization of the projection (see Section 2) suggests that it may well be discrete at the level of a particular cortical area. This raises the possibility that the cholinergic input may be involved in the task-dependent, selective activation of particular cortical areas in the waking state (see Fig. 11). Certainly the changes elicited by ACh in relation to the enhancement of stimulus-selective responses and the signal-to-noise level would be entirely compatible with this view. If in addition to this there is an interaction between ACh and VIP in terms of the neuronal effects of these substances and possibly in relation to cortical blood flow (e.g., Lundberg *et al.*, 1982), then we have a mechanism for producing an activity-dependent localized modulation of the global pattern of change produced by the cholinergic input to a particular cortical area.

The other two modulatory inputs to neocortex also exhibit lamina-specific patterns of innervation and in the squirrel monkey these show a pattern in visual cortex that differs from those present in other cortical regions (Morrison *et al.*, 1982). Following from the detailed consideration given to visual cortex above, I shall concentrate on this area here. The data bear direct comparison with the illustrations in Fig. 1. In the case of the noradrenergic input, fibers appear to be most dense in layers V and VI, absent in layer IV, and sparse in layers I–III. The serotonergic fibers are present in maximum density in layer IV, sparse in layers V and VI, and relatively dense in the superficial layers. This suggests areas of overlap and distinction in the laminar pattern of innervation made by the three systems. Broadly speaking, both noradrenaline and 5HT seem to exert inhibitory effects when applied iontophoretically to cortical cells (Krnjević and Phillis, 1963c; Stone, 1973; Olpe, 1981; Videen *et al.*, 1984; Sillito and Kemp, unpublished observations), which is consistent with the data obtained by stimulating the locus coeruleus (Taylor and Stone, 1980; Olpe *et al.*, 1980) and raphe nuclei (Olpe, 1981). Although some facilitatory effects have been reported (Reader, 1978; Videen *et al.*, 1984), these appear to occur only in a small minority of cases. There is, however, evidence from the hippocampal slice that suggests that noradrenaline may block the calcium-dependent potassium channels (Madison and Nicoll, 1982; Haas and Konnerth, 1983), which introduces the possibility of a pattern of facilitation rather more subtle than that seen with the probable dual action of ACh on both the "M" current and the calcium-dependent potassium channel. The facilitation might thus only be apparent under certain very specific conditions where the cell was responding in a frequency- and time-dependent fashion that would be limited by this channel. However, the presence of both noradrenaline and ACh may, because of a complementary action on the calcium-dependent potassium channel, reveal a much more significant effect on neuronal responsiveness than that seen with either alone. There has been a persistent suggestion that noradrenaline produces a change in signal-to-noise level (Moises *et al.*, 1981; Kasamatsu and Heggelund, 1982), a view that would be compatible with an action on the calcium-activated potassium channel. However, in cortex at least, this effect does not seem to be distinguishable from that which would follow from a slight hyperpolarization of a cell with a background discharge (Videen *et al.*, 1984), a fact supported by evidence showing that it can be mimicked by GABA (e.g., Foote *et al.*, 1975). This is slightly puzzling and suggests that further work needs to be carried out on the effects of noradrenaline on cortical cell responsiveness. Both the noradrenergic and serotonergic fibers appear to innervate dendritic shafts and spines (Parnavelas *et al.*, 1985) and both can promote glycogenolysis via effects on cyclic AMP (Quach *et al.*, 1978, 1982; Magistretti and Schorderet, 1985). The role of VIP in relation to cyclic AMP-mediated glycogenolysis in neocortex, raises the possibility that the VIP-containing cells may also provide a mechanism for modulating the global effects of the serotonergic and noradrenergic systems. There is evidence to support this possibility for noradrenaline, which seems to interact synergistically with VIP in raising cyclic AMP levels, but not for 5HT (Magistretti and Schorderet, 1985). The suggestion then is that the VIP cells could provide the fine tuning of the set states established in the neocortical circuitry by all three extrinsic modulatory inputs. From this viewpoint, one can identify a number of potential functional distinctions in the range of influence exerted. The most obvious general effect of the cholinergic input seems to be on signal-to-noise ratio and the enhancement of response selectivity, which, as suggested above, the VIP cells may amplify on a local basis. There is the further possibility of a role for an ACh–VIP interaction in relation to cortical blood flow. Conversely, the noradrenergic influence may be more relevant in terms of effects on metabolism, although with the potential to influence neuronal responsiveness via a component of the mechanism influenced by ACh, but likewise modulated locally by the VIP cells. Similar comments could apply to the serotonergic input although there is no basis at present for an interaction with VIP. Another facet of recent evidence in relation to 5HT raises the potential for a further type of interaction here. This is the suggestion that cholinergic terminals in layer IV of cortex have 5HT type 2 receptors (Quirion *et al.*, 1985) and hence that there may be a modulation of the functional effect of the cholinergic influence by the serotonergic system.

6. Cholinergic Influences in Plasticity, Memory, and the Potential Cholinergic Deficit in Alzheimer's Disease

Alzheimer's disease involves a progressive and global intellectual impairment with severe memory deficit and has been clearly associated with a loss of the cholinergic input to neocortex (Davies and Maloney, 1976; Rossor *et al.*, 1984) and loss of neurons in the NBM region (Whitehouse *et al.*, 1982). This has led to the view that the cholinergic lesion is the factor precipitating the disease process, with the further implication that problems of Alzheimer patients provide a demonstration of those processes that are dependent on the cholinergic input. However, it is far from clear that this is the case. The brain of Alzheimer patients shows abundant neurofibrillary tangles and neocortical senile plaques, and a loss of GABAergic and somatostatin-containing neurons, and deficits in the nor-adrenergic, serotonergic, and cholinergic projections to cortex (Adolfsson *et al.*, 1979; Bondareff *et al.*, 1982; Rossor *et al.*, 1984; Mann *et al.*, 1985). Thus, the loss of the cholinergic input can hardly be considered in isolation in relation to Alzheimer patients. Indeed, it is now becoming apparent that the loss of the transmitter-specific extrinsic modulatory inputs to cortex may be secondary to the loss of the cortical target cells of these elements (Mann *et al.*, 1985; Morrison *et al.*, 1985). There are for example strong correlations between cortical plaque and tangle counts and the loss of cells in the NBM region, the locus coeruleus, and the raphe nuclei (Arendt *et al.*, 1984; Mann *et al.*, 1985). Hence, the primary lesion may be in cortex and not in the cholinergic input; indeed, there is some experimental evidence to support the possibility (Pearson *et al.*, 1983; Sofraniew and Pearson, 1985). The secondary effects of the wide-ranging disturbance may be very complex. The discussion above would give rise to the view that the loss of the modulatory inputs is likely to be followed by a wide-ranging disturbance of the patterns of cortical metabolism and blood flow and this does seem to be the case (Farkas *et al.*, 1982; Foster *et al.*, 1983; Lamarca and Fibiger, 1984). These changes will obviously compound those that follow from the damage to the neural circuitry. Thus, with the evidence now available, it seems unwise to rely on data from Alzheimer patients to provide any real insight into the function of the cholinergic system and likewise over-optimistic to anticipate that a drug enhancing cholinergic function will produce any dramatic remission of symptoms in advanced cases of the disease, although undoubtedly a cholinergic deficit is one component of the disease process.

Despite the above comments, there do seem to be grounds for considering the cholinergic input to be capable of producing long-term changes in cell properties and possibly for having a role in plasticity and memory. The effects of ACh on neocortical cell excitability can be long-lasting (Sillito and Kemp, 1983), particularly if associated with a current-induced spike discharge (Woody *et al.*, 1978; Schwartz and Woody, 1979). This has led to the view that the cholinergic input might be a cofactor involved in the plasticity seen in the neonate visual cortex (Sillito, 1983). An involvement of the cholinergic system would help resolve some of the dilemma surrounding the conflicting data for the role of the noradrenergic input (Daw *et al.*, 1985), and recently Bear and Singer (1985)

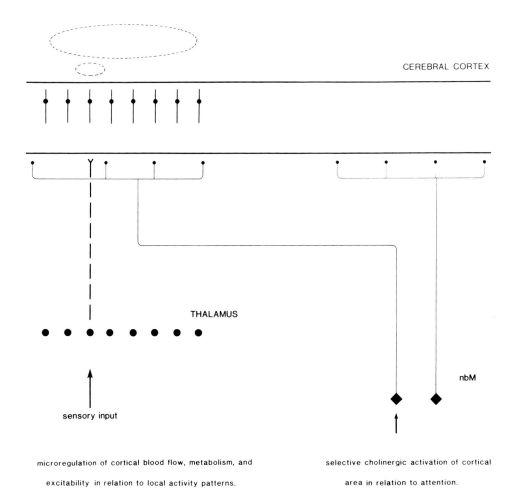

Figure 11. Hypothetical interaction between the extrinsic cholinergic input from basal forebrain to cortex of the cat, and the intrinsic VIP-containing cells. It is postulated that the cholinergic input is involved in the task-dependent selective activation of a cortical area or areas, and that the VIP-containing cells produce a localized modulation of this activation in terms of the specific pattern of input or neural processing engaging the region in question. In addition, the control exerted by the VIP cells over blood flow and metabolism ensures that these parameters are matched to the neural processes. The cholinergic input may interact synergistically with the VIP released by the bipolars in relation to the control of blood flow. Similar arguments may apply to the other modulatory systems. There is for example evidence to favor a synergistic interaction between VIP and noradrenaline in the control of cortical metabolism.

have provided evidence to support the role of both these systems in the neo-cortical response to monocular deprivation in kittens. Following from Singer and Rauschecker's (1982) speculation about the role of Hebb synapses, it seems likely that the potentiation of the response to an excitatory synaptic input pre-cipitated by the ACh-induced conductance changes would provide the essential gating influence allowing the critical level of depolarization postulated to be necessary for synaptic modification. While this type of change may be a long way from providing any insight into the processes underlying memory, there are behavioral data now that necessitate a serious consideration of the role of cholinergic processes in memory.

7. Overview

Although there is now a considerable and diverse literature concerning the cholinergic input to neocortex, it is possible to isolate several main themes with respect to its potential functional organization. First, it appears to have the potential to be discrete with respect to cortical area, raising the possibility that it might be involved in the task-dependent selective activation of a given region. Second, although it seems to exert an influence over a wide range of pre- and postsynaptic processes, the bias of its overall influence would seem to lie in the direction of increasing the signal-to-noise ratio of the neuronal response to a specific input. The range of different effects in terms of lamina and synaptic location may be concerned with establishing a particular "functional set" in the neocortical circuit that determines the shift in state required for the alert and operational condition in contrast to the nonoperational/sleeping condition. Third, the issue of the interaction between ACh and VIP, and the relation of this to the function of the noradrenergic and serotonergic inputs, suggests a pattern of influence over the three modulatory systems that is complementary with respect to the modulation of neural activity, metabolism, and blood flow. In this the three modulatory systems are seen as producing global changes within a given cortical area, while the VIP bipolars produce an activity-dependent local-ized modulation of this influence that fine tunes the effects to take note of the specific pattern of influence engaging the neocortical area in question. This idea is summarized in Fig. 11 for the cholinergic input in relation to sensory cortex. The remarkable thing that emerges is that the pattern of influence is on one level very complex and subtle, and yet on another it is suggestive, even if in a preliminary sense, of a group of changes that have the logical force of being almost self-evident.

8. References

Adolfsson, R., Gottfries, C. G., Roos, B. E., and Winblad, B., 1979, Changes in brain catecholamines in patients with dementia of the Alzheimer type, *Br. J. Psychiatry* **135**:216–223.

Arendt. T., Bigl, V., Tennstedt, A., and Arendt, A., 1984, Correlation between cortical plaque count and neuronal loss in the nucleus basalis in Alzheimer's disease, *Neurosci. Lett.* **48**:81–85.

Aston-Jones, G., and Bloom, F. E., 1981, Activity of norepinephrine-containing locus coeruleus neurons in behaving rats anticipates fluctuations in the sleep–waking cycle, *J. Neurosci.* **1**:876–886.

Bear, M. F., and Singer, W., 1985, The effects of basal forebrain lesions on ocular dominance plasticity in kitten striate cortex, *Neurosci. Lett. Suppl.* **22**:S354.

Bear, M. F., Carnes, K. M., and Ebner, F. E., 1985, An investigation of cholinergic circuitry in cat striate cortex using acetylcholinesterase histochemistry, *J. Comp. Neurol.* **234**:411–430.

Ben-Ari, Y., Krnjević, K., Reinhardt, W., and Ropert, N., 1981, Intracellular observations on the disinhibitory action of acetylcholine in the hippocampus, *Neuroscience* **6**:2475–2484.

Benardo, L. S., and Prince, D. A., 1982a, Cholinergic excitation of mammalian hippocampal cells, *Brain Res.* **249**:315–331.

Benardo, L. S., and Prince, D. A., 1982b, Ionic mechanisms of cholinergic excitation in mammalian hippocampal pyramidal cells, *Brain Res.* **249**:333–344.

Bigl, V., Woolf, N. J., and Butcher, L. L., 1982, Cholinergic projections from the basal forebrain to frontal, parietal, temporal, occipital, and cingulate cortices: A combined fluorescent tracer and acetylcholinesterase analysis, *Brain Res. Bull.* **8**:727–749.

Bondareff, W., Mountjoy, C. Q., and Roth, M., 1982, Loss of neurons of origin of the adrenergic projection to cerebral cortex (nucleus locus coeruleus) in senile dementia, *Neurology* **32**:164–168.

Brown, D. A., and Adams, P. R., 1980, Muscarinic suppression of a novel voltage sensitive K^+ current in a vertebrate neurone, *Nature* **283**:673–676.

Butcher, L. L., Talbot, K., and Bilezikjian, L., 1975, Acetylcholinesterase neurons in dopamine-containing regions of the brain, *J. Neural. Transm.* **37**:127–153.

Cole, A. E., and Nicoll, R. A., 1984, The pharmacology of cholinergic excitatory responses in hippocampal pyramidal cells, *Brain Res.* **305**:283–290.

Davies, P., and Maloney, A. J., 1976, Selective loss of central cholinergic neurones in Alzheimer's disease, *Lancet* **2**:1403.

Daw, N. W., Videen, T. O., Robertson, T., and Rader, R. K., 1985, An evaluation of the hypothesis that noradrenaline affects plasticity in the developing visual cortex, in: *The Visual System* (A. Fine and J. S. Levine, eds.), Liss, New York, pp. 133–144.

Dingledine, R., 1984, Hippocampus: Synaptic pharmacology, in: *Brain Slices* (R. Dingledine, ed.), Plenum Press, New York, pp. 87–112.

Eckenstein, F., and Baughman, R. W., 1984, Two types of cholinergic innervation in the cortex, one co-localised with vasoactive intestinal polypeptide, *Nature* **309**:153–155.

Eckenstein, F., and Thoenin, A., 1983, Cholinergic neurons in the rat cerebral cortex demonstrated by immunohistochemical localisation of choline acetyltransferase, *Neurosci. Lett.* **36**:211–215.

Farkas, T., Ferris, S. H., Wolf, A. P., DeLcon, M. J., Christman, D. R., Reisberg, B., Alvai, A., Fowler, J. S., George, A. E., and Reivich, M., 1982, ^{18}F-2-deoxy-2-fluoro-D-glucose as a tracer in the positron emission tomographic study of senile dementia, *Am. J. Psychiatry* **139**:352–353.

Fitzpatrick, D., and Diamond, I. T., 1980, Distribution of AChE in the geniculo-striate system: Evidence for the origin of the reaction product in the lateral geniculate body, *J. Comp. Neurol.* **194**:703–720.

Foote, S. L., Freedman, R., and Oliver, A. P., 1975, Effects of putative neurotransmitters on neuronal activity in monkey auditory cortex, *Brain Res.* **86**:229–242.

Foster, N. L., Chase, T. N., Fedio, P., Patronas, N. J., Brooks, R. A., and DiChiro, G., 1983, Alzheimer's disease: Focal cortical changes shown by positron emission tomography, *Neurology* **33**:961–965.

Gorry, J. D., 1963, Studies on the comparative anatomy of the ganglion basale of Meynert, *Acta Anat.* **55**:51–104.

Grieve, K. L., Murphy, P. C., and Sillito, A. M., 1985, The actions of VIP and ACh on the visual responses of neurones in the striate cortex, *J. Pharmacol.* **85**:235.

Haas, H. L., and Konnerth, A., 1983, Histamine and noradrenaline decrease calcium-activated potassium conductance in hippocampal pyramidal cells, *Nature* **303**:432–434.

Halliwell, J. V., and Adams, P. R., 1982, Voltage-clamp analysis of muscarinic excitation in hippocampal neurons, *Brain Res.* **250**:71–92.

Hebb, C. O., 1957, Biochemical evidence for the neural function of acetylcholine, *Physiol. Rev.* **37**:196–220.

Hebb, C. O., Krnjević, K., and Silver, A., 1963, Effect of undercutting on the acetylcholinesterase and choline acetyltransferase activity in cat's cerebral cortex, *Nature* **198**:692.

Hedreen, J. C., Uhl, G. R., Bacon, S. J., Fambrough, D. M., and Price, D. L., 1984, Acetylcholinesterase-immunoreactive axonal network in monkey visual cortex, *J. Comp. Neurol.* **226**:246–254.

Henderson, Z., 1981, A projection from acetylcholinesterase containing neurones in the diagonal band to the occipital cortex of the rat, *Neuroscience* **6**:1081–1088.

Henderson, Z., 1986, Is there a link between choline acetyltransferase-containing neurones and butyrylcholinesterase in rat cerebral cortex?, *Trends Neurosci.* **9**(1):20.

Hounsgaard, J., 1978, Presynaptic inhibitory action of acetylcholine in area CA1 of the hippocampus, *Exp. Neurol.* **62**:787–797.

Houser, C. R., Crawford, G. D., Barber, P. R., Salvaterra, P. M., and Vaughn, J. E., 1983, Organisation and morphological characteristics of cholinergic neurones: An immunocytochemical study with a monoclonal antibody to choline acetyltransferase, *Brain Res.* **266**:97–119.

Houser, C. R., Crawford, G. D., Salvaterra, P. M., and Vaughn, J. E., 1985, Immunocytochemical localization of choline acetyltransferase in rat cerebral cortex: A study of cholinergic neurons and synapses, *J. Comp. Neurol.* **234**:17–34.

Johnston, M. V., McKinney, M., and Coyle, J. T., 1981, Neocortical cholinergic innervation: A description of extrinsic and intrinsic components in the rat, *Exp. Brain Res.* **43**:159–172.

Jones, E. G., Burton, H., Saper, C. B., and Swanson, L. W., 1976, Midbrain diencephalic and cortical relationships of the basal nucleus of Meynert and associated structures in primates, *J. Comp. Neurol.* **167**:385–420.

Jordon, L. M., and Phillis, J. W., 1972, Acetylcholine inhibition in the intact and chronically isolated cerebral cortex, *Br. J. Pharmacol.* **45**:584–593.

Kasamatsu, T., and Heggelund, P., 1982, Single cell responses in cat visual cortex to visual stimulation during iontophoresis of noradrenaline, *Exp. Brain Res.* **45**:317–327.

Kawatani, M., Rutigliano, M., and De Groat, W. C., 1985, Selective facilitatory effect of vasoactive intestinal polypeptide (VIP) on muscarinic firing in vesical ganglia of the cat, *Brain Res.* **336**:223–234.

Kemp, J. A., Murphy, P. C., and Sillito, A. M., 1981, Cholinergic influences on the response properties of cells in the cat visual cortex, *J. Physiol. (London)* **320**:16–17P.

Kimura, H., McGeer, P. L., Peng, J. H., and McGeer, E. G., 1981, The central cholinergic system studied by choline acetyltransferase immunohistochemistry in the cat, *J. Comp. Neurol.* **200**:151–201.

Kristt, D.A., McGowan, R. A., Martin-MacKinnon, N., and Solomon, J., 1985, Basal forebrain innervation of rodent neocortex: Studies using acetylcholinesterase histochemistry, Golgi and lesion studies, *Brain Res.* **337**:19–39.

Krnjević, K., and Phillis, J. W., 1963a, Acetylcholine sensitive cells in the cerebral cortex, *J. Physiol. (London)* **166**:296–327.

Krnjević, K., and Phillis, J. W., 1963b, Pharmacological properties of acetylcholine-sensitive cells in the cerebral cortex, *J. Physiol. (London)* **166**:328–350.

Krnjević, K., and Phillis, J. W., 1963c, Actions of certain amines on cerebral cortical neurones, *Br. J. Pharmacol.* **20**:471–490.

Krnjević, K., Pumain, R., and Renaud, L., 1971, The mechanism of excitation by acetylcholine in the cerebral cortex, *J. Physiol. (London)* **215**:247–268.

Lamarca, M. V., and Fibiger, H. C., 1984, Deoxyglucose uptake and choline acetyltransferase activity in cerebral cortex following lesions of the nucleus basalis magnocellularis, *Brain Res.* **307**:366–369.

Lamour, Y., Dutar, P., and Jobert, A., 1982, Excitatory effect of acetylcholine on different types of neurons in the first somatosensory neocortex of the rat: Laminar distribution and pharmacological characteristics, *Neuroscience* **7**:1483–1494.

Lamour, Y., Dutar, P., and Jobert, A., 1983, A comparative study of two populations of acetylcholine-sensitive neurons in rat somatosensory cortex, *Brain Res.* **289**:157–167.

Lee, T. J.-F., Saito, A., and Berezin, I., 1984, Vasoactive intestinal polypeptide-like substance: The potential transmitter for cerebral vasodilation, *Science* **224**:898–901.

Lehmann, J., and Fibiger, H. C., 1978, Acetylcholinesterase in the substantia nigra and caudate–putamen of the rat: Properties and localization in dopaminergic neurons, *J. Neurochem.* **30**:615–624.

Lehmann, J., Nagy, I., Atmadja, S., and Fibiger, H. C., 1980, The nucleus basalis magnocellularis: The origin of a cholinergic projection to the neocortex of the rat, *Neuroscience* **5**:1161–1174.

Lemann, W., and Saper, C. B., 1985, Evidence for a cortical projection to the magnocellular basal nucleus in the rat: An electron microscopic axonal transport study, *Brain Res.* **334**:339–343.

Levey, A. I., Wainer, B. H., Mufson, E. J., and Mesulam, M.-M., 1983, Co-localisation of acetylcholinesterase and choline acetyltransferase in rat cerebrum, *Neuroscience* **9**:9–22.

Levey, A. I., Wainer, B. H., Rye, D. B., Mufson, E. J., and Mesulam, M.-M., 1984, Choline acetyltransferase-immunoreactive neurons intrinsic to rodent cortex and distinction from acetylcholinesterase-positive neurons, *Neuroscience* **13**:341–353.

Levitt, P., and Moore, R. Y., 1978, Noradrenaline innervation of the neocortex in the rat, *Brain Res.* **139**:219–232.

Lidov, H. G. W., Grzanna, R., and Molliver, M. E., 1980, The serotonin innervation of the cerebral cortex in the rat—An immunochemical analysis, *Neuroscience* **5:**207–227.

Livingstone, M. S., and Hubel, D. H., 1981, Effects of sleep and arousal on the processing of visual information in the cat, *Nature* **291:**554–561.

Lundberg, J. M., Anggard, A., and Fahrenkrug, J., 1982, Complementary role of vasoactive intestinal polypeptide (VIP) and acetylcholine for cat submandibular gland blood flow and secretion. III. Effects of local infusions, *Acta Physiol. Scand.* **114:**329–337.

McKinney, M., Coyle, J. T., and Hedreen, J. C., 1983, Topographic analysis of the innervation of the rat neocortex and hippocampus by the basal forebrain cholinergic system, *J. Comp. Neurol.* **217:**103–121.

Madison, D. V., and Nicoll, R. A., 1982, Noradrenaline blocks accommodation of pyramidal cell discharge in the hippocampus, *Nature* **299:**636–638.

Magistretti, P. J., and Schorderet, M., 1985, Norepinephrine and histamine potentiate the increase in cyclic adenosine 3':5'-monophosphate elicited by vasoactive intestinal polypeptide in mouse cerebral cortical slices: Mediation by α_1-adrenergic and H_1-histaminergic receptors, *J. Neurosci.* **5:**362–368.

Magistretti, P. J., Morrison, J. H., Shoemaker, W. J., Sapin, U., and Bloom, F. E., 1981, Vasoactive intestinal polypeptide induces glycogenolysis in mouse cortical slices: A possible regulatory mechanism for the local control of energy metabolism, *Proc. Natl. Acad. Sci. USA* **78:**6535–6539.

Mann, D. M. A., Yates, P. O., and Marcyniuk, B., 1985, Correlation between senile plaque and neurofibrillary tangle counts in cerebral cortex and neuronal counts in cortex and subcortical structures in Alzheimer's disease, *Neurosci. Lett.* **56:**51–55.

Mesulam, M.-M., Mufson, E. J., Levey, A., and Wainer, B. H., 1983a, Cholinergic innervation of cortex by the basal forebrain: Cytochemistry and cortical connection of the septal area, diagonal band nuclei, nucleus basalis (substantia innominata) and hypothalamus in the rhesus monkey, *J. Comp. Neurol.* **214:**170–197.

Mesulam, M.-M., Mufson, E. J., Wainer, B. H., and Levey, A. I., 1983b, Central cholinergic pathways in the rat: An overview based on an alternative nomenclature (Ch1–Ch6), *Neuroscience* **10:**1185–1201.

Mesulam, M.-M., Mufson, E. J., Levey, A. I., and Wainer, B. H., 1984a, Atlas of cholinergic neurones in the forebrain and upper brainstem of the macaque based on monoclonal ChAT immunohistochemistry and acetylcholinesterase histochemistry, *Neuroscience* **12:**669–686.

Mesulam, M.-M., Rosen, A. D., and Mufson, E. J., 1984b, Regional variations in cortical cholinergic innervation: Chemoarchitectonics of acetylcholinesterase containing fibres in the macaque brain, *Brain Res.* **311:**245–258.

Miller, J. P., Rall, W., and Rinzel, J., 1985, Synaptic amplification by active membrane in dendritic spines, *Brain Res.* **325:**325–330.

Moises, H. C., Waterhouse, B. D., and Woodward, D. J., 1981, Locus coeruleus stimulation potentiates Purkinje cell responses to afferent input: The climbing fiber system, *Brain Res.* **222:**43–64.

Moore, R. Y., Halaris, A. E., and Jones, B. E., 1978, Serotonin neurons of the midbrain raphe: Ascending projections, *J. Comp. Neurol.* **180:**417–438.

Morrison, J. H., Foote, S. L., Molliver, M. E., Bloom, F. E., and Lidov, H. G. W., 1982, Noradrenergic and serotonergic fibers innervate complementary layers in monkey primary visual cortex—An immunohistochemical study, *Proc. Natl. Acad. Sci. USA* **79:**2401–2405.

Morrison, J. H., Magistretti, P. J., Benoit, R., and Bloom, F. E., 1984, The distribution and morphological characteristics of the intracortical VIP positive cell: An immunohistochemical analysis, *Brain Res.* **292:**269–282.

Morrison, J. H., Rogers, J., Scherr, S., Benoit, R., and Bloom, F., 1985, Somatostatin immunoreactivity in neuritic plaques of Alzheimer's patients, *Nature* **314:**90–92.

Mufson, E. J., Levey, A., Wainer, B., and Mesulam, M.-M., 1982, Cholinergic projections from the mesencephalic tegmentum to neocortex in rhesus monkey, *Soc. Neurosci. Abstr.* **8:**135.

Olpe, H. R., 1981, The cortical projection of the dorsal raphe nucleus: Some electrophysiological and pharmacological properties, *Brain Res.* **216:**61–71.

Olpe, H. R., Glatt, A., Laszlo, J., and Schellenberg, A., 1980, Some electrophysiological and pharmacological properties of the cortical noradrenergic projection of the locus coeruleus in the rat, *Brain Res.* **186:**9–19.

Parent, A., Boucher, R., and O'Reilly-Fromentin, J., 1981, Acetylcholinesterase-containing neurons in cat pallidal complex: Morphological characteristics and projections to the neocortex, *Brain Res.* **230:**356–361.

Parnavelas, J. G., Moises, H. C., and Speciale, S. G., 1985, The monoaminergic innervation of the rat visual cortex, *Proc. R. Soc. London Ser. B* **223**:319–329.

Pearson, R. C. A., Sofroniew, M. V., Eckenstein, F., Cuello, A. C., and Powell, T. P. S., 1983, Retrograde degeneration of identified cholinergic neurones in the basal forebrain of the rat, *Neurosci. Lett. Suppl.* **14**:S277.

Perkel, D. H., and Perkel, D. J., 1985, Dendritic spines: Role of active membrane in modulating synaptic efficacy, *Brain Res.* **325**:331–335.

Peters, A., and Kimerer, L. M., 1981, Bipolar neurons in rat visual cortex: A combined Golgi–electron microscope study, *J. Neurocytol.* **10**:921–946.

Phillis, J. W., and York, D., 1967, Cholinergic inhibition in the cerebral cortex, *Brain Res.* **5**:317–320.

Price, J. L., and Stern, R., 1983, Individual cells in the nucleus basalis–diagonal band complex have restricted axonal projections to the cerebral cortex in the rat, *Brain Res.* **269**:352–354.

Quach, T. T., Rose, C., and Schwartz, J. C., 1978, (^{3}H)-glycogen hydrolysis in brain slices: Responses to neurotransmitters and modulation of noradrenaline receptors, *J. Neurochem.* **30**:1335–1341.

Quach, T. T., Rose, C., Duchemin, A. M., and Schwartz, J. C., 1982, Glycogenolysis induced by serotonin in brain: Identification of a new class of receptor, *Nature* **298**:373–375.

Quirion, R., Richard, J., and Dam, T. V., 1985, Evidence for the existence of serotonin type-2 receptors on cholinergic terminals in rat cortex, *Brain Res.* **333**:345–349.

Reader, T. A., 1978, The effects of dopamine, noradrenaline and serotonin in the visual cortex of the cat, *Experientia* **34**:1586–1588.

Ribak, C. E., and Kramer, W. G., 1982, Cholinergic neurons in the basal forebrain of the cat have direct projections to the sensory motor cortex, *Exp. Neurol.* **75**:453–465.

Rosser, M. N., Iversen, L. L., Reynolds, G. P., Mountjoy, C. Q., and Roth, M., 1984, Neurochemical characteristics of early and late onset types of Alzheimer's disease, *Br. Med. J.* **288**:961–964.

Rovira, C., Ben-Ari, Y., Cherubini, E., Krnjević, K., and Ropert, N., 1983, Pharmacology of the dendritic action of acetylcholine and further observations on the somatic disinhibition in the rat hippocampus in situ, *Neuroscience* **8**:97–106.

Saper, C. B., 1984, Organisation of cerebral cortical afferent systems in the rat. II. Magnocellular basal nucleus, *J. Comp. Neurol.* **222**:313–342.

Schwartz, B. E., and Woody, C. D., 1979, Correlated effects of acetylcholine and cyclic guanosine monophosphate on membrane properties of mammalian neocortical neurons, *J. Neurobiol.* **10**:465–488.

Segal, M., 1982, Multiple actions of acetylcholine at a muscarinic receptor studied in the rat hippocampal slice, *Brain Res.* **246**:77–87.

Shute, C. C. D., and Lewis, P., 1967, The ascending cholinergic reticular system: Neocortical, olfactory and subcortical projections, *Brain* **90**:497–519.

Sillito, A. M., 1977, Inhibitory processes underlying the directional specificity of simple, complex and hypercomplex cells in the cat's visual cortex, *J. Physiol. (London)* **271**:699–720.

Sillito, A. M., 1979, Inhibitory mechanisms influencing complex cell orientation selectivity and their modification at high resting discharge levels, *J. Physiol. (London)* **289**:33–53.

Sillito, A. M., 1983, Plasticity in the visual cortex, *Nature* **303**:477–478.

Sillito, A. M., 1984, Functional considerations of the operation of GABAergic inhibitory processes in the visual cortex, in: *The Cerebral Cortex*, Vol. 2 (A. Peters and E. G. Jones, eds.), Plenum Press, New York, pp. 91–117.

Sillito, A. M., 1985, Inhibitory circuits and orientation selectivity in the visual cortex, in: *Models of the Visual Cortex* (D. Rose and V. Dobson, eds.), Wiley, New York, 396–407.

Sillito, A. M., and Kemp, J. A., 1983, Cholinergic modulation of the functional organisation of the cat visual cortex, *Brain Res.* **289**:143–155.

Singer, W., 1979, Central-core control of visual cortex functions, in: *The Neurosciences Fourth Study Program* (F. O. Schmidt and F. G. Worden, eds.), Rockefeller University Press, New York, pp. 1093–1110.

Singer, W., and Rauschecker, J. P., 1982, Central core control of developmental plasticity in the kitten visual cortex. II. Electrical activation of mesencephalic and diencephalic projections, *Exp. Brain Res.* **47**:223–233.

Sofroniew, M. V., and Pearson, R. C. A., 1985, Degeneration of cholinergic neurones in the basal nucleus following kainic or N-methyl-D-aspartic acid application to the cerebral cortex in the rat, *Brain Res.* **339**:186–190.

Spehlmann, R., 1971, Acetylcholine and the synaptic transmission of non-specific impulses to the visual cortex, *Brain* **94**:139–150.

Spehlmann, R., Daniel, J. C., and Smathers, C. C., 1971, Acetylcholine and the synaptic transmission of specific impulses to the visual cortex, *Brain* **94**:125–138.

Stichel, C. C., and Singer, W., 1985, Organisation and morphological characteristics of choline acetyltransferase containing fibres in the visual thalamus and striate cortex of the cat, *Neurosci. Lett.* **53**:155–160.

Stone, T. W., 1972, Cholinergic mechanisms in the rat somatosensory cortex, *J. Physiol. (London)* **225**:485–499.

Stone, T. W., 1973, Pharmacology of pyramidal tract cells in the cerebral cortex: Noradrenergic and related substances, *Arch. Pharmacol.* **278**:333–346.

Szerb, J. C., 1967, Cortical acetylcholine release and electroencephalographic arousal, *J. Physiol (London)* **192**:329–343.

Taylor, D. A., and Stone, T. W., 1980, The action of adenosine on noradrenergic neuronal inhibition induced by stimulation of the locus coeruleus, *Brain Res.* **183**:367–376.

Trulson, M. E., and Jacobs, B. L., 1979, Raphe unit activity in freely moving cats: Correlation with level of behavioral arousal, *Brain Res.* **163**:135–150.

Ungerstedt, U., 1971, Stereotaxic mapping of the monoamine pathways in the rat brain, *Acta Physiol. Scand.* **82**(Suppl. 367):1–48.

Valentino, R. J., and Dingledine, R., 1981, Presynaptic inhibitory effect of acetylcholine in the hippocampus, *J. Neurosci.* **1**:784–792.

Videen, T. O., Daw, N. W., and Radar, R. K., 1984, The effect of norepinephrine on visual cortical neurones in kittens and adult cats, *J. Neurosci.* **4**:1607–1617.

Wahle, P., Sanides-Bucholtz, C., Eckenstein, F., and Albus, K., 1984, Concurrent visualisation of choline acetyltransferase-like immunoreactivity and retrograde transport of neocortically injected markers in basal forebrain neurons of cat and rat, *Neurosci. Lett* **44**:223–228.

Wainer, B. H., Bolam, J. P., Freund, T. F., Henderson, Z., Totterdell, S., and Smith, A. D., 1984, Cholinergic synapses in the rat brain: A correlated light and electron microscopic immunohistochemical study employing a monoclonal antibody against choline acetyltransferase, *Brain Res.* **308**:69–76.

Wallingford, E., Ostdahl, D., Zarzecki, P., Kaufman, P., and Somjen, G., 1973, Optical and pharmacological stimulation of visual cortical neurones, *Nature New Biol.* **242**:210–212.

Wenk, H., Bigl, V., and Meyer, U., 1980, Cholinergic projections from magnocellular nuclei of the basal forebrain to cortical areas in rats, *Brain Res. Rev.* **2**:295–316.

Whitehouse, P. J., Price, D. L., Struble, R. G., Clark, A. W., Coyle, J. T., and DeLong, M. R., 1982, Alzheimer's disease and senile dementia: Loss of neurons in the basal forebrain, *Science* **215**:1237–1239.

Woody, C. D., Schwartz, B. E., and Gruen, E., 1978, Effects of acetylcholine and cyclic GMP on input resistance of cortical neurones in awake cats, *Brain Res.* **158**:373–395.

Yamamoto, C., and Kawai, N., 1967, Presynaptic action of acetylcholine in thin sections from the guinea pig dentate gyrus *in vitro*, *Exp. Neurol.* **19**:176–187.

5

Acetylcholinesterase in the Cortex

DONALD A. KRISTT

1. Introduction

Acetylcholinesterase (AChE) is a ubiquitous, stable, and readily demonstrable enzyme in the mammalian CNS. Although this "specific" cholinesterase is associated with sites and cells involved in cholinergic neurotransmission, many AChE-containing structures in brain are probably noncholinergic. Some of these are cholinoceptive, i.e., are postsynaptic to cholinergic inputs. In other areas, the role of AChE remains to be clarified, so that one cannot equate AChE-stained elements with cholinergic connectivity without further qualification (Butcher, 1977; Koelle, 1955; Krnjević, 1967; Lehman and Fibiger, 1979). Until quite recently, little attention was given to cortical AChE neuronal systems, either intrinsic or extrinsic. This state of affairs probably reflected the low level of AChE in neocortex as compared to brain stem or basal forebrain. However, in the last several years, histochemical and biochemical studies have begun to provide new information in this area. The work suggests that AChE-reactive elements are not only useful morphological handles enabling distinction between different cortical regions, but appear to reflect an important functional aspect of neocortical organization as well.

The goal of this chapter is to describe the organization of neuronal somata and fibers in cerebral neocortex that exhibit AChE-dependent staining. It will

DONALD A. KRISTT • Stanford University Medical Center, Division of Neuropathology, Stanford, California 94305. *Present address:* Department of Pathology, Division of Neuropathology, University of Maryland School of Medicine, Baltimore, Maryland 21201.

be important to interpret these enzymotectonic observations in terms of relevant biochemical, pharmacological, and physiological information on cortical cholinergic connectivity. Consideration will also be given to the maturation of AChE-rich cortical elements. As a starting point, a brief review of what is known about the chemical properties of AChE and its histochemical demonstration in brain may be helpful. Since relatively few studies have examined AChE in neocortex, much of the focus of this review will be on the rat, an animal being studied in the author's laboratory. Findings in other rodents, cat, and man are generally similar, but differences do exist and will be discussed.

2. Biochemistry of AChE

Acetylcholinesterase (acetylcholine acylhydrolase, EC 3.1.1.7) is a glycoprotein (Rieger and Vigny, 1976) that is bound to neuronal membranes (Shute and Lewis, 1966; Pannese *et al.*, 1974; Tennyson *et al.*, 1967; Davis and Koelle, 1978; Rotundo, 1984). Evidence for secretion into the extracellular compartment has also been presented (Jenssen *et al.*, 1978; Somogyi *et al.*, 1975). AChE exists in several molecular forms (see review by Massoulie and Bon, 1982). Although these forms differ in terms of molecular weight and solubility, immunological studies suggest that they represent the same molecular components exhibiting different degrees of aggregation (Adamson, 1977). In addition, several forms may have a collagenlike tail (Massoulie and Bon, 1982). The occurrence of the tailed (A, collagenase-sensitive) form in the cholinoparval cerebellum but not in the cholinergic neostriatum (Rieger *et al.*, 1980) raises the possibility that different forms subserve different functions in the CNS. In the brain of the adult mammal, and throughout much of development, the forms with poor water solubility predominate (Rieger and Vigny, 1976). This has had important advantages in the histochemical demonstration of the enzyme in brain sections. However, the presence of reaction product in the rough endoplasmic reticulum (RER) of *immature* CNS neurons (Kasa and Bansaghi, 1979; Kristt, 1979b, 1983) has suggested that even the newly synthesized, more soluble monomeric forms are being demonstrated at the site of synthesis (Huther and Luppa, 1979). The Golgi apparatus and cell surface are other sites of localization (Lewis and Shute, 1966; Davis and Koelle, 1978; Kristt, 1979b, 1983).

This subcellular distribution suggests that the processing of AChE is similar to that for other cell surface glycoproteins (Robbins, 1982). Recent biochemical evidence also indicates that glycosylation occurs in the RER (Gisiger *et al.*, 1978; Rotundo, 1984).

Many neurons contain *nonspecific cholinesterase* (ChE) as well. In rat, ChE is predominantly a propionylcholinesterase (EC 3.1.1.8, ProChE) (Myers, 1953). In some species, enzymes that have a substrate preference for butyrylcholinesterase (BuChE) are more abundant. Koelle and co-workers have made observations that are consistent with their suggestion that in some neurons BuChE/ProChE may be the precursor of AChE (Koelle *et al.*, 1979). However, the generality of this relationship has been questioned (Massoulie and Bon, 1982).

Although AChE predominates in rat diencephalon and forebrain (Graybiel and Berson, 1980; Craybiel and Ragsdale, 1978; Butcher and Hodge, 1976; Parent and Butcher, 1976; Kristt, 1983; Sakai *et al.*, 1983), BuChE/ProChE activity may possibly be high enough to affect the interpretation of histochemical preparations in some brain regions early in development (Silver, 1974; Rieger and Bigny, 1976; Kostovic and Goldman-Rakic, 1983). Nonspecific cholinesterases do not appear to contribute significantly to neuronal ChE reactivity in neocortex at any age (Kristt, 1979a, rat, mouse; Krnjević and Silver, 1966, cat), although vascular staining has been noted (Kozik and Szczech, 1977).

3. Histochemistry of AChE

In 1949, Koelle and Friedenwald introduced the thiocholine method to demonstrate tissue sites believed to be rich in AChE (Koelle and Friedenwald, 1949). The histochemical localization of AChE is indirect and depends on the catalytic activity of the enzyme. Consequently, many factors in the cellular environment that influence the catalytic reaction can affect the histochemical outcome. This method has gone through many modifications (e.g., Couteaux and Taxi, 1952; Karnovfsky and Roots, 1964; Tsuji, 1974; Geneser-Jensen and Blackstadt, 1971), and has a wide variety of applications. For instance, it has been useful in investigating organization (Paxinos and Watson, 1982; Kristt, 1979b, 1983; Graybiel and Berson, 1980; Graybiel and Ragsdale, 1978; Sakai *et al.*, 1983), development (Nadler *et al.*, 1974; Kasa and Bansaghi, 1979; Krnjević and Silver, 1966; Butcher and Hodge, 1976; Kozik and Szczech, 1977; Shipley and Adamek, 1982; Kristt, 1979a,c, 1983; Kristt and Waldman, 1981, 1982; Ishii, 1957; Krmpotic-Nemanic *et al.*, 1983), and plasticity in the nervous system (Kristt and Waldman, 1981; Chen *et al.*, 1983; Lynch *et al.*, 1976; Nadler *et al.*, 1977). The distribution of AChE-containing somata and fibers (Paxinos and Watson, 1982; Kristt, 1983; Kristt *et al.*, 1985; Arimatsu *et al.*, 1981; Jacobowitz and Palkovits, 1974; Graybiel and Ragsdale, 1978; Koelle, 1955; Parent and Butcher, 1976) has been the subject of several recent studies and the subcellular distribution of the enzyme has been well documented (see below). A detailed treatment of histochemical reactions and procedures involved can be found in several other works (Silver, 1974; Lewis and Shute, 1978; Pearse, 1980; Tsuji, 1974; Tsuji and Larabi, 1983). A combination of pharmacological and histological strategies has been found useful in characterizing cells in many sites, particularly where the background AChE fiber staining is intense (Lynch *et al.*, 1972; Butcher and Hodge, 1976). However, these techniques offer no additional advantage for neocortex (Satoh *et al.*, 1983). At the latter site, this worker has found osmication to be useful in highlighting cell characteristics (e.g., overnight 0.5–2% osmium tetroxide). Immunocytochemical techniques have recently been applied to the localization of AChE in the CNS (Hedreen *et al.*, 1984). While the latter are unlikely to supplant the histochemical approaches for most applications, certain experimental problems may require the higher levels of specificity and confidence that the immunocytochemical methods afford.

In a practical vein, several further comments are germane regarding the procedures and controls used in the author's laboratory that have afforded good histochemical preparations at the light and electron microscopic levels as well as reasonable assurance of the specificity of the reaction.

Differences in the quality of fixation are relevant to what can be visualized histochemically. Fine fiber detail requires the best fixation. Staining of even moderately positive somata is less sensitive to fixation quality. A wide variety of aldehyde fixation protocols are satisfactory. However, fixatives that achieve best ultrastructural preservation for a given species and age have produced the best histochemical results. Perfusion is clearly superior to immersion, and must itself have been maximally effective. Fixed brains are soaked in a sucrose-containing phosphate buffer solution (5–30%), then cut on a sliding microtome and directly deposited in the incubation solution. The incubation solution has the following composition: acetylthiocholine iodide, 1.160 g/liter; glycine, 0.748 g/liter; copper sulfate, 0.500 g/liter; sodium acetate, 4.100 g/liter. These ingredients are solubilized by heating to 38°C. Final pH is adjusted to 5.6. Sections are continuously agitated during incubation.

Incubation time and section thickness are two important and related variables that must be assessed for each application. Although long incubation times (e.g., 12–16 hr) have usually been discouraged because of the possibility of diffusion artifacts, this need not always be a concern if tissue has been well fixed. In such tissue, cut at 75–100 μm a 12-hr incubation produces the same pattern of distribution and relative intensities as 2- to 4-hr incubations, but the patterns are more clearly demonstrable with longer incubations. For fiber patterns in neocortex, the longer incubations emphasize the patterning, without impairing the delicacy of the staining of individual fibers; in poorly fixed material, diffusion will occur. For thinner sections, there is generally little need for prolonged incubations, except at very immature stages of brain growth. Performing the final coloring reaction with potassium ferricyanide (Hatchett's Brown) as a sep-

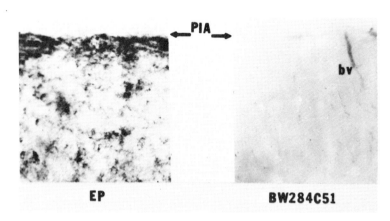

Figure 1. Effect of inhibitors on acetylcholinesterase (AChE)-dependent staining in neocortex. Ethopropazine (EP) inhibits pseudocholinesterases; fibers in the subpial region are well stained for AChE. BW284C51 specifically inhibits AChE; the only stained structures are small blood vessels (bv). The superficial layers of somatosensory cortex are illustrated in both panels, ×200. From Kristt (1979a) with permission.

arate step also minimizes diffusion artifacts, and improves the crispness of stained membranes. Tsuji has made a similar observation, and analyzed the chemical bases of this phenomenon (Tsuji, 1974; Tsuji and Larabi, 1983).

Since the thiocholine methods generally detect AChE as well as nonspecific cholinesterase (i.e., propionyl- and butyrylcholinesterases), a number of control reactions need to be performed to interpret the results. These include the use of specific inhibitors added to the incubation medium and/or to a substrateless preincubation solution. In my experience, "preincubation" with available inhibitors has not been necessary. Ethopropazine can be used to inhibit nonspecific cholinesterases. Bayliss and Todrick (1956) recommend this drug over iso-OMPA, because the latter, an irreversible inhibitor, resulted in inhibition that varied markedly as a function of time of contact. AChE can be specifically inhibited by BW284C51 (Austin and Berry, 1953; Fig. 1). Eserine and a number of other compounds, such as the organophosphates [e.g., diisopropyl fluorophosphate, DFP (Goodman and Gilman, 1975; Pearse, 1980)], will inhibit both AChE and nonspecific cholinesterases. Distinguishing nonspecific-cholinesterase-containing structures is also facilitated by using substrates other than acetylthiocholine (e.g., butyrylithiocholine or propionylthiocholine) often in conjunction with AChE inhibitors (Shute and Lewis, 1967).

4. Organization of the Neocortex

A few comments on the cellular and connectivity organization of neocortex are approriate here as background for the biochemical and histochemical observations presented below, although other chapters in this work deal in considerable detail with this subject.

Neocortex is not homogeneous in terms of cell types, organization of inputs and connections, and the distribution of these different elements. On the other hand, there are general rules of organization that do provide some unity. Attempts to find a common structural thread have been based on the laminar patterns of different cell types and fibers (Brodmann, 1909; Campbell, 1905; Lorente de Nó, 1949). Radial relationships (columnar organization) have also received some attention (Powell and Mountcastle, 1959; Hubel and Wiesel, 1962). It is not surprising, then, that functionally differentiated fields have been identified that can be consistently recognized based on a number of structural criteria. Thalamocortical relations are useful in delineating functionally related areas with different cytoarchitecture (Divac, 1979). Similarly, because the substantial input from basal forebrain is probably the major determinant of AChE enzymotectonics (see below), histochemical analysis of AChE in neocortex may also delineate functionally related areas. It will be important to determine how these AChE-stained domains relate to the parcellation based on cytoarchitectonics and thalamocortical connectivity.

The maturation of laminar and columnar organizational features of neocortex also follows a general plan (for reviews see Lund, 1978; Kristt, 1984). The differences that occur in the spatiotemporal aspects of this developmental sequence distinguish various cortical regions from one another.

5. Biochemistry of Cholinergic and Cholinesterase-Rich Cortical Circuitry

The regional and laminar localization of AChE has been evaluated in a limited number of biochemical studies in rat and cat. The regional distribution of the enzyme does not appear to be uniform between fields or within a particular field. For instance, somatosensory cortex appears to have higher levels and to release greater amounts of AChE on stimulation than visual cortex (Phillis, 1968a; Collier and Mitchell, 1966; Bartolini *et al.*, 1972). However, it should be pointed out that even cortical regions with relatively "high" levels of enzyme have minimal absolute concentrations of AChE. Cortex as a whole exhibits substantially lower levels of activity than seen in caudate and putamen in every mammalian species examined. For instance, rat caudate nucleus has a concentration of AChE (nmoles/μg protein per hr) that is approximately 18 times greater than parietal cortex (Hoover *et al.*, 1978); in man, caudate AChE levels are 50-fold greater than in cerebral cortex (Okinaka *et al.*, 1961). Indeed, due to these very low levels—and even lower levels in infancy (Ishii, 1957)—the early postnatal changes in distribution of AChE-stained elements in cortex had not been detected. As noted above, some improvements in histochemical procedures have increased the sensitivity of these methods, so that more information on enzymotectonics and their maturation are now becoming available. The more specific cholinergic enzymatic marker, choline acetyltransferase (ChAT), is eight times lower in rat parietal cortex as compared to caudate (Hoover *et al.*, 1978).

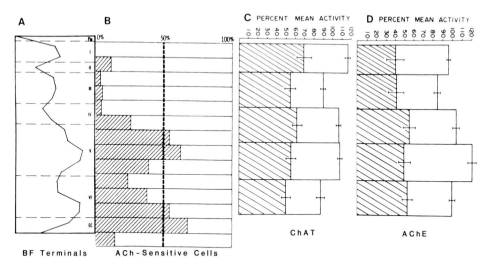

Figure 2. Comparison of laminar distribution of anterogradely labeled cortical afferents from basal forebrain (BF), with the physiologically determined distribution of ACh-sensitive cells, and laminar differences in concentration of ChAT and AChE. (A) Laminar distribution of autoradiographic grains resulting from an injection of radiolabeled amino acids into the basal forebrain nuclei (Saper, 1984). (B) Laminar distribution of cells responsive to iontophoretically applied ACh (Lamour *et al.*, 1983). (C) Biochemically determined laminar concentrations of ChAT in normal rats and those with kainate lesions of basal forebrain (hatched areas) (Johnston *et al.*, 1981). (D) Biochemically determined distribution of AChE (Johnston *et al.*, 1981). From Saper (1984), Johnston *et al.* (1981), and Lamour *et al.* (1983) with permission.

Laminar variations in enzyme levels have also been examined in rat by two laboratories. In Pope's study (1952), serial tangential, frozen sections were biochemically evaluated from primary somtosensory cortex of the rat. Highest levels of AChE were seen in layer I; layers IV and VIa had the lowest. Within layer V enzyme levels in the superficial depths were marginally increased over deeper levels in this lamina. In layer VI, VIb was marginally higher. Another more recent study on rat sensorimotor cortex used a laminar "shave" method to obtain samples of AChE in each cortical layer (Johnston *et al.,* 1981). However, the intralaminar distribution cannot be inferred from these data. This study also compared the distribution of AChE and ChAT. They found that both AChE and ChAT were lowest in layers IV and VI (Fig. 2). Although the general pattern of distribution was similar for these two enzymes, some differences are apparent. Highest concentrations of ChAT were seen in layer I, whereas AChE peaked between 1000 and 1400 μm (probably layer V). It is not clear how this difference should be interpreted, but noncholinergic roles for AChE in cortex ought to be considered (Silver, 1974; Kristt, 1983; Greenfield *et al.,* 1981; Nachmansohn, 1975; Burn and Rand, 1959; Altschuler *et al.,* 1983; Vincent *et al.,* 1983). To examine the question of the relation of these enzyme levels to the cholinergic innervation of neocortex, lesion experiments were also performed (Johnston *et al.,* 1981). In response to excitotoxin lesions in the nucleus basalis, both AChE and ChAT levels are not only reduced, but laminar differences in the concentration of these enzymes are lost. The significance of this finding in terms of the origin of AChE circuitry is considered below. At this point, these observations suggest another important conclusion: *the laminar patterning of AChE-rich extrinsic inputs is apt predominantly to reflect the cholinergic innervation of neocortex.*

Although this is a useful generalization, we must bear in mind that 20–30% of the cholinergic circuitry in neocortex is of unknown origin and that some AChE may not be related to cholinergic neurotransmission. Further, the biochemical approaches entail intrinsic limitations that should influence the interpretation of the data. The depth bins used are rather large because of technical constraints. Also, in Pope's 1952 study, a cylinder of tissue limited to a single field was used, so the generality of the findings needs to be established; as noted below, primary somatosensory cortex is enzymotectonically distinctive. In the report of Johnston *et al.* (1981), the technique involves a series of samples from progressively more lateral fields, so that field–field differences may further obscure some details of the distribution by an averaging phenomenon.

6. Pharmacology and Physiology of Cholinergic Cortical Circuitry

Two approaches have been used to identify putative cholinoceptive elements in relation to the laminar architecture of neocortex. One is pharmacophysiologic and the other is pharmacoautoradiographic.

Physiologic studies using iontophoretic techniques have found evidence for cholinoceptive elements in cortex. Receptors are predominantly muscarinic in character, but have nicotinic features as well. They are concentrated in several layers, particularly in V and VIb (Krnjević and Phillis, 1963; Spehlmann *et al.,*

1971; Spehlmann, 1971; Mitchell, 1963; Stone, 1972; Lamour *et al.*, 1983). These data agree well with the biochemical data and the histochemical findings (cf. Figs. 2–4).

However, pharmacological studies using autoradiographic techniques suggest different conclusions. Cholinergic receptor ligand binding studies have consistently indicated a concentration of binding sites in layers I, IV, and VI in adult rats (Kuhar and Yamamura, 1976; Wamsley *et al.*, 1980), mainly layer IV (Kristt and Kasper, 1983) or layer III (Rotter *et al.*, 1979) in infants (Fig. 3). A range of receptor antagonists and agonists have been employed. Although it is possible that the discrepancy may be resolvable based on the misinterpretation of cytoarchitectonics in thin, submaximal cryostat sections of cortex, several points would militate against this argument. First, a number of laboratories have independently come to the same conclusion regarding localization (Kuhar and Yamamura, 1976; Wamsley *et al.*, 1980; Kristt and Kasper, 1983). Second, in infant rats where layer IV can be clearly identified using a number of criteria (see below) that are easily recognizable in thin frozen sections, a prominent peak of antagonist binding (i.e., [³H]-QNB) was observed in layer IV (Fig. 3; Kristt and Kasper, 1983). Also, recent work defining high- and low-affinity muscarinic cholinergic binding have shown that the peak in layer IV is mostly the high-affinity type. Low-affinity binding predominates in layer III (Wamsley *et al.*, 1980). The latter has been proposed to be relevant to neurotransmission (Birdsall *et al.*, 1978; Birdsall and Hulme, 1976). A preliminary autoradiographic ultrastructural study using a muscarinic ligand ([³H]-PBCM) did report a significant fraction of grains over cortical synapses (Kuhar *et al.*, 1981) although a laminar analysis was not employed. If this election microscopic observation can be confirmed for layer IV, then the discrepancy between the pharmacoautoradiographic and other approaches to the laminar organization of the cortical cholinergic innervation remains puzzling. However, two points may be relevant to consider at this time. First, binding with the ligand may be a necessary but not sufficient condition for a functional receptor. Second, ligand-binding receptors are apt to be diffusely distributed on the neuron (M. Kuhar, personal communication). Although preferential concentration of binding sites on some parts of a neuron may occur—and presumably relate to laminar patterning in cortex—these distributional heterogeneities may not reflect the connectivity of the cell.

7. General Enzymotectonics of Neocortex

Although biochemical studies have provided information on some important issues, the organization of AChE-rich cell and fiber systems in neocortex can best be delineated in histochemical preparations. Any review of the latter subject must recognize the important and enduring contribution of Krnjević and Silver (1965, 1966) in their early studies on cat.

Histochemically stained sections of cortex show a number of features that most fields have in common. Characteristic regional differences in the laminar staining patterns also enable one to distinguish individual cortical fields (Fig. 4). However, when field-specific variations occur, they usually represent additions

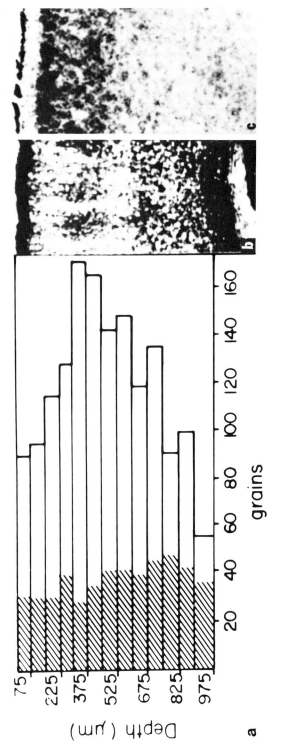

Figure 3. (a) Autoradiographic analysis of muscarinic ligand binding in infant rat neocortex. Histogram compares the grain distribution between two pups: one has been treated with the muscarinic antagonist QNB alone (outer histogram), and the other with atropine + QNB (hatched). Approximately 25,000 μm^2 of tissue was examined to prepare the histogram for each animal. Note prominent concentration (peak) of grains between 300 and 400 μm. Scale also applies to b and c. (b) AChE-stained somatosensory cortex of a third 6-day-old rat. The "bottoms" of discrete AChE-positive foci, at approximately 450 μm, mark the deep margin of layer IV (see text). (c) Cresyl violet (Nissl)-stained somatosensory cortex in the same 6-day-old rat examined for outer histogram a; 4-μm-thick frozen section. The arrow marks the approximate level of layer IV, which coincides with the bottom of the cell-dense cortical plate at this age. This demonstrates that both the AChE-positive foci and the peak of muscarinic receptor binding are localized to the deep sublamina of the cortical plate, i.e., primordial layer IV. From Krist and Kasper (1983).

to, rather than subtractions from, this basic plan. In most fields in rat cortex, at least two tangential bands of intense fiber staining are apparent. One occurs in layer I (Fig. 4; Kristt, 1979a,b) and the other in the superficial extent of layer V. Visual cortex in the monkey may have his latter plexus in lamina IVc of Brodmann; layer V is extremely thin in this field (Hedreen *et al.,* 1984). The

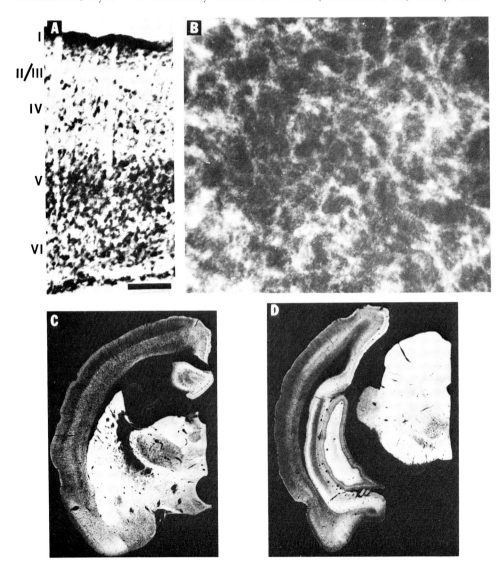

Figure 4. AChE histochemical staining of neocortex. (A) Laminar distribution of AChE-stained elements in rat somatosensory cortex. Bar = 200 μm. (B) AChE-stained fibers and fiber bundles in layer I (subpial band) of rat neocortex as viewed in tangential section. Negative image print. Within plane there is conspicuous absence of a directional preference among the fibers. This photograph also illustrates the fine fiber detail possible using improvements in the histochemical procedure. ×150. (C, D) Two different coronal levels of adult rat brain stained for AChE, showing features that in A can be seen quite generally throughout the cortex. C is more rostral and passes through somatosensory cortex. ×7.

histochemical data, then, are in good agreement with the results of biochemical studies noted above. These AChE-positive fibers are organized into dense tangled plexuses, in which most member fibers are not grouped according to any discernible orientation (Fig. 4B). Autoradiographic observations indicate that these layers receive the bulk of imputs from basal forebrain (Fig. 2; Saper, 1984). Human cortex exhibits similar AChE enzymotectonics except that the AChE band in layer I is deep in this lamina (Kostovic *et al.*, 1980; Kostovic, 1982), rather than being superfically placed, as in rat, mouse, and cat (Kristt, 1979a–c; Kristt and Waldman, 1982; Krnjević and Silver, 1965). Golgi studies show a comparable difference in the localization of the fiber-dense band in layer I between man (Marin-Padilla, 1970) and rat (Kristt, 1978). This suggests that cholinergic/AChE-rich fibers form a major component of this plexus in these species.

A sparser array of fibers is seen in deep layer VI. These are generally oriented in the coronal plane or as short arcs (Fig. 5). Less dense and generally uniform staining of fibers is seen at other cortical depths.

In cats (Krnjević and Silver, 1965, 1966), layer I staining is variable; it is intense in the walls of the sulci, but negligible over the gyral convexity. The midcortical band of staining in the cat appears to predominantly involve layer V, in which stained somata—thought to be cholinoceptive (Krnjević and Phillis,

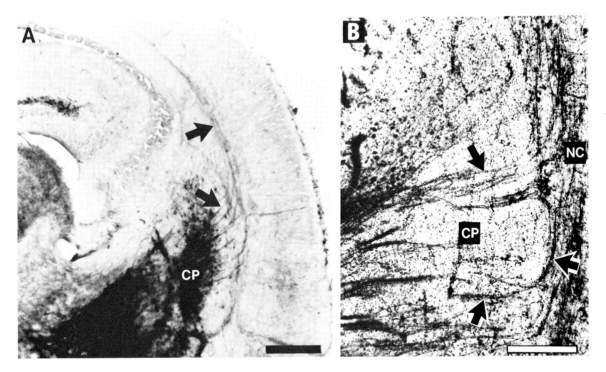

Figure 5. Coronal section of rat showing arcing segments of AChE-rich basal forebrain inputs to somatosensory cortex. (A) AChE, postnatal day 4. Bar = 500 μm. (B) Golgi, postnatal day 8. Bar = 200 μm. From Kristt *et al.* (1985) with permission.

1963; Jordan and Phillis, 1972; Lamour *et al.*, 1983)— and a dense plexus of fibers were noted. In cat, as in our material, AChE-positive neurons were seen at the bottom of cortex in layer VI. It was proposed (Krnjević and Silver, 1965, 1966) that in the cat these layer VI polymorph cells give rise to cholinergic corticocortical association fibers (U-fibers). In rat, these layer VI cells are believed to contribute AChE-rich inputs to layer I (Lamour *et al.*, 1983; Kristt, 1979b) and some of these cells project to thalamus (Wise, 1975). However, these fibers do not form a distinct U-fiber system. Some of these minor differences between the cat and the rat presumably reflect modifications in AChE-associated cholinergic cortical circuitry attendant on developing a gyrencephalic neocortex. (The rat is lissencephalic.)

Immunocytochemical studies on ChAT localization have revealed a *diffuse* distribution of "puncta" (Houser *et al.*, 1983; Kimura *et al.*, 1981). These puncta appear to correlate with stained terminals at the ultrastructural level. Since the biochemical data do suggest that ChAT is laminarly distributed, as is AChE, technical factors may be impairing the immunocytochemical demonstration of these patterns of distribution. Some difference of opinion exists regarding the occurrence of ChAT-containing intrinsic somata. This issue will be dealt with in another part of this chapter.

In appropriately prepared sections (see above), a number of AChE-stained cells are noted (Fig. 6). These cells all appear to be neuronal, and not glial. As elsewhere in the brain, cortical neurons exhibit two types of staining patterns (Krnjević and Silver, 1965). For one, a rim of AChE reaction product highlights the somal perimeter and may extend along the proximal dendrites, outlining them as well. Although in previous work individual "puncta" have not been demonstrated because of the diffusion of reaction product that usually takes place, this rim pattern has usually been considered to represent a cholinesterase-positive innervation (Krnjević and Silver, 1965) and not intrinsic reactivity of the stained cell, i.e., presynaptic, not postsynaptic AChE. Using a mildly extracting plastic embedding medium (Quetol), we have been able to resolve this rim of stain into discrete foci that are quite similar in appearance to immunocytochemically demonstrated puncta (Fig. 6). Although we have not examined this material ultrastructurally, the interpretation of this pattern of cell staining as cholinesterase-receptive appears justified. Large pyramidal neurons of layer V in cat often exhibit this "superficial" type of staining (Krnjević and Silver, 1966). Physiological (Jordon and Phillis, 1972; Lamour *et al.*, 1983; Krnjević and Phillis, 1963) and biochemical data (Feldberg and Vogt, 1948) suggest that they are cholinoceptive, too. In contrast, some neurons stain more diffusely and contain reaction product within the perikaryon—as we have confirmed ultrastructurally (Kristt, 1979b; Fig. 7)—that extends out into dendrites. The latter are exemplified by the small nonpyramidal neurons seen at all cortical depths (Johnston *et al.*, 1981). In some fields, e.g., primary somatosensory cortex in rat, the latter are concentrated in layer VIb, providing one distinguishing landmark for this field (Fig. 17). Some of these neurons may be cholinergic (Houser *et al.*, 1983) and contribute axons to layer I (Kristt, 1979b). Layer I contains many positive somata postnatally (Fig. 16; Kristt, 1979a, rat; Duckett and Pearse, 1968, man; Krnjević and Silver, 1966, cat) as discussed below.

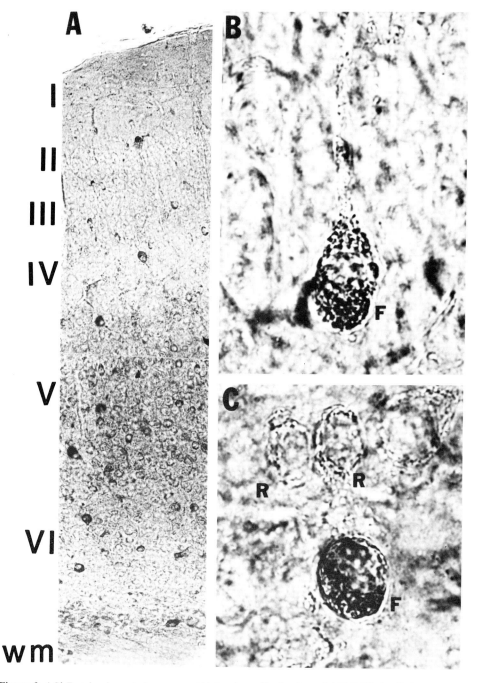

Figure 6. AChE-stained cortical neurons. (A) Laminar distribution of AChE-filled cells in somato-sensory cortex of rat (×150). Two patterns of cell staining are seen. In one (B), reaction product is seen to fill the perikaryon and extend out into the proximal dendrites of the cell. Such cells are seen to contain reaction product within the RER when examined ultrastructurally ("filled cells," F). ×1230. In the other (C), a thin rim of stain invests the periphery of the cell ("rimmed cells," R). ×1230. wm, white matter.

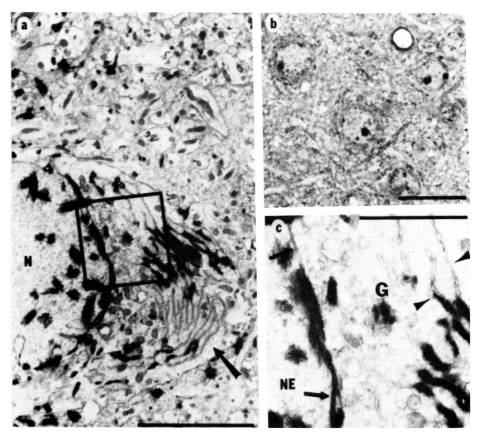

Figure 7. (a) Electron micrograph of AChE-stained layer VIb neuron from 16-day-old rat. Reaction product is noncrystalline; a nonspecific crystalline material is seen over nucleus of this and some other cells as well. Arrow, RER; N, nucleus. Bar = 5 μm. (b) Light micrograph of layer VIb neurons for comparison. Toluidine blue, 1.5 μm. AChE reaction product is fine, black material. Bar = 25 μm. (c) Higher magnification of box in (a). AChE reaction product is noncrystalline and appears in rough endoplasmic reticulum (RER) (arrowheads), nuclear envelope (NE), and possibly Golgi complex (G). Bar = 2 μm. From Kristt (1979b) with permission.

8. Ultrastructural Distribution of AChE

The distribution of ultrastructurally detectable, AChE-dependent reaction product in neocortex is quite similar to that reported for neurons in other regions in the CNS (Shute and Lewis, 1966; Lewis and Shute, 1966; Tennyson *et al.,* 1967; Kristt, 1979b, 1983; Villani *et al.,* 1977; Satoh *et al.,* 1983; Klinar and Brzin, 1977; Kasa, 1971). Although we have only examined young and infant rats, the light microscopic similarities suggest that the findings will also be applicable to adult animals.

Reaction product is associated with intracellular and extracellular elements. In cells seen heavily stained for AChE at the light microscopic level, electron microscopic examinations demonstrate intraneuronal reaction product. In such neurons, reaction product is found at a number of sites within the nuclear envelope, RER, and Golgi apparatus (Fig. 7). While this is the distribution of AChE in putative cholinergic neurons such as the anterior horn cell (Navaratnam and Lewis, 1970; Lewis and Shute, 1966), caution must be used in inferring that a neuron is cholinergic based on the localization of AChE at these sites. For instance, the neurons of the infant rat ventrobasal complex (VB) were found to exhibit this pattern of intracellular distribution transiently (Kristt, 1983), although all other indicators suggest these neurons are not cholinergic or significantly cholinoceptive at any age (Hoover *et al.*, 1978; Jacobowitz and Palkovits,

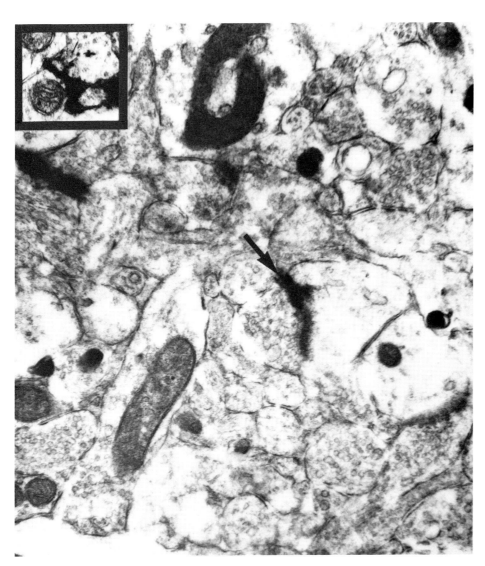

Figure 8. Extracellular distribution of AChE as seen with the electron microscope. Reaction product is associated with the lateral margins of the synaptic cleft (arrow). ×15,800. Inset: Small axon in layer IV is enveloped by a cuff of AChE associated with the axolemma. ×17,200.

1974; Arimatsu *et al.*, 1981; Kristt, 1983; Satoh *et al.*, 1983; Kobayashi *et al.*, 1978; Morley *et al.*, 1979; Kuhar *et al.*, 1980). It is probable that the immature Purkinje cell is another example of this phenomenon (Olschowka and Vijayan, 1980). A reasonable interpretation would be that many neurons in neocortex are synthesizing AChE; whether they are indeed cholinergic or cholinoceptive must await combined immunocytochemical and histochemical approaches. In infant brains, dendritic processes in layer I occasionally contain AChE associated with cytoskeletal elements. The latter may relate to the transport of AChE distally in the neuron.

In the extracellular compartment, reaction product is characteristically found surrounding small-caliber axons (Fig. 8). Again, although this is usually a characteristic of cholinergic neurons (Shute and Lewis, 1966), putative noncholinergic neurons of the infant rat VB show this characteristic as well (Kristt, unpublished observations).

Occasionally, one sees reaction product on the lateral margins of the synaptic cleft. These histochemically tagged synapses were not numerous (Fig. 8). As will be detailed below, immature rat somatosensory cortex contains dense plexuses of AChE-positive fibers that are believed to originate in the ventrobasal thalamus (VB). In 16-day-old rats, our preliminary unpublished work suggested that AChE-stained synapses in layer IV of SmI account for approximately 5% of synapses, a figure commensurate with the density of thalamocortical synapses originating in the VB found in other studies using different techniques (Garey and Powell, 1971; Colonnier, 1968). On the other hand, it is likely that this is an underestimation of VB afferents, since the histochemically determined density of AChE-rich thalamocortical afferents is apt to be lower than the density as determined autoradiographically. We do not have information at the present time on other laminae or ages. Although this density of AChE-associated synapses in layer IV of immature SmI may possibly represent a special case, the occurrence of AChE-tagged synapses is common throughout cortex.

9. Sources of Cortical AChE

In understanding the organization of the AChE-rich innervation of neocortex, it will be important to identify the component fiber systems (e.g., based on their cell bodies of origin) and the contribution of each component to the overall staining patterns. Histochemical and early biochemical studies found a loss of AChE and ChAT following cortical undercutting (Krnjević *et al.*, 1970; Green *et al.*, 1970) or subcortical lesions (Lehman *et al.*, 1980; Wenk *et al.*, 1980; Johnston *et al.*, 1979, 1981; Kelly and Moore, 1978; Hebb *et al.*, 1963). The percentage reduction varied somewhat, but generally compelled workers to expect that a substantial extrinsic AChE-rich cholinergic input to neocortex existed, as well as the more minor intrinsic cholinergic AChE-containing elements.

Several origins for the extrinsic inputs have been suggested based on histochemical, biochemical, and pharmacological strategies. It has been proposed that direct projections form the brain-stem reticular formation to cortex exist (Pepeu and Mantegazzini, 1964; Collier and Mitchell, 1966; Shute and Lewis,

1967; Phillis, 1968a; Bartolini *et al.*, 1972). Other evidence indicated the basal forebrain as a possible source for these inputs (Krnjević and Silver, 1965, 1966; Shute and Lewis, 1967; Das, 1971; Divac, 1975, 1981; Heimer and Wilson, 1975; Kieviet and Kuypers, 1975; Jones *et al.*, 1976; Henderson, 1981; Lehmann *et al.*, 1980; Kitt *et al.*, 1982; Bigl *et al.*, 1982; Ribak and Kramer, 1982; McKinney *et al.*, 1983; Mesulam *et al.*, 1983; Saper, 1984; Kristt *et al.*, 1985).

Shute and Lewis (1967), using histochemical and lesion strategies, made observations that appeared to support these two extracortical sources of the AChE-rich innervation. From all of this work, there was no clear consensus as to the relative contributions from each of the proposed sources. Nor was information on the patterns of distribution in cortex of these inputs available.

Most recently, biochemical studies have been able to rectify this situation. It now appears that in adult rat neocortex 50–70% of ChAT activity originates in basal forebrain inputs (Johnston *et al.*, 1981; Kelly and Moore, 1978; Green *et al.*, 1970). These projections are likely to be AChE-positive (Johnston *et al.*, 1981). This last inference would have two implications. First, the vast majority of AChE-positive fibers that we observe histochemically in neocortex are derived from basal forebrain. Second, these histochemically detected fibers are likely to reflect the organization of a major component of cholinergic circuitry in neocortex. This last conclusion has additional experimental support. Lesions of the basal forebrain made with an excitotoxin for cholinergic neurons—which should not affect corticopetal fibers of passage—or electrolytically, or by cortical undercutting eliminate a major proportion of AChE-rich fibers in cortex (Johnston *et al.*, 1979, 1981; Wenk *et al.*, 1980; Kristt *et al.*, 1985; Lehmann *et al.*, 1980). The views on the actual organization of this innervation differ and will be dealt with in another section.

Histochemical (Shute and Lewis, 1967, 1967), physiological, pharmacological (Phillis, 1968a, Pepeu and Mantegazzini, 1964; Collier and Mitchell, 1966; Bartolini *et al.*, 1972), and anatomical (Vincent *et al.*, 1983) findings suggested the existence of AChE-stained, cholinergic brain-stem afferents. But newer observations suggest that the proportional contribution of brain-stem AChE-rich inputs to neocortex are probably small. This conclusion is supported by two histochemical experiments. In the first, midbrain hemisections were made unilaterally and changes in staining in SmI cortex were assessed (Kristt and Waldman, 1981). No effect of the lesion could be detected in cortex of either hemisphere stained for AChE. The second experiment involved administering a catecholamine neurotoxin and its rationale was based on a number of earlier observations. First, it had been shown that the locus coeruleus projects extensively over much of neocortex (Moore and Bloom, 1978; Lindvall and Björklund, 1974), even in young animals (Kristt and Silverman, 1980; Lidov *et al.*, 1978). This group provides the major noradrenergic innervation of cortex. In infant rats, ultracytochemical, biochemical, and retrograde tracing data indicate that the coerulear cortical innervation is relatively dense (Coyle and Molliver, 1977; Kristt, 1979d; Kristt and Silverman, 1980; Kristt *et al.*, 1980). The second background observation made by several workers is that noncholinergic, catecholaminergic neurons of the locus coeruleus and substantia nigra contained high levels of AChE (Butcher, 1977; Palkovits and Jacobowitz, 1974; Koelle, 1955). This is evident even in young rats (Fig. 9). Since substantia nigra neurons send axons to neostriatum that appear to be AChE-rich (Emson and Lindvall, 1979; Marshall *et al.*, 1983), we wondered whether coerulear neurons have a substantial density of AChE-positive fibers in cortex. To examine this question, infant rats were used. The noradrenergic neurotoxin 6-hydroxydopamine was administered at an age when it passes the blood–brain barrier and at a dose to produce a persistent 90% decrement in cortical norepinephrine (Jonsson and Sachs, 1976; Schmidt and Bhatnagar, 1979). In animals we have treated in this fashion, the coerulear input to neocortex (Kristt and Silverman, 1980) can no longer be demonstrated by retrograde transport of horseradish peroxidase, suggesting that coerulear input to cortex is substantially eliminated. Yet, in preparations treated for AChE, no effects on the organization or intensity of this innervation were apparent (unpublished observations). Similarly, neurotoxic interruption of the mesotelencephalic dopaminergic projections also did not detectably influence the AChE staining of receptive limbic cortical areas (Marshall *et al.*, 1983). In short, the proportional contribution and intracortical distribution of AChE-containing brain-stem afferents are unknown presently. However, the contribution from this source is apt to be small.

Another source of extrinsic AChE-positive innervation can be detected only transiently during development and appears to be derived from thalamus. More on this subject below.

The possibility has been raised that intrinsic cholinergic circuits exist, derived from cell bodies located within neocortex. There are three parts to this issue. First, we need to consider whether there are intrinsic AChE-synthesizing somata in neocortex. Second, are AChE-synthesizing cortical neurons cholinergic? Third, if we assume such neurons are present in cortex, do they primarily form local or distant connections? It has very clearly been shown that AChE-

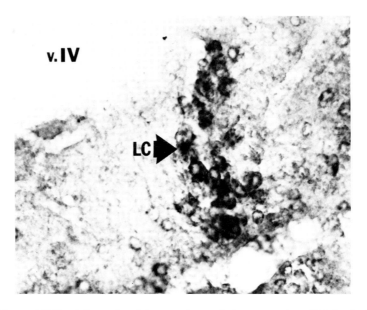

Figure 9. Dense AChE-staining cells of the noradrenergic locus coeruleus (LC) in the infant rat. The fourth ventricle (v. IV) is seen in the upper left corner. ×250.

rich neurons showing dense perikaryal AChE staining (Fig. 6) are present in most neocortical regions in several mammals including cat, rat, monkey, and man (Krnjević and Silver, 1965; Johnston *et al.*, 1981; Kristt, 1979b; Kristt *et al.*, 1985; Okinaka *et al.*, 1961). For these cells, dense staining of proximal dendrites is also seen (Kristt, 1979b). This pattern of cell staining has been traditionally felt to be indicative of a cholinergic neuron. As noted in another section, these latter cells do appear to be synthesizing AChE based on ultrastructural observations. Since several different cell types that lack cholinergic markers stain this way—e.g., locus coeruleus (Butcher, 1977; fig. 9), VB (Kristt, 1983)—interpretation of these histochemical data is moot. From these findings alone we can conclude only that cortex contains *"cholinesterase-synthesizing"* cells. Some workers require the further histochemical criterion for a cholinergic neuron that its axon stain for AChE as well as the perikaryon (e.g., Shute and Lewis, 1966). But this too can be questioned, as discussed elsewhere in this chapter. Further, it appears that many AChE-positive neurons are not immunoreactive for ChAT (Levey *et al.*, 1983; Wainer *et al.*, 1984), but rather AChE colocalizes with GABA immunoreactivity (Wainer *et al.*, 1984). Independent replication of those last findings using other antibodies against ChAT, would be important in confirming this fundamental aspect of cortical organization. A this time, serious consideration must be given to the possibility that many AChE-containing intrinsic cortical neurons are noncholinergic.

The biochemical data we reviewed earlier suggest that the majority of cholinergic circuits in neocortex are probably extrinsic in origin. However, several different experimental approaches consistently have shown that a substantial level of cholinergic markers, including AChE, persist after various types of cortical deafferentation such as undercutting (Johnston *et al.*, 1981; Lehmann *et al.*, 1980; Green *et al.*, 1970; Kristt *et al.*, 1985). These biochemical and histochemical results generally have been felt to support the possibility of intrinsic cholinergic circuitry. On the other hand, one group has suggested that residual cholinergic activity is attributable to cholinergic vascular innervation (Satch *et al.*, 1983).

In a physiological study using chronically isolated cat cerebral cortex (Jordan and Phillis 1972), data were presented that strongly support the existence of intracortical cholinergic neurons that form synapses in superficial cortex. This conclusion would be consonant with biochemical findings (reviewed above), histochemical observations in cat (Krnjević and Silver, 1965), the histochemically detectable organization of residual AChE-stained elements in rat cortex following deafferenting lesions (Johnston *et al.*, 1979, 1981; Kristt *et al.*, 1985), and immunocytochemistry in rat (Houser *et al.*, 1983; Kimura *et al.*, 1980). The absence of ChAT-immunoreactive cells in some studies (e.g., Armstrong *et al.*, 1983, rat; Satoh *et al.*, 1983, rat, same antibody; Sofroniew *et al.*, 1982, rat, different antibody) is therefore perplexing. Before we rule out the existence of intrinsic cholinergic cortical neurons on such evidence, a number of technical concerns must be addressed. These include sensitivity, specificity of the immunocytochemical procedures, the existence of multiple forms of the enzyme (Benishin and Carroll, 1983), and biologically active naturally occurring inhibitors of the enzyme (Cozzari and Hartman, 1983) that could affect the immunocytochemical outcome. In regard to sensitivity, there may be considerable variations between antibodies or the immunocytochemical techniques utilizing them. For instance, while studying the rat nucleus basalis, one laboratory found that 100% of AChE-staining neurons were ChAT-immunoreactive (Eckenstein and Sofroniew, 1983) while other workers have found only 73% to be ChAT-positive (Levey *et al.*, 1983). Further, the antibody used by Sofroniew *et al.* (1982) does not appear to detect "puncta" on cholinoceptive neurons as does the antibody used by Houser *et al.* (1983).

In brief, interpreting ChAT immunocytochemical staining is a complex issue that needs to be more completely evaluated. Whatever the outcome of this polemic, I believe that there is sufficient evidence to conclude that AChE-synthesizing neurons are present in cortex, and probably ramify locally within their field. The functional significance of these AChE-positive intrinsic elements may have to be reinterpreted as new information becomes available.

Another series of observations indicate that these intrinsic, AChE-rich cortical neurons ramify locally in their fields. In adult rats, it was found that lesions that remove almost all of the AChE-reactive fibers in a small region of neocortex leave layer I least affected (Kristt *et al.*, 1985).* The source of this fiber staining that persists in layer I following these lesions could be intrinsic since some lesions completely isolated a cylindrical zone of cortex extending from pia to white matter from all directions (save for narrow perivascular strips) (Fig. 10). Admittedly, it is still possible that some extrinsically derived fibers enter cortex and travel pialwards in a radial plane, so that they are not intercepted by the knife blade. Such fibers, if they originate in basal forebrain, would be expected to ramify mostly in layer V (Saper, 1984) with some additional branching in layer I. However, layer V had very few residual fibers after such circular lesions, as opposed to layer I. One conclusion, then, is that layer I was still well innervated by AChE-positive cells *within* the region encompassed by the lesion, i.e., layer I may reflect intrinsic connectivity. It would be of value to investigate other noncortical sources, aside from basal forebrain, in these circular lesion preparations. The preparation may afford the opportunity to examine small contributions from AChE-rich afferents that normally may be masked by the dense basal forebrain innervation.

Developmental studies in the rat also suggest an intracortical source for these putative layer I inputs (Kristt, 1979b). In infant rat cortex, there are neurons in layer VI that project their axons toward the pial surface and terminate in layer I; these are the so-called Martinotti cells (Fig. 17; Ramón y Cajal, 1911, 1960; Astrom, 1967; Marin-Padilla, 1972; Meller *et al.*, 1969; Kristt, 1979b). It has been suggested that they play a crucial role in cortical ontogenesis by forming an intracortical circuit (Marin-Padilla, 1978). In many cortical fields, these neurons are densely stained for AChE (Figs. 6 and 17). The stained cells are already in evidence at birth in some cortical regions. Although there is a continuously advancing front of basal forebrain-originating AChE fibers growing adpially, fibers in layer I are present several days earlier than they are in deeper laminae (Kristt, 1979a). Cajal–Retzius cells in layer I are also AChE-stained in this period, but are too sparse to account for much of this fiber staining (Kristt, 1979a, rat;

---

* The biochemical study by Johnston *et al.* (1981) did not detect this effect, but that may be due to the large 350-μm-depth bins; the subpial band of staining is only about 25–50 μm wide.

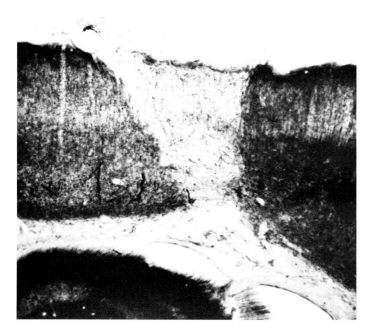

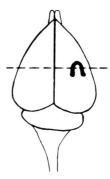

Figure 10. Effect of pia-to-white-matter U-lesion in cortex on AChE staining in adult rat. Note dramatic loss of fibers in center of lesion, with relatively greater preservation of fibers in layer I in comparison to other laminae. Lateral margins are well stained. ×32. Diagram at right shows orientation of knife cut and dashed line indicates plate of section. From Kristt *et al.* (1985) with permission.

Krnjević and Silver, 1966, cat; Duckett and Pearse, 1968, man). It has been suggested that these early arriving fibers in layer I derive from the AChE-synthesizing somata in layer VIb (Kristt, 1979b).

10. Organization of the AChE-Rich Innervation from Basal Forebrain

As noted above, the major source of cortical AChE-rich inputs derives from the AChE-rich cell bodies of the basal forebrain. Such cells were observed in the diagonal band, hypothalamus and substantia innominata, and ventral pallidum. These neurons form a series of contiguous but poorly delineated aggregates of AChE-rich neurons in basal forebrain (Armstrong *et al.*, 1983; Das, 1971; Divac, 1975, 1981; Gorry, 1963, Hayaraman, 1980; Heimer and Wilson, 1975; Jacobowitz and Palkovits, 1974; Jones, 1975; Kelly and Moore, 1978; Kimura *et al.*, 1980; Mesulam and Van Hoesen, 1976; Parent and Butcher, 1976; Ribak and Kramer, 1982; Saper, 1984). Most of these cells exhibit ChAT immunoreactivity and lesions of this region reduce cortical levels of both AChE and cholinergic markers (Armstrong *et al.*, 1983; Bigl *et al.*, 1982; Candy *et al.*, 1981; Eckenstein and Sofroniew, 1983; Houser *et al.*, 1983; Johnston *et al.*, 1979, 1981; Jones *et al.*, 1976; Kievet and Kuypers, 1975; Kimura *et al.*, 1980; Kristt *et al.,* 1985; Krnjević and Silver, 1966; Lehmann *et al.,* 1980; Luskin and Price, 1982; Mesulam *et al.,* 1983; Saper, 1984; Whitehouse *et al.,* 1981). In addition to a laminar organization for these inputs, earlier workers, using lesion and antero- and retrograde pathway tracing techniques, have adduced the basic spatial relationship between cortex and the AChE-rich (cholinergic) basal forebrain nuclear cell groups. It has been consistently noted that in several mammalian species there is a rostrocaudal topographical relationship (Saper, 1984; Jones *et al.,* 1976; Lehmann *et al.,* 1980; Wenk *et al.,* 1980; Mesulam *et al.,* 1983). One prominent exception has been noted, viz. the innervation of parts of occipital cortex which derives from neurons in the anterior components of the basal forebrain complex (e.g., the diagonal band). However, this exception can be more easily understood by considering the distribution of fibers in each of the different pathways basal forebrain fibers follow to neocortex (Fig. 11). The latter issue has been the subject of two recent papers in the rat. One study used retro- and anterograde pathway tracing techniques (Saper, 1984) and the other used a combination of AChE-histochemical, lesion, and Golgi techniques (Kristt *et al.,* 1985). The results in both studies are remarkably congruent. They show that medial cortex and occipital cortex are innervated by a bundle of rostrocaudally running fibers (the *medial pathway*). Lesions in this pathway result in a substantial loss of staining caudal to the lesion in cingulate and medial occipital fields (Fig. 12). Reaction product is seen to accumulate on the rostral side of the cut.

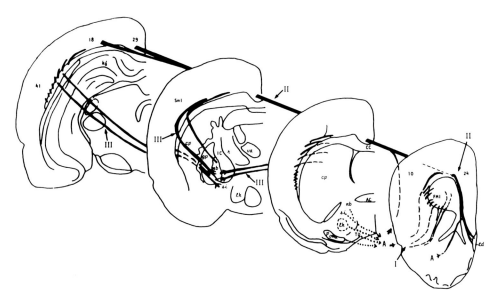

Figure 11. Reconstructed representation of the three proposed pathways from basal forebrain to neocortex based on AChE-dependent staining and lesions: I, anterior; II, medial; III, lateral. Origin of a pathway is traceable to a general region, not to specific cell groups, as indicated by arrowheads. Region A contains a number of AChE-rich cell groups that are likely to be contributing to pathways I and II. The cell groups are indicated by dotted-line arrows directed at "A." Dashed lines indicate fibers that are passing through the thickness of a particular section. Cortical field SmI contains the barrel field. Numerical field designations after Krieg (1946). Schematics modified from Konig and Klippel (1974). From Kristt *et al.* (1985) with permission.

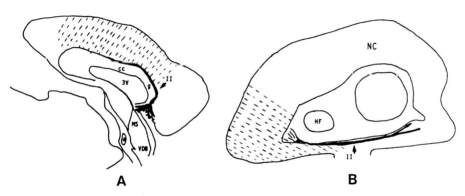

Figure 12. Composite drawings showing effects of lesions on AChE-stained proximal components of the medial pathway (see Fig. 11). The drawings show AChE-stained fibers/fascicles (dark lines) connecting basal forebrain with neocortex. Each drawing was traced from an optical projection of a single section at age 4 days (A) and adult (B). At each of the illustrated regions of cerebrum, lesions (arrows) were made in another set of adult rats. Areas showing decreased AChE staining following lesioning are hatched. (A) Sagittal section, rostral-right, 4-day-old rat. Persistent staining caudally reflects caudolateral orientation of fibers in this pathway. (B) Horizontal section, rostral-right, adult rat. Note loss of staining involves medial occipital cortex. cc, corpus callosum; g, genu, cc; HF, hippocampal formation; MS, medial septal nucleus; NC, neocortex; 3V, third ventricle; VDB, diagonal band, ventral limb. From Kristt *et al.* (1985) with permission.

The organization of fibers innervating lateral and frontopolar cortex is quite different. These fibers emanate from the AChE-rich basal forebrain nuclei to reach layer VI of cortex (Fig. 11). The fibers run for short distances in this lamina before ascending toward the pia. Lesion studies suggest that these fibers terminate predominantly in layer V where they form a dense plexus. Antero-grade tracing experiments using radiolabeled amino acids similarly suggest a concentration of basal forebrain inputs in layer V of most cortical fields (Fig. 2). This work also suggests terminal field dimensions for individual basal forebrain neurons of approximately 1.5 mm (Saper, 1984). Lesion studies suggested a figure of 1–2 mm (Kristt *et al.*, 1985). Additionally, sagittal knife cuts have much less of an effect than coronal cuts. This suggests that the fibers appear to run for longer distances in a roughly rostrocaudal dimension than in the mediolateral plane, i.e., a roughly oval shape to the terminal field with the major axis close to a rostrocaudal orientation. Some fibers also appear to terminate in layer I as well ("subpial band," Kristt, 1979a; Kristt *et al.*, 1985; Saper, 1984), but other AChE-rich inputs, e.g., intrinsic, are apt to contribute to this latter stratum, as considered above. Observations suggesting a limited tangential extent for the terminal zones of basal forebrain afferents to lateral and anterior cortex are supported by double retrograde labeling experiments from several laboratories (Saper, 1984; Luskin and Price, 1982; Bigl *et al.*, 1982; Price and Stern, 1983). In contrast, one study has suggested that at least 16% of basal forebrain neurons have a more widespread distribution of intracortical collaterals, based on double-labeled cell frequency (McKinney *et al.*, 1983). The apparent anomaly of these last data has been attributed to technical factors in their experimental design (Saper, 1984).

The physiologic implication for this pattern of innervation is that a single basal forebrain neuron interacts with a relatively small population of cortical neurons. This raises several questions that are dealt with in the final section of this chapter.

11. Development of AChE Innervation to Neocortex

Although developmental events have been alluded to at several points, it will be of value to consider in a more systematic way the maturation of the patterns of cell and fiber staining in neocortex.

Two temporal–spatial developmental gradients exist. One is the progression of AChE staining—predominantly in fibers—across the neocortex as a whole. In light of the predominant contribution of basal forebrain to this innervation, it is not surprising that this progression moves in lockstep with the maturation of the basal forebrain projections to neocortex. The regional organization of the basal forebrain projection system is reflected in the regional timetable for maturation.

As noted above, there are apparently three sets of AChE-rich basal forebrain afferents that provide the innervation of neocortex. These are (1) the medial system; (2) the anterior system; and (3) the lateral system. Earliest fibers reach the cortex at two points, more or less synchronously. Axons from the medial pathway initially invade anterior medial cortex, while the lateral pathway fibers first appear in the anterior lateral part of frontal cortex (Fig. 13). This is the picture at 18–20 days of gestation in rat (Kristt, unpublished observations) and at 41–50 days of gestation in the cat (Krnjević and Silver, 1966) and 18–22 weeks of gestation in man (Kostovic, 1983). In relation to this site in frontal cortex, the fibers progressively appear more medially and caudally within the lateral and anterior territories. The medial system progresses along a more regular rostral–caudal vector.

In addition to these geographic patterns of fiber in growth, there is a stereotyped progression within a single cortical region. This generally follows an inside-out format with the deepest layers being stained at earliest ages. As noted above, there is one prominent exception to this developmental scheme. Fiber staining in the subpial band (Kristt 1979a) of layer I appears before stained fibers can be detected in layers II and III (Fig. 14); stained fibers appear in the latter between days 4 and 5 postnatally in the rat (cf. Figs. 14 and 15). Similar findings have been noted in the cat (Krnjević and Silver, 1965). The development of human cortex is similar (Kostovic et al., 1980). AChE-positive somata are also evident early in development. They are initially concentrated in layer I as Cajal–Retzius cells and layer VI as Martinotti cells (Figs. 16 and 17). In rat, by the end of the first week postnatally, stained somata are seen at most other depths as well (Fig. 6). Although the absolute time course differs somewhat between species, the stagewise progression is similar (Krnjević and Silver, 1966, cat; Krmpotic-Nemanic et al., 1980, 1983; Kostovic, 1982, man).

There is another point of similarity among these mammalian species that I would like to emphasize. In immature neocortex of rat, cat, man, and mouse, synaptogenesis (Cragg, 1975; Kristt, 1978, 1979d; Kristt and Molliver, 1976,

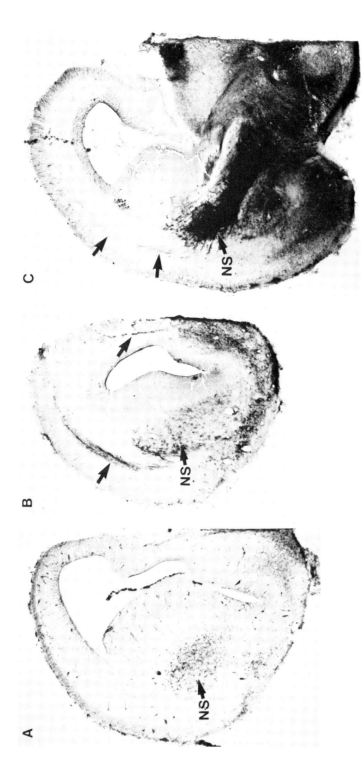

Figure 13. AChE-stained coronal sections of fetal cerebrum at (A) 17 days of gestation and (B, C) 19 days of gestation. Note initial fibers (arrows) enter cortex from basal forebrain medial pathway and anterior pathways. Lateral pathway appears in cortex along a rostrocaudal gradient. NS, neostriatum. ×22.

Molliver *et al.*, 1973; Kristt *et al.*, 1980) and AChE staining (Krnjević and Silver, 1966; Kristt, 1979a; Kristt and Kasper, 1983; Kostovic *et al.*, 1980; Krmpotic-Nemanic *et al.*, 1980) are laminar, i.e., consistently concentrated in specific cell layers of immature cortex (Fig. 15). In neonatal rat this is particularly striking at postnatal day 6, where the two bands of intense AChE neuropil staining correspond to depths (or strata) of relatively high synapse density (Kristt, 1979d;

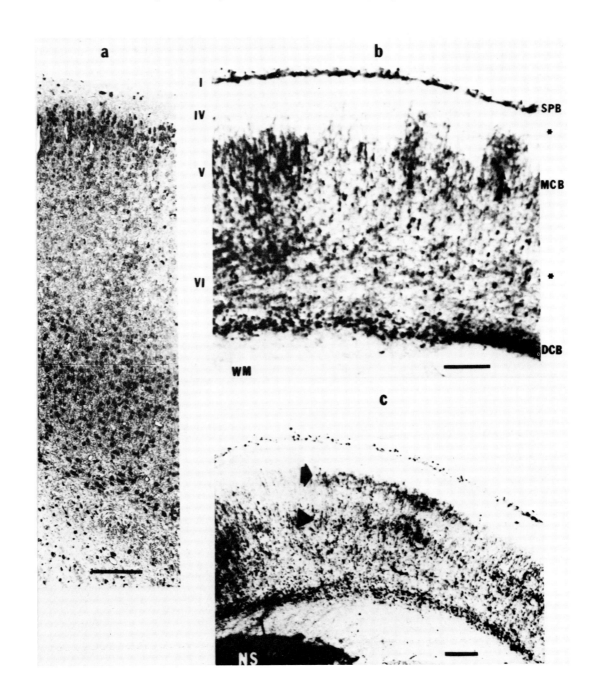

Kristt and Molliver, 1976; Kristt *et al.*, 1980). There are a number of possible explanations for the congruence of an AChE-rich neuropil with particular synapse-dense strata. For instance, a transient developmental phenomenon among certain classes of neurons is possible. This has been seen, for instance, in several neuronal types outside of neocortex, as explained below. This stimulates the speculation that AChE may have a role in the maturation of cortical circuitry. Such a suggestion would be compatible with the thought that cells in layers I and VI—frequently AChE-synthesizing in the infant—play a basic role in the developing organization of neocortex (Marin-Padilla, 1978; Kristt, 1979b). Another possibility is that cholinergic axons are forming synapses in these AChE-rich strata. This is a reasonable suggestion if we accept two propositions: (1) cholinergic synapses probably exist in immature neocortex (Coyle and Yamamura, 1976) as they do in the adult (Collier and Mitchell, 1966; Feldberg and Vogt, 1948; Hebb and Silver, 1956; Krnjević and Phillis, 1963; Stone, 1972; Jordan and Phillis, 1972; Lamour *et al.*, 1983) and (2) cholinergic synapses are more likely to occur in AChE-rich rather than AChE-poor sites (Gerebtzoff, 1959; Kobayashi *et al.*, 1978) or laminae. Current information suggests that both options probably appertain, with putative cholinergic inputs to layers I and V and a transient, presumably noncholinergic input in layer IV in some fields (see below). However, synaptological studies with specific cholinergic markers still need to be performed to confirm these suggestions.

12. Transient AChE in Cortex

Although the above description of developmental events is applicable for most cortical fields, primary somatosensory cortex (SmI) exhibits a number of developmental features that are unique to it. Because SmI represents such a substantial proportion of rodent neocortex, it is worth giving special attention to these exceptional features. Additionally, in manifesting a developmental pro-

Figure 14. Somatosensory cortex of 3-day-old rat stained for AChE. (a) Toluidine blue-stained section, 1.5 μm thick. Not processed for histochemistry. Pia is toward top margin of photograph. Bar = 100 μm. (b) Coronal section stained for AChE. Three bands of relatively intense AChE staining are present: subpial (SPB), midcortical (MCB), and deep cortical (DCB). SPB consists of a dark tangential band of fiber staining in which AChE-positive cells are frequently observed. Cells are similar to those illustrated in Fig. 16. They are better seen in (c), where the fiber staining is less conspicuous. At this age, MCB consists mostly of fiber staining in the primordium of layer IV. Note intermittent foci of staining, that represent barrels. Scattered cells are also stained in the primordium of layer V. DCB consists of a lamina of AChE-positive cells at the bottom of layer VI (cf. Fig. 17) and fiber staining (Fig. 5). Laminar designations to left are approximately in center of the respective primordial lamina. Asterisks to right denote the boundaries of the MCB. Ventrolateral = right margin of picture; dorsomedial = left margin. wm, white matter. Bar = 200 μm. (c) Coronal section of somatosensory cortex stained for AChE in region presumed to be SmII. MCB appears as two parallel tangential lines of fiber staining. Upper line is in layer IV and more heavily stained than the lower line in layer V. Darkly stained cells are particularly prominent in the subpial band in layer I but are also apparent in primordial layers V and VI. Compare the intensity of staining in neostriatum (NS) at bottom of picture. Dorsomedial, right margin; ventrolateral, left margin. Bar = 200 μm. From Kristt (1979a) with permission.

gression for AChE-stained elements that differs from other regions of cortex, SmI may provide some clues for noncholinergic functions of AChE during maturation.

A characteristic aspect of rat SmI is the aggregation of somata in layer IV, known as "barrels" (Fig. 18). Recent attention was drawn to this special cytoarchitectural characteristic of whisking rodents by the work of Woolsey and Van der Loos (1970) in mice. Barrels probably represent a morphological expression of the functional columnar organization of neocortex alluded to above. In many regards, the maturation and organization of barrel "fields" in SmI of rats and mice are closely related (Kristt, 1979a; Kristt and Waldman, 1982); differences

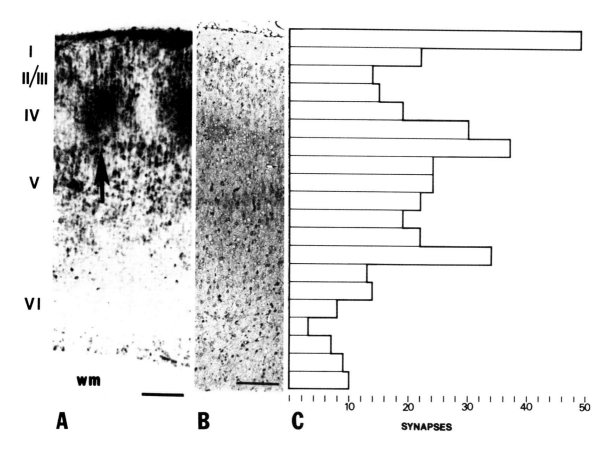

Figure 15. Somatosensory cortex of 6-day-old rat. (A) Arrow points to the center of one of a series of darkly staining foci in layer IV. The distribution, location, and dimensions of these zones suggest an overlap with the "specific" thalamocortical projection to the barrel fields of SmI. The subpial band is more densely stained than at earlier ages. Numerous positive somata are seen in layer V of the midcortical band and in layer VI of the deep cortical band, but their outlines are generally indistinct at this magnification without counterstain (cf. Fig. 17). wm, white matter. Bar = 200 μm. (B) Toluidine blue section, 1.5 μm thick, of region corresponding to that illustrated in A; material not processed for AChE histochemistry. Note that at approximately 400 μm deep, there is a slight intensification of neuropil staining. This marks the primordium of layer IV, which contains developing barrel neurons of SmI. The white matter is approximately at the same depth as in A. Bar = 200 μm. (C) Laminar synapse distribution in neocortex of rat at postnatal day 6. Area of inspected tissue in each 50-μm depth class = 875 μm². N = 395 synapses. Note that synapses with AChE-rich fibers are concentrated in layers I and IV. From Kristt (1979a) and Kristt and Molliver (1976) with permission.

do exist and have been well considered in many other studies (Welker and Woolsey, 1975; Woolsey *et al.*, 1975). For our purposes here, the differences are quite minor and are noted in Table I.

The barrels in the rat first become apparent between postnatal (P) day 2 and 3, depending on the method used to demonstrate them. AChE staining of fibers in the barrel centers of rat can be histochemically detected by P3 (Fig. 14); in the mouse at P4–5, but fewer fibers are seen in the latter (Kristt, 1979a; Kristt and Waldman, 1982).

The staining initially appears as periodic foci in layer IV consisting of a few intertwined or highly branched fibers (Kristt, 1979a; Kristt and Waldman, 1982).

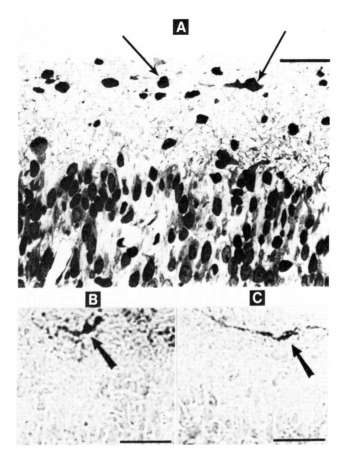

Figure 16. AChE-stained cells in layer I of newborn rat. (A) Higher magnification of marginal zone and upper cortical plate. In the sparsely cellular marginal zone, two types of cells are apparent; one has a globular soma and the other a more fusiform or club-shaped soma (marked with arrows). The globular neuron on the left corresponds to the AChE-positive cell in B; the club-shaped cell on the right corresponds to the AChE-stained cell in C. (We cannot exclude the possibility that the globular cell is an "on-end" view of more fusiform neurons.) The absence of AChE staining in the immature neurons of the upper cortical plate is well seen by comparing A with B and C. Bar = 30 μm and overlies pia. (B) AChE-positive Cajal–Retzius cell in the marginal zone. Arrow indicates soma. Bar = 25 μm. (C) AChE-positive Cajal–Retzius cell in the marginal zone. Arrow indicates soma. Bar = 25 μm. From Kristt (1979a) with permission.

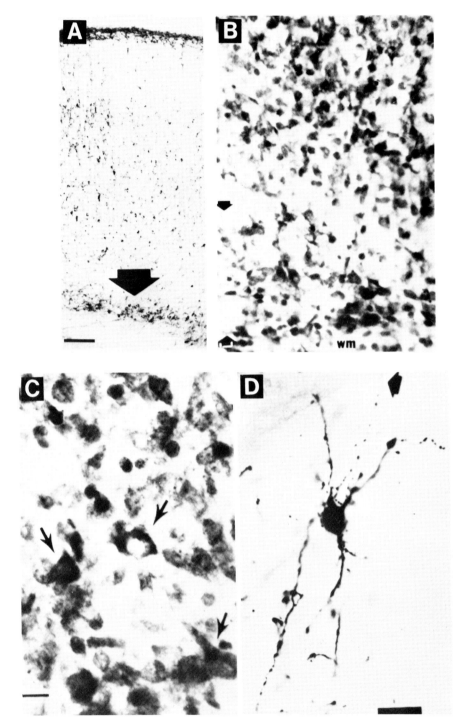

Figure 17. AChE-filled neurons in layer VIb of rat. (A) AChE-stained cortex following undercut, highlights cell staining in layer VIb (arrow). (B, C) Counterstained AChE-reacted section shows in comparison with A that most cells in layer VI are unstained. Reaction product fills processes of some cells in layer VIb. wm, white matter. (D) Golgi impregnation of layer VIb cell with ascending axon. From Kristt (1979b) with permission.

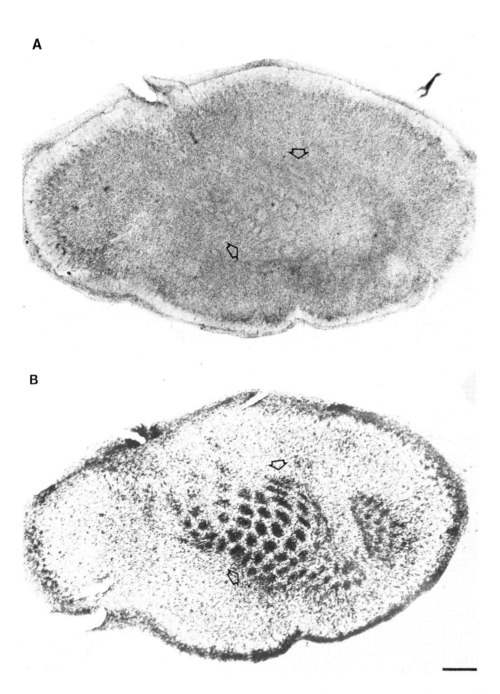

Figure 18. Barrels in SmI cortex stained for AChE and Nissl in two successive (A,B) tangential sections through layer IV of 6-day-old rat. Several regions of the barrel field are stained. Note that only centers appear AChE positive; sides and septa are much paler. Arrows indicate same rows in both pictures. Section thickness: AChE, 80 μm; cresyl violet, 40 μm. Bar = 0.5 mm.

Table I. Comparison of AChE-Stained[a] Barrels in Mice and Rats[b]

	AChE-stained (max. diam., μm)	Shape	Wall (μm)[c]	Onset (days postnatal)
Mouse	200–250 or	Circular	40	4–5
	300 × 120	Oval		
Rat	250–300	Circular	BB 60–100 BR 200	3

[a] Based on tangential sections through layer IV and SmI at postnatal day 6–7.
[b] Abbreviations: diam., diameter of major and minor axes; BB, distance between barrels in a row; BR, distance between rows.
[c] Unstained for AChE.

Within a few days' time, a regular array of cylindrical foci of AChE-rich fibers is seen (cf. Figs. 14 and 18). In rats, the staining is so intense by P6 and the fibers so fine that individual fibers cannot be resolved at the light microscopic level (Fig. 15); these foci have a soft, "smudged" appearance. Somata in layer IV are, however, not noticeably reactive. The dimensions of these foci suggest that they fill the centers and generally conform to the shape defined by the cellular sides of the barrels (Table I, Fig. 18).*

It has been suggested that AChE-rich foci that overlap the barrel centers in SmI are composed of axons derived from VB (Kristt, 1979a,c, 1983; Kristt and Waldman, 1981). Based on other methods to detect thalamic inputs, it appears that VB sends fibers into the barrels by P2–4 in rats and mice (Waite, 1977; Killackey and Belford, 1979; Kristt and Silverman, 1981; Wise and Jones, 1978; Ivy and Killackey, 1982). The finding in mouse of AChE-positive fibers after this time (Kristt and Waldman, 1982) probably does not reflect ingrowth of another set of AChE-rich afferents, but only our inability to detect the fibers histochemically at an earlier age in mouse. This interpretation is consistent with our observations that the AChE-staining density in mouse is generally lower than in rat. The latter phenomenon is likely due to either lower AChE per fiber in mouse, fewer fibers, a lag in anterograde transport, or an intracellular environment that interferes with the histochemical reaction. Based on differences in packing density between the barrels of mouse and rat—the density is higher in rat—it has been speculated that there may be fewer trigeminal afferents related to a given sinus hair on the face of the mouse (Welker and Woolsey, 1975). The differential density and lighter staining of AChE-positive fibers could influence initial detection. These considerations, incidently, raise the more general point that caution is warranted in equating onset of detectable staining in AChE-stained afferents with the actual time course of ingrowth. Independent evidence in each instance is needed to establish the extent of a correlation. In any event, the time frame for the onset of AChE staining of barrel afferents in the mouse is consistent

* In mouse, the barrels are "hollow" in that the cell density centrally is less than that at the sides. The septa between the barrels are also relatively hypocellular. In adult rat, the barrel centers from anterior SmI are hollow, whereas the large barrels of the posteromedial barrel subfield have a more evenly distributed cell density between the sides and centers. In infant rats, the posterior barrels are also relatively hollow (Fig. 18).

with the early phases of ingrowth of VB afferents into the barrels, even if the initial fibers cannot be histochemically detected in this rodent; in rat, the developmental correspondence is excellent.

In thalamus (Kristt, 1983), the putative cells of origin for the barrel afferents are also AChE-rich during the period the barrels are stained (Fig. 19), despite the evidence suggesting that VB is not cholinergic (Jacobowitz and Palkovits, 1974; Arimatsu *et al.*, 1981; Kimura *et al.*, 1981) or significantly cholinoceptive (Kobayashi *et al.*, 1978; Morley *et al.*, 1979; Kuhar *et al.*, 1980). Most neurons in VB and the barrels lose most of their AChE reactivity in the third week postnatally; the VB precedes cortex by several days (Figs. 20 and 21).

In favorable histochemical reactions for AChE, one can also see that the elaborate branching of AChE-positive fibers in the barrels is similar to that seen in several types of preparations demonstrating thalamocortical afferents (Kristt and Waldman, 1982; Landry and Deschenes, 1981; Lorente de Nó, 1949; Steffen, 1976). Electrolytic lesions of VB (Fig. 22) eliminate barrel AChE staining ipsilaterally, an effect that extensive lesions of basal forebrain inputs do not duplicate (McGowan *et al.*, 1983). In neonatal animals where lesions were inadvertently placed medial, dorsal, lateral, or ventral to VB, no loss of barrel staining was seen (Kristt and Waldman, 1981). Thalamus immediately adjacent to VB, vz. the reticular, ventrolateral, central lateral, posterior, and ventral medial nuclei, were slightly damaged by these lesions (Kristt and Waldman, 1981) but somata in these nuclei do not appear to be synthesizing AChE during the first postnatal week (Kristt, 1983). Also in relation to potential inputs from the basal forebrain, preliminary observations suggest that these are still infragranular

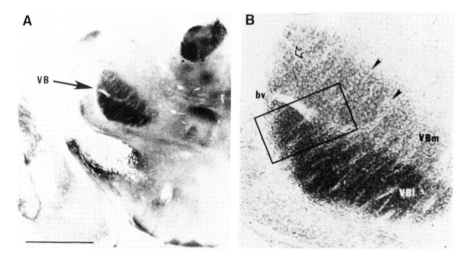

Figure 19. AChE-stained coronal sections of ventrobasal complex in thalamus of 6-day-old rat. VB is still relatively heavily stained in comparison to surrounding thalamus. (A) Note clear distinction in staining intensity between VBl and VBm. In some areas, AChE-positive somata are clustered into bands separated by thin unstained zones. (B) Higher-magnification view of the VB. Zones of somata are separated by fine AChE-negative arciform bands (arrowheads). Circular or polygonal clusters of cells within a zone (open arrow) are occasionally noted, particularly in the dorsomedial portion of the nucleus. Within area of rectangle, virtually all cells were AChE-positive when examined in 4-μm-thick plastic sections. bv, blood vessel. From Kristt (1983) with permission.

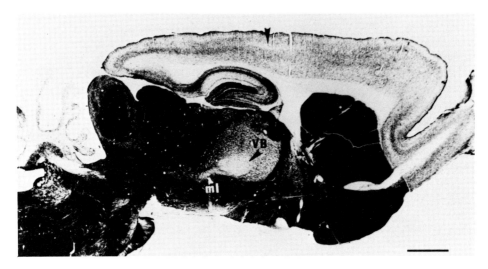

Figure 20. Sagittal section of adult rat cerebrum showing distinct pallor of layer IV in somatosensory cortex and the hyporeactivity of VB among thalamic structures. ml, medial lemniscus. Bar = 1 μm. From Kristt (1983) with permission.

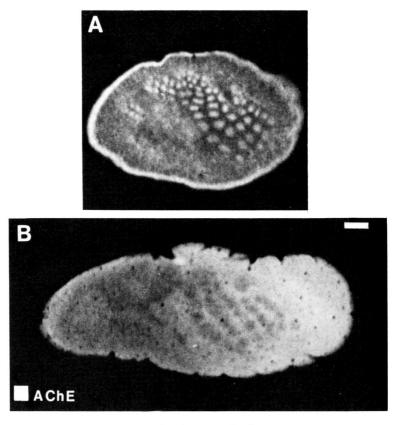

Figure 21. Maturation of the barrel field in layer IV of primary somatosensory cortex as seen in tangential, negative-image photographs of AChE-stained material. (A) Rat, postnatal day 6; (B) adult rat. Bar = 0.5 mm. From Kristt and Waldman (1986) with permission.

in their distribution in SmI by P3; yet, at this stage the barrels are quite distinctly stained in the rat (Fig. 14). Biochemical data are also consistent with the conclusion that little detectable basal forebrain input is present during the first postnatal week (Coyle and Yamamura, 1976). This contrasts with the finding that AChE-positive fibers in the barrels show organizational alterations following damage to the sensory periphery that parallels responses seen using other markers for thalamic inputs and cells (Van der Loos and Woolsey, 1973; Weller and Johnson, 1975; Woolsey and Wann, 1976; Jeanmonod *et al.*, 1977; Killackey and Belford, 1980; Pidoux *et al.*, 1980). For instance, neonatal destruction of a single row of mystacial vibrissae results in an elongated tangential domain of AChE positivity that corresponds in location to the affected row, but lacks discrete

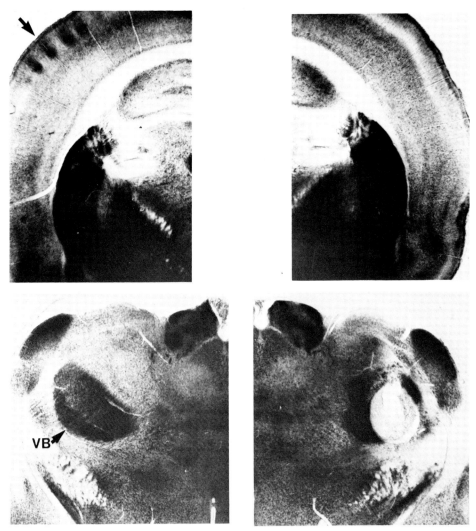

Figure 22. Effects of electrolytic lesions of VB thalamus on ipsilateral staining in layer IV of somatosensory cortex. Rat, postnatal day 6. (Top) Coronal sections through somatosensory cortex and barrel field. (Bottom) Sections at more posterior levels through VB. Note loss of distinct foci in layer IV, i.e., barrel centers no longer stain for AChE, although other layers are well stained, particularly the forebrain input receptive zone in layer V. Contralateral side is normally stained. ×15.

barrel foci (Fig. 23). With further destruction of all vibrissal rows, the elongated bars of AChE fiber staining in cortex preserved the row locations, i.e., fusing of arcs or bridging of rows was not seen (Kristt and Waldman, 1981). Similar results have been reported using succinic dehydrogenase histochemistry (Killackey and Belford, 1980), which appears to preferentially stain cortical VB terminals (Killackey and Belford, 1979). Hence, the AChE-positive inputs to barrel cortex respond to altered peripheral input, as do cells and afferents in the somatosensory system. Although it is possible that a nonthalamic input may be constrained in its intracortical distribution by the abnormal organization of neurons and afferents in the barrels resulting from vibrissal damage, the weight of all the evidence above would not support this alternative. In addition, as can be seen from Fig. 14, layer IV in SmII also is densely stained for AChE by P3. In agreement with our hypothesis, this can be explained by a previous observation showing that collaterals from VB neurons innervate this field too (Jones, 1975).

In conclusion, the AChE-rich innervation of the barrel field in immature rats and mice appears to derive from the transiently positive neurons of the VB.

As alluded to above, in the rat and mouse, the picture of AChE staining in cortex persists until P16–28. In rats, the barrel centers exhibit an absolute reduction in the reactivity of fibers (Fig. 21). There is not an equivalent loss of fibers and terminal based on Golgi, axon, anterograde transport, degeneration, and histochemical staining for thalamic terminals (Lorente de Nó, 1949; Steffen, 1976; Waite, 1977; Killackey and Belford, 1979; Wise and Jones, 1978; Killackey and Leshin, 1975; Caviness *et al.*, 1976). Consequently, either new nonstained fibers have displaced the AChE-rich positive inputs or the fibers terminating in the barrel centers—predominantly from VB thalamus—have lost their complement of AChE, or perhaps both processes occur. Based on present evidence, it is likely that the primary events involve loss of staining in VB afferents to these barrels. A dilutional effect may also contribute to the loss of staining and should still be considered. In recent work, GABA-(transaminase)-stained nonpyramidal neurons in layer IV are associated with dense GABA-t staining of fibers in the barrel centers. This GABA-t-positive fiber plexus in the barrels appears as the AChE reactivity disappears (Kristt and Waldman, 1986; Fig. 24). Another line of evidence consistent with the view that AChE-rich barrel inputs (putatively thalamic in origin) may be "reoganized" during development derives from studies on the mouse (Kristt and Waldman, 1982). In this rodent, the distribution of AChE-rich fibers within the barrel changes between P16 and P21. The bottom of the barrel in deep layer IV loses its AChE staining; the superficial part of the barrel at the layer III–IV boundary continues to show an AChE-rich fiber plexus (Fig. 25). This pattern of fiber distribution could be due to displacement by late-arriving fibers, e.g., GABAergic inputs (Kristt and Waldman, 1986). On the other hand, virtually every VB neuron is transiently positive for AChE, and a very high proportion—possibly the entire cell population—are afferent to SmI (Kristt, 1983; Saporta and Kruger, 1977). Consequently, it is likely that the transience of AChE synthesis in VB noted above—rather than significant reorganization of VB afferents in layer IV—primarily accounts for the changing pattern of SmI staining during development in both rat and mouse.

In adult rat, the barrels are still visualizable despite the loss of AchE-stained fibers in their centers. After P19–21, the septa are moderately stained by fibers ascending radially so that the barrels are negatively stained images of cylindrical

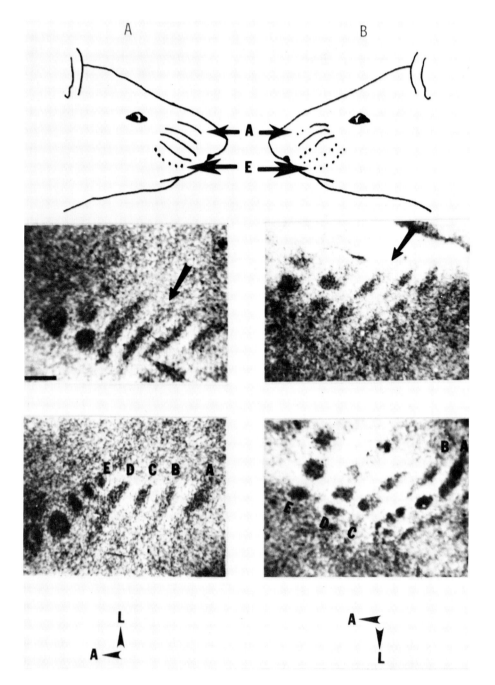

Figure 23. AChE-dependent staining of one of the barrel subfields following neonatal coagulation of the large mystacial vibrissae, contralaterally. Two experiments are shown. In both A and B, sequential 80-μm tangential sections through layer IV of SmI; rat, postnatal day 6. Line drawings after Killackey *et al.* (1978). (A) Coagulation of vibrissal rows A–D (line drawing). In SmI, the usually discrete foci of staining in rows A–D (arrow = row C) are replaced by solid bars of AChE positivity. The bars replicate the normal spatial orientation of each row. Bar = 0.5 mm. (B) Second case of vibrissal coagulation involving muzzle rows A, B, and C (line drawing). Rows A and C were incompletely destroyed, so that partial "fusion" of barrel AChE foci within a cortical row is seen. From Kristt and Waldman (1981) with permission.

spaces (Fig. 21). If one views these in tangential sections, the overall organization of the barrel field can be readily appreciated. In sagittal sections of adult rat brain passing through VB, one can see that layer IV of SmI exhibits meager AChE reactivity; in thalamus, VB stands alone as a palely stained structure (Fig. 20).

If this transient AChE synthesis is not related to cholinergic neurotransmission, what alternative function could it serve? It is tempting to relate the expression of AChE to developmental events in VB or cortex. Since it appears most intensely during the phase when processes of VB neurons are being elaborated and cell interactions are being initiated, these events may involve AChE. The surface localization of the glycoprotein would be appropriate for this type of role. *In vitro* studies in different cell lines have also linked AChE to a noncholinergic mechanism of process outgrowth and/or cell adhesion (Adler *et al.*, 1976; Cherbas *et al.*, 1977; Bartos and Glinos, 1976; Rieger *et al.*, 1980b). Repeated neonatal exposure *in vivo* to an irreversible cholinesterase inhibitor (DFP) reduces surface density of synapses in VB at P11 by 70–75%. In these treated animals, there is no statistically significant decrease in brain or body weights and the VB is cytologically and architectonically well developed (Kristt, unpublished observations). It can be seen that observations from rather different experimental systems seem to point to the same possible role for AChE in the genesis or regulation of early intercellular relationships. However, it is doubtful that AChE plays a role in the formation of the actual junctional specialization during synaptogenesis. To function in the latter context, the molecule would have to

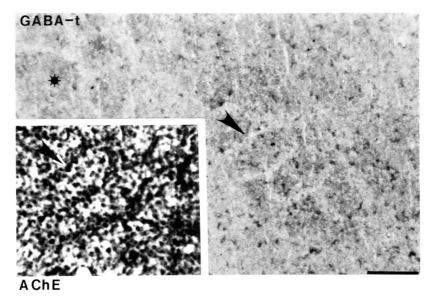

Figure 24. Comparison of AChE-stained barrels in anterior subfield (inset, left) with GABA-transaminase-stained tangential section through same region. Both sections are from an adult rat. Notice that the AChE staining is predominantly associated with fiber bundles delineating the septa between barrels, whereas GABA-t-stained processes fill the barrels, and presumably are derived from intrinsic cells. Bar = 250 μm.

be structurally modified since AChE stainability progressively diminishes as synaptogenesis procedes (cf. Kristt, 1983; Mathews and Faciane, 1977).

These observations on the thalamocortical innervation to SmI are not entirely unique. Transient AChE reactivity of neocortical inputs to different fields and in several species has been recorded (Kostovic and Goldman-Rakic, 1983;

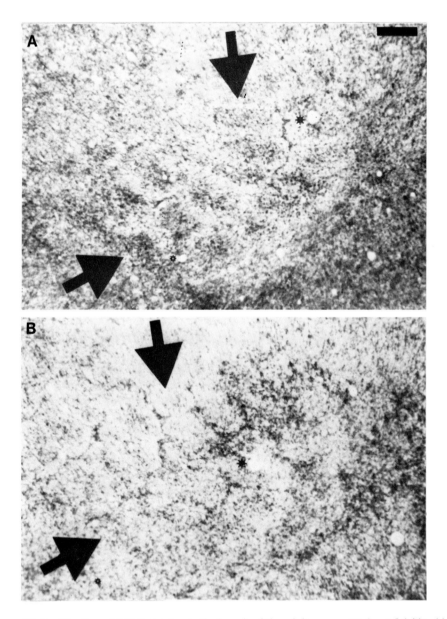

Figure 25. Stratification of AChE staining in the barrels of the adult mouse. (A) Superficial level in barrel (300 μm below pia). Note AChE in barrel centers. (B) AChE is concentrated in the periphery of barrel at deeper levels in layer IV (460 μm deep to pia). Bar = 450 μm.

Krmpotic-Nemanic *et al.*, 1980; Kostovic and Rakic, 1984; Robertson *et al.*, 1985). Additionally, various sites in the CNS, besides cerebral cortex, exhibit a brief period of AChE synthesis (Silver, 1974; Filogamo and Marchisio, 1971; Kasa and Csillik, 1964; Kasa *et al.*, 1966; Phillis, 1968b). Transient synthesis by immature neurons of other unexplained proteins also has been noted (Ali *et al.*, 1983). Perhaps the transient expression of AChE is part of a more general neuromaturational phenomenon. Clearly, the developmental significance of these events needs to be more critically examined.

13. Potential Functional Implications of the AChE-Rich Innervation of Neocortex

As noted above, the majority of AChE-positive fibers innervating neocortex probably are involved in cholinergic neurotransmission and originate from the basal forebrain. It has been proposed based on several lines of evidence reviewed elsewhere (e.g., Bigl *et al.*, 1982; Coyle *et al.*, 1983; Drachman and Leavitt, 1974) that the putative cholinergic innervation of neocortex in man plays a role critical to cognitive function. Similarly, in animals, certain learning functions have been claimed to be dependent on the cholinergic cell groups of the basal forebrain (Friedman *et al.*, 1983). If this role requires integrating neuronal activity over a

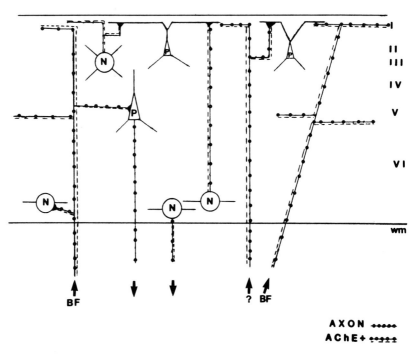

Figure 26. Diagram of proposed organization of AChE-rich cortical connectivity in rat. P, pyramidal cell; N, nonpyramidal cell; wm, white matter; BF, basal forebrain AChE-rich neurons.

broad region of cortex, the small domains of termination of these inputs—as described above—would seem puzzling. There are two possible, but speculative, options to potentially resolve this problem. First, Jones and Powell (1970) have shown that circuitry exists for progressive convergence of polymodal information from primary sensory cortical fields to more remote association zones. Consequently, the basal forebrain/cholinergic innervation of just these latter areas could have a substantial impact on human cognitive brain function, since cognition seems sensitive to the normal function of these convergence zones in man (Critchley, 1953). The first option, then, is that integration occurs at the cortical level, with modulation of activity in the convergence zones by basal forebrain inputs.

Alternatively, the integration may occur intranuclearly within the component groups of the basal forebrain cholinergic, AChE-rich, cortical projection system. Preliminary support for this possibility derives from recent Golgi studies that show small clusters of short axon collaterals originating near the perikaryon of these basal forebrain neurons (Kristt et al., 1985). Such collaterals could provide a basis for intranuclear synaptic interactions.

In the way of a concluding overview, it may well be of value to briefly comment on possible functional relationships of the various AChE-stained elements in cortex described above. Physiologic studies have suggested that somata in layer V of sensory-motor cortex possess receptors with predominantly muscarinic properties. The dense concentration of cholinergic afferents in this lamina derived predominantly from the basal forebrain (Saper, 1984; Kristt et al., 1985) indicate that these cells are probably postsynaptic to these inputs, and may well be the principal cholinoceptive elements in neocortex. Considerable cholinergic connectivity is apt to involve distal neuronal processes localized in layer I as well. In this lamina an important input component may be derived from sources outside of basal forebrain, perhaps from intrinsic cholinergic neurons, the brain stem or other cell groups providing nonspecific cortical afferents. Somata in layer VIb are also likely cholinergic synaptic targets for basal forebrain and possibly intrinsic fibers. These laminae, postulated to have rich cholinergic connectivity, are sites of relatively high levels of ChAT and AChE. Layers I and VI contain a high density of cholinergic receptor ligand binding sites; the absence of such preferential binding in layer V is unresolved at present. Some possible arrangements for AChE-rich putative cholinergic cortical connectivity, based on present knowledge, are presented in schematic form in Fig. 26. Connectivity is undoubtedly more complex, but this schematic at least is a starting point for future analysis of cortical cholinergic circuitry. As a final cautionary note, it should be borne in mind that a number of observations indicate that cortical AChE, although predominantly associated with cholinergic neurotransmission, may have other equally important roles in ensuring the normal maturation, function, and integrity of neocortex cerebri. Future investigations on AChE will need to refine our understanding of the multifaceted activities of this interesting substance.

ACKNOWLEDGMENTS. Personal work reviewed above was supported by grants from the National Institutes of Health and the National Science Foundation.

14. References

Adamson, E. D., 1977, Acetylcholinesterase in mouse brain, erythrocytes and muscle, *J. Neurochem.* **28:**605–615.

Adler, R., Teitelman, G., and Suburo, A. M., 1976, Cell interactions and the regulation of cholinergic enzymes during neural differentiation in vitro, *Dev. Biol.* **50:**48–57.

Ali, M., Mujoo, K., and Sahib, M. K., 1983, Synthesis and secretion of alpha-fetoprotein and albumin by newborn rat brain cells in culture, *Dev. Brain Res.* **6:**47–55.

Altschuler, R. A., Paralkkal, N. H., and Fex, J., 1983, Localization of enkephalin-like immunoreactivity in acetylcholinesterase-positive cells in the guinea-pig lateral superior olivary complex that project to the cochlea, *Neuroscience* **9:**621–630.

Arimatsu, Y., Seto, A., and Amano, T., 1981, An atlas of bungarotoxin binding sites and structures containing AChE in the mouse CNS, *J. Comp. Neurol.* **198:**603–632.

Armstrong, D. M., Saper, C. B., Levey, A. I., Wainer, B. H., and Terry, R. D., 1983, Distribution of cholinergic neurons in rat brain: Demonstrated by the immunocytochemical localization of choline acetyltransferase, *J. Comp. Neurol.* **216:**53–68.

Astrom, K. E., 1967, On the early development of the isocortex in fetal sheep, in: *Developmental Neurology* (C. G. Bernhard and J. P. Schade, eds.), Elsevier, Amsterdam, p. 1059.

Austin, L., and Berry, W. K., 1953, Two selective inhibitors of cholinesterase, *Biochem. J.* **54:**695–700.

Bartolini, A., Weisenthal, L., and Domino, E., 1972, Effect of photic stimulation on acetylcholine release from cat cerebral cortex, *Neuropharmacology* **11:**113–122.

Bartos, E. M., and Glinos, A. D., 1976, Properties of growth-related acetylcholinesterase in a cell line of fibroblastic origin, *J. Cell. Biol.* **69:**638.

Bayliss, F. J., and Todrick, A., 1956, The use of a selective acetylcholinesterase inhibitor in the estimation of pseudocholinesterase activity in rat brain, *Biochem. J.* **62:**62–67.

Benishin, C. G., and Carroll, P. T., 1983, Multiple forms of choline-O-acetyltransferase in mouse and rat brain: Solubilization and characterization, *J. Neurochem.* **41:**1030–1039.

Bigl, V., Wolf, N. J., and Butcher, L., 1982, Cholinergic projections from the basal forebrain to frontal, parietal, temporal, occipital, and cingulate cortices: A combined fluorescent tracer and acetylcholinesterase analysis, *Brain Res. Bull.* **8:**727–749.

Birdsall, N. J. M., and Hulme, E. C., 1976, Biochemical studies on muscarinic acetylcholine receptors, *J. Neurochem.* **27:**7–16.

Birdsall, N. J. M., Bergen, A. S. V., and Hulme, E. C., 1978, The binding of agonists to brain muscarinic receptors, *Mol. Pharmacol.* **14:**723–736.

Brodmann, K., 1909, *Vergleichende Lokalisationlehre der Grosshirnrinde in ihren Prinzipien dargestellt auf Grund des Zellenbaues,* Barth, Leipzig.

Burn, J. H., and Rand, M. J., 1959, Sympathetic post-ganglionic mechanisms, *Nature* **184:**163–165.

Butcher, L. I., 1977, Nature and mechanisms of cholinergic–monoaminergic interactions in the brain, *Life Sci.* **21:**1207–1226.

Butcher, L. I., and Hodge, G. K., 1976, Postnatal development of acetylcholinesterase in the caudate–putamen nucleus and substantia nigra of rats, *Brain Res.* **106:**223–240.

Campbell, A. W., 1905, *Histological Studies on the Localization of Cerebral Function,* Cambridge University Press, London.

Candy, J. M., Perry, R. H., Perry, E. K., and Thompson, J. E., 1981, Distribution of putative cholinergic cell bodies and various neuropeptides in the substantia innominata region of the human brain, *J. Anat.* **133:**123–124.

Caviness, V. S., Jr., Frost, D. O., and Hayes, N. L., 1976, Barrels in somatosensory cortex of normal and Reeler mutant mice, *Neurosci. Lett.* **3:**7–14.

Chen, L. L., Van Hoesen, G. W., Barnes, C. L., and West, J. R., 1983, Enhanced acetylcholinesterase staining in the hippocampal perforant pathway zone after combined lesions of the septum and entorhinal cortex, *Brain Res.* **272:**353–359.

Cherbas, P., Cherbas, L., and Williams, C. M., 1977, Induction of acetylcholinesterase activity by beta-ecdysone in a drosophila cell line, *Science* **197:**275–277.

Collier, B., and Mitchell, J., 1966, The central release of acetylcholine during stimulation of the visual pathway, *J. Physiol. (London)* **184:**239–254.

Colonnier, M., 1968, Synaptic patterns on different cell types in the different laminae of the cat visual cortex, *Brain Res.* **9:**268–287.

Couteaux, R., and Taxi, J., 1952, Recheriches histochimiques sur la distribution des activities chol-inesterasiques, *Arch. Anat. Microscop. Morph. Exp.* **41**:352–392.

Coyle, J. T., and Molliver, M. E., 1977, Major innervation of newborn rat cortex by monoaminergic neurons, *Science* **196**:444–446.

Coyle, J. T., and Yamamura, H. I., 1976, Neurochemical aspects of the ontogenesis of cholinergic neurons in the rat brain, *Brain Res.* **118**:429–440.

Coyle, J. T., Price, D. L., and DeLong, M. R., 1983, Alzheimer's disease: a disorder of cortical cholinergic innervation, *Science* **29**:1184–1190.

Cozzari, C., and Hartman, B. K., 1983, An endogenous inhibitory factor for choline acetyltransferase, *Brain Res.* **276**:109–117.

Cragg, B. G., 1975, The development of synapses in the visual system of the cat, *J. Comp. Neurol.* **160**:147–166.

Critchley,M., 1953, *The Parietal Lobes*, Arnold, London.

Das, G. D., 1971, Projection of the interstitial nerve cells surrounding the globus pallidus: a study of retrograde changes following cortical ablations in rabbits, *Z. Anat. EntwGesh* **133**:135–160.

Davis, R., and Koelle, G. B., 1978, Electron microscope localization of acetylcholinesterase and butyrylcholinesterase in the superior cervical ganglion of the cat, *J. Cell Biol.* **78**:785–790.

Divac, I., 1975, Magnocellular nuclei of the basal forebrain project to neocortex, brain stem, and olfactory bulb. A review of some basic correlates, *Brain Res.* **93**:385–398.

Divac, I., 1979, Pattern of subcortico-cortical projections as revealed by somatopetal horseradish tracing, *Neuroscience* **4**:455–461.

Divac, I., 1981, Cortical projections of the magnocellular nuclei of the basal forebrain: A re-inves-tigation, *Neuroscience* **6**:983–984.

Drachman, D. A., and Leavitt, J., 1974, Human memory and the cholinergic system—A relationship to aging, *Arch. Neurol.* **30**:113–121.

Duckett, S., and Pearse, A. G. E., 1968, The cells of Cajal–Retzius in the developing human brain, *J. Anat.* **102**:183–187.

Eckenstein, F., and Sofroniew, M. V., 1983, Identification of central cholinergic neurons containing both choline acetyltransferase and acetylcholinesterase and of central neurons containing only acetylcholinesterase, *J. Neurosci.* **3**:2286–2291.

Emson, P. C., and Lindvall, O., 1979, Distribution of putative neurotransmiters in the neocortex, *Neuroscience* **4**:1–30.

Feldberg, W., and Vogt, M., 1948, Acetylcholine synthesis in different regions of the CNS, *J. Physiol. (London)* **107**:372–381.

Filogamo, G., and Marchisio, P. C., 1971, Acetylcholine system and neural development, *Neuroscience* **4**:29–64.

Friedman, E., Lerrer, B., and Kuster, J., 1983, Loss of cholinergic neurons in the rat neocortex produces deficits in passive avoidance learning, *Pharmacol. Biochem. Behav.* **19**:309–312.

Garey, L. J., and Powell, T.P. S., 1971, An experimental study of the termination of the lateral geniculate–cortical pathway in the cat and monkey, *Proc. Soc. London Ser. B.* **179**:41–63.

Geneser-Jensen, F. A., and Blackstadt, T. W., 1971, Distribution of acetylcholinesterase in the hippocampal region of the guinea pig, *Z. Zellforsch,* **114**:460–481.

Gerebtzoff, M. A., 1959, *Cholinesterases: A Histochemical Contribution to the Solution of Some Functional Problems*, Pergamon Press, Elmsford, N. Y.

Gisiger, V., Vigny, M., Gautron, J., and Reiger, F., 1978, Acetylcholinesterase of rat sympathetic ganglion: Molecular forms. Localization and effects of denervation, *J. Neurochem.* **30**:501–516.

Goodman, L. S., and Gilman, A., 1975, *The Pharmacological Bases of Therapeutics*, 5th ed., Macmillan Co., New York.

Gorry, J. D., 1963, Studies on the cooperative anatomy of the ganglion basale of Meynert, *Acta Anat.* **55**:51–104.

Graybiel, A. M., and Berson, D. M., 1980, Histochemical localization and different connections of subdivisions on the lateralis posterior–pulvinar complex and related thalamic nuclei in the cat, *Neuroscience* **5**:12–38.

Graybiel, A., and Ragsdale, C., Jr., 1978, Histochemically distinct compartments in the striatum of human, monkey, and cat demonstrated by acetylcholinesterase staining, *Proc. Natl. Acad. Sci. USA* **75**:5723–5726.

Green, J. R., Halpeen, L. M., and Van Niel, S., 1970, Choline acetylase and acetylcholinesterase changes in chronic isolated cerebral cortex of cat, *Life Sci.* **9**:481–488.

Greenfield, S. A., Stein, J. F., Hodgson, A. J., and Chubb, I. W., 1981, Depression of nigral pars compacta cell discharge by exogenous acetylcholinesterase, *Neuroscience* **6:**2287–2295.

Hayaraman, A., 1980, Anatomical evidence for cortical projections from the striatum in the cat, *Brain Res.* **195:**29–36.

Hebb, C. O., and Silver, A., 1956, Choline acetylase in the central nervous system of man and some other mammals, *J. Physiol. (London)* **134:**718–728.

Hebb, C. O., Krnjević, K., and Silver, A., 1963, Effect of undercutting on the acetylcholinesterase and choline acetyltransferase activity in the cat's cerebral cortex, *Nature* **198:**692.

Hedreen, J. C., Uhl, G. R., Bacon, S. J., Fambrough, D. M., and Price, D. L., 1984, Acetyl-cholinesterase-immunoreactive axonal network in monkey visual cortex, *J. Comp. Neurol.* **226:** 246–254.

Heimer, L., and Wilson, R. D., 1975, The subcortical projections of the allocortex: Similarities in the neural associations of the hippocampus, the piriform cortex, and neocortex, in: *Golgi Centennial Symposium* (M. Santini, ed.), Raven Press, New York, pp. 177–193.

Henderson, A., 1981, A projection from acetylcholinesterase-containing neurons in he diagonal band to the occipital cortex of the rat, *Neuroscience* **6:**1081–1088.

Hoover, B., Muth, A., and Jacobowitz, D. M., 1978, A mapping of the distribution of acetylcholine, choline acetyltransferase and acetylcholinesterase in discrete areas of rat brain, *Brain Res.* **153:**295–306.

Houser, L. R., Cranford, G. D., Barbor, R. P., Salvaterra, P. M., and Vaughn, J. E., 1983, Organization and morphological characteristics of cholinergic neurons: An immunocytochemical study with a monoclonal antibody to choline acetyltransferase, *Brain Res.* **260:**97–119.

Hubel, D. H., and Wiesel, T. N., 1962, Receptive fields, binocular interaction and functional architecture in the cat's visual cortex, *J. Physiol. (London)* **160:**106–154.

Huther, G., and Luppa, H., 1979, The multiple forms of brain acetylcholinesterase. III. Implications for the histochemical demonstration of acetylcholinesterase, *Histochemistry* **63:**115–123.

Ishii, Y., 1957, The histochemical studies of cholinesterase in the central nervous system. II. His-tochemical alteration of cholinesterase of the brain of rats from fetal life to adults, *Arch. Histol. Okoyama* **12:**613–637.

Ivy, G. O., and Killackey, H. P., 1982, Ephemeral cellular segmentation in the thalamus of the neonatal rat, *Dev. Brain Res.* **2:**1–17.

Jacobowitz, D. M., and Palkovits, M., 1974, Topographic atlas of catecholamine and actylcholines-terase containing neurons in the rat brain, *J. Comp. Neurol.* **157:**13–28.

Jeanmonod, D., Rice, F. L., and Van Der Loos, H., 1977, Mouse somatosensory cortex: Development of the alteration in the barrel field which is caused by injury to the vibrissal follicles, *Neurosci. Lett.* **6:**151–156.

Jessen, K. R., Chubb, I. W., and Smith, A. D., 1978, Intracellular localization of acetylcholinesterase in nerve terminals and capillaries of the rat superior cervical ganglion, *J. Neurocytol.* **7:**145–154.

Johnston, M. V., McKinney, M., and Coyle, J. T., 1979, Evidence for a cholinergic projection to neocortex from neurons in the basal forebrain, *Proc. Natl. Acad. Sci. USA* **10:**5392–5396.

Johnston, M. V., Young, A. C., and Coyle, J. T., 1981, Laminar distribution of cholinergic markers in neocortex, *J. Neurosci. Res.* **6:**597–607.

Jones, E. G., 1975, Possible determinants of the degree of retrograde neuronal labeling with horse-radish peroxidase, *Brain Res.* **85:**249–254.

Jones, E. G., and Powell, T. P. S., 1970, An anatomical study of converging sensory pathways within the cerebral cortex of the monkey, *Brain* **93:**793–820.

Jones, E. G., Burton, H., Saper, C. B., and Swanson, L. W., 1976, Midbrain diencephalic and cortical relationships of the basal nucleus of Meynert and associated structures in primates, *J. Comp. Neurol.* **167:**385–420.

Jonsson, G., and Sachs, C., 1976, Regional changes in [³H]-noradrenaline uptake, catecholamine, and catecholamine synthetic and catabolic enzymes in rat brain following neonatal 6-hydroxy-dopamine treatment, *Med. Biol.* **54:**286–297.

Jordan, L. M., and Phillis, J. W., 1972, Acetylcholine inhibition in the intact and chronically isolated cerebral cortex, *Br. J. Pharmacol.* **45:**584–595.

Karnovsky, M. S., and Roots, L., 1964, A 'direct-coloring' thiocholine method for cholinesterases, *J. Histochem. Cytochem.* **12:**219–221.

Kasa, P., 1971, Ultrastructural localization of choline acetyltransferase and acetylcholinesterase in central and peripheral nervous tissue, *Prog. Brain Res.* **34:**337.

Kasa, P., and Bansaghi, K., 1979, Development of neurons containing acetylcholinesterase and choline acetyltransferase in dispersed cell culture of rat cerebellum, *Histochemistry* **61**:263–270.

Kasa, P., Csillik, B., Joo, F., and Knyihar, E., 1966, Histochemical and ultrastructural alterations in the isolated archicerebellum of the rat, *J. Neurochem.* **13**:173–178.

Kasa, P., and Csillik, B., 1964, Histochemical studies on the effect of nerve degeneration in the cerebellar cortex, *2nd Int. Congr. Histochem. Cytochem.* pp. 195–196.

Kelly, P. H., and Moore, K. E., 1978, Decrease of neocortical choline acetyltransferase after lesion of the globus pallidus in the rat, *Exp. Neurol.* **61**:479–484.

Kieviet, J.,and Kuypers, H. G. J., 1975, Basal forebrain and hypothalamic connections to the frontal and parietal cortex in rhesus monkey, *Science* **187**:660–662.

Killackey, H. P., and Leshin, S., 1975, The organization of specific thalamocortical projections to the posteromedial barrel subfield of the rat somatic sensory cortex, *Brain Res.* **86**:469–472.

Killackey, H. P., and Belford, G. R., 1979, The formation of different patterns in the somatosensory cortex of the neonatal rat, *J. Comp. Neurol.* **183**:285–304.

Killackey, H. P., and Belford,G. R., 1980, Central correlates of peripheral pattern alterations in the trigeminal system of the rat, *J. Comp. Neurol. 183:*205–210.

Killackey, H. P., Ivy, G. O., and Cunningham, T. J., 1978, Anomalous organization of SMI somatotopic map consequent to vibrissal removal in the newborn rat, *Brain Res.***155**:136–140.

Kimura, H., McGeer, P. L., Peng, F., and McGeer, E. G., 1980, Choline acetyltransferase-containing neurons in rodent brain demonstrated by immunocytochemistry, *Science* **208**:1057–1059.

Kimura, H., McGeer, P. L., Peng, F., and McGeer, E. G., 1981, The central cholinergic system, studied by choline acetyltransferase immunohistochemistry in the cat, *J. Comp. Neurol.* **200**:151–201.

Kitt, C. A., Price, D. L., DeLong, M. R., Strubble, R. G., Mitchell, S. J., and Hedreen, J. C., 1982, The nucleus basalis of Meynert, projections to the cortex, amygdala and hippocampus, *Soc. Neurosci. Abstr.* **8**:212.

Klinar, B., and Brzin, M., 1977, Cytochemical localization of acetylcholinesterase in the rat striatum, *Acta Histochem.* **58**:223–231.

Kobayashi, R. M., Palkovits, M., Hruska, R. E., Rothschild, R., and Yamamura, H. I., 1978, Regional distribution of muscarine cholinergic receptors in rat brain, *Brain Res.* **154**:13–23.

Koelle, G. B., 1955, The histochemical localization of cholinesterases in the central nervous system of the rat, *J. Pharmacol. Exp. Ther.* **114**:167.

Koelle, G. B., and Friedenwald, J. S., 1949, A histochemical method for localizing cholinesterase activity, *Proc. Soc. Exp. Biol. Med.* **70**:617–622.

Koelle, G. B., Rickard, K. K., and Ruch, G. A., 1979, Interrelationships between ganglionic acetylcholinesterase and non-specific cholinesterase of the cat and rat, *Proc. Natl. Acad. Sci. USA* **76**:6012–6016.

Konig, J., and Klippel, A., 1974, *The Rat Brain: A Stereotaxic Atlas of the Forebrain and Lower Parts of the Brain Stem*, Krieger, New York.

Kostovic, I., 1982, Distribution of acetylcholinesterase reactive cell bodies and fibers in the frontal granular cortex of the human brain, *Soc. Neurosci. Abstr.* **8**:933.

Kostovic, I., 1983, Prenatal development of the nucleus basalis/Meynert/and related fiber systems in man, *Soc. Neurosci. Abstr.* **9**:850.

Kostovic, I., and Goldman-Rakic, P. S., 1983, Transient cholinesterase staining in the mediodorsal nucleus of the thalamus and its connectors in the developing human and monkey brain, *J. Comp. Neurol.* **219**:431–447.

Kostovic, I., and Rakic, P., 1984, Development of prestriate visual projections in the monkey and human fetal cerebrum revealed by transient cholinesterase staining, *J. Neurosci.* **4**:25–42.

Kostovic, I., Kelovic, Z., Krmpotic-Nemanic, J., and Kracum, I., 1980, Development of the human somatosensory cortex: Laminar distribution and vertical organization of the acetylcholinesterase positive fibers during fetal life, *Neurosci. Lett. Suppl.* **5**:484.

Kozik, M. B., and Szczech, J., 1977, The histoenzymic activity of gyrus cinguli in the course of postnatal ontogeny of the rat, *Folia Histochem. Cytochem.* **15**:277–288.

Krieg, W. J. S., 1946, Connections of the cerebral cortex. I. The albino rat. A topography of the cortical areas, *J. Comp. Neurol.* **84**:221–275.

Kristt, D. A., 1978, Neuronal differentiation in somatosensory cortex of the rat. I. Relationship to synaptogenesis in the first postnatal week, *Brain Res.* **150**:467–486.

Kristt, D. A., 1979a, Development of neocortical circuitry: Histochemical localization of acetylcholinesterase in relation to the cell layers of rat somatosensory cortex, *J. Comp. Neurol.* **186**:1–16.

Kristt, D. A., 1979b, Acetylcholinesterase-containing neurons of layer VIb in immature neocortex: Possible component of an early formed intrinsic cortical circuit, *Anat. Embryol.* **157**:221–226.

Kristt, D. A., 1979c, Somatosensory cortex: Acetylcholinesterase staining of barrel neuropil in the rat, *Neurosci. Lett.* **12**:177–182.

Kristt, D. A., 1979d, Development of neocortical circuitry: Quantitative ultrastructural analysis of putative monoaminergic synapses, *Brain Res.* **178**:69–88.

Kristt, D. A., 1983, Acetylcholinesterase in the ventrobasal thalamus: Transcience and patterning during ontogenesis, *Neuroscience* **10**:923–939.

Kristt, D. A., 1984, Development of connections within sensory cortex, in: *Development, Organization and Processing in Somatosensory Pathways* (W. D. Willis and M. J. Rowe, eds.), Liss, New York, pp. 69–77.

Kristt, D. A., and Kasper, E. K., 1983, High density of cholinergic muscarinic receptors accompanies high density acetylcholinesterase-staining in layer IV of infant rat somatosensory cortex, *Dev. Brain Res.* **8**:373–376.

Kristt, D. A., and Molliver, M. E., 1976, Synapses in newborn rat cerebral neocortex: A quantitative ultrastructural study, *Brain Res.* **108**:180–186.

Kristt, D. A., and Silverman, J. D., 1980, Catecholaminergic cell groups innervating infant rat somatosensory cortex, *Neurosci. Lett.* **16**:181–186.

Kristt, D. A., and Silverman, J. D., 1981, Horseradish peroxidase pellets implanted into infant neocortex: Some technical consideration, *Neurosci. Lett.* **26**:203–208.

Kristt, D. A., and Waldman, J. V., 1981, The origin of the acetylcholinesterase-rich afferents to layer IV of infant somatosensory cortex: A histochemical analysis following lesions, *Anat. Embryol.* **163**:31–41.

Kristt, D. A., and Waldman, J. V., 1982, Developmental reorganization of acetylcholinesterase-rich inputs to somatosensory cortex of the mouse, *Anat. Embryol.* **164**:331–342.

Kristt, D. A., and Waldman, J. V., 1986, Late postnatal changes in rat somatosensory cortex: Temporal and spatial relationships of GABA-T and AChE histochemical reactivity, *Anat. Embryol.* **174**:115–122.

Kristt, D. A., Shirley, M. S., and Kasper, E., 1980, Monoaminergic synapses in infant mouse neocortex: Comparison of cortical fields in seizure-prone and resistant mice, *Neuroscience* **5**:883–891.

Kristt, D. A., McGowan, R. A., Jr., Martin-MacKinnon, N., and Solomon, J., 1985, Basal forebrain innervation of rodent neocortex: Studies using acetylcholinesterase histochemistry, Golgi and lesion strategies, *Brain Res.* **337**:19–39.

Krmpotic-Nemanic, J., Kostovic, I., Kelovic, Z., and Nemanic, D., 1980, Development of acetylcholinesterase (AChE) staining in human fetal auditory cortex, *Acta Otol-Laryngol.* **89**:388–392.

Krmpotic-Nemanic, J., Kostovic, I., Kelovic, Z., Nemanic, D., and Mrzljak, L., 1983, Development of the human fetal auditory cortex: Growth of afferent fibres, *Acta Anat.* **116**:69–73.

Krnjević, K., 1967, Chemical transmission and cortical arousal, *Anesthesiology* **28**:100–105.

Krnjević, K., and Phillis, J. W., 1963, Acetylcholine-sensitive cells in the cerebral cortex, *J. Physiol. (London)* **166**:296–327.

Krnjević, K., and Silver, A., 1966, Acetylcholinesterase in the developing forebrain, *J. Anat.* **100**:63–89.

Krnjević, K., Reiffenstein, R. J., and Silver, A., 1970, Chemical sensitivity of neurons in long-isolated slabs of cat cerebral cortex, *Electroencephalogr. Clin. Neurophysiol.* **29**:269–282.

Kuhar, M. J., and Yamamura, H. I., 1976, Localization of cholinergic muscarinic receptors in rat brain by light microscopic autoradiography, *Brain Res.* **110**:229–243.

Kuhar, M. J., Birdsall, N. J. M., Burgen, A. S. V., and Hulme, E. C., 1980, Ontogeny of muscarinic receptors in rat brain, *Brain Res.* **184**:375–384.

Kuhar, M. J., Taylor, N., Wamsley, J., Hulme, E. C., and Birdsall, N. J. M., 1981, Muscarinic cholinergic receptor localization in brain by electron microscopic autoradiography, *Brain Res.* **216**:1–9.

Lamour, Y., Dutar, P., and Jobert, A., 1983, A comparative study of two populations of acetylcholine-sensitive neurons in rat somatosensory cortex, *Brain Res.* **289**:157–167.

Landry, P., and Deschenes, M., 1981, Intracortical arborizations and receptive fields of identified ventrobasal thalamocortical afferents to the primary somatic sensory cortex in the cat, *J. Comp. Neurol.* **199**:345–372.

Lehmann, J., and Fibiger, H. C., 1979, Acetylcholinesterase and the cholinergic neuron, *Life Sci.* **25**:1939–1947.

Lehmann, J., Nagy, J. I., Atmadja, S., and Fibiger, H. C., 1980, The nucleus basalis magnocellularis: The origin of a cholinergic projection to the neocortex of the rat, *Neuroscience* **5**:1161–1174.

Levey, A. I., Wainer, B. H., Mufson, E. J., and Mesulam, M.-M., 1983, Localization of acetylcholinesterase and choline acetyltransferase in the rat cerebrum, *Neuroscience* **9**:9–22.

Lewis, P. R., and Shute, C. C. D., 1966, The distribution of cholinesterase in cholinergic neurons demonstrated with the electron microscope, *J. Cell. Sci.* **1**:381–390.

Lewis, P. R., and Shute, C. C. D., 1978, Cholinergic pathways in CNS, in: *Handbook of Psychopharmacology* (L. L. Iversen, S. O. Iversen, and S. H. Snyder, eds,), Vol. 9, Plenum Press, New York, pp. 315–355.

Lidov, H. G. W., Molliver, M. E., and Zecevic, N. R., 1978, Characterization of the monoaminergic innervation of immature rat neocortex: A histofluorescence analysis, *J. Comp. Neurol.* **181**: 663–680.

Lindvall, O., and Björklund, A., 1974, The organization of the ascending catecholamine neuron systems in the rat brain, *Acta Physiol. Scand. Suppl.* **412**:1–48.

Lorente de Nó, R., 1949, *Physiology of the Nervous System*, 3rd ed. (J. F. Fulton, ed.), Oxford University Press, London, pp. 288–330.

Lund, R. D., 1978, *Development and Plasticity of the Brain: An Introduction*, Oxford University Press, London.

Luskin, M. B., and Price, J. L., 1982, The distribution of axon collaterals from the olfactory bulb and the nucleus of the horizontal limb of the diagonal band to the olfactory cortex, demonstrated by double-retrograde labeling techniques, *J. Comp. Neurol.* **209**:249–263.

Lynch, G., Lucas, P. A., and Deadwyler, S. A., 1972, The demonstration of acetylcholinesterase-containing neurons within the caudate nucleus of the rat, *Brain Res.* **45**:617–621.

Lynch, G., Gall, C., Rose, G., and Cotman, C., 1976, Changes in the distribution of the dentate gyrus associational system following unilateral or bilateral entorhinal lesions in the adult rat, *Brain Res.* **110**:57–71.

McGowan, R. A., Solomon, J., Martin-MacKinnon, N., and Kristt, D. A., 1983, Acetylcholinesterase-rich projections to neocortex. II. Areal distribution, laminar staining and barrel innervation studied with lesions, *Soc. Neurosci. Abstr.* **9**:215.

McKinney, M., Coyle, J. T., and Hedreen, J. C., 1983, Topographic analysis of the innervation of the rat neocortex and hippocampus by the basal forebrain cholinergic system, *J. Comp. Neurol.* **217**:103–121.

Marin-Padilla, M., 1970, Pre-natal and early postnatal ontogenesis of the human motor cortex: A Golgi study. I. The sequential development of cortical layers, *Brain Res.* **23**:167–183.

Marin-Padilla, M., 1972, Pre-natal ontogenic history of the neocortex of cat (Felis domestica). A Golgi study. II. Developmental differences and their significance, *Z. Anat. Entwicklungsgesch.* **136**:135–142.

Marin-Padilla, M., 1978, Dual origin of the mammalian neocortex and evolution of the cortical plate, *Anat. Embryol.* **152**:109–126.

Marshall, J. F., Van Oordt, K., and Kozlowski, M. R., 1983, Acetylcholinesterase associated with dopaminergic innervation of the neostriatum: Histochemical observations of a heterogenous distribution, *Brain Res.* **274**:283–289.

Massoulie, J., and Bon, S., 1982, The molecular forms of cholinesterase and acetylcholinesterase invertebrates, *Annu. Rev. Neurosci.* **5**:57–106.

Mathews, M. A., and Faciane, C. L., 1977, Electron microscopy of the development of synaptic patterns in the ventrobasal complex of the rat, *Brain Res.* **13**:197–215.

Meller, K., Breipohl, W., and Glees, P., 1969, Ontogeny of the mouse motor cortex. The polymorph layer or layer IV. A Golgi and electron microscopic study, *Z. Zellforsch.* **99**:443–458.

Mesulam, M.-M., and Van Hoesen, G. W., 1976, Acetylcholinesterase-rich projections from the basal forebrain of the rhesus monkey to neocortex, *Brain Res.* **109**:152–157.

Mesulam, M.-M., Mufson, E. J., Levey, A. I., and Wainer, B. H., 1983, Cholinergic innervation of cortex by the basal forebrain: Cytochemistry and cortical connections of the septal area, diagonal band nuclei, nucleus basalis (substantia innominata) and hypothalamus in the rhesus monkey, *J. Comp. Neurol.* **214**:170–197.

Mitchell, J. F., 1963, The spontaneous and evoked release of acetylcholine from the cerebral cortex, *J. Physiol. (London)* **165**:98–116.

Molliver, M. E., Kostovic, I., and Van der Loos, H., 1973, The development of synapses in cerebral cortex of the human fetus, *Brain Res.* **50**:403–407.

Moore, R. Y., and Bloom, F. E., 1978, Central catecholamine neuron systems: Anatomy and physiology of the dopamine systems, *Annu. Rev. Neurosci.* **1:**129–170.

Morley, B. J., Kemp, G. E., and Salvatore, P., 1979, Alpha-bungarotoxin binding sites in the CNS, *Life Sci.* **24:**859–872.

Myers, D. K., 1953, Studies on cholinesterase. IX. Species variation in the specificity pattern of the pseudo cholinesterase, *Biochem. J.* **55:**67–79.

Nachmansohn, D., 1975, *Chemical and Molecular Bases of Nerve Activity,* Academic Press, New York, pp. 1–227.

Nadler, J. V., Matthews, D., Cotman, C., and Lynch, G., 1974, Development of cholinergic innervation in the hippocampal formation of the rat. II. Quantitative changes in choline acetyltransferase and acetylcholinesterase activities, *Dev. Biol.* **36:**142–154.

Nadler, J. V., Cotman, C., V., and Lynch, G. S., 1977, Histochemical evidence of altered development of cholinergic fibers in the rat dentate following lesions. I. Time course after complete unilateral entorhinal lesion at various ages, *J. Comp. Neurol.* **171:**561–588.

Navaratnam, V., and Lewis, P. R., 1970, Cholinesterase-containing neurones in the spinal cord of the rat, *Brain Res.* **18:**411–425.

Okinaka, S., Yoshikawa, M., Uono, M., Muro, T., Mozai, T., Ihata, A., Tanabe, H., Ueda, S., and Tomonaga, M., 1961, Distribution of cholinesterase activity in the human cerebral cortex, *Am. J. Physiol. Med.* **40:**135–145.

Olschowka, J. A., and Vijayan, V. K., 1980, Postnatal development of cholinergic transmitter enzymes in the mouse cerebellum: Biochemical light microscopic and electron microscopic cytochemical investigations, *J. Comp. Neurol.* **191:**77–101.

Palkovits, M., and Jacobowitz, D., 1974, Topographic atlas of catecholamine and acetylcholinesterase containing neurons in the rat brain, *J. Comp. Neurol.* **157:**29–42.

Pannese, E., Luciano, L., Iurato, S., and Reale, E., 1974, The localization of acetylcholinesterase activity in the spinal cord of the adult fowl studied by electron microscope histochemistry, *Histochemistry* **39:**1–13.

Parent, A., and Butcher, L. L., 1976, Organization and morphologies of acetylcholinesterase-containing neurons in the thalamus and hypothalamus of the rat, *J. Comp. Neurol.* **170:**205–226.

Paxinos, G., and Watson, C., 1982, *The Rat Brain in Stereotaxic Coordinates,* Academic Press, New York.

Pearse, A. G., 1980, *Histochemistry: Theoretical and Applied,* Vol. 2, 3rd ed., Churchill Livingstone, Edinburgh.

Pepeu, G., and Mantegazzini, P., 1964, Midbrain hemisection effect on cortical acetylcholine in the cat, *Science* **145:**1069–1070.

Phillis, J. W., 1968a, Acetylcholine release from the cerebral cortex: Its role in cortical arousal, *Brain Res.* **7:**378–389.

Phillis, J W., 1968b, Acetylcholinesterase in the feline cerebellum, *J. Neurochem.* **15:**691–698.

Pidoux, B., Diebler, M. F., Savy, C. L., Farka, E., and Verley, R., 1980, Cortical organization of the postero-medial barrel-subfield in mice and its organization after destruction of vibrissal follicles after birth, *Neuropathol. Appl. Neurobiol.* **6:**93–107.

Pope, A., 1952, Quantitative distribution of dipeptidase and acetylcholine esterase in architectonic layers of rat cerebral cortex, *J. Neurophysiol.* **15:**115–130.

Powell, T. P. S., and Mountcastle, V. B., 1959, Some aspects of the functional organization of the cortex of the postcentral gyrus of the monkey: A correlation of findings obtained in a single unit analysis with cytoarchitecture, *Bull. Johns Hopkins Hosp.* **105:**133–162.

Price, J. L., and Stern, R., 1983, Individual cells in the nucleus basalis–diagonal band complex have restricted axonal projections to the cerebral cortex in the rat, *Brain Res.* **269:**352–356.

Ramón y Cajal, S., 1911, *Histologie du Système Nerveux,* Vol. 2, Maloine, Paris.

Ramón y Cajal, S., 1960, *Studies on Vertebrate Neurogenesis* (translated by L. Guth), Thomas, Springfield, Ill., pp. 325–350.

Ribak, C. E., and Kramer, W. G., III, 1982, Cholinergic neurons in the basal forebrain of the cat have direct projections to the sensorimotor cortex, *Exp. Neurol.* **75:**453–465.

Rieger, F., and Vigny, M., 1976, Solubilization and physicochemical characterization of rat brain acetylcholinesterase: Development and maturation of its molecular forms, *J. Neurochem.* **27:**121–129.

Rieger, F., Chetelat, R., Nicolet, M., Kamal, L., and Poullet, M., 1980a, Presence of tailed asymmetric forms of acetylcholinesterase in the central nervous system of vertebrates, *FEBS Lett.* **121:**169–174.

Robbins, P. W., 1982, The processing of cell-surface glycoproteins, in: *Molecular Genetic Neuroscience* (F. O. Schmitt, S.J. Bird, and F. E. Bloom, eds.), Raven Press, New York, pp. 161–169.

Robertson, R. T., Tijerina, A. A., and Gallivan, M. E., 1985, Transient patterns of acetylcholinesterase activity in visual cortex of the rat: Normal development and the effects of neonatal monocular enucleation, *Dev. Brain Res.* **21**:203–211.

Rotter, A., Field, P. M., and Raisman, G., 1979, Muscarinic receptors in the central nervous system of the rat. III. Postnatal development of binding of [^{3}H] propylbenzilylcholine mustard, *Brain Res. Rev.* **1**:185–206.

Rotundo, R. L., 1984, Asymmetric acetylcholinesterase is assembled in the Golgi apparatus, *Proc. Natl. Acad. Sci. USA* **81**:479–483.

Sakai, S. T., Stanton, G. B., and Tanaka, D., Jr., 1983, The ventral lateral thalamic nucleus in the dog: Cytoarchitecture, acetylthiocholinesterase histochemistry, and cerebellar afferents, *Brain Res.* **271**:1–10.

Saper, C. B., 1984, Organization of the cerebral cortex afferent systems in the rat. I. Magnocellular basal nucleus, *J. Comp. Neurol.* **222**:313–342.

Saporta, S., and Kruger, L., 1977, The organization of thalamocortical relay neurons in the rat ventrobasal complex studied by the retrograde transport of horseradish peroxidase, *J. Comp. Neurol.* **174**:187–208.

Satoh, K., Armstrong, D. M., and Fibiger, H. C., 1983, A comparison of the distribution of central cholinergic neurons as demonstrated by acetylcholinesterase, pharmacohistochemistry and choline acetyltransferase immunohistochemistry, *Brain Res. Bull.* **11**:693–720.

Schmidt, R. H., and Bhatnagar, R. K., 1979, Assessment of the effect of neonatal subcutaneous hydroxy-dopamine on noradrenergic and dopaminergic innervations of the cerebral cortex, *Brain Res.* **166**:309–320.

Shipley, M. T., and Adamek, G. D., 1982, Connections of the newborn rat olfactory bulb, *Soc. Neurosci. Abstr.* **8**:822.

Shute, C. C. D., and Lewis, P. R., 1966, Electron microscopy of cholinergic terminals and actylcholinesterase-containing neurones in the hippocampal formation of the rat, *Z. Zellforsch.* **69**:334–343.

Shute, C. C. D., and Lewis, P. R., 1967, The ascending cholinergic reticular system: Neocortical, olfactory, and subcortical projections, *Brain* **90**:497–519.

Silver, A., 1974, *The Biology of Cholinesterases*, North Holland, Amsterdam, pp. 379–386.

Sofroniew, M. V., Eckenstein, F., Thoenen, H., and Cuello, A. C., 1982, Topography of choline acetyltransferase-containing neurons in the forebrain of the rat, *Neurosci. Lett.* **33**:7–12.

Somogyi, P., Chubb, I. W., and Smith, A. D., 1975, A possible structural basis for the extracellular release of acetylcholinesterase, *Proc. R. Soc. London Ser. B* **191**:271–283.

Spehlmann, R., 1971, Acetylcholine and the synaptic transmission of non-specific impulses to the visual cortex, *Brain* **94**:139–150.

Spehlmann, R., Daniels, J. C., and Smathers, C. C., Jr., 1971, Acetylcholine and the synaptic transmission of specific impulses to the visual cortex, *Brain* **94**:125–138.

Steffen, H., 1976, Golgi-stained barrel-neurons in the somatosensory region of the mouse cerebral cortex, *Neurosci. Lett.* **2**:57–59.

Stone, T. W., 1972, Cholinergic mechanisms in the rat somatosensory cerebral cortex, *J. Physiol. (London)* **225**:485–499.

Tennyson, V. M., Brzin, M., and Duffy, P., 1967, Electron microscope cytochemistry and microgasometric analysis of cholinesterase in the nervous system, *Prog. Brain Res.* **29**:41–61.

Tsuji, S., 1974, On the chemical basis of thiocholine methods for demonstration of acetylcholinesterase activities, *Histochemistry* **42**:99–110.

Tsuji, S., and Larabi, Y., 1983, A modification of thiocholine–ferricyanide method of Karnovsky and Roots for localization of acetylcholinesterase activity without interference of Koelle's copper thiocholine iodide precipitate, *Histochemistry* **78**:317–323.

Van der Loos, H., and Woolsey, T. A., 1973, Somatosensory cortex: Structural alterations following early injury to sense organs, *Science* **179**:395–398.

Villani, L., Ciani, F., and Contestabile, A., 1977, Ultrastructural pattern of acetylcholinesterase distribution in the cerebellar cortex of the quail, *Anat. Embryol.* **152**:29–41.

Vincent, S. R., Satoh, K., Armstrong, D. M., and Fibiger, H. C., 1983, Substance P in the ascending cholinergic reticular system, *Nature* **306**:688–691.

Wainer, B. H., Levey, A. I., Rye, D. B., Bluemke, A., Mufson, E. J., and Mesulam, M.-M., 1984, Different populations of rat cortical neurons stain for choline acetyltransferase and acetylcholinesterase, *Soc. Neurosci. Abstr.* **10:**809.

Waite, P. M. E., 1977, Normal nerve fibers in the barrel region of developing and adult mouse cortex, *J. Comp. Neurol.* **173:**165–174.

Wamsley, J., Zarbin, M., Birdsall, N., and Kunar, M. J., 1980, Muscarinic cholinergic receptors: Autoradiographic localization of high and low affinity agonist-binding sites, *Brain Res.* **200:**1–12.

Welker, C., and Woolsey, T. A., 1975, Structure of layer IV in the somatosensory neocortex in the rat: Description and comparison with the mouse, *J. Comp. Neurol.* **158:**47–454.

Weller, W. L., and Johnson, J. I., 1975, Barrels in cerebral cortex altered by receptor disruption in newborn, but not five-day-old mice, *Brain Res.* **83:**504–508.

Wenk, H., Bigl, V., and Meyer, U., 1980, Cholinergic projections from magnocellular nuclei of the basal forebrain to cortical areas in rats, *Brain Res. Rev.* **2:**295–316.

Whitehouse, P. J., Price, D. L., Clark, A. W., Coyle, J. T., and DeLong, M. R., 1981, Alzheimer disease: Evidence for selective loss of cholinergic neurons in the nucleus basalis, *Am. J. Neurol.* **10:**122–126.

Wise, S. P., 1975, The laminar organization of certain afferent and efferent fiber systems in rat somatosensory cortex, *Brain Res.* **90:**139–142.

Wise, S. P., and Jones, E. G., 1978, Developmental studies of thalamocortical and commissural connections in the rat somatic sensory cortex, *J. Comp. Neurol.* **178:**187–208.

Woolsey, T. A., and Van der Loos, H., 1970, The structural organization of layer IV in the somatosensory region (SI) of mouse cerebral cortex, *Brain Res.* **17:**205–242.

Woolsey, T. A., and Wann, J. R., 1976, Areal changes in mouse cortical barrels following vibrissal damage at different postnatal ages, *J. Comp. Neurol.* **170:**53–66.

Woolsey, T. A., Welker, C., and Schwartz, R. H., 1975, Comparative anatomical studies of the SmI face cortex with special reference to the barrels, *J. Comp. Neurol.* **164:**79–84.

6

GABA–Peptide Neurons of the Primate Cerebral Cortex
A Limited Cell Class

E. G. JONES, S. H. C. HENDRY, and J. DeFELIPE

1. Introduction

The presence in the mammalian cerebral cortex of the classical neurotransmitter, γ-aminobutyric acid (GABA), and its synthesizing enzyme, glutamic acid decarboxylase (GAD), has been known for a relatively long time (Awapara *et al.*, 1950; Roberts and Fenkel, 1950; Albers and Brady, 1959). In recent years, immunocytochemistry has revealed the existence of a large population of neurons immunoreactive for both GAD and GABA in the cortex of a wide variety of mammals (Ribak, 1978; Hendry and Jones, 1986; Emson and Hunt, 1981; Hendrickson *et al.*, 1981; Peters *et al.*, 1982; Hendry *et al.*, 1983a; Houser *et al.*, 1983b, 1985; Bear *et al.*, 1985; Lin *et al.*, 1985). Recent quantitative assessments in the monkey cortex indicate that approximately 25% of the neuronal population in any cortical area is GABA- or GAD-immunoreactive (Hendry *et al.*, 1987). The point has also been made (Jones and Hendry, 1986; Fig. 1) that probably all the morphological varieties of intrinsic cortical neurons, except the

E. G. JONES, S. H. C. HENDRY, and J. DeFELIPE • Department of Anatomy and Neurobiology, University of California, Irvine, California 92717. *Present address of J.D.:* Unidad de Neuroanatomia, Instituto Cajal, CSIC, 28006 Madrid, Spain.

population of small, putatively excitatory, dendritic-spine-covered neurons of layer IV, are GABA-immunoreactive. The several varieties of pyramidal neurons in the cortex are undoubtedly excitatory also and a good case can be made for their use of glutamate as a transmitter (Cotman *et al.,* 1981; Streit, 1984; Donoghue *et al.,* 1985).

The presence of neuroactive brain–gut peptides was first reported in the mammalian cerebral cortex in a number of radioimmunoassay or immunocytochemical studies from 1976 to 1978 (Carraway and Leeman, 1976; Hökfelt *et al.,* 1976; Said and Rosenberg, 1976; Uhl and Snyder, 1976; Dockray, 1976; Muller *et al.,* 1977; Hökfelt *et al.,* 1978; Paxinos *et al.,* 1978; Sachs *et al.,* 1977). Since then, the presence of a dozen or more neuropeptides has been reported, commonly on the basis of radioimmunoassay (RIA), but usually RIA has been followed by immunocytochemistry, which has documented the existence of immunoreactivity for the peptide (or a closely similar antigen) in neurons and/or fibers of the cortex. Table I lists the cortical neuropeptides thus far identified and indicates the distribution of cells or fibers immunoreactive for them. On current evidence, cells immunoreactive for many peptides appear to be widely distributed to all cortical areas; those immunoreactive for certain others are found in more restricted areas.

Given the large numbers of cortical peptides and the wide distribution of cells immunoreactive for them, it would not have been surprising if their presence defined a considerable variety of new cortical cell types. Indeed, the majority of workers studying cortical cells by immunocytochemistry for the peptides, have attempted to place cells immunoreactive for each peptide into particular categories defined by the conventional morphological terms bipolar, multipolar, bitufted, and so on (McDonald *et al.,* 1982a–d; Peters *et al.,* 1983; McGinty *et*

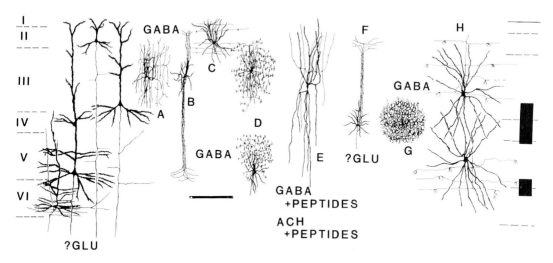

Figure 1. Morphological types of cells identifiable in monkey cerebral cortex, based on studies of Jones (1975) on sensory-motor areas. Cells at left are typical pyramidal cells of layers II–VI which are likely to use glutamate as a transmitter. Cells A–H are intrinsic neurons. All except the small spiny, putatively excitatory cell (F) of layer IV are proven or likely to be GABAergic. Long, stringy cell (E) is typical cell type that colocalizes GABA and neuropeptides or (in rat) acetylcholine and neuropeptides. A, cell with axonal arcades; B, double bouquet cell; C, H, basket cells; D, chandelier cells; G, neurogliaform cell.

al., 1984; Morrison *et al.*, 1983; Emson and Hunt, 1985). However, in studying somatostatin (SRIF)- and neuropeptide Y (NPY)-immunoreactive cortical cells (Hendry *et al.*, 1984a), we noted that none of these morphological terms adequately defined the cells. The cells could have a wide variety of dendritic field configurations if only the staining of the proximal dendrites was considered. (Incomplete staining of the total dendritic field is a feature of many immunocytochemical studies of cerebral neurons.) However, when more complete staining was achieved, all NPY- and SRIF-immunoreactive cells, irrespective of the configurations of their proximal dendrites, extended elongated vertical processes through several layers of the cortex. Subsequent studies of cortical cells immunoreactive for other neuropeptides (Jones *et al.*, 1987), and a review of reports in the literature, have led us to conclude that all the known cortical neuropeptides are contained in a limited cell class that can best be described as having a small rounded soma and a variable number of elongated, "stringy" vertical processes (Figs. 2–4).

In addition to seemingly belonging to a single morphological class, the cortical cells immunoreactive for known neuropeptides share a further feature in common. It has been determined that many, perhaps all, show colocalization of immunoreactivity for classical neurotransmitters or their biosynthetic enzymes. In 1984 four reports appeared on this subject: Eckenstein and Baughman in the rat cortex identified certain cells showing colocalization of immunoreactivity for vasoactive intestinal polypeptide (VIP) and choline acetyltransferase (ChAT); Schmechel *et al.*, reported colocalization of SRIF and GAD immunoreactivity in the rat, cat, and monkey cortex; Somogyi *et al.*, identified cells immunoreactive for SRIF and GABA or for CCK and GABA in the cat cortex and hippocampus; Hendry *et al.*, identified cells immunoreactive for SRIF and GAD, CCK and GAD, or NPY and GAD in the monkey and cat cortex and

Table I. Known Neocortical Transmitters[a]

	Extrinsic (in afferent fibers)		Intrinsic (in cortical neurons)	
	General (to all areas)	Regional (to some areas)	General	Regional
GABA	+	−	+ + + +	−
ACh	+ +	−	+ +	−
5HT	+ + +	−	−	−
NA	+ + +	−	−	−
DA	−	+ +	−	−
Glu/Asp	(+ +)[b]	−	(+ + +)	−
CCK	−	+	+ + +	−
NPY	−	−	+ + +	−
SRIF	−	−	+ + +	−
VIP	−	−	+ +	−
SP	−	+	+ + +	−
DYN	−	−	+ +	−
CRF	−	−	−	+
NT	−	+	−	−
CGRP	−	−	−	+

[a] From Jones and Hendry (1986).
[b] Entries in parentheses: likely, not proven conclusively.

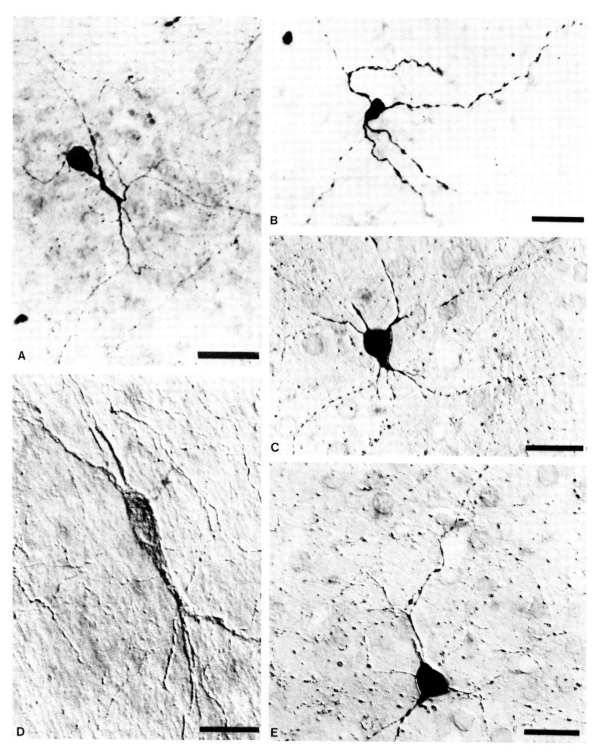

Figure 2. Variable forms of somatostatin-immunoreactive cells in cerebral cortex of rat (A, D) and monkey (B, C, E). From Hendry *et al.* (1984a). Bars = 25 μm.

showed quantitatively that at least 95% of cells immunoreactive for any of these peptides were also immunoreactive for GAD. We had previously shown that at least 24% of SRIF-positive cells in monkey cortex were also NPY-positive (Hendry *et al.*, 1984b). More recently, we have increased this percentage to close to 100% and, in addition, we have been able to determine that several cortical peptides are almost invariably colocalized with GABA and/or GAD (Jones and Hendry, 1986; Hendry *et al.*, 1987; Jones *et al.*, 1987).

The characteristic morphology of the presumed peptidergic neurons of the

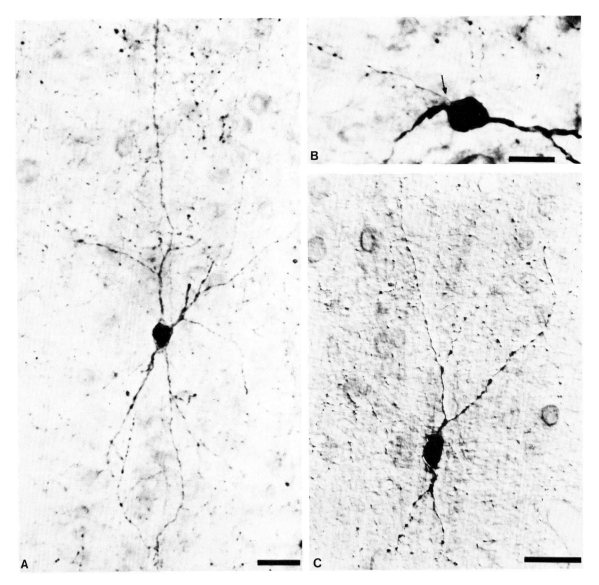

Figure 3 Variable forms of neuropeptide Y-immunoreactive cells in monkey cortex. From Hendry *et al.* (1984a). Bars = 25 μm (A, C), 10 μm (B).

cortex, their almost invariable colocalization with a classical transmitter, and the appearance in them of more than one type of peptide appear to make them a unique group. In what follows, we present many of the data upon which this assessment is based and deal with its potential implications for the organization and function of the cerebral cortex.

2. Observations

2.1. Pyramidal Neurons Are Not Immunoreactive for Known Peptides

The pyramidal neurons (Fig. 1) appear to form between 50 and 60% of the total cell population in any cortical area; these figures are essentially estimates,

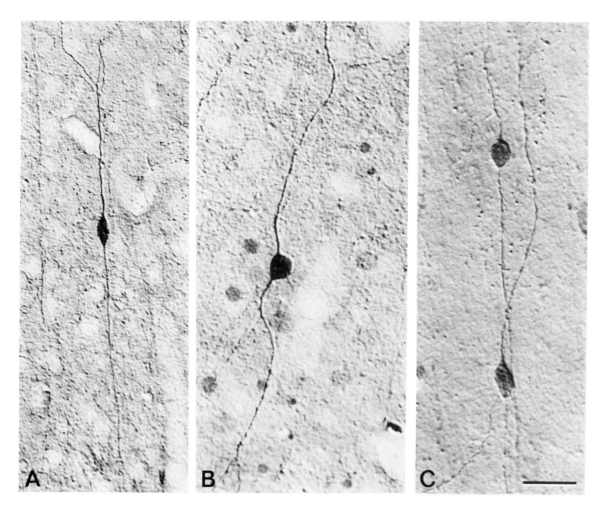

Figure 4. Cholecystokinin (A, B)- and vasoactive intestinal polypeptide (C)-immunoreactive cells in rat cortex. Bar = 25 μm.

as no extensive quantifications of their numbers have yet been done (but see Peters, this volume). Pyramidal neurons are the cells that give rise to the majority of, and in most areas all, the output connections of a cortical area (see Jones, 1984). These output connections include those to neighboring and distant cortical areas, to cortical areas in the contralateral hemisphere, and to the large variety of subcortical structures to which the cortex projects. The pyramidal cells are also major contributors to intracortical circuitry by means of their extensive systems of axon collaterals. Wherever they have been studied, the immediate effect of stimulation of pyramidal cell axons or their collaterals is the induction of excitatory postsynaptic potentials in cells with which they synapse, though this may be succeeded by profound inhibition.

There is a strong body of circumstantial evidence to suggest that the acidic amino acid glutamate (or possibly aspartate) is the transmitter utilized by pyramidal cell axon terminals. This evidence rests primarily upon: the reduced specific uptake of these two materials (which share the same high-affinity uptake system) by synaptosomes in cortical projection targets after decortication; the specific retrograde axoplasmic transport of $[^3H]$-D-aspartate in pyramidal cell axons (see Streit, 1984). The demonstration of immunoreactivity for phosphate-dependent glutaminase or aspartate aminotransferase in pyramidal neurons (Donoghue et al., 1985), though supportive of the idea that these cells are glutamergic or aspartergic, is inconclusive since it could simply reflect the involvement of glutamate and aspartate in the normal, non-transmitter-related metabolism of the cells.

Neuropeptide immunoreactivity has never been convincingly reported in pyramidal neurons. Some workers have certainly described peptide-immunoreactive cell bodies as "pyramidal" in shape. But this is insufficient for the most experienced workers for whom a true pyramidal neuron can only be defined by the presence of its stereotyped apical and basal dendritic systems covered in dendritic spines and an axon that descends vertically toward the white matter. No putatively peptide-immunoreactive neurons described as pyramidal in the literature have ever been stained much beyond the proximal portions of their dendrites and, thus, the rigid morphological criteria have not been met. In our own studies, we have never stained peptide-immunoreactive cells that we could feel comfortable about classifying as pyramidal. Moreover, at the electron microscopic level we have never detected a peptide-immunoreactive dendritic spine, though it has been possible to stain small dendrites of comparable caliber, and virtually all peptide-immunoreactive synapses that we have studied in the cortex are of the symmetric variety (Fig. 5), quite unlike the asymmetric synapses of pyramidal cell axon collaterals (Winfield et al., 1981; McGuire et al., 1984). Finally, peptide-positive cell bodies invariably receive both symmetric and asymmetric synaptic contacts, like most nonpyramidal cell bodies but unlike pyramidal cell bodies, which receive symmetric contacts only (see Hendry et al., 1983a, 1984b).

One point about peptide immunoreactivity and pyramidal cells that needs mentioning is the observation of Roberts et al., (1985) to the effect that SRIF immunoreactivity coexists with neurofibrillary tangles in human cortical neurons in Alzheimer's disease. Neuropathological studies almost universally describe tangles as being confined to pyramidal neurons and this has been our own experience. Nor have we been able to demonstrate colocalization of tangles and immunoreactivity for SRIF or several other peptides in our cases. The results

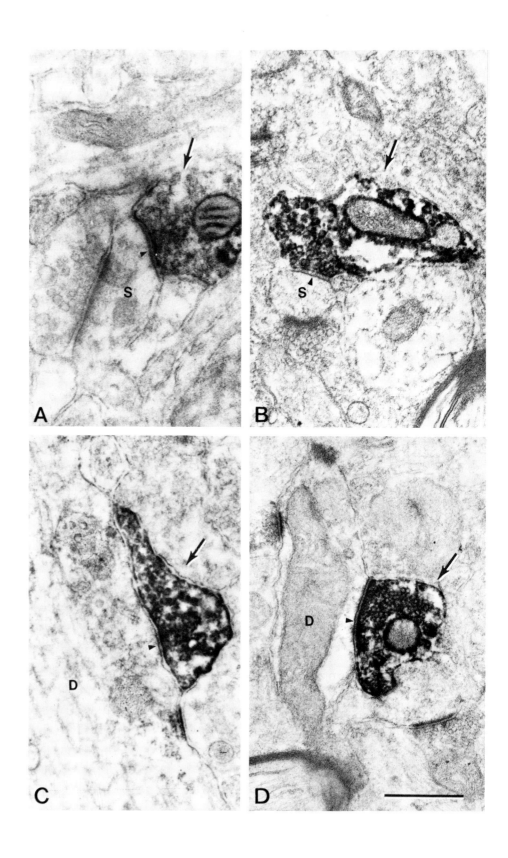

of Roberts *et al.*, (1985) may reflect expression of a peptide in pyramidal cells that normally do not do so, or the hitherto unremarked presence of tangles in peptidergic, nonpyramidal neurons. But independent corroboration appears desirable.

2.2. GABA Neurons Make Up a Large Proportion of Cortical Neurons

Any section of the monkey cortex when stained immunocytochemically for GABA or GAD, reveals that a large proportion of the cortical neuronal population is immunoreactive for these compounds (Fig. 6). Stained cells appear in all layers of all areas with, qualitatively speaking, the largest number in the middle layers, particularly layer IV of the sensory areas. By using relatively thin sections, stained in a manner that maximizes penetration of and staining by the immunoreagents, it is possible to count accurately the GABAergic cell population from area to area (Hendry *et al.*, 1987). In cynomolgus monkeys, counts have been made in 50-μm-wide rectangular, vertical traverses extending from the pia mater to the white matter across areas 17 and 18 of visual cortex, the parietal fields areas 5 and 7, the temporal fields 21 and 22, motor cortex, and orbitofrontal cortex (Table II). These counts reveal a remarkable constancy of GABA-immunoreactive cell numbers from area to area, with a notable increase only in area 17. All areas except area 17 average approximately 30 to 40 GABA- or GAD-immunoreactive cells per 50-μm-wide traverse. In area 17 the number is approximately 54 to 58. When these numbers are compared, either with our own counts of the total, Nissl-stained neuronal population (Table II) or with the counts made by Rockel *et al.* (1980) in rhesus monkeys, it is apparent that GABAergic neurons form approximately 25% of the cell population in any area except the visual in which the consistently higher total cell population ensures that the GABA population falls to approximately 20%.

2.3. GABA Neurons Belong to Several Varieties of Cortical Intrinsic Neuron

Among the large cortical GABAergic population, there are a variety of morphological types of neuron (Fig. 1). All, however, are nonpyramidal, all lack significant populations of dendritic spines, and all their axons seem to be intrinsic to the cortex and form symmetrical synaptic contacts with flattenable synaptic vesicles (Hendry *et al.*, 1983a, 1984b). These are all features of the nonspiny types of cortical interneuron. There has been some difficulty in defining further whether all or only some of the morphological forms of nonspiny intrinsic neuron are GABA- or GAD-immunoreactive since it is rare for the total dendritic tree or complete axonal ramification to be stained. Among the six or so nonspiny forms of cortical interneuron, two at least stand out as being almost certainly GABAergic, even in the absence of dendritic staining much beyond the primary

Figure 5. Neuropeptide Y (A)-, somatostatin (B, D)-, and cholecystokinin (C)-immunoreactive terminals (arrows) making symmetric synaptic contacts (arrowheads) on dendritic spines (S) or dendritic shafts (D) in monkey cortex. Bar = 0.5 μm.

branches. These are the basket cells because of their large somal size, dendritic and axonal morphology, and the chandelier cells because of the unique site of termination of their axons. A review of the dendritic fields of other GABA-immunoreactive neurons, so far as the fields can be stained (Houser *et al.*, 1983b), suggests that possibly all the other types of nonspiny cortical intrinsic neuron are also GABAergic, though it is hard to document this conclusively. Among the types recognizable in studies of GABA and GAD localization are those with small rounded somata from which long thin dendrites arise singly or in tufts and turn vertically, giving the cell a bipolar or bitufted appearance (Fig. 7). The somata of these cells appear to be most common in layer II and the superficial part of layer III, and at the junction of layers V and VI. There is reason to believe (see below and Fig. 1) that this GABAergic cell type is the cortical cell type that contains all or most of the known cortical neuropeptides.

The concentration of the somata of these elongated GABA cells in superficial and deep strata correlates quite well with the positions in most monkey cortical areas of two strata of somata that are specifically labeled by transport of [³H]-GABA injected into individual cortical layers (Somogyi *et al.*, 1981; DeFelipe and Jones, 1985). When this material is injected into layer II and the superficial part

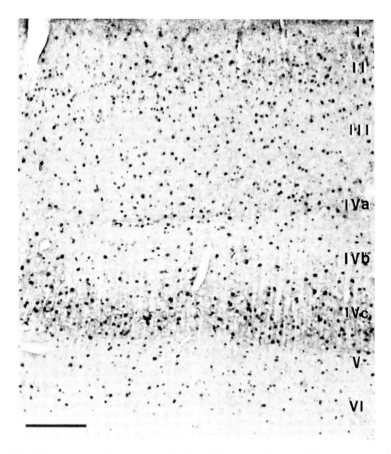

Figure 6. GABA-immunoreactive neurons distributed through all layers of the monkey visual cortex in a 10-μ-thick section. Bar = 0.5 μm.

Table II. Number of GABA Positive Cells per 50-μm-Wide Traverse (Means of 80–100 Traverses) in Monkey Cortex[a]

	Area 17	Area 18	Area 5	Areas 1–2	Area 3b	Area 4
Animal 1	54.2 ± 2.9	38.4 ± 5.0	38.1 ± 3.2	10.4 ± 3	31.6 ± 3.3	40.0 ± 2.5
Animal 2	54.1 ± 3.1	36.8 ± 5.4	41.7 ± 3.9	39.8 ± 3.1	38.4 ± 2.9	39.7 ± 3.0
Animal 3	57.7 ± 4.5	39.7 ± 4.0	38.6 ± 2.5	39.5 ± 2.8	28.5 ± 4.0	40.4 ± 2.8
Mean	56.2 ± 3.1	38.4 ± 5.1	39.4 ± 3.1	39.8 ± 2.9	32.8 ± 6.1	39.7 ± 2.9
		Total number of cells per 50 μm-wide traverse				
Range	309.0–314.7	152.0–156.1	153.1–154.5	149.7–154.3	152.7–154.9	148.9–151.7
Mean	311.6 ± 19.3	155.1 ± 8.1	153.7 ± 6.4	153.0 ± 7.2	153.66 ± 6.1	150.4 ± 6.1

[a] From Hendry *et al.* (1987).

of layer III, small nonpyramidal cell somata are labeled in layers V and VI, in a small focus immediately deep to the injection focus, but not in intervening layers (Fig. 8A). Conversely, injection of [³H]-GABA into layers V and VI leads to somal labeling in a focus in layer II and the superficial part of layer III, again without somal labeling in intervening layers (Fig. 8B).

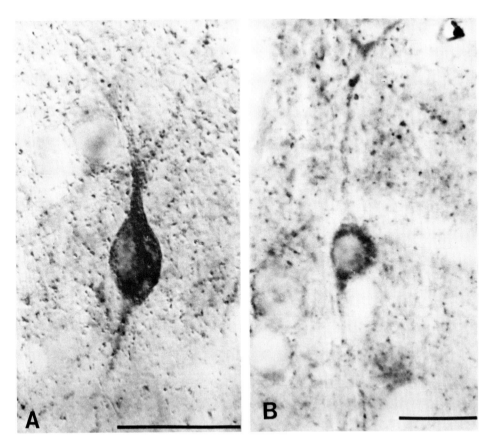

Figure 7. Neurons immunoreactive for GAD in monkey cortex. These cells have the form typical of GABA neurons that colocalize immunoreactivity for neuropeptides. Bars = 10 μm.

The common interpretation of this remarkably specific, columnar pattern of interlaminar labeling is that it is based upon high-affinity terminal uptake and retrograde axoplasmic transport of the [³H]-GABA to the parent somata of axons that interconnect layers II–III with V–VI, and vice versa. The blockade of the effect by intracortical injections of colchicine (DeFelipe and Jones, 1985) supports this. Electron microscopic examination of the autoradiographically labeled, linear profiles that connect injection site and labeled somata, however, reveals labeled dendrites as well as labeled axons. Thus, cells with vertical dendrites as well as axons appear to be involved in the phenomenon and somal labeling may be due to a combination of retrograde axonal and dendritic transport. The elongated GABA neurons of layers II–III and V–VI are obvious candidates to form the basis for this specific translaminar transport of [³H]-

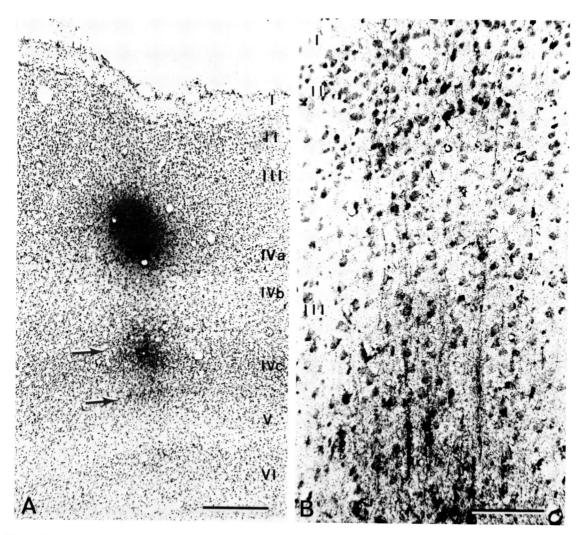

Figure 8. Selective retrograde labeling of neurons by [³H]-GABA. Cells in layers IVc and V of monkey visual cortex (A) are labeled after an injection in layers III–IVa. Cells in layers II–III of monkey motor cortex (B) are labeled after an injection in layer V. From DeFelipe and Jones (1985). Bars = 0.5 μm.

GABA. Their morphology is appropriate, as also is the general belief that this form of transmitter-specific retrograde labeling is a feature of neurons using the transmitter normally (see Streit, 1984).

2.4. All Cortical Neuropeptide Neurons Have a Similar Morphology

The following neuropeptides have been localized by immunocytochemistry in neuronal somata of cerebral cortex in a number of mammalian species (Table I): CCK, NPY, SRIF and its longer precursors, substance P (SP), dynorphin (DYN), VIP, corticotropin-releasing factor (CRF), calcitonin gene-related peptide (CGRP). Immunoreactivity for all of those mentioned has been observed in the rat but only CCK, NPY, SRIF, and SP have been so far localized in the higher primate cortex. There is, however, evidence from RIA for the presence of most of the others in monkeys and man.

Our own observations in monkeys, cats, rats, and several other mammalian species suggest that all cells immunoreactive for any of the cortical neuropeptides have an overall similarity in their morphology, irrespective of the species. In what follows, therefore, we shall make the tentative assumption that when cells immunoreactive for peptides hitherto not stained in the primate cortex are discovered, they will resemble not only their counterparts in other species but also the cells immunoreactive for other peptides in the primate cortex.

Several features distinguish cortical neuropeptide cells. All have small rounded somata, perhaps among the smallest of all cortical neurons. The somata are found in all layers but tend to be concentrated in layer II and the superficial part of layer III, and in layer VI and the immediately underlying white matter (Fig. 9), particularly in monkeys and man. In some areas, additional concentrations of somata can sometimes be found in other layers. In the monkey visual cortex, for example, a significant concentration of SP-immunoreactive somata occurs in layer V as well (Fig. 10). The cells have slender dendrites that can arise in extremely variable numbers from any part of the surface of the soma at any angle. Where, as is common in many immunocytochemical preparations, only the proximal portions of the dendrites are stained, the cells may appear to adopt a variety of shapes. Thus, in the literature one finds cortical peptide cells described variously as bipolar, bitufted, multipolar, stellate, and so on, and even as pyramidal cells. After examining large numbers of peptide-immunoreactive cells in our own preparations with the staining of secondary and tertiary dendrites enhanced, along with the photographs of the better stained cells in the literature, we have been led to the following conclusion. Verticality of dendrites is the *sine qua non* of these cells. Irrespective of how many dendrites arise from a soma and irrespective of their angles of origin, all will branch and/or turn into a vertical set of processes that traverse two or more layers of the cortex perpendicularly. The terminal portions of the processes may branch relatively profusely. Thus, two major plexuses tend to be set up, one in the supragranular layers and one in the infragranular layers and underlying white matter (Fig. 11). Layer IV is in some areas, particularly the visual, notably devoid of a peptidergic plexus, though in others a third subsidiary plexus may be set up there (Fig. 11).

Putative axons of the peptide-immunoreactive cells have often been identified in light micrographs and synaptic terminals typical of those normally found on axons are common at the electron microscopic level (Fig. 5). The linkup between "axon" and terminals has not been made, however, and many processes labeled in the literature as axons are unconvincing. Because of the considerable variability in the dimensions and branching patterns of processes emerging from peptide-immunoreactive cells in cerebral cortex, some cells, whose processes are adequately stained, give the impression of having multiple "axons." It is not yet

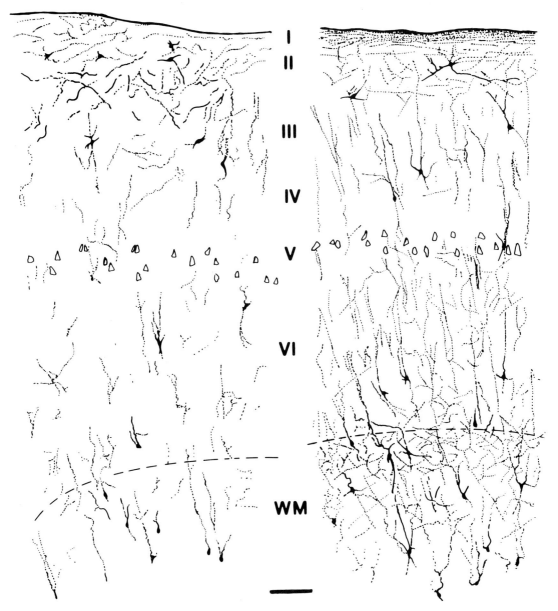

Figure 9. Camera lucida drawing showing distributions of somatostatin (left)- and neuropeptide Y-immunoreactive fibers and cells in monkey motor cortex. Betz cells of layer V are outlined but were not labeled. From Hendry *et al.* (1984a). wm, white matter. Bar = 250 μm.

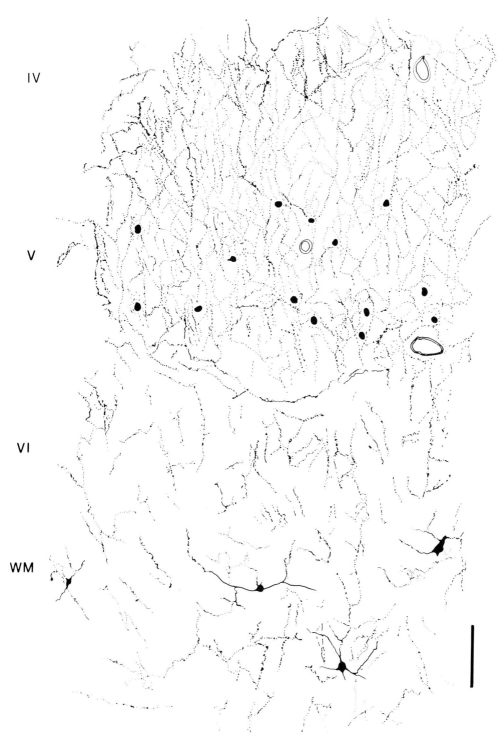

IV

V

VI

WM

Figure 10. Camera lucida drawing of substance P-immunoreactive cells and fibers in deeper layers of monkey visual cortex. Cells without stained processes in layer V colocalize GABA immunoreactivity; cells with long stained processes in layer VI and white matter colocalize NPY immunoreactivity. wm, white matter. Bar = 100 μm.

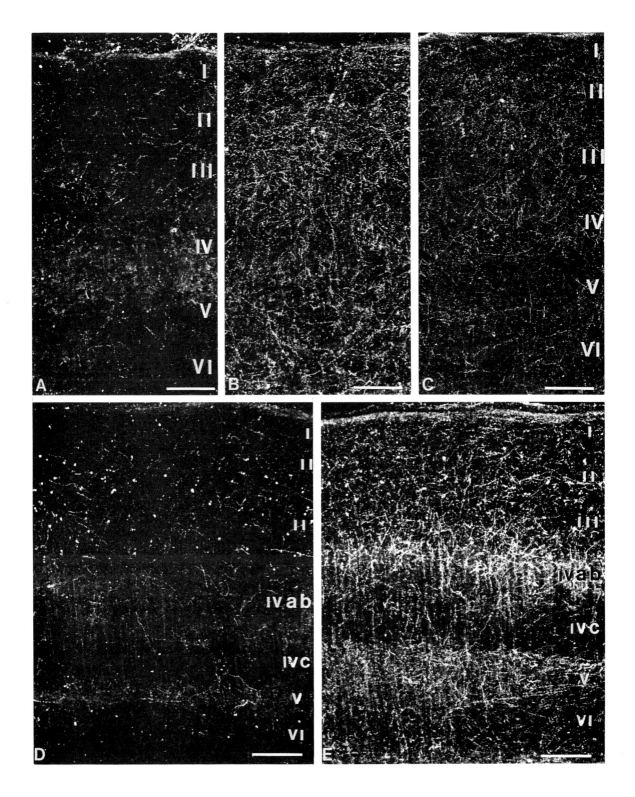

clear, therefore, whether these cells have conventional axons or multiple presynaptic processes.

There have been occasional reports of a small number of peptide-immunoreactive neurons projecting axons outside cerebral cortex in rats. These reports are based upon retrograde labeling of the immunoreactive cell somata by fluorescent dyes injected into certain of the subcortical targets of the cortex. If correct, they imply the existence of a population of pyramidal neurons immunoreactive for peptides or nonpyramidal projection neurons. In our studies, we have not been able to confirm either implication and have not been able to label cortical peptidergic neurons retrogradely from injections of tracers in cortical or subcortical sites. We believe it likely that contamination of the plexus of peptidergic processes in the white matter deep to the cortex may account for the reports of extrinsic peptidergic projections from the cortex. This plexus is always evident in white matter overlain by cortex but disappears from deep or exposed white matter such as the internal capsule and corpus callosum (Hendry et al., 1984b). The fact that most cortical peptide cells are also immunoreactive for GABA or GAD (see below) is also against their projecting subcortically since no known subcortical projections are GABAergic.

The intracortical immunoreactive terminals of all peptide neurons are very similar. They are small, contain synaptic vesicles that flatten or become pleomorphic in the usual fixatives, and in the vast majority of cases, irrespective of the peptide localized, make typical symmetric membrane contacts. Points of contact have been demonstrated on large and small dendrites of both pyramidal and nonpyramidal neurons and on dendritic spines (Fig. 5). The peptide-immunoreactive cells themselves, including those in the white matter beneath the cortex, receive modest numbers of other, usually nonpeptidergic synapses.

Among other forms of contact made by peptide-immunoreactive terminals are some in which membrane specializations are lacking, as proven by serial thin sectioning of the whole terminal. Such terminals tend to lie closely adjacent to other nonimmunoreactive synapses (Fig. 12). Non-vesicle-containing portions of CCK-immunoreactive cells in particular may also have intimate appositions, without membrane specializations with other nerve cells or with the basal lamina of a small intracortical blood vessel (Fig. 13). A small number of SRIF- and NPY-immunoreactive terminals have been observed to make asymmetric synaptic contacts. In these, the immunoreactive material is mainly in large dense-core vesicles (Fig. 14), rather than diffusely throughout the cytosol as in the far more common immunoreactive terminals that make symmetric contacts. Whether the few terminals with asymmetric contacts arise from the same cells as the more common terminals or from some other set of cells or come from an extrinsic afferent fiber source has not been determined. Nor has it been decided if these large dense-core vesicles simply contain another peptide with amino acid sequences closely similar to those of NPY and SRIF and thus cross-reacting with the antisera used.

Figure 11. Somatostatin (A, C, D)- and neuropeptide Y (B, E)-immunoreactive plexuses in monkey somatosensory (A, B), parietal (C), and visual (D, E) cortex. From Hendry et al. (1984a). Bars = 200 μm.

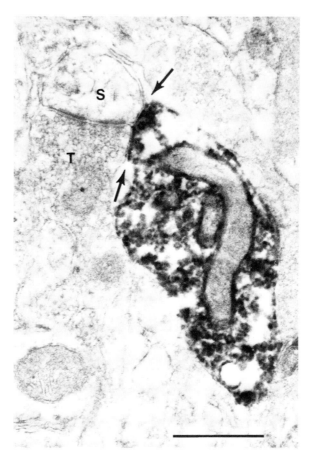

Figure 12. Neuropeptide Y-immunoreactive terminal closely adjacent (arrows) to a nonimmuno-reactive terminal (T) ending in an asymmetric synapse on a dendritic spine (S). No evident morphological specialization was formed by the NPY terminal even in serial sections. From Hendry *et al.* (1984a). Bar = 0.25 μm.

2.5. Many Peptide-Immunoreactive Cortical Neurons Are Immunoreactive for GABA

In the monkey we have made a systematic effort to quantify the proportions of neurons that show colocalization of peptides with classical neurotransmitters, particularly GABA (Figs. 15 and 16). Where certain neuropeptides such as VIP have proven refractory to immunocytochemical staining in the monkey cortex, we have studied these in rats only. In our first reports we noted that at least 90% of all CCK-, SRIF-, and NPY-immunoreactive cortical neurons also colocalized immunoreactivity for GAD (Hendry *et al.*, 1984b). Furthermore, a significant number of SRIF-immunoreactive neurons showed colocalization of NPY immunoreactivity (Hendry *et al.*, 1984a). As these studies have continued, it has become evident that the population of neurons colocalizing these and other substances is particularly high. The current status of work on the monkey (Hendry *et al.*, 1987) (Fig. 16) is that virtually all CCK neurons are also GABA- and

GAD-immunoreactive. In the rat, some also show VIP immunoreactivity. Approximately 95% of NPY neurons and 95% of SRIF neurons colocalize GABA and GAD. Virtually 100% of SRIF neurons also colocalize NPY and vice versa. About 90–95% of SP neurons (100% of those in layer V) colocalize GABA and GAD. The remaining 5–10% (mainly in layer VI and the white matter) colocalize SRIF and NPY (Fig. 10).

It appears, therefore, that not only are most of the neurons immunoreactive for the peptides studied to date also GABAergic but also that they often contain other peptides as well. It is not known yet if the peptides such as dynorphin, hitherto not stained in the monkey cortex, are also contained in GABA neurons. As mentioned earlier, however, cortical cells immunoreactive for these other peptides in rats are morphologically very similar to those that show colocalization of peptide and GABA immunoreactivity in the monkey. A similar question also arises about acetylcholine. Its synthetic enzyme, ChAT, is colocalized with VIP in an unspecified number of neurons in the rat cortex (Eckenstein and Baughman, 1984). There, the ChAT-immunoreactive cells have the long, stringy morphology typical of peptidergic cells throughout the cortex (Houser *et al.*, 1983a).

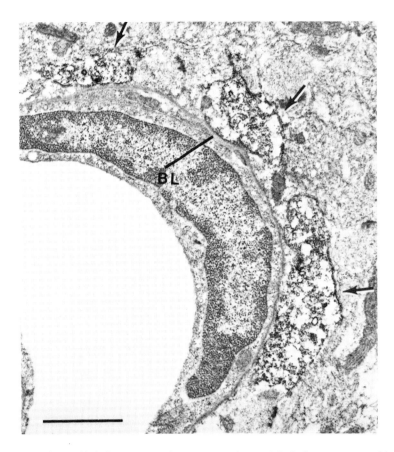

Figure 13. Cholecystokinin-immunoreactive processes (arrows) in intimate contact with the basal lamina (BL) of a capillary in monkey cortex. Bar = 0.5 μm.

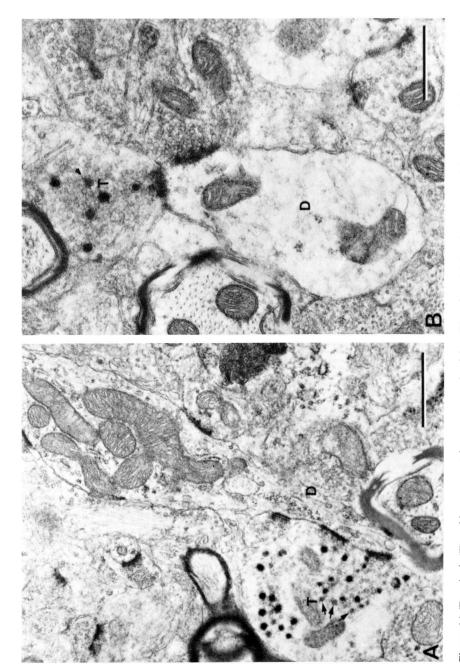

Figure 14. Terminals (T) making asymmetric synapses on dendrites (D) and containing dense-core vesicles apparently immunoreactive for neuropeptide Y (A) and somatostatin (B) in monkey cortex. Nonimmunoreactive dense-core vesicles are indicated by arrows. From Hendry *et al.* (1984a). Bars = 1 μm.

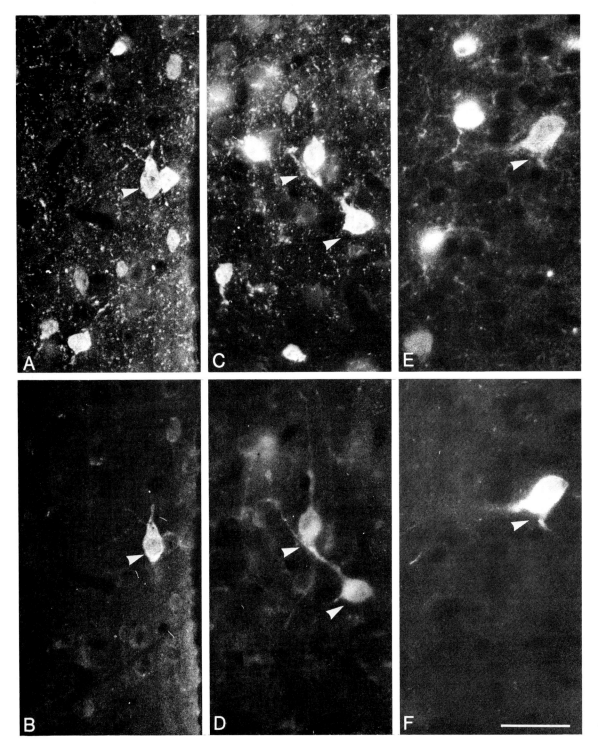

Figure 15. Pairs of fluorescence photomicrographs from sections of monkey cortex stained immunocytochemically for GABA and somatostatin (A, B), for GABA and cholecystokinin (C, D), and for GABA and neuropeptide Y (E, F). A small proportion of the GABA-immunoreactive cells are also immunoreactive for the peptide. Bar = 10 μm.

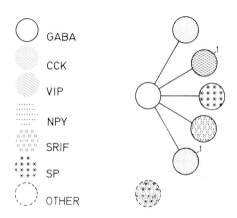

GABA

CCK

VIP

NPY

SRIF

SP

OTHER

Figure 16. Combinations of GABA and neuropeptide immunoreactivity demonstrated to date in neocortex. "1" indicates combinations demonstrated only in rats. "Other" indicates a small population of neurons showing peptide immunoreactivity only but may contain another classical neurotransmitter. From Jones and Hendry (1986).

In addition, some VIP-positive cells in the rat costain for GABA and GAD (Hendry and Jones, unpublished). Are GAD and ChAT colocalized? That is a question for which there was no answer at the time of writing.

2.6. All GABA Neurons Are Not Immunoreactive for Known Peptides

Although the majority of peptide-positive cortical neurons in the monkey are also GAD- and GABA-positive, the converse is by no means true. By our counts, approximately 70–75% of the GABA-positive neurons do not costain for a known peptide. In addition, at least two morphological classes of GABA neuron are ruled out as staining for a known peptide. The basket cells cannot be peptide-immunoreactive since no somata larger than 10 μm have ever been stained for a known peptide. Basket cells in monkeys normally have somata 20–50 μm in diameter. The chandelier cells are also ruled out for no chains of peptide-immunoreactive axon terminals have ever been demonstrated light or electron microscopically on the initial segments of pyramidal cell axons. While it is possible that certain other forms of putatively GABAergic nonpyramidal cell are also peptide-immunoreactive, the small size and elongated, "stringy" morphology of all the peptide neurons thus far identified place them best among a limited, perhaps single cell class. In Golgi preparations, the type example, in our opinion, is the cell often described as bipolar or bitufted, although obvious bipolar cells are rare in primates and there appear to be gradations in form from one to the other.

It would be foolish to suggest that cortical GABA neurons that do not show immunoreactivity for known peptides, do not contain neuroactive peptides. Probably many new agents of this type remain to be discovered and it is likely that some will turn up in basket or chandelier cells or in other types of cortical GABA neuron. Furthermore, it is still possible that these cells normally express such small amounts of the known peptides that they simply fail to stain for them. Perhaps, under certain conditions of stimulation, they may be induced to express these peptides in sufficiently large amounts to be stained immunocytochemically. If the known peptides are not expressed at all by certain cells because of failure of transcription, perhaps these cells can be induced to transcribe the appropriate mRNAs under novel conditions.

Presynaptic innervation can regulate levels of transmitters, transmitter-synthesizing enzymes, receptors, and the abundance of related mRNAs in the peripheral nervous system (Ip and Zigmond, 1984; Black *et al.*, 1984, 1985; Roach *et al.*, 1985). There is reason to believe that comparable effects are operational in the CNS: In our studies of visual cortex of adult monkeys subjected to monocular visual deprivation for 9–11 weeks, we have found that immunoreactive staining for GABA, GAD, and SP declines markedly in deprived ocular dominance columns (Fig. 17). The reduction in staining is not simply a decline in intensity but an actual reduction in the number of stained cells in comparison with adjacent nondeprived columns. NPY-immunoreactive staining is unaffected (Hendry and Jones, 1986; Jones and Hendry, 1986). This indicates that GABA levels can be down-regulated through a reduction in immunoreactive GAD and, moreover, that sensory experience appears to control levels of one peptide expressed by the same cells. Our results show further that levels of immunoreactivity for a calcium/calmodulin-dependent protein kinase, CaM kinase II (Bennett *et al.*, 1983; DeRiemer *et al.*, 1984; Browning *et al.*, 1985), are actually upregulated in the deprived cells (Hendry *et al.*, 1985; Hendry and Kennedy, 1986), suggesting that the GABA–GAD–SP effect may be mediated by second messengers associated with changes in intracellular phosphoproteins (Nestler *et al.*, 1984; Nishizuka, 1984; Berridge and Irvine, 1984).

2.7. Can Different Classes of GABA–Peptide Cortical Neurons Be Identified?

Although in our opinion division of the peptide-immunoreactive neurons of the neocortex into classes on morphological grounds is artificial, there appear to be classes that can be distinguished either by the constellation of peptides they contain (usually in association with GABA), or in terms of the synaptic targets of their axons. In an earlier section we indicated that most cortical SRIF neurons colocalize NPY and vice versa. However, neither of these appears to show CCK or VIP immunoreactivity. Most SP cells colocalize GABA and not NPY but the layer VI–white matter population colocalizes NPY and not GABA. Other combinations are evident in Fig. 16. Conceivably, these various combinations simply reflect the presence of a population of GABA neurons in which all the known cortical peptides are potentially present but that differential modulations of their levels occur. This seems unlikely since certain combinations, e.g., CCK and/or VIP with NPY and/or SRIF, have never been found. Possibly this is reflected in the tendency for CCK and VIP cells (Fig. 4) to have fewer vertical processes than NPY and SRIF cells (Figs. 2 and 3).

Differential targeting of their synaptic terminals may be one convenient way of distinguishing classes of cortical peptidergic neurons. Although extensive quantification has not yet been carried out, preliminary evidence suggests that the bulk of SRIF- and NPY-immunoreactive synapses are formed on distal dendritic branches and on dendritic spines of pyramidal neurons. CCK- and VIP-immunoreactive synapses, on the other hand, appear to terminate on more

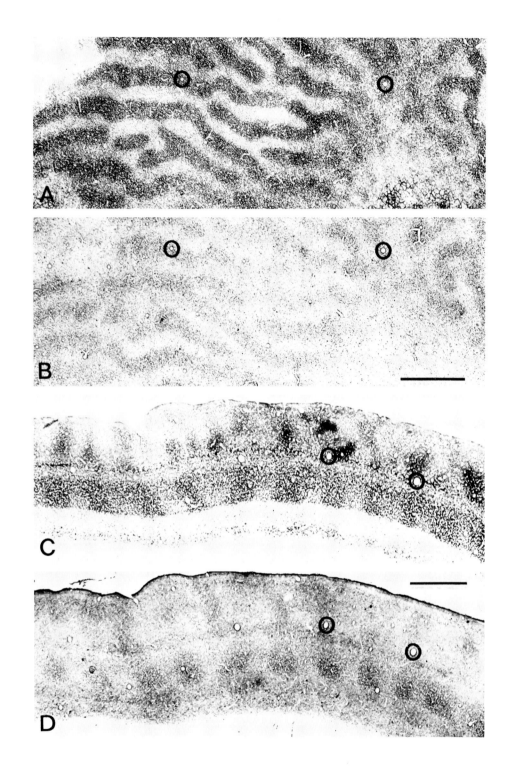

proximal dendrites of pyramidal neurons (Hendry *et al.*, 1983a, 1984a). SP-immunoreactive synapses appear to be found at all three sites (Jones *et al.*, 1987). To what extent these qualitative impressions will stand the test of rigorous quantification remains to be seen. However, for the present they seem to offer a more reliable means of characterizing the peptidergic cortical neurons along lines that probably have more functional significance than morphology alone.

3. What Are the Functions of Cortical Peptide Neurons?

Most of the neuropeptides mentioned here have been iontophoresed onto neocortical or hippocampal neurons and they have usually been reported to increase resting levels of discharge and to induce excitatory postsynaptic potentials, with accompanying changes in membrane conductance. The responses can be almost as rapid as those induced by such potent excitatory agents as aspartate or glutamate. On occasion, inhibition and complex mixed effects have been reported, especially with SRIF. Any effects that the neuropeptides might have on cortical neuronal receptive fields have not been reported.

Given the colocalization of at least the better known cortical peptides with GABA, it is hard to explain how their release from a GABAergic terminal might induce excitation in the postsynaptic cell without postulating some special type of mechanism. In this context, it may be noted that there is no evidence yet to indicate that peptides released from a GABAergic synapse necessarily act directly at that synaptic site. They could, for example, be acting back on receptors located on the terminal from which they are released and might possibly regulate GABA release. This suggestion arises from the indications that the opioid peptides, acting through receptors located on presynaptic terminals, can inhibit the release of catecholamines, ACh, and other peptides (Bloom, 1983) and from evidence that NPY acts presynaptically in reducing orthodromically induced population spikes in hippocampal neurons (Colmers *et al.*, 1985).

Peptides released from GABA terminals could, of course, exert their effects over wide distances, perhaps affecting populations of neurons removed from the active synapse. Populations of neurons in amphibian sympathetic ganglia appear to be affected in this way by an LHRH (luteinizing hormone-releasing hormone)-like peptide coreleased with ACh (Jan and Jan, 1982).

Other potential actions of neuropeptides in cerebral cortex include the regulation of vascular perfusion and trophic effects. NPY and VIP are strongly vasoactive (Edvinsson, 1985) and VIP coreleased with ACh from parasympathetic terminals in the submandibular gland leads to vasodilatation, increased blood

---

Figure 17. Pairs of alternate sections from visual cortex of monkeys subjected to monocular deprivation for 11 weeks. The same blood vessels are circled in each pair. (A, B) Tangential sections through layer IV showing cytochrome oxidase staining (A) and GABA immunoreactivity (B) reduced in deprived ocular dominance strips. (C, D) Vertical sections showing reduction in cytochrome oxidase staining (C) and in substance P immunoreactivity (D) in deprived ocular dominance columns. Bars = 1 μm.

flow, and, thus, to enhancement of the secretomotor effect of ACh (Lundberg *et al.*, 1980). NPY is a vasoconstrictor and, thus, the two together might be effective in the control of cortical vascular perfusion (McCulloch, 1983), perhaps activity mediated. No experiments relevant to this, however, have yet been reported.

Some neuropeptides appear to have trophic actions akin to those of the polypeptide growth factors, e.g., nerve growth factor and epidermal growth factor. SP, VIP, and vasopressin stimulate DNA synthesis and mitogenesis in mesodermal cells and in cultured cell lines (Brenneman *et al.*, 1984; James and Bradshaw, 1984; Nilsson *et al.*, 1985). Some of the polypeptide growth factors also contain amino acid sequences closely similar to those of known neuropeptides (Gimenez-Gallego *et al.*, 1985). In the peripheral nervous system, certain neuropeptides such as VIP and secretin seem to be capable of inducing tyrosine hydroxylase in sympathetic postganglionic neurons (Ip *et al.*, 1982; Ip and Zigmond, 1984). Hence, long-term modulations of nerve cell chemistry may be one of the more important functions of the peptides.

In the neocortex there are indications that levels of certain peptides may be altered in demented states. NPY and SRIF levels decline in cortex of cases of Alzheimer's disease (Davies *et al.*, 1980; Rossor *et al.*, 1980) and SRIF falls in the frontal cortex of Parkinsonian patients with dementia. In Alzheimer's disease there is also a large decrease in markers for ACh but interestingly no decline in those for GABA with which SRIF and NPY are normally colocalized. The latter suggests a differential regulation of GABA and the peptides in this disease. Whether the decline in the two peptides then deprives the cortex of essential trophic agents that in turn cause the destruction of cholinergic neurons and terminals, is a question for the future.

4. Conclusions

The neuropeptide-containing neurons of the neocortex are a less heterogeneous group than commonly supposed. As judged by immunocytochemistry, virtually all of those known appear to be contained in a limited type of GABAergic intrinsic neuron. One, VIP, may be more commonly found in a cholinergic neuron that shares the morphological features of the GABA–peptide class. The vast majority of cortical neurons, including all the pyramidal neurons and most varieties of GABAergic intrinsic neuron, are not immunoreactive for known peptides.

The roles of the neuropeptides in cortical function are not known and conjectures range from actions close to those of the classical transmitters to those relating to control of levels of activity in populations of neurons and control of regional cortical blood flow, and ideas of actions of a trophic nature which although ill-defined may yield clues as to the role of peptides in cortical disease.

ACKNOWLEDGMENT. Personal work reported here was supported by USPHS Grant NS 21377 from the National Institutes of Health.

5. References

Albers, R. W., and Brady, R. O., 1959, The distribution of glutamate decarboxylase in the nervous system of the rhesus monkey, *J. Biol. Chem.* **234:**926–928.

Awapara, J., Landau, A. J., Fuerst, R., and Seale, B., 1950, Free γ-aminobutyric acid in brain, *J. Biol. Chem.* **187:**35–39.

Bear, M. F., Schmechel, D. E., and Ebner, F. F., 1985, Glutamic acid decarboxylase the striate cortex of normal and monocularly deprived kittens, *J. Neurosci.* **5:**1262–1275.

Bennett, M. K., Erondu, N. E., and Kennedy, M. B., 1983, Purification and characterization of a calmodulin-dependent protein kinase that is highly concentrated in brain, *J. Biol. Chem.* **258:**12735–12744.

Berridge, M. J., and Irvine, R. F., 1984, Inositol triphosphate, a novel second messenger in cellular signal-transduction, *Nature* **312:**315–321.

Black, I. B., Adler, J. E., Dreyfus, C. F., Jonakait, G. M., Katz, D. M., LaGamma, E. F., and Markey, K. M., 1984, Neurotransmitter plasticity at the molecular level, *Science* **225:**1266–1270.

Black, I. B., Chkaraishi, D. M., and Lewis, E. J., 1985, Trans-synaptic increase in RNA coding for tyrosine hydroxylase in a rat sympathetic ganglion, *Brain Res.* **339:**151–153.

Bloom, F. E., 1983, The endorphins: A growing family of pharmacologically pertinent peptides, *Annu. Rev. Pharmacol. Toxicol.* **23:**151–170.

Brenneman, D. E., Eider, L. E., and Seigel, R. E., 1984, Vasoactive intestinal peptide increases activity-dependent neuronal survival in developing spinal core cultures, *Soc. Neurosci. Abstr.* **10:**1050.

Browning, M. D., Huganir, R., and Greengard, P., 1985, Protein phosphorylation and neuronal function, *J. Neurochem.* **45:**11–23.

Carraway, R., and Leeman, S. E., 1976, Characterization of radioimmunoassayable neurotensin in the rat, *J. Biol. Chem.* **251:**1045–1052.

Colmers, W. F., Lukowiak, K., and Pitman, Q. J., 1985, Neuropeptide Y reduces orthodromically evoked population spike in rat hippocampal CA1 by a possibly presynaptic mechanism, *Brain Res.* **346:**404–408.

Cotman, C. W., Foster, A., and Lanthorn, T., 1981, An overview of glutamate as a neurotransmitter, *Adv. Biochem. Psychopharmacol.* **27:**1–27.

Davies, P., Katzman, R., and Terry, R., 1980, Reduced somatostatin-like immunoreactivity in cerebral cortex from cases of Alzheimer's disease and Alzheimer senile dementia, *Nature* **288:**279–280.

DeFelipe, J., and Jones, E. G., 1985, Vertical organization of γ-aminobutyric acid-accumulating intrinsic neuronal systems in monkey cerebral cortex, *J. Neurosci.* **5:**3246–3260.

DeFelipe, J., Hendry, S. H. C., and Jones, E. G., 1986, A correlative electron microscopic study of basket cells and large GABAergic neurons in the monkey sensory-motor cortex, *Neuroscience* **17:**991–1009.

DeRiemer, S. A., Kaczmarek, L. K., Lai, Y., McGuiness, T. L., and Greengard, P., 1984, Calcium/calmodulin-dependent protein phosphorylation in the nervous system of Aplysia, *J. Neurosci.* **4:**1618–1625.

Dockray, G. J., 1976, Immunochemical evidence of cholecystokinin like peptides in brain, *Nature* **264:**568–570.

Donoghue, J. P., Wenthold, R. J., and Altschuler, R. A., 1985, Localisation of glutaminase-like and aspartate aminotransferase-like immunoreactivity in neurons of cerebral neocortex, *J. Neurosci.* **5:**2597–2609.

Eckenstein, F., and Baughman, R. W., 1984, Two types of cholinergic innervation in cortex, one co-localized with vasoactive intestinal polypeptide, *Nature* **314:**153–155.

Edvinsson, L., 1985, Functional role of perivascular peptides in the control of cerebral circulation, *Trends Neurosci.* **8:**126–131.

Emson, P. C., and Hunt, S. P., 1981, Anatomical chemistry of the cerebral cortex, in: *The Organization of the Cerebral Cortex* (F. O. Schmitt, F. C. Worden, G. Adelman, and S. G. Dennis, eds.), MIT Press, Cambridge, Mass., pp. 325–345.

Emson, P. C., and Hunt, S. P., 1985, Peptide-containing neurons of the cerebral cortex, in: *Cerebral Cortex*, Vol. 2 (E. G. Jones and A. Peters, eds.), Plenum Press, New York, pp. 145–172.

Gimenez-Gallego, G., Rodkey, J., Bennett, C., Rios-Candelore, M., DeSalvo, J., and Thomas, K., 1985, Brain-derived acidic fibroblast growth factor: Complete amino acid sequence and homologies, *Science* **230**:1385–1388.

Hendrickson, A. E., Hunt, S. P., and Wu, J.-Y., 1981, Immunocytochemical localization of glutamic acid decarboxylase in monkey striate cortex, *Nature* **292**:605–606.

Hendry, S. H. C., and Jones, E. G., 1986, Reduction in number of immunostained GABA neurons in deprived-eye dominance columns of monkey area 17, *Nature* **320**:750–753.

Hendry, S. H. C., and Kennedy, M. B., 1986, Altered immunoreactivity for a calcium/calmodulin-dependent kinase in neurons of monkey striate cortex deprived of visual input, *Proc. Natl. Acad. Sci. USA* **83**:1536–1540.

Hendry, S. H. C., Houser, C. R., Jones, E. G., and Vaughn, J. E., 1983a, Synaptic organization of immunocytochemically identified GABA neurons in monkey sensory-motor cortex, *J. Neurocytol.* **12**:639–660.

Hendry, S. H. C., Jones, E. G., and Beinfeld, M. C., 1983b, Cholecystokinin-immunoreactive neurons in rat and monkey cerebral cortex make symmetric synapses and have intimate associations with blood vessels, *Proc. Natl. Acad. Sci. USA* **80**:2400–2404.

Hendry, S. H. C., Jones, E. G., DeFelipe, J., Schmechel, D., Brandon, C., and Emson, P. C., 1984a, Neuropeptide containing neurons of the cerebral cortex are also GABAergic, *Proc. Natl. Acad. Sci. USA* **81**:6526–6530.

Hendry, S. H. C., Jones, E. G., and Emson, P. C., 1984b, Morphology, distribution and synaptic relations of somatostatin- and neuropeptide Y-immunoreactive neurons in rat and monkey neocortex, *J. Neurosci.* **4**:2497–2517.

Hendry, S. H. C., Jones, E. G., and Kennedy, M. B., 1985, Modulation of GABA, substance P and protein kinase immunoreactivities in monkey striate cortex following eye removal, *Soc. Neurosci. Abstr.* **11**:16.

Hendry, S. H. C., Jones, E. G., and Yan, J., 1987, Proportions of GABA immunoreactive neurons in different areas of monkey cerebral cortex, *J. Neurosci.* in press.

Hökfelt, T., Meyerson, B., Nilsson, G., Pernow, B., and Sachs, C., 1976, Immunohistochemical evidence for substance P containing nerve endings in the human cortex, *Brain Res.* **104**:181–186.

Hökfelt, T., Elde, R., Johansson, O., Ljungdahl, Å., Schultzberg, M., Fuxe, K., Goldstein, M., Nilsson, G., Pernow, B., Terenius, L., Garten, D., Jeffcoate, S. L., Rehfeld, J., and Said, S., 1978, Distribution of peptide-containing neurones, in: *Psychopharmacology: A Generation of Progress* (M. A. Lipton, A. DiMascio, and K. F. Killam, eds.), Raven Press, New York, pp. 39–66.

Houser, C. R., Crawford, C. D., Barber, R. P., Salvaterra, P. M., and Vaughn, J. E., 1983a, Organization and morphological characteristics of cholinergic neurons: An immunocytochemical study with a monoclonal antibody to choline acetyltransferase, *Brain Res.* **266**:97–119.

Houser, C. R., Hendry, S. H. C., Jones, E. G., and Vaughn, J. E., 1983b, Morphological diversity of immunocytochemically identified GABA neurons in monkey sensory motor cortex. *J. Neurocytol.* **12**:617–638.

Houser, C. R., Crawford, G. D., Salvaterra, P. M., and Vaughn, J. E., 1985, Immunocytochemical localization of choline acetyltransferase in rat cerebral cortex: A study of cholinergic neurons and synapses, *J. Comp. Neurol.* **234**:17–33.

Ip, N. Y., and Zigmond, R. E., 1984, Pattern of presynaptic nerve activity can determine the type of neurotransmitter regulating a postsynaptic event, *Nature* **311**:472–474.

Ip, N. Y., Ho, C. K., and Zigmond, R. E., 1982, Secretin and vasoactive intestinal polypeptide acutely increase tyrosine 3-monooxygenase in the rat superior cervical ganglion, *Proc. Natl. Acad. Sci. USA* **79**:7566–7569.

James, R., and Bradshaw, R. A., 1984, Polypeptide growth factors, *Annu. Rev. Biochem.* **53**:259–292.

Jan, L. Y., and Jan, Y. N., 1982, Peptidergic transmission in sympathetic ganglia of the frog, *J. Physiol. (London)* **327**:219–246.

Jones, E. G., 1975, Varieties and distributions of non-pyramidal cells in the sensory-motor cortex of the squirrel monkey, *J. Comp. Neurol.* **160**:205–268.

Jones, E. G., 1984, Identification and classification of intrinsic circuit elements in the neocortex, in: *Dynamic Aspects of Neocortical Function* (G. M. Edelman, W. E. Gall, and W. M. Cowan, eds.), Wiley, New York, pp. 7–40.

Jones, E. G., and Hendry, S. H. C., 1986, Colocalization of GABA and neuropeptides in neocortical neurons, *Trends Neurosci.* **9**:71–76.

Jones, E. G., DeFelipe, J., Hendry, S. H. C., and Maggio, J. E., 1987, Tachykinin immunoreactivity in neurons of monkey cerebral cortex. *J. Neurosci.* in press.

Lin, C.-S., Lu, S. M., and Schmechel, D. E., 1985, Glutamic acid decarboxylase immunoreactivity in layer IV of barrel cortex of rat and mouse, *J. Neurosci.* **5:**1934–1939.

Lundberg, A., Anggard, A., Fahrenkrug, J., Hökfelt, T., and Mutt, V., 1980, Vasoactive intestinal polypeptide in cholinergic neurons of exocrine glands: Functional significance of co-existing transmitters for vasodilation and secretion, *Proc. Natl. Acad. Sci. USA* **77:**1651–1655.

McCulloch, J., 1983, Peptides and the microregulation of bloodflow in the brain, *Nature* **304:**129.

McDonald, J. K., Parnavelas, J. G., Karamanlidis, A., Brecha, N., and Koenig, J. I., 1982a, The morphology and distribution of peptide-containing neurons in the adult and developing visual cortex of the rat. I. Somatostatin, *J. Neurocytol.* **11:**809–824.

McDonald, J. K., Parnavelas, J. G., Karamanlidis, A., and Brecha, N., 1982b, The morphology and distribution of peptide-containing neurons in the adult and developing visual cortex of the rat. II. Vasoactive intestinal polypeptide, *J. Neurocytol.* **11:** 825–837.

McDonald, J. K., Parnavelas, J. G., Karamanlidis, A., Brecha, N., and Rosenquist, G., 1982c, The morphology and distribution of peptide-containing neurons in the adult and developing visual cortex of the rat. III. Cholecystokinin, *J. Neurocytol.* **11:**881–895.

McDonald, J. K., Parnavelas, J. G., Karamanlidis, A., and Brecha, N., 1982d, The morphology and distribution of peptide-containing neurons in the adult and developing visual cortex of the rat. IV. Avian pancreatic polypeptide, *J. Neurocytol.* **11:**985–995.

McGinty, J. F., van der Kooy, D., and Bloom, F. E., 1984, The distribution and morphology of opioid peptide immunoreactive neurons in the cerebral cortex of rats, *J. Neurosci.* **4:**1104–1117.

McGuire, B. A., Hornung, J.-P., Gilbert, C. D., and Wiesel, T. N., 1984, Patterns of synaptic input to layer 4 of cat striate cortex, *J. Neurosci.* **4:**3021–3033.

Morrison, J. H., Benoit, R., Magistretti, P. J., and Bloom, F. E., 1983, Immunohistochemical distribution of pro-somatostatin-related peptides in cerebral cortex, *Brain Res.* **262:**344–351.

Muller, J. E., Straus, E., and Yalow, R. S., 1977, Cholecystokinin and its COOH-terminal octapeptide in the pig brain, *Proc. Natl. Acad. Sci. USA* **74:**3035–3037.

Nestler, E. J., Walaas, S. I., and Greengard, P., 1984, Neuronal phosphoproteins: Physiological and clinical implications, *Science* **225:**1357–1364.

Nilsson, J., von Euler, A. M., and Dalsgaard, C.-J., 1985, Stimulation of connective tissue cell growth by substance P and substance K, *Nature* **315:**61–63.

Nishizuka, Y., 1984, Turnover of inositol phospholipids and signal transduction, *Science* **225:**1365–1370.

Paxinos, G., Emson, P. C., and Cuello, A. C., 1978, The substance P projections to the frontal cortex and the substantia nigra, *Neuroscience* **7:**127–131.

Peters, A., Proskauer, C. C., and Ribak, C., 1982, Chandelier cells in rat visual cortex, *J. Comp. Neurol.* **206:** 397–416.

Peters, A., Miller, M., and Kimerer, L. M., 1983, Cholecystokinin-like immunoreactive neurons in rat cerebral cortex, *Neuroscience* **8:** 431–448.

Ribak, C., 1978, Aspinous and sparsely-spinous stellate neurons contain glutamic acid decarboxylase in the visual cortex of rats, *J. Neurocytol.* **7:**461–476.

Roach, A. H., Adler, J. E., Krause, J., and Black, I. E., 1985, Depolarization regulates the level of preprotachykinin messenger RNA in the cultured superior cervical ganglion, *Soc. Neurosci. Abstr.* **11:**669.

Roberts, E., and Fenkel, S., 1950, γ-Aminobutyric acid in brain: Its formation from glutamic acid, *J. Biol. Chem.* **187:**55–63.

Roberts, G. W., Crow, T. J., and Polak, J. M., 1985, Location of neuronal tangles in somatostatin neurons in Alzheimer's disease, *Nature* **314:**92–94.

Rockel, A. J., Hiorns, R. W., and Powell, T. P. S., 1980, The basic uniformity in structure of the neocortex, *Brain* **103:**221–244.

Rossor, M. N., Emson, P. C., Mountjoy, C. W., Roth, M., and Iversen, L. L. 1980, Reduced amounts of immunoreactive somatostatin in the temporal cortex in senile dementia of the Alzheimer type, *Neurosci. Lett.* **20:** 373–377.

Sachs, C., Hökfelt, T., Meyerson, B., Elde, R., and Rehfeld, J., 1977, Peptide neurons in human cerebral cortex—II, in: *11th World Congress of Neurology* (W. A. den Hartog, G. W. Gruyn, and A. P. J. Heijstee, eds.), Excerpta Medica, Amsterdam, pp. 1–3.

Said, S. I., and Rosenberg, R. N., 1976, Vasoactive intestinal polypeptide: Abundant immunoreactivity in neural cell lines and normal tissue, *Science* **192:**907–908.

Schmechel, D. E., Vickrey, B. G., Fitzpatrick, D., and Elde, R. P., 1984, GABAergic neurons of mammalian cerebral cortex: Widespread subclass defined by somatostatin content, *Neurosci. Lett.* **47:**227–232.

Somogyi, P., Cowey, A., Halász, N., and Freund, T. F., 1981, Vertical organization of neurons accumulating [^{3}H]-GABA in visual cortex of rhesus monkey, *Nature* **294:**761–763.

Somogyi, P., Hodgson, A. J., Smith, A. D., Nunzi, M. G., Gorio, A., and Wu, J.-Y., 1984, Different populations of GABAergic neurons in the visual cortex and hippocampus of cat contain somatostatin- or cholecystokinin-immunoreactive material, *J. Neurosci.* **4:**2590–2603.

Streit, P., 1984, Glutamate and aspartate as transmitter candidates for systems of the cerebral cortex, in: *Cerebral Cortex*, Vol. 2 (E. G. Jones and A. Peters, eds.), Plenum Press, New York, pp. 119–143.

Uhl, G. R., and Snyder, S. H., 1976, Regional and subcellular distributions of brain neurotensin, *Life Sci.* **19:**1827–1832.

Winfield, D. A., Brooke, R. N. L., Sloper, J. J., and Powell, T. P. S., 1981, A combined Golgi–electron microscopic study of the synapses made by the proximal axon and recurrent collaterals of a pyramidal cell in the somatic sensory cortex of the monkey, *Neuroscience* **6:**1217–1230.

Number of Neurons and Synapses in Primary Visual Cortex

ALAN PETERS

1. Introduction

Of all cortical areas, primary visual cortex has been the one to attract the overwhelming attention of neurophysiologists, largely because the stimuli necessary to activate it can be readily offered to an animal in a reproducible fashion to evoke well-defined responses from the constituent neurons. This activity on the part of neurophysiologists has induced neuroanatomists, and more recently neurophysiologists themselves, to examine the neurons present in visual cortex in attempts to ascertain how the various neuronal types are synaptically related to each other and to the extrinsic inputs that impinge upon them. In addition, visual cortex, and in particular area 17 of the rat, has been a favorite object for those interested in the neurotransmitters used by various neuronal types, while in cat visual cortex others have tried to determine how different transmitters affect the response properties of neurons. Much of these data have been presented in Volume 2 of this series.

This concentration of attention on visual cortex has also provided the stimulus for a somewhat milder effort to attempt to analyze its neuronal composition, to determine how many neurons are available for processing the information received by the cortex, what proportions of pyramidal and nonpyramidal cells

---

ALAN PETERS • Department of Anatomy, Boston University School of Medicine, Boston, Massachusetts 02118.

are present, and how many synapses are involved. The purpose of the present chapter is to summarize and examine the results of the numerical analyses of area 17, some of which have been reviewed previously by Colonnier and O'Kusky (1981).

2. Concentration of Neurons

2.1. Monkey

The most recent analysis of the composition of macaque visual cortex is that of O'Kusky and Colonnier (1982). They used material from adult monkeys that had been fixed by perfusion, after which the tissue was osmicated and embedded in plastic. The counts of neurons were made from semithin sections. Neuronal nuclei were used as the test objects and account was taken of the shrinkage that occurred during tissue processing. As shown in Table I, O'Kusky and Colonnier (1982) estimated that in area 17 of both *Macaca mulatta* and *M. fascicularis* there are about 120,000 neurons per mm^3 of tissue and about 200,000 neurons beneath 1 mm^2 of cortical surface, 28% of which are in layers I–III, 45% in layer IV, and 27% in layers V–VI.

In another study, Rockel *et al.* (1980) used a different approach, and counted the number of neurons contained in a 30-μm-wide strip of cortex in a 25-μm-thick paraffin section passing through the depth of the cortex. This was part of a comparative study of the numbers of neurons in different cortical areas of a variety of species, and the brains, except for the human ones, were fixed by perfusion with 10% formalin. Blocks were further fixed in 70% alcohol and 2% acetic acid before being embedded in paraffin. In those preparations from visual cortex of the macaque, Rockel *et al.* (1980) estimated there are 267.9 ± 13.7 neurons contained in a 30 × 25-μm strip. From this it can be calculated, as shown in Table I, that there are some 357,000 neurons beneath 1 mm^2 of cortical surface. This is higher than the figure calculated by O'Kusky and Colonnier (1982), but Rockel *et al.* (1980) did not take into account the shrinkage produced by tissue processing, although they estimated the linear shrinkage to be 18%. Powell and Hendrickson (1981) have subsequently taken this shrinkage into account, and determined that corrections for shrinkage lead to an estimated 218 neurons in a column of macaque area 17 measuring 30 × 30 μm. This would give a figure of 240,000 neurons beneath 1 mm^2 of cortical surface. By comparison, in frozen sections of macaque visual cortex in which they believe no shrinkage to occur, Powell and Hendrickson (1981) find 175 neurons in a 30 × 30-μm strip, equivalent to 194,000 neurons beneath 1 mm^2 of cortical surface. As can be seen in Table I, these values are compatible with those of O'Kusky and Colonnier (1982).

Chow *et al.* (1950) have also calculated the numerical density of neurons in macaque area 17, using the brains of two immature specimens fixed in 10% formalin and embedded in nitrocellulose. They estimated the number of neurons per 0.0005 mm^3 of area 17 to be 79. This gives 160,000 neurons/mm^3.

Other data on macaque area 17 come from the comparative study of Cragg (1967), who determined the densities of neurons in the visual and motor areas of a number of species. The brains he examined were fixed by perfusion with formalin, except for the human brains, and frozen sections cut. He considers that in such sections there is no shrinkage during the tissue processing. In the three specimens of *M. mulatta* examined by Cragg (1967), he estimates there to be between 104,000 and 126,700 neurons/mm^3. Assuming the thickness of 1.59 mm for this cortex given by O'Kusky and Colonnier (1982), this would be equivalent to 182,000 neurons beneath 1 mm^2 of cortical surface (Table I).

Less attention has been paid to visual cortex of other monkeys, but from the data given by Rockel *et al.* (1980), it would appear that the number of neurons in area 17 of galago, marmoset, squirrel monkey, baboon, and chimpanzee (and man) is equal to that in macaque. Further in all of these primates, the number of neurons in their 25 × 30-μm strips is about double that in similar strips through other cortical areas examined. This includes area 18, for in frozen sections of macaque cortex Powell and Hendrickson (1981) found only 79.5 neurons per 30 × 30-μm strip of area 18, compared with 173.4 neurons in monocular region and 176.0 neurons in binocular region of macaque area 17.

2.2. Cat

Using the same approach employed by O'Kusky and Colonnier (1982) for the macaque, Beaulieu and Colonnier (1982, 1985b) have examined area 17 of the cat, paying attention to both the binocular [interhemispheric face of the lateral (marginal) gyrus] and the monocular (upper lip of splenial sulcus) regions. They found the number of neurons per mm^3 to be about the same in these regions, namely 48,000 and 50,000 neurons/mm^3 (see also Beaulieu and Colonnier, 1985b). Due to differences in thickness of the binocular (1.62 mm) and monocular (1.24 mm) regions, however, the binocular region has about 78,000 neurons beneath 1 mm^2 of cortical surface, and the monocular region about 62,000 neurons (see Table I).

These values are comparable with those obtained by Cragg (1975) from examining frozen sections of cat visual cortex. Cragg (1975) assumed no shrinkage, and found 42,500 neurons/mm^3. This estimate is very similar to the one obtained by Cragg (1967) in his comparative study of visual cortices, when he determined the neuronal density to be 34,000–49,000 neurons/mm^3.

Again, these values are significantly lower than the ones obtained by Rockel *et al.* (1980). In their strip of 25 × 30 μm passing through cat visual cortex, they estimated a mean of 109.8 neurons to be present. This equals 146,000 neurons beneath 1 mm^2 of cortical surface, and using the figure of 1.5 mm for cortical thickness shown in Fig. 5 of Rockel *et al.* (1980) for cat area 17, this would give about 98,000 neurons/mm^3.

2.3. Rabbit

The only studies that appear to have estimated the density of neurons in rabbit visual cortex are those of Vrensen *et al.* (1977) and Cragg (1967). Vrensen *et al.* (1977) perfused brains from newborn and adult Dutch belted rabbits. They then osmicated the tissue and embedded it in Epon. Their neuronal counts were

Table I. Numbers of Neurons in Area 17

	No. of neurons per mm³	No. of neurons beneath 1 mm² of cortical surface	Cortical thickness measured	Reference
Macaque	119,000	202,000	1.59 mm	O'Kusky and Colonnier (1982)
	104,000–127,000	182,000[a]	—	Cragg (1967)
	—	357,000[b]	1.5 mm	Rockel et al. (1980)
	160,000[e]	194,000[d]	1.8 mm	Powell and Hendrickson (1981)
		—	1.4 mm	Chow et al. (1950)
Cat				
Binocular	48,013[c]	78,440	1.62 mm	Beaulieu and Colonnier (1983)
Monocular	50,006[c]	61,900	1.24 mm	
	42,500	—	—	Cragg (1975)
	34,000–49,400	—	—	Cragg (1967)
	97,500[f]	146,000[b]	1.5 mm	Rockel et al. (1980)
Rabbit	38,000[g]	80,000	2.1 mm	Vrensen et al. (1977)
	41,000–47,000	—	—	Cragg (1967)
Rat	80,725	120,280	1.49 mm	Peters et al. (1985)
	—	144,000[b]	1.0 mm	Rockel et al. (1980)
	76,300[h]	—	—	Warren and Bedi (1982)

Species				Reference
	44,300[i]	60,000	1.34 mm	Knox (1982)
	—	98,824[j]	1.1 mm	Werner et al. (1982)
	—	39,496[k]	1.74 mm	Werner et al. (1982)
	32,000–54,000	—	—	Cragg (1967)
	—	—	1.15–1.33 mm	Winkelmann et al. (1972)
Mouse	214,000	150,000[b]	0.7 mm	Rockel et al. (1980)
	194,000[l]	141,000	0.73 mm	Heumann et al. (1977)
	87,000–107,400	—	—	Cragg (1967)
Man	182,000	345,000[b]	1.9 mm	Rockel et al. (1980)
	28,000–51,900	—	—	Cragg (1967)
	97,200	150,000[m]	1.93 mm	Sholl (1959)
			—	Sharrif (1953)

[a] Calculated on the basis of a thickness of 1.59 mm.
[b] Calculated from the number of neurons in a 30-μm strip of a 25-μm thick section.
[c] Calculated by applying a correction of 14.8% for linear shrinkage.
[d] Value calculated from the neurons in 30 × 30 μm of a frozen section.
[e] Calculated from their value of 79 neurons per 0.0005 mm^3 of tissue.
[f] Calculated on the thickness of cortex given in their Fig. 5.
[g] Calculated using the given thickness of 2.1 mm.
[h] 200-day-old rats—layers II–IV.
[i] 3-month-old SHR rats.
[j] Number of neurons counted in paraffin sections.
[k] Number corrected to account for shrinkage in processing.
[l] Calculated from the thickness of 0.73 mm given by the authors.
[m] Calculated from the number of neurons in a cylinder of 400 μm^2 area.

made on 1-μm-thick sections, and they calculated the neuronal density in 7-month-old rabbits to be 38,000 neurons per mm^3 of tissue. Accepting the cortical depth of about 2.1 mm they cite, this leads to an estimate of 80,000 neurons beneath 1 mm^3 of cortical surface (Table I).

The above value is in reasonable agreement with the estimate of 41,000–47,000 neurons/mm^3 obtained in Cragg's (1967) comparative study.

2.4. Rat

The most recent estimate of the number of neurons in rat visual cortex is that obtained by Peters *et al.* (1985). They fixed brains by perfusion and used semithin plastic sections in an approach similar to that used by O'Kusky and Colonnier (1982) and Beaulieu and Colonnier (1983) to examine monkey and cat visual cortices. Peters *et al.* (1985) estimate there are some 120,000 neurons beneath 1 mm^2 of cortical surface in rat area 17, and about 80,700 neurons/mm^3. These authors also determined the numbers of neurons in each cortical layer lying beneath 1 mm^2 of cortical surface, and were able to check their results by showing that the number of large pyramidal cells estimated to be present in layer V was in agreement with the number of large apical dendritic profiles counted in tangential sections cut at the level of layer IV.

The estimate of Peters *et al.* (1985) for the number of neurons per unit volume is very similar to that of Warren and Bedi (1982)—76,300 neurons/mm^3—in their study of the packing density of neurons in layers II–IV of 200-day-old rats.

However, there are great differences between these values and those obtained by Cragg (1967), Knox (1982), and Werner *et al.* (1982). Using frozen sections, Cragg (1967) estimated between 32,000 and 54,000 neurons/mm^3 in rat area 17, and Knox (1982) obtained a value of 44,000 neurons/mm^3. Knox (1982) used plastic-embedded and perfused tissue, and counted only neurons containing nucleoli 1.2 μm in diameter. In their study, Werner *et al.* (1982) employed paraffin sections, and they estimated 99,000 neurons/mm^3 to be present in these sections. However, when they corrected this value to account for a linear shrinkage of 16%, and a volumetric shrinkage of 60%, the number of neurons per mm^3 decreased to 39,000. As will be discussed later, it can be questioned whether the volumetric shrinkage is really so great.

In their study of rat area 17, Rockel *et al.* (1980) estimated 107.8 neurons to be present in a strip 25 × 30 μm passing through the depth of the cortex. This translates into 144,000 neurons beneath 1 mm^2 of cortical surface, which, like their values for monkey and cat, appears to be high. However, if the same correction used by Powell and Hendrickson (1981) for monkey cortex is applied to rat cortex, it would give 87 cells in a 25 × 30-μm strip, or 116,000 neurons beneath 1 mm^2 of cortical surface, a figure similar to that obtained by Peters *et al.* (1985).

2.5. Mouse

Heumann *et al.* (1977) have estimated primary visual cortex of the mouse to contain 194,000 neurons per mm^3 of tissue, and since they give a cortical thickness of 0.7 mm for mouse area 17, this would mean about 141,000 neurons beneath 1 mm² of cortical surface. This value is not too different from that obtained by Rockel *et al.* (1980), who found 112.2 neurons in their 25 × 30-μm strip, which would give 150,000 neurons beneath 1 mm² of cortical surface. As shown in the previous sections, however, the uncorrected values of Rockel *et al.* (1980) are consistently high, but even so, it is difficult to reconcile the above data with that of 92,400 neurons per mm³ of mouse area 17 obtained by Cragg (1967).

2.6. Man

Clearly, of all species, the neuronal concentration in area 17 is most difficult to estimate in man, because of the problem in obtaining adequately preserved material. Consequently, the estimates of neuronal number for human area 17 are likely to be the most inaccurate ones. Rockel *et al.* (1980) have estimated 258.9 neurons to be present in a 25 × 30-μm strip, giving a value of about 345,000 neurons beneath 1 mm² of cortical surface, and on the basis of their neuronal thickness of about 1.9 mm, some 182,000 neurons/mm³. This is quite different from the estimates of between 27,900 and 51,900 neurons/mm³ obtained by Cragg (1967), the value of 150,000 neurons beneath 1 mm² of cortical surface (78,000 neurons/mm³) that can be derived from the data given by Sholl (1959), and the figure of 97,200 neurons/mm³ estimated by Sharrif (1953).

2.7. Discussion

When the accumulated data for each species are examined, it is seen that there can be great variations between the number of neurons either in 1 mm³ of visual cortex, or beneath 1 mm² of cortical surface estimated by different investigators. These differences can be attributed to a number of factors, including use of different counting methods, ignoring or taking into account the shrinkage that occurs during the preparation of the tissue, and perhaps uncertainty about how to compensate for shrinkage.

If the values obtained by Rockel *et al.* (1980) are ignored for the present, it seems that of the visual cortices the greatest concentration of neurons is in area 17 of the monkey, in which there are relatively consistent values of between 182,000 and 240,000 neurons beneath 1 mm² of cortical surface, and 104,000–160,000 neurons/mm³. The values for cat cortex are also relatively compatible. They are 62,000–78,000 neurons beneath 1 mm² of cortical surface, and 42,000–50,000 neurons/mm³. These values for the cat are very similar to those that have been obtained for rabbit visual cortex.

The estimates for rat visual cortex are much more diverse, and range from an upper value of 76,000–81,000 neurons/mm³ obtained by two research groups, to values about half that, namely 32,000–54,000, by two other groups. It would be easy to suggest that these differences can be attributed to different methods of procedure and to the different counting methods employed, but Peters *et al.* (1985), Warren and Bedi (1982), and Knox (1982) all employed tissue fixed by perfusion and embedded in epoxy resin, so it is surprising that values obtained by Knox (1982) are only half of those obtained by the two other groups. There is also great diversity in the estimates of neuronal concentrations in the mouse visual cortex and in human visual cortex.

To turn now to the values obtained by Rockel *et al.* (1980), the interest of these authors was to compare the numbers of neurons in strips of paraffin sections of equal dimensions (30 × 25 μm) passing through the entire depth of the neocortices of different species of animals. They concluded that with the exception of area 17 of visual cortices, in different functional areas (motor, somatic sensory, visual, frontal, parietal, and temporal) of a number of primates, the number of neurons in 25 × 30-μm strips is the same (about 110 neurons), indicating a basic uniformity in the neocortices of mammals. In the binocular part of area 17 of primates, on the other hand, they counted some 2.5 times more neurons in similar strips. Their data for visual cortices of rat, cat, and macaque are shown in Table II.

In Table I the data of Rockel *et al.* (1980) have been converted into numbers of neurons lying beneath 1 mm^2 of cortical surface. As expected, the conversion still supports their contention that while the numbers of neurons beneath 1 mm^2 of cortical surface are the same in area 17 of the cat, rat, and mouse, the values for macaque and man are about 2.5 times greater. However, this conversion of their data, enabling comparison with other estimates, shows that their values are generally greater than those produced by other investigators. But as shown by Powell and Hendrickson (1981), when frozen sections are examined, or account is taken of the shrinkage that occurs in the preparation of paraffin sections, then the values for at least macaque visual cortex become similar to those reported by O'Kusky and Colonnier (1982) and Cragg (1967). And indeed even if the data of Rockel *et al.* (1980) and of Colonnier and his co-workers (O'Kusky and Colonnier, 1982; Beaulieu and Colonnier, 1983) are considered separately (Table II), there is still agreement that there are 2.5 times more neurons beneath a unit of cortical surface in the macaque than in the cat. However, Beaulieu and Colonnier (1985b) have recently emphasized that while the monocular portion of area 17 in cat visual cortex has about the same number of neurons beneath 1 mm^2 of cortical surface as both area 18 and the cortex of the posteromedial suprasylvian area (PMLS), the binocular region has a greater number of neurons beneath 1 mm^2 of cortical surface. This is due to the presence of a greater number of neurons in all layers except layers III and VIb. An important point to emerge from this detailed study is that even though the number of neurons beneath 1 mm^2 of cortical surface is similar, in the monocular portion of area 17, in area 18, and in PMLS, there are significant differences both in the thicknesses of individual layers and in the neuronal packing densities among these areas.

Table II. Comparison of Numbers of Neurons in Different Visual Cortices

	No. of neurons per 25 × 30-μm strip[a]	No. of neurons per mm^3[b]	Neurons beneath 1 mm^2 of cortical suface
Macaque	267.9	104,000–126,700	202,000[c]
Cat	109.8	42,000–49,000	78,000[d]
Rat	107.8	32,000–54,000	

[a] From Rockel *et al.* (1980).
[b] From Cragg (1967).
[c] From O'Kusky and Colonnier (1982).
[d] From Beaulieu and Colonnier (1983).

The conclusion of Rockel *et al.* (1980) that primate area 17 contains more neurons than other areas is also supported by the earlier data of Sholl (1959), who determined the numbers of neurons in cylinders of cortex with cross-sectional areas of 400 μm^2. In his data for human cortex, Sholl (1959) states there are 60 neurons in such a cylinder of human striate cortex, as compared with 32 neurons in parastriate cortex, and 23 in precentral gyrus. However, it should also be pointed out that for cat cortex Sholl (1959) gives a figure of 55 neurons in a cylinder through visual cortex, and 29 in a cylinder from sigmoid gyrus, suggesting that even in the cat, visual cortex has more neurons than sensorimotor cortex.

Apart from Rockel *et al.* (1980), the other investigator who has examined the cerebral cortices of different species in a comparative fashion is Cragg (1967). The data he produced on visual cortices are also given in Table II. Cragg's data are in terms of the number of neurons per mm^3, but since the thickness of visual cortex in monkey and cat binocular regions, and in rat area 17, are not too different (see Table I), Cragg's data can be compared with those of Rockel *et al.* (1980). Cragg's (1967) data also indicate that macaque visual cortex has more than twice as many neurons per unit volume than visual cortex of cat and rat. To ascertain the validity of this conclusion, we have taken 1-μm-thick plastic sections from blocks of area 17 of rat, cat, and monkey, using brains fixed by perfusion with glutaraldehyde and formaldehyde, and made camera lucida drawings to show the locations of all neuronal profiles containing nuclei in strips 300 μm wide passing through the entire depth of the cortex. The resulting drawings are shown in Fig. 1. The strip through rat area 17 has 276 neuronal profiles, that through cat area 17 has 232 profiles, and the one through monkey area 17 has 327 profiles. Interestingly, the neurons in monkey area 17 are smaller than those in area 17 of rat and cat, so that the differences in neuronal packing density between monkey area 17 and area 17 of rat and cat must be even greater than the profile counts indicate. Thus, these drawings support the contention that monkey area 17 contains significantly more neurons than area 17 of either rat or cat.

Finally, if the distribution of neurons in the various layers of visual cortices of rat, cat, and monkey is examined, it becomes evident that the most prominent difference is in the percentage of total neurons contained in layer IV (see Fig. 1). Thus, when the available data for the number of neurons beneath 1 mm^2 of cortical surface are compared, it is found that in rat visual cortex only 23% of the neurons are contained in layer IV (Peters *et al.*, 1985), while in cat the proportion increases to 34% in the binocular region and 36% in the monocular region (Beaulieu and Colonnier, 1983, 1985b), and to 45% in monkey area 17 (O'Kusky and Colonnier, 1982), a reflection of the proportion of neurons available to receive the main thalamic input from the lateral geniculate nucleus terminating in layer IV.

3. Total Numbers of Neurons

Knowing the number of neurons beneath 1 mm^2 of surface in area 17, and the total surface area it occupies, it is possible to estimate the total number of neurons involved in primary visual processing in different animals.

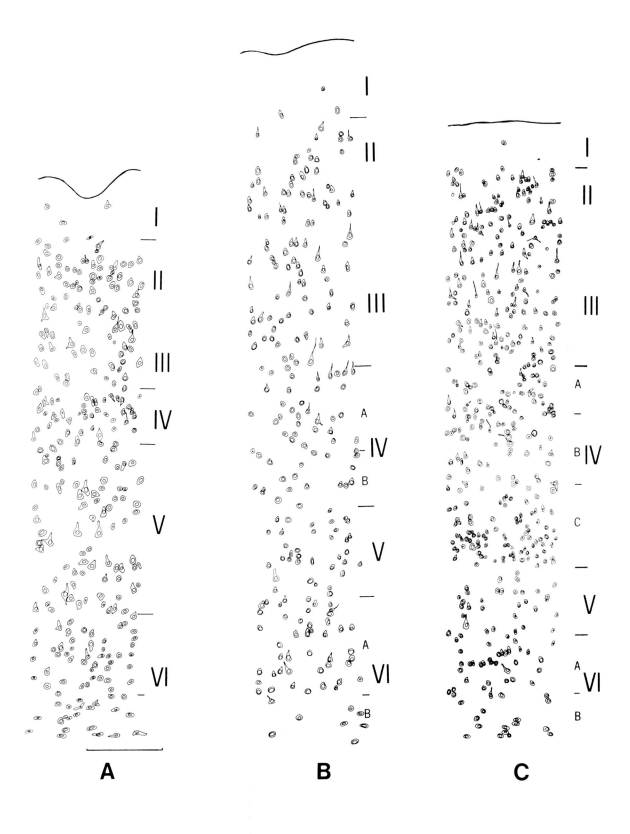

I
II
III
IV
V
VI

A

I
II
III
IV
A
B
V
A
VI
B

B

I
II
III
A
B IV
C
V
A
VI
B

C

For the macaque, the literature pertaining to the surface area occupied by area 17 has been reviewed by O'Kusky and Colonnier (1982) in their Table 7. They show that the estimates vary from 1450 mm^2 determined by Clark (1942) to a low value of 576 mm^2 calculated by Popoff (1929). Other more recent estimates are 1379 mm^2 (Cowey, 1964), 1320 mm^2 (Daniel and Whitteridge, 1961), 1090 mm^2 (Van Essen and Maunsell, 1980), 841 mm^2 (O'Kusky and Colonnier, 1982), and 645 mm^2 (Chow et al., 1950). As in the estimates of neuronal concentrations, it is difficult to know that effect shrinkage has had on these estimates, and so perhaps the best approximations of the total numbers of neurons in macaque primary visual cortex are those obtained from the data of Chow et al. (1950) and O'Kusky and Colonnier (1982), who have calculated both neuronal densities and area of primary visual cortex in the same preparations, for in their studies shrinkage would affect both values in a parallel fashion.

Chow et al. (1950) calculate there is an average of 79 neurons per 0.0005 mm^2 of macaque visual cortex, and given their figures of an average thickness of 1.4 mm, and a surface area of 645 mm^2, it can be estimated that there are 145,000,000 neurons in area 17 of one hemisphere (Table III). This is similar to the estimate of 161,000,000 neurons determined by O'Kusky and Colonnier (1982).

In their study of cat visual cortex, Beaulieu and Colonnier (1983) did not measure the area of surface occupied by area 17, but used the data of Tusa et al. (1978) to estimate the total number of neurons. Tusa et al. (1978) give the area occupied by area 17 in one hemisphere as 380 mm^2, which is similar to the value of 310 mm^2 obtained by Van Essen and Maunsell (1980). Correlating these values with the estimate of 78,440 neurons beneath 1 mm^2 of cortical surface obtained by Beaulieu and Colonnier (1983) for the binocular region, cat area 17 can be estimated to contain between 24,300,000 and 29,000,000 neurons in each hemisphere.

The area occupied by area 17 has also been examined in the rat. Thus, from physiological studies Espinoza and Thomas (1983) estimate area VI to occupy 7.1 mm^2, while Peters et al. (1985) estimate the area from histological preparations to be 9.4 mm^2, similar to the area of 9.0 mm^2 obtained by measuring the area depicted in the article by Schober and Winkelmann (1975). Using the estimate obtained by Peters et al. (1985) of 120,000 neurons beneath 1 mm^2 of cortical surface (Table I) and a value of 9.4 mm^2 for the area, rat area 17 would contain a total of 1,130,000 neurons (Table III). This estimate is not too different from that obtained by using the uncorrected figure of 98,824 neurons/mm^3 obtained by Werner et al. (1982), their thickness of 1.1 mm for the paraffin-embedded cortex (Table I), and the area of 9.0 mm^2 for area 17 of visual cortex shown in work from the same laboratory by Schober and Winkelmann (1975).

Figure 1. Camera lucida drawing of 300-μ-wide strips of 1-μm-thick plastic sections of area 17 in (A) rat, (B) cat, and (C) monkey (*Macaca mulatta*), to show the distribution of neuronal profiles containing nuclei. In these specimens, rat area 17 is 1.5 mm deep, cat area 17 is 1.65 mm deep, and that of the monkey is 1.59 mm deep. The numbers of neuronal profiles in the 300-μm-wide strips, which pass through the entire depth of the cortex, are: rat, 276; cat, 232; monkey, 327. Note the small size of the neurons in the monkey as compared with the rat and cat. Bar = 250 μm.

Table III. Total Number of Neurons in Primary Visual Cortex of One Hemisphere

	Area of area 17	Total number of neurons	Source
Macaque	645 mm^2	145 × 10^6	Chow *et al.* (1950)
	841 mm^2	161 × 10^6	O'Kusky and Colonnier (1982)
Cat	310–380 mm^2	24–29 × 10^6	Beaulieu and Colonnier (1983), Tusa *et al.* (1978), Van Essen and Maunsell (1980)
Rat	9.4 mm^2	1.1 × 10^6	Peters *et al.* (1985)
	9.0 mm^2	0.98 × 10^6	Werner *et al.* (1982), Schober and Winkelmann (1975)

Using these values leads to an estimate of 978,000 for the total number of neurons in area 17 of one rat hemisphere (Table III).

From this data then, it seems that in rat area 17 contains about 1 × 10^6 neurons, in cat 24–30 × 10^6 neurons, and in macaque 145–160 × 10^6 neurons. These differences largely reflect the differences in the surface area of visual cortex in these three species, although in the monkey the number is further increased due to the greater packing density of the neurons.

Insufficient information is available to make similar estimates for visual cortices of mouse, rabbit, and man, although based upon data extrapolated from a number of sources, Colonnier and O'Kusky (1981) calculate that the total number of neurons in primary visual cortex of man may be on the order of 538 × 10^6.

4. Pyramidal and Nonpyramidal Cells

4.1. Rat Visual Cortex

The most complete analysis of the neuronal composition of rat area 17 is that by Peters *et al.* (1985). These investigators carried out their analysis using four perfused brains. Pieces of area 17 were osmicated, embedded in Araldite, and sectioned in the vertical plane, such that the plane of section passed parallel to the apical dendrites of the pyramidal cells. From each visual cortex they took a thin section for electron microscopy and then an immediately adjacent 1-μm-thick section stained with toluidine blue for light microscopy. The sections passed through the entire depth of the cortex, and a drawing was made of the thick section to show all neurons containing nuclei, for the nuclei were the test objects used to determine total neuronal populations. Then using the drawings as maps, the adjacent thin sections were examined in the electron microscope and all of the profiles of the neurons containing nuclei were examined and photographed. This allowed the neuronal profiles to be classified as belonging to either pyramidal or nonpyramidal cells, the classification being made on the basis of both the forms of the axosomatic synapses and the cytological features of the cell bodies. The forms of the axosomatic synapses provided the primary clue as to whether the cells were either pyramidal or nonpyramidal ones, for while nonpyramidal cells in rat visual cortex have both symmetric and asymmetric axosomatic synapses (see Fig. 2), the pyramidal cells possess only symmetric ones (see Colonnier, 1981; Peters and Kara, 1985a,b; Peters and Jones in Volume 1 of this series). Further distinction between neuronal types was based on the cytological features of the cell bodies, and this made it possible to further classify the profiles of the nonpyramidal cells as belonging either to bipolar cells or to multipolar cells (see Peters and Kara, 1985b). It was not possible to recognize different varieties of multipolar cells, or of nonpyramidal cells in layer I and layer VIb, since this can only be done by knowing the forms of the dendritic trees and of the axonal plexuses of the neurons, information not available from this type of preparation. However, based upon the sizes of the profiles, the bipolar and multipolar cells in layers II–VIa were further classified as belonging to either small or large varieties.

As stated, the neuronal nuclei were used as the test objects counted, and from their dimensions the concentrations of various types of neurons present in the different cellular layers were determined using Abercrombie's (1946) formula. Table IV, based on data from Peters *et al.* (1985), shows the total numbers of neurons and percentages of pyramidal cells, bipolar cells, and multipolar cells present in the layers of rat area 17 beneath 1 mm^2 of cortical surface. As can be seen, there is a total of 120,280 neurons beneath 1 mm^2 of cortical surface (also see Table I). Eighty five percent of these neurons are believed to be pyramidal cells, about one-third of which are in layer II/III. Layers IV and VIa, both of which have small pyramidal cells, each contain about 25% of the pyramidal cell population, while the remaining 17% of the pyramidal cells are in layer V.

Peters *et al.* (1985) estimate that nonpyramidal cells account for 15% of the total neuronal population of rat area 17. Both layers I and VIb contain only nonpyramidal cells, and together account for 35% of all nonpyramidal cells. The remaining 65% of the nonpyramidal cell population is in layers II–VIa, with the greatest concentration in layer II/III (see Fig. 3). Of the nonpyramidal cells in layer II/III, there are about equal numbers of bipolar cells and multipolar cells, and support for the conclusion that bipolar cells are most common in layer II/III of rat visual cortex comes from studies that have been carried out using an antibody to vasoactive intestinal polypeptide (VIP). This antibody largely reacts with bipolar cells (e.g., see McDonald *et al.*, 1982; Morrison *et al.*, 1984; Connor and Peters, 1984) and shows bipolar cells to be most common in layer II/III.

The only other studies that have attempted to ascertain the proportions of pyramidal and nonpyramidal cells in rat visual cortex have been those of Winfield *et al.* (1980) and Werner *et al.* (1982). Winfield *et al.* (1980) also used electron microscopy to identify cell types, and examined visual and motor cortices of a number of species, including rat. Using the types of axosomatic synapses and cytological features as criteria, they distinguished between pyramidal cells, and large and small varieties of nonpyramidal (stellate) cells, and determined the proportions of these cell types by examining profiles of some 100 neuronal cell

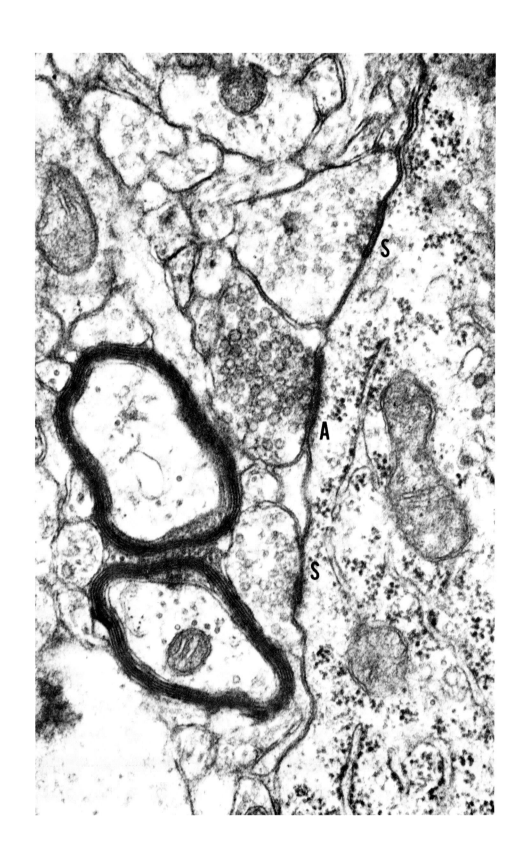

bodies that contained nuclei in tissue specimen from three rats. They estimate that in rat area 17 the proportion of pyramidal cells is between 62 and 72%, small nonpyramidal cells 23–33%, and large nonpyramidal cells 3–8%. Thus, they find nonpyramidal cells to account for a much larger percentage of the population than did Peters *et al.* (1985).

The study carried out by Werner *et al.* (1982) employed light microscopic sections stained by the Nissl method, and they distinguished between neuronal types on the basis of the amount of perikaryal cytoplasm and the nuclear characteristics of the cells. On this basis, Werner *et al.* (1982) concluded that about 82% of neurons in layers II–VI of rat area 17 are pyramidal cells. However, in layer IV they suggest that the majority of neurons are small stellate cells, which presumably correspond to the small pyramidal cells with thin apical dendrites that are so abundant in layer IV of rat visual cortex (see Peters and Kara, 1985a). The conclusion of Werner *et al.* (1982), that about 82% of neurons in rat area 17 are pyramidal cells, is essentially in agreement with the results of Peters *et al.* (1985), who estimated 85%. Both these estimates of pyramidal cell proportions are higher than the 62–72% determined by Winfield *et al.* (1980). The results of these studies on rat visual cortex are summarized in Table V, in which the data have been modified to show only the proportions of pyramidal versus nonpyramidal cells, since the various groups of authors have subdivided the nonpyramidal population in different ways.

Additional information about the nonpyramidal cell population of rat visual cortex can be obtained from the observations of Wolff and Chronwall (1982), who injected tritiated GABA into rat visual cortex to ascertain which neurons are GABAergic in function. They found the GABA-accumulating cells to constitute a heterogeneous group of neurons, which seem to correspond to the nonpyramidal cells with spine-free or sparsely spinous dendrites. Such neurons are contained in the group designated as multipolar cells by Peters *et al.* (1985). Wolff and Chronwall (1982) determined that in rat visual cortex about 10% of the neurons are GABA-accumulating, a value in agreement with the estimate of Peters *et al.* (1985) that multipolar neurons account for 10.4% of all neurons in rat visual cortex (Table IV).

4.2. Other Visual Cortices

Winfield *et al.* (1980) have examined the proportions of pyramidal and nonpyramidal cells in a number of other cortices. As stated above, they based their analyses upon the appearance of about 100 neurons in electron micrographs of the cortices and in this manner determined the proportions of pyramidal cells, large stellate cells, and small stellate cells. In cat area 17, Winfield *et al.* (1980) estimated the following percentages: pyramidal cells, 66–67%; large stellate cells, 5%; small stellate cells, 28–29%. Monkey visual cortex had a similar distribution of these cell types (Table V), so Winfield *et al.* (1980) conclude that in rat, cat, and monkey visual cortex, the proportions of these three neuronal

Figure 2. Electron micrograph from rat area 17, to show symmetric (S), and asymmetric (A) synapses on the surface of a nonpyramidal cell in layer II/III. ×60,000.

281

NEURON AND SYNAPSE NUMBERS

types is of the same order; they suggest that this points to a basic similarity between visual (and motor) cortices across species (see Table V).

The figures of Winfield *et al.* (1980) are similar to those reported by Tömböl (1974) for cat visual cortex. Since she worked in the same laboratory as Winfield *et al.* (1980), Tömböl (1974) used the same classification of neurons into pyramidal cells, large stellate cells, and small stellate cells, and gives the proportions of these cell types as 60, 7, and 33%, respectively. It is interesting, however, that from an extrapolation of the data provided by Tömböl (1974), 79% of the total population of small stellate cells she encountered were contained in layer IV of cat visual cortex. In monkey visual cortex, Mates and Lund (1983) examined electron micrographs to ascertain the proportions of those neurons with spiny dendrites and only symmetric synapses on their perikarya, i.e., the spiny stellate cells, as opposed to neurons with smooth dendrites and some asymmetric synapses on their cell bodies in layer 4C. Distinguishing between neuronal types on these bases, Mates and Lund (1983) estimate that in layer 4C of monkey visual cortex, spiny stellate cells account for about 95% of the neuronal population, and cells with smooth dendrites (nonpyramidal cells) account for 3–7% of the neurons. This percentage for spiny stellate cells is somewhat greater than the 86% determined by Tigges *et al.* (1977) for layer IV of monkey visual cortex. Other information about the nonpyramidal cell content of cat and monkey visual cortex comes from the study of Fitzpatrick *et al.* (1983) on glutamic acid decarboxylase (GAD)-immunoreactive neurons. These authors estimate that in cat and squirrel monkey visual cortex, 8 to 15% of the neurons (nonpyramidal neurons) are GAD-positive.

These data for layer IV of cat and monkey visual cortex, along with those obtained by Peters *et al.* (1985) for rat visual cortex, are summarized in Table VI, in which the relative percentages of spiny neurons and smooth stellate cells are given. It should be emphasized that for purposes of comparison, spiny neurons include those neurons with spiny dendrites and only symmetric synapses on their cell bodies, since although cat and monkey layer IV contains spiny stellate cells, most of the spiny cells in layer IV of rat visual cortex appear to have thin apical dendrites (Peters and Kara, 1985a). These spiny neurons contrast with the smooth stellate cells, or nonpyramidal cells whose dendrites have few if any spines and have cell bodies with both symmetric and asymmetric synapses. For the most part, such smooth neurons are GABAergic. Comparison of these data suggests that the data obtained by Tömböl (1974) present too high

Table IV. Number of Neurons Under 1 mm² Surface in Rat Area 17[a]

Layer	Total number of neurons	Percentage distribution of neurons of each type			
		Pyramids	Bipolar cells	Multipolar cells	Other
I	940	—	—	—	0.8%
II–III	38,970	27.6%	2.4%	2.5%	—
IV	27,370	21.1%	0.7%	0.9%	—
V	20,900	15.1%	1.1%	1.1%	—
VIa	26,550	21.3%	0.3%	0.5%	—
VIb	5,550	—	—	—	4.6%
Total	120,280	85.1%	4.5%	5.0%	5.4%

[a] Peters *et al.* (1985).

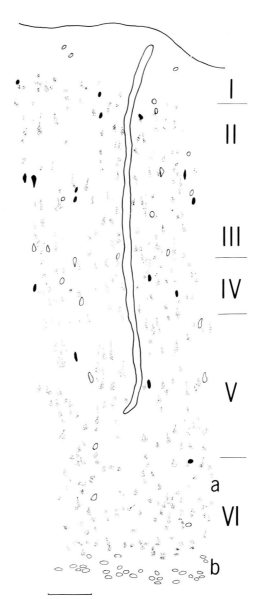

Figure 3. Drawing of a 1-μm-thick section taken through the depth of area 17 in the rat to show the locations of all neuronal cell bodies containing nuclei. The adjacent thin section was examined in the electron microscope to determine whether the cell bodies belonged to pyramidal cells, bipolar cells, or multipolar cells. Those neurons identified as pyramidal cells are shown by stippling; bipolar cells are shown in solid black; other nonpyramidal cells are shown in outline. There is a large blood vessel passing through the cortex. The boundaries between the cell layers are indicated on the drawing. Bar = 100 μm.

**Table V. Proportions of Pyramidal and Nonpyramidal Cells in Visual Cortex
(All Layers)**

	Pyramidal cells	Nonpyramidal cells	Source
Rat	85%	15%	Peters *et al.* (1985)
	82%	18%	Werner *et al.* (1982)
	62–72%	28–38%	Winfield *et al.* (1980)
Cat	66–67%	33–34%	Winfield *et al.* (1980)
	59%	41%	Tömböl (1974)
Monkey	62%	38%	Winfield *et al.* (1980)

Table VI. Percentages of Neurons in Layer IV of Visual Cortex

	Smooth stellate cells	Spiny neurons	Source
Rat	7%	93%	Peters *et al.* (1985)
Cat	79%	21%	Tömöl (1974)
Monkey	5%	95%	Mates and Lund (1983)
	14%	86%	Tigges *et al.* (1977)
	8–15%	85–92%	Fitzpatrick *et al.* (1983)

a proportion of smooth stellate cells for layer IV of cat visual cortex, and with respect to Tömböl's (1974) data as a whole, the estimates of Winfield *et al.* (1980) propose that the high proportion of small stellate (nonpyramidal) cells encountered was due to the fact that Tömböl (1974) restricted the sampling to only neuronal profiles with nucleoli. Because of their smaller-diameter nuclei, this would tend to favor the small stellate cells as compared with the other two cell types. However, as can be seen from Tables V and VI, the estimates of both Winfield *et al.* (1980) and Tömböl (1974) for the proportions of nonpyramidal cells in area 17 are much higher than estimates obtained by other investigators.

5. Densities of Synapses

Studies of the densities of synapses in visual cortex have necessarily involved electron microscopy, and each investigator has had to employ stereological methods to determine synaptic numbers per unit volume. The stereological formulas used have varied, and as shown recently by Colonnier and Beaulieu (1985), use of different formulas to determine the true densities of synapses from their profiles in thin sections can lead to somewhat different results, as can the method used to ascertain the sizes of the densities at the synaptic junctions, the objects most frequently counted (see Mayhew, 1979). The other fact to note is that most investigators have determined total numbers of synapses per unit volume, making no attempt to differentiate between asymmetric and symmetric synapses, and it is the determinations of total synaptic populations per unit volume of mature visual cortex that will first be considered in this section. The few studies estimating the proportions of asymmetric and symmetric synapses will be considered separately.

5.1. Counts of Total Numbers of Synapses

5.1.1. Monkey

The most recent investigation of the number of synapses in monkey visual cortex is that by O'Kusky and Colonnier (1982), the same one in which they also determined the numbers of neurons. O'Kusky and Colonnier (1982) estimate that there is an average of 276×10^6 synapses per mm^3 of cortical tissue in monkey area 17, with small peaks of density in layer II–III and in layer IVc. Dividing this number of synapses by the average number of neurons in 1 mm^3 of cortex (see Table I), O'Kusky and Colonnier (1982) calculate there is an average of 2300 synapses/neuron. In a later article, Beaulieu and Colonnier (1985a) suggest that because of the stereological formula they used earlier (O'-Kusky and Colonnier, 1982), this ratio should be increased by as much as 50% (see Colonnier and Beaulieu, 1985) and that a more valid estimate of the number of synapses per mm^3 of monkey area 17 is 414 × 10^6, giving 3450 synapses/neuron (see Table VII). Both of these estimates are lower than the one obtained by Cragg (1967), who calculated 620 × 10^6 synapses/mm^3 and 5600 synapses/neuron.

5.1.2. Cat

In their recent study of cat area 17, Beaulieu and Colonnier (1985a) estimate that on average there is a total of 284 × 10^6 synapses/mm^3, with values of 286 × 10^6 synapses/mm^3 for the binocular segment and 281 × 10^6 synapses/mm^3 for the monocular segment. These values lead to an estimate of an average of 5800 synapses/neuron. The number of synapses per unit volume determined by Beaulieu and Colonnier (1985a) is very similar to the value of 276 × 10^6 synapses/mm^3 determined by Winfield (1981, 1983). In contrast to these estimates, however, Cragg (1975) earlier obtained a value of 406 × 10^6 synapses/mm^3 in adult cat area 17; with a synapse-to-neuron ratio of 9800 (Table VII). This is about twice the value obtained by Beaulieu and Colonnier (1985a).

5.1.3. Rabbit

The only study in which synaptic density has been estimated in rabbit visual cortex appears to be that of Vrensen *et al.* (1977). They estimated 673 × 10^6 synapses/mm^3 in 7-month-old rabbits, and a synapse-to-neuron ratio of 17,700

Table VII. Numbers of Synapses in Visual Cortex

	No. of synapses per mm^3	Synapses per neuron	Source
Macaque	276 × 10^6	2.3 × 10^3	O'Kusky and Colonnier (1982)
	414 × 10^6	3.4 × 10^3	Beaulieu and Colonnier (1985a)
	620 × 10^6	5.6 × 10^3	Cragg (1967)
Cat	284 × 10^6	5.8 × 10^3	Beaulieu and Colonnier (1985a)
	276 × 10^6	—	Winfield (1981, 1983)
	406 × 10^6	9.8 × 10^3	Cragg (1975)
Rabbit	673 × 10^6	17.7 × 10^3	Vrensen *et al.* (1977)
	211 × 10^6	5.5 × 10^3	Recalculated by Mayhew (1979)
Rat	946 × 10^6	12.5 × 10^3	Warren and Bedi (1984)
	750 × 10^6	13.5 × 10^3	Thomas *et al.* (1980)
	320 × 10^6	—	Cragg (1967)
Mouse	660 × 10^6	7 × 10^3	Cragg (1967)

(Table VII). This value is considerably higher than those obtained in monkey and cat (see Table VII). Vrensen *et al.* (1977) state that they calculated the synaptic densities in rabbit cortex using the formula of de Hoff (1966), but do not give the measurements upon which the derivation of the number of synapses per unit volume was based. An odd fact is that Mayhew (1979) uses earlier data on rabbit visual cortex published by Vrensen and de Groot (1973) as an illustration of how to calculate synaptic densities by employing Abercrombie's (1946) formula, and using their data calculates 211×10^6 synapses/mm^3 for rabbit visual cortex. This brings the estimate of synaptic numbers for rabbit visual cortex much closer to those calculated by others for monkey and cat visual cortex.

5.1.4. Rat

Surprisingly, there appear to be few publications dealing with the synaptic density in visual cortex of the mature rat, although a number of reports have dealt with changes in various synaptic parameters with age, experience, and nutrition. Warren and Bedi (1982, 1984) determined the synaptic density in 200-day-old rats as part of their study on the effects of undernourishment on development, and found 946×10^6 synapses per mm^3 of cortical tissue in layers II–IV, and a synapse-to-neuron ratio of 12,490 (Table VII), and in a similar study Thomas *et al.* (1980) estimated that in 6-month-old rats, the synaptic density in visual cortex is 750×10^6/mm^3, and the synapse-to-neuron ratio is 13.5×10^3 (Table VII). Since these values have been obtained by the same group of investigators, it is not surprising that they are similar and the only value that can be used for comparison is that quoted by Cragg (1967), who states that Gray gave figures that would lead to an estimate of 320×10^6 synapses/mm^3.

5.1.5. Mouse

In mouse visual cortex the only data seem to be those of Cragg (1967), who estimates the number of synapses to be 660×10^6/mm^3, and a synapse-to-neuron ratio of 7000.

5.2. Symmetric and Asymmetric Synapses

The most complete study in which separate counts of asymmetric and symmetric synapses have been made appears to be that of Beaulieu and Colonnier (1985a) in area 17 of cat visual cortex. As shown in Table VII, they find a total of 284×10^6 synapses in 1 mm^3 of cortical tissue and estimate that 84% of these are asymmetric synapses and 16% symmetric synapses. Of the total number of asymmetric synapses, Beaulieu and Colonnier (1985a) find about 79% of them to be with dendritic spines, and 21% with dendritic shafts. In contrast, only 0.1% of the symmetric synapses involve dendritic spines, while 62% are with dendritic shafts and 7% with neuronal cell bodies.

Winfield (1983) has also made differential counts of asymmetric and symmetric synapses in cat visual cortex, and of a total of 276×10^6 synapses/mm^3 (Table VII), he found only 6% to be of the symmetric variety. This is lower than the average of 16% estimated by Beaulieu and Colonnier (1985a). But as they point out, there are differences between individual cats, and the value of 6% for the symmetric synapses determined by Winfield (1981) is close to the low end of their scale, for in one of their cats they estimated that only 8% of synapses in the binocular region of area 17 are symmetric.

Very little information about the distribution of asymmetric and symmetric synapses in rat area 17 seems to be available, beyond that provided by Peters and Feldman (1976) for layer IV. Peters and Feldman (1976) did not estimate synapses per unit volume in layer IV of rat visual cortex, but examined the distribution of synapses relative to the profiles of postsynaptic elements in thin sections. They found 87% of the synapses to be asymmetric, and 13% symmetric in form. Of the asymmetric synapses, 85% involved dendritic spines and 15% dendritic shafts; for the symmetric synapses, 86% were with dendritic shafts, 8% with dendritic spines, and 6% with neuronal perikarya. This distribution is not too unlike that determined by Beaulieu and Colonnier (1985a) for cat visual cortex.

5.3. Discussion

As shown in Table VII, there is sufficient variability between the estimates found by individual investigators to make it difficult to ascertain if there are real differences both in the number of synapses per mm^3 of visual cortex and in the average numbers of synapses per neuron between species. However, Beaulieu and Colonnier (1985a) suggest that their data indicate a greater number of synapses both per volume of tissue and per neuron in area 17 of the cat than in area 17 of the monkey. This contention seems to be supported by the results of Cragg (1967, 1975), who, although he obtained higher values than Colonnier and his co-workers, also found greater numbers of synapses in cat than in monkey. The data of Warren and Bedi (1984) and of Thomas et al. (1980) would further indicate that both synaptic density and number of synapses per neuron are greater in rat visual cortex than in either cat or monkey, but on the other hand the estimate of Cragg (1967) that there are 320×10^6 synapses per mm^3 of rat visual cortex would suggest the contrary.

6. General Discussion

A striking fact to emerge from this review of the existing numerical data on the composition of area 17, is how diverse the results obtained by different investigators are, even when examining visual cortex of the same species. Part of the diversity in estimating numbers of neurons present in unit volumes of cortex can be attributed to how the tissue was fixed and how it was prepared for sectioning. Both of these processes can lead to changes in the volume of cortical tissue as compared to the fresh state. The volumetric problems begin with the fixation of the brain. All of the investigators quoted in this review fixed the brains by perfusion (except for the human brains), but they used a variety of fixatives, and we have no knowledge of how different fixatives change the volume of the fresh brain. Other volumetric changes occur in preparation of the fixed tissue for sectioning and this always appears to lead to some shrinkage, except perhaps when frozen sections are prepared, and of the embedding procedures those employing osmication followed by embedding in epoxy resins probably result in less shrinkage than paraffin embedding. But both epoxy and paraffin embedding result in some shrinkage of the fixed tissue, and although some investigators have ignored this shrinkage, others have attempted to account for it. This has usually been done by measuring the depth of the cortex before and after embedding. For example, O'Kusky and Colonnier (1982), who discuss their correction for shrinkage at length, found that the linear shrinkage in depth was about 16% in their preparations of monkey visual cortex. This led them to assume that compared to freshly fixed tissue their surface measurements decreased by 29%, and their volumetric ones by 41%. This assumes that shrinkage during tissue preparation is equal in all dimensions. However, it seems that this has not been ascertained, and we have frequently observed that in excessively shrunken cortical tissue the cell bodies of neurons become flattened in the vertical direction and apical dendrites of pyramidal cells become undulated. This would indicate that the shrinkage in depth is greater than the shrinkage in the tangential or horizontal direction. In any case, corrections for, or lack of corrections for, shrinkage occurring in tissue preparation can radically change the numerical data and make comparisons between the results of various investigators difficult.

A good example of the effects of shrinkage in the estimation of the total number of neurons in a given volume of tissue is provided by Powell and Hendrickson (1981). Assuming no shrinkage to take place during the preparation of frozen sections, in such sections 30 μm thick, they estimated there are 175 neurons in a 30-μm-wide strip passing through the depth of area 17 in monkey. On the other hand, Powell and his colleagues (Rockel *et al.*, 1980) found previously that in 30-μm-thick paraffin sections, which Powell and Hendrickson (1981) calculate to have undergone 18% linear shrinkage as compared to the frozen sections, there are 270 neurons in a 25-μm-wide strip, which would be the equivalent of 374 neurons in a 30-μm-wide strip of a 30-μm-thick paraffin section. Thus, failure to take into account shrinkage occurring during paraffin embedding led to an overestimate of the neuronal concentration. As shown in Table I, when correction is made for the shrinkage occurring during paraffin embedding, the original estimates of neuronal concentration made by Rockel *et al.* (1980) for monkey area 17 become significantly reduced, and the corrected value leads to the estimated numbers beneath unit areas of monkey area 17 becoming very similar to those obtained in that same cortex by O'Kusky and Colonnier (1982). If a similar compensation for shrinkage is also applied to the value obtained by Rockel *et al.* (1980) for rat visual cortex, the corrected value also comes close to that of Peters *et al.* (1985) for the number of neurons beneath 1 mm² of cortical surface. For cat area 71, on the other hand, even when corrected, the estimate of Rockel *et al.* (1980) still comes nowhere near the estimate obtained by Beaulieu and Colonnier (1983). Some possible reasons for this difference in the estimates for cat area 17 are considered by Beaulieu and Colonnier (1983).

Taking these effects of shrinkage into account, it seems that reasonable estimates for the number of neurons within 1 mm³ of area 17 are about 120,000 in the monkey, about 50,000 in the cat, and about 75,000 in the rat. In the rabbit, the concentration of neurons seems to be somewhat similar to the cat, while in mouse area 17 the neurons are much more tightly packed (see Table I).

To estimate the total number of neurons in area 17, it is necessary to determine the total number of neurons beneath 1 mm² of cortical surface, and then extrapolate this figure to the surface area occupied by area 17. Problems of shrinkage again occur when the surface area of visual cortex is estimated by reconstruction using serial sections through the brain, and this is probably the major reason why the estimates of the surface area of monkey area 17 range from 576 mm² to 1450 mm², as shown by O'Kusky and Colonnier (1982). Surprisingly though, the two sets of investigators who have estimated both the neuronal concentration in monkey area 17, and its surface area (Chow et al., 1950; O'Kusky and Colonnier, 1982), arrive at a similar conclusion, that the total number of neurons in this area is about 155 million for monkey visual cortex (Table III). In cat area 17, Beaulieu and Colonnier (1983) estimate 24–30 million neurons, while in rat, the data of Peters et al. (1985) and of Werner et al. (1982) and Schober and Winkelmann (1975) lead to estimates of about 1 million neurons in area 17. To a large extent, these differences in total number of neurons in area 17 of rat, cat, and monkey must reflect the differences in the sizes of the brains, and certainly the differences in the surface area of cortex, but the consequence is that cortex of the cat, for example, has some 25 times more neurons for processing visual information than the rat.

To return to the question of how many neurons are beneath a unit area of cortical surface, on the basis of the total neurons counted in 30-μm-wide strips of 25-μm-thick sections passing through the depth of cortex, Rockel et al. (1980) concluded that except for area 17 of primates there is a basic uniformity between species. The conclusion was based on the fact that in such strips from motor, somatic sensory, primary visual, frontal, parietal and temporal cortices of a number of species, they counted about 110 neurons to be present. The only exception occurred in the binocular region of area 17 in primates, where they found about 2.5 times more neurons. The data obtained by others (Tables I and II) would certainly uphold the observation that there are significantly more neurons beneath a unit area of cortical surface in monkey area 17 as compared with other species, but not that there is a basic uniformity among other species.

The proposition that there is a "basic" uniformity among cortices from a variety of species has been extended by Powell and his co-workers (see Winfield et al., 1980; Powell, 1981) to suggest that the proportions of pyramidal and nonpyramidal cells are also similar across species. This, as stated earlier, is based on the study by Winfield et al. (1980), who examined neuronal profiles in thin sections from motor and visual cortices of monkey, cat, and rat. Other studies suggest that the proportion of stellate (nonpyramidal) cells estimated by Winfield et al. (1980) is too high, but more studies are necessary before definite statements can be made about whether the proportion of nonpyramidal cells present in different species is similar.

When the data for the average number of synapses per average neuron are considered (Table VII), the surprising fact is not so much that individual investigators do not entirely agree about how many synapses are formed by the average neuron, but how many synapsing axon terminals each neuron receives, for the numbers are in the thousands. It must also be remembered that these are average estimates and that some neurons like the large layer V pyramids probably form many more synapses than, for example, the small nonpyramidal cells, or the layer II pyramidal cells with their shorter apical dendrites. The other point to note is that if the asymmetric synapses are excitatory and the symmetric synapses inhibitory in function, as the present available evidence suggests (see Peters and Jones, Volume 1 of this series), then the differential analyses of the frequency of asymmetric versus symmetric synapses indicate that about 85–90% of the synapses received by neurons are asymmetric or excitatory ones, and that for pyramidal cells about 80% of these synapses are received by their dendritic spines. Some symmetric synapses are also formed with dendritic spines, but the majority (60–80%) of symmetric synapses involve dendritic shafts, and a relatively small proportion of them are axosomatic. However, as far as pyramidal cells are concerned, symmetric synapses are the only ones formed on their cell bodies, axon hillocks, and initial axon segments (see Peters, Chapter 10 in Volume 1 of this series). There is increasing evidence that such synapses are GABAergic in function (see Houser *et al.*, Volume 2 of this series), and the preponderance of inhibitory synapses close to the site of initiation of the action potential probably means that, relatively, their influence over neuronal activity is enhanced. In part, this is supported by the fact that orientation and direction selectivity of cortical neurons are under GABAergic control (see Sillito, Volume 2 of this series).

If, as the data in Table VII indicate, the average cortical neuron receives several thousand synapses, the question arises as to the origin of the synapses. The data are sparse as to how many synapses in visual cortex are from extrinsic sources, but without doubt one of the strongest inputs to visual cortex is the thalamic input that terminates in layer IV, and in cat area 17 the data obtained by LeVay and Gilbert (1976) suggest that about 30% of the total number of axon terminals forming asymmetric synapses in layer IV originate from the lateral geniculate body. Even assuming that 30% of all axon terminals forming asymmetric synapses in each layer have an extrinsic origin, then about 70% of all axon terminals forming asymmetric synapses must have an intrinsic origin; in other words, they arise from those collateral branches of axons and remain in the portion of cortex containing the parent cell body. On the other hand, for those neurons forming symmetric synapses, which are inhibitory and GABAergic, there is no evidence that the axons leave the cortex, for all GABAergic axon terminals seem to have an origin intrinsic to the cortex.

If these data can be accepted, then it follows that the average neuron in area 17 must have an axon that produces at least a thousand terminals that form intrinsic synapses. This is difficult to believe when one examines Golgi-impregnated material, but seems more reasonable when neurons filled intracellularly with HRP are examined. Then the neurons are seen to have luxuriant axonal plexuses, and those of pyramidal cells ramify and extend for long distances (see Parnavelas, and Martin, Volume 2 of this series), frequently forming boutons at 2-μm intervals (Martin and Whitteridge, 1984), so that there can be some 500 boutons for each millimeter or axonal length.

These numerical data are clearly important for an eventual understanding of how visual cortex functions, and the surprising fact is how little attention has been paid to this kind of analysis. However, when one considers the large number of neurons present in area 17, and the vast numbers of synapses impinging upon each neuron, we are bound to question whether we will even be able to understand how primary visual cortex processes the information it receives. If we attempt to consider area 17 as a whole, the task seems formidable, and for the present it is much more profitable to attempt to analyze area 17 on the basis that it has a highly ordered structure and contains a mosaic of repeating units that span the depth of the cortex. Evidence that this is so comes from neurophysiological studies, which have demonstrated the existence of vertically oriented groups of neurons, the functional columns, in which the constituent neurons respond well to similar stimulus parameters. Thus, in monkey area 17 some columns of neurons respond to the specific orientation of bars, others respond preferentially to information derived from one eye (e.g., Hubel and Wiesel, 1977), and still others respond to specific colors (e.g., Michael, 1981). Yet these functional columns all occupy the same cortical space, so that any one neuron in area 17 may be contained within more than one type of functional column, and possibly all three types. This suggests that there should be an underlying anatomical substrate in the cortex, consisting of a mosaic of vertically oriented modules of neurons each of which is smaller, or as small as the smallest of the functional columns themselves. The smallest functional columns appear to be the ones concerned with orientation, which shifts over very short distances, indicating that the columns may be only 20–50 μm wide (see Hubel and Wiesel, 1977). But the color columns are also small, and Michael (1981) suggests that they are generally 100–250 μm wide. The only vertically oriented anatomical units so far described that are of a comparable size are groups of layer V pyramidal cells, whose apical dendrites cluster together to form a regular pattern readily visible in tangential sections of area 17 taken at the level of layer IV. Such sections show the clusters of apical dendrites to have a center-to-center spacing of 30–50 μm (see Fleischhauer *et al.*, 1972; Feldman and Peters, 1974; Feldman, Volume 1 of this series). How many other pyramidal neurons through the depth of the cortex are associated with these clusters of layer V pyramidal cells has not yet been ascertained, but it could be derived from the numerical data presently available, once the exact spacing between the clusters has been determined. Data about how many inhibitory, nonpyramidal, neurons using GABA as their neurotransmitter are associated with the groups of pyramidal neurons could also be obtained. However, at present it would be difficult to ascertain the distribution of different types of inhibitory neurons through the cortex, for it is not yet possible to display all of these neurons and then distinguish between the various types. Yet this information must be obtained if we are to understand the anatomical basis for the manner in which visual cortex processes information, because it seems that the inhibitory neurons are the ones largely responsible for allowing individual neurons, as well as groups of neurons, to respond in a discrete fashion (see Sillito, Volume 2 of this series).

The preceding is not meant to imply that the clusters of layer V pyramidal cells are the anatomical substrate for the functional columns. Rather, they are used as an example of a regularly repeating anatomical unit and to point out that any postulate of cortical function must take into account the composition of the cortex in terms of how many neurons are present, the proportions of various types of neurons, and how they are distributed.

ACKNOWLEDGMENTS. The author wishes to thank Dan Kara for his help in preparing the chapter, and Dr. Bert Payne for carefully reading the manuscript. Mary Alba and Janet Harry are thanked for their patience in typing the several versions of the chapter. Work from our laboratory was supported by NIH Grants NS 07016 and AG 00001.

7. References

Abercrombie, N., 1946, Estimation of nuclear population from microtome sections, *Anat. Rec.* **94:**239–247.

Beaulieu, C., and Colonnier, M., 1983, The numbers of neurons in the different laminae of the binocular and monocular regions of area 17 in the cat, *J. Comp. Neurol.* **217:**337–344.

Beaulieu, C., and Colonnier, M., 1985a, A laminar analysis of the number of round-asymmetric and flat-symmetric synapses on spines, dendritic trunks, and cell bodies in area 17 of the cat, *J. Comp. Neurol.* **231:**180–189.

Beaulieu, C., and Colonnier, M., 1985b, A comparison of the number of neurons in individual laminae of cortical areas 17, 18 and posteromedial suprasylvian (PMLS) area in the cat, *Brain Res.* **339:**166–170.

Chow, K., Blum, J. S., and Blum, R. A., 1950, Cell ratios in the thalamocortical visual system of *Macaca mulatta, J. Comp. Neurol.* **92:**227–239.

Clark, W. E. L., 1942, The cells of Meynert in the visual cortex of the monkey, *J. Anat.* **76:**369–376.

Colonnier, M., 1981, The electron-microscopic analysis of the neuronal organization of the cerebral cortex, in: *The Organization of the Cerebral Cortex* (F. O. Schmitt, F. G. Worden, and S. G. Dennis, eds.), MIT Press, Cambridge, Mass., pp. 125–152.

Colonnier, M., and Beaulieu, C., 1985, An empirical assessment of stereological formulae applied to the counting of synaptic disks in the cerebral cortex, *J. Comp. Neurol.* **231:**175–179.

Colonnier, M., and O'Kusky, J., 1981, Le nombre de neurones et de synapses dans le cortex visuel de différentes espèces, *Rev. Can. Biol.* **40:**91–99.

Connor, J. R., and Peters, A., 1984, Vasoactive intestinal polypeptide-immunoreactive neurons in rat visual cortex, *Neuroscience* **12:**1027–1044.

Cowey, A., 1964, Projection of the retina on to striate and prestriate cortex in the squirrel monkey, *Saimiri sciureus, J. Neurophysiol.* **27:**366–393.

Cragg, B. G., 1967, The density of synapses and neurones in the motor and visual areas of the cerebral cortex, *J. Anat.* **101:**639–654.

Cragg, B. G., 1975, The development of synapses in the visual system of the cat, *J. Comp. Neurol.* **160:**147–166.

Daniel, P. M., and Whitteridge, D., 1961, The representation of the visual field on the cerebral cortex in monkeys, *J. Physiol. (London)* **159:**203–221.

de Hoff, R. T., 1966, Measurement of number and average size in volume, in: *Quantitative Microscopy* (R. T. de Hoff and F. N. Rhines, eds.), McGraw–Hill, New York, pp. 128–148.

Espinoza, S. G., and Thomas, H. C., 1983, Retinotopic organization of striate and extrastriate visual cortex in the hooded rat, *Brain Res.* **272:**137–144.

Feldman, M. L., and Peters, A., 1974, A study of barrels and pyramidal dendritic clusters in the cerebral cortex, *Brain Res.* **77:**55–76.

Fitzpatrick, D., Lund, J. S., and Schmechel, D., 1983, Glutamic acid decarboxylase immunoreactive neurons and terminals in the visual cortex of monkey and cat, *Soc. Neurosci. Abstr.* **9:**616.

Fleischhauer, K., Petsche, H., and Wittkowski W., 1972, Vertical bundles of dendrites in the neocortex, *Z. Anat. Entwicklungsgesch.* **136:**213–223.

Heumann, D., Leuba, G., and Rabinowicz, T. 1977, Postnatal development of the mouse cerebral neocortex. II. Quantitative cytoarchitectonics of visual and auditory areas, *J Hirnforsch.* **18**:483–500.

Hubel, D. H., and Wiesel, T. N., 1977, Functional architecture of macaque monkey visual cortex, *Proc. R. Soc. London Ser. B* **198**:1–59.

Knox, C. A., 1982, Effects of aging and chronic arterial hypertension on the cell populations in the neocortex and archicortex of the rat, *Acta Neuropathol.* **56**:139–145.

LeVay, S., and Gilbert, C. D., 1976, Laminar patterns of geniculocortical projection in the cat, *Brain Res.* **113**:1–19.

McDonald, J. K., Parnavelas, J. G., Karamanlidis, A. N., and Brecha, N., 1982, The morphology and distribution of peptide-containing neurons in the adult and developing visual cortex of the rat. II. Vasoactive intestinal polypeptide, *J. Neurocytol.* **11**:825–837.

Martin, K. A. C., and Whitteridge, D., 1984, Form, function and intracortical projections of spiny neurones in the striate visual cortex of the cat, *J. Physiol. (London)* **353**:463–504.

Mates, S. L., and Lund, J. S., 1983, Neuronal composition and development in lamina 4C of monkey striate cortex, *J. Comp. Neurol.* **221**:60–90.

Mayhew, T. M., 1979, Stereological approach to the study of synapse morphometry with particular regard to estimating number in volume and on a surface, *J. Neurocytol.* **8**:123–138.

Michael, C. R., 1981, Columnar organization of color cells in monkey's striate cortex, *J. Neurophysiol.* **46**:587–604.

Morrison, J. H., Magistretti, P. J., Benoit, R., and Bloom, F. E., 1984, The distribution and morphological characteristics of the intracortical VIP-positive cells: An immunohistochemical analysis, *Brain Res.* **292**:269–282.

O'Kusky, J., and Colonnier, M., 1982, A laminar analysis of the number of neurons, glia and synapses in the visual cortex (area 17) of adult macaque monkeys, *J. Comp. Neurol.* **210**:278–290.

Peters, A., and Feldman, M. L., 1976, The projection of the lateral geniculate nucleus to area 17 of the rat cerebral cortex. I. General description, *J. Neurocytol.* **5**:63–84.

Peters, A., and Kara, D. A., 1985a, The neuronal composition of area 17 of rat visual cortex. I. The pyramidal cells, *J. Comp. Neurol.* **234**:218–241.

Peters, A., and Kara, D. A., 1985b, The neuronal composition of area 17 of rat visual cortex. II. The nonpyramidal cells, *J. Comp. Neurol.* **234**:242–263.

Peters, A., Kara, D. A., and Harriman, K. M., 1985, The neuronal composition of area 17 of rat visual cortex. III. Numerical considerations, *J. Comp. Neurol.* **238**:263–274.

Popoff, I., 1929, Uber einige Grossenverhaltnisse der Affenhirne, *J. Psychol. Neurol.* **38**:82–90.

Powell, T. P. S., 1981, Certain aspects of the intrinsic organization of the cerebral cortex, in: *Brain Mechanisms and Perceptual Awareness* (O. Pompeiano and C. Ajmone Marsan, eds.), Raven Press, New York, pp. 1–19.

Powell, T. P. S., and Hendrickson, A. E., 1981, Similarity in number of neurons through the depth of the cortex in the binocular and monocular parts of area 17 of the monkey, *Brain Res.* **216**:409–413.

Rockel, A. J., Hiorns, R. W., and Powell, T. P. S., 1980, The basic uniformity in structure of the neocortex, *Brain* **103**:221–244.

Schober, W., and Winkelmann, E., 1975, Der visuelle Kortex der Ratte: Cytoarchitektonic und stereotaktische Parameter, *Z. Mikrosk. Anat. Forsch.* **89**:431–446.

Sharrif, G. A., 1953, Cell counts in the primate cerebral cortex, *J. Comp. Neurol.* **98**:318–400.

Sholl, D. A., 1959, A comparative study of the neuronal packing density in the cerebral cortex, *J. Anat.* **93**:143–158.

Thomas, Y. M., Peeling, A., Bedi, K. S., Davies, C. A., and Dobbing, J., 1980, Deficits in synapse-to-neuron ratios due to early undernutrition show evidence of catch up in later life, *Experientia* **35**:556–557.

Tigges, M., Bos, J., Tigges, J., and Bridges, E., 1977, Ultrastructural characteristics of layer IV neuropil in area 17 of monkeys, *Cell Tissue Res.* **182**:39–59.

Tömböl, T., 1974, An electron microscopic study of the neurons of the visual cortex, *J. Neurocytol.* **3**:525–531.

Tusa, R. J., Palmer, L. A., and Rosenquist, A. C., 1978, The retinotopic organization of area 17 (striate cortex) in the cat, *J. Comp. Neurol.* **177**:213–236.

Van Essen, D. C., and Maunsell, J. H. R., 1980, Two-dimensional maps of the cerebral cortex, *J. Comp. Neurol.* **191**:255–281.

Vrensen, G., and de Groot, D., 1973, Quantitative stereology of synapses: A critical investigation, *Brain Res.* **58**:25–35.

Vrensen, G., de Groot, D., and Nunes-Cardozo, J., 1977, Postnatal development of neurons and synapses in the visual and motor cortex of rabbits: A quantitative light and electron microscopic study, *Brain Res. Bull.* **2**:405–416.

Warren, M. A., and Bedi, K. S., 1982, Synapse-to-neuron ratios in the visual cortex of adult rats undernourished from about birth until 100 days of age, *J. Comp. Neurol.* **210**:59–64.

Warren, M. A., and Bedi, K. S., 1984, A quantitative assessment of the development of synapses and neurons in the visual cortex of control and undernourished rats, *J. Comp. Neurol.* **227**:104–108.

Werner, L, Wilke, A., Blodner, R., Winkelmann, E., and Brauer, K., 1982, Topographical distribution of neuronal types in the albino rat's area 17: A qualitative and quantitative Nissl study, *Z. Mikrosk. Anat. Forsch.* **96**:433–453.

Winfield, D. A., 1981, The postnatal development of synapses in the visual cortex of the cat and the effects of eyelid closure, *Brain Res.* **206**:166–171.

Winfield, D. A., 1983, The postnatal development of synapses in the different laminae of the visual cortex in the normal kitten and in kitten with eyelid suture, *Dev. Brain Res.* **9**:155–169.

Winfield, D. A., Gatter, K. C., and Powell, T. P. S., 1980, An electron microscopic study of the types and proportions of neurons in the cortex of the motor and visual areas of the cat and rat, *Brain* **103**:245–258.

Winkelmann, E., Kunz, G., and Winkelmann, A., 1972, Untersuchungen zur laminaren Organisation des Cortex cerebri der Ratte unter besonderer Berücksichtigung der Sehrinde (Area 17), *Z. Mikrosk. Anat. Forsch.* **85**:353–364.

Wolff, J. R., and Chronwall, B. M., 1982, Axosomatic synapses in the visual cortex of adult rat: A comparison between GABA-accumulating and other neurons, *J. Neurocytol.* **11**:409–425.

Electrophysiology of Hippocampal Neurons

PHILIP A. SCHWARTZKROIN and
ALAN L. MUELLER

1. Introduction

There is perhaps more information available today regarding the properties of hippocampal pyramidal cells than of any other CNS cell type except the spinal cord motoneuron. The hippocampus, with the associated dentate granule cell region, has been studied intensively with electrophysiological techniques. The reasons for such interest and study are several, ranging from the technical accessibility of hippocampal neurons to their hypothesized role in learning and memory (see Isaacson and Pribram, 1975; Swanson *et al.*, 1982; Seifert, 1983).

1.1. Theta Activity

Perhaps the earliest electrophysiological observation that demanded further study of hippocampus was the high-voltage "theta" (θ) rhythm recorded in the electroencephalogram (EEG) of rodents (Green *et al.*, 1960). The large amplitude of this 4- to 10-Hz sinusoidal activity is particularly evident when electrodes are

PHILIP A. SCHWARTZKROIN • Department of Neurological Surgery and Department of Physiology and Biophysics, University of Washington, Seattle, Washington 98195. ALAN L. MUELLER • Department of Neurological Surgery, University of Washington, Seattle, Washington 98195. *Present address:* Abbott Laboratories, Abbott Park, Illinois 60064.

inserted directly into hippocampus, but may at times be large enough to dominate the cortically recorded EEG. Studies have shown that at least one form of the hippocampal θ rhythm is: (1) dependent on the input from medial septal nucleus and diagonal band of Broca (Petsche *et al.,* 1962); (2) cholinergically mediated (blocked by the muscarinic antagonist, atropine) (Kramis *et al.,* 1975); and (3) reflective of a behavioral state corresponding to "intentional" movement (Vanderwolf *et al.,* 1975). The θ rhythm is rather complex, however, inasmuch as: (1) an atropine-insensitive component has been described (Kramis *et al.,* 1975); and (2) there are apparently two separate hippocampal generators of the potential (in the regio superior and fascia dentate), which are 180° out of phase with each other (Winson, 1974; Bland *et al.,* 1975). The behavioral significance of θ activity is the subject of considerable controversy (Winston, 1974; Isaacson and Pribram, 1975; Vanderwolf *et al.,* 1975; Swanson *et al.,* 1982).

1.2. Field Potentials

What is most clear from the recordings of hippocampal θ activity is that the field potentials generated in hippocampus are unusually large, measuring in millivolts rather the usual cortical tens or hundreds of microvolts. Such potentials are apparently due to the uniform parallel alignment of pyramidal and granule cell somata and dendrites, and the en passant synapses made by most hippocampal afferents that trigger near-simultaneous activation of a large population of hippocampal neurons. Field potentials evoked by afferent stimulation have been described in a number of different studies (Andersen and Lømo, 1966; Lømo, 1971a; Andersen *et al.,* 1971b, 1973; Andersen, 1975). Stimulation of the primary inputs to hippocampal cells (e.g., perforant path input to dentate; mossy fiber input to CA3; Schaffer collateral input to CA1; commissural input to all three regions) results in field potential reflections of synaptic excitation and in field potential "envelopes" of action potential discharge. The so-called "population EPSP" (excitatory postsynaptic potential) is seen as a slow positivity when recorded at the level of the cell bodies, but as a negativity when recorded at the site of the dendritic generation (active sink). When afferent input is sufficiently intense to discharge synchronous activity in hippocampal neurons, the result is a field potential "population spike" that has been shown to reflect in its amplitude the number and synchrony of discharging neurons (Andersen *et al.,* 1971a). The population spike can reach amplitudes of 10–20 mV. Although hippocampal inhibition is a major effect of afferent stimulation, there is less agreement as to whether any field potential component accurately reflects IPSP (inhibitory postsynaptic potential) activity.

1.3. Functional Role

The functional significance of these large hippocampal fields is unclear, just as are the roles played by hippocampus in an animal's behavior. A variety of hypotheses have been developed to describe the behavioral role of hippocampus, for it has been repeatedly demonstrated that: (1) lesions of hippocampus result in significant alterations in behavioral abilities; (2) hippocampal neurons discharge in a complex behavior-dependent fashion; and (3) hippocampus is particularly seizure-prone (Green and Petsche, 1961; Swanson *et al.*, 1982). Results of lesion studies in animals have been interpreted to implicate hippocampus as a spatial and/or cognitive map (O'Keefe and Nadel, 1978), as the site of response inhibition (Douglas, 1975), and as an essential operator in short-term memory (Olton *et al.*, 1979) or recognition memory (Gaffan, 1974). Human studies tend to support the hypothesis that hippocampus is involved in memory processes (Squire, 1982).

Many of the human studies of hippocampus have resulted from surgical procedures to alleviate intractable seizure activity (Scoville and Milner, 1957). Focal temporal discharges are often localized to the mesial temporal lobe structures (Lieb *et al.*, 1981). Hippocampus also has an extremely low threshold for afterdischarge or seizures elicited from direct electrical or drug-induced stimulation.

The mechanisms underlying epileptiform activity, the behavioral role of hippocampal neurons, and the large field events so peculiar to the hippocampal formation can only be understood as the cellular properties and connectivities of hippocampal neurons are elucidated. Thus, although there is a wealth of literature dealing with the gross electrophysiological, pathological, and behavioral involvement of hippocampus, the remainder of this chapter will focus on single-cell and microcircuitry studies.

2. Electrotonic Structure

A number of laboratories have made an attempt to investigate the electrotonic structure of the various hippocampal cell types. These studies have depended heavily on the theoretical work of Rall and co-workers, who developed the so-called "equivalent cylinder" model of neuronal structure (Rall, 1969, 1974, 1977; Rall and Rinzel, 1973). This model has enabled the investigator to calculate some basic characteristics of a neuron's electrical structure without having to measure directly all the relevant parameters. To do this, however, the model makes a number of simplifying assumptions about the properties of the neuron and its surroundings (e.g., uniformity of membrane properties, insignificance of local extracellular resistances). Studies of hippocampal cells have derived electrotonic parameters both from modeling techniques based on equivalent cylinder assumptions, and also from methods in which cell structure is directly measured using anatomical data.

Careful studies of electrotonic structure have been carried out on the CA1 pyramidal cell, the CA3 pyramidal cell, and the dentate granule cell (Turner and Schwartzkroin, 1980, 1983; T. H. Brown *et al.*, 1981; Johnston, 1981; Brown and Johnston, 1983; Durand *et al.*, 1983). Some data are available describing an interneuron cell type from the CA1 region. Virtually all these studies have been carried out in recent years using the hippocampal slice preparation from rat and guinea pig, building on the early observations of Kandel *et al.* (1961) in *in vivo* preparations. Two main approaches have been used: (1) Strictly electrophysiological data have been obtained and fitted to the equivalent cylinder model to calculate parameters of interest (T. H. Brown *et al.*, 1981; Johnston, 1981; Durand *et al.*, 1983); and (2) intracellular cell staining and subsequent morphological reconstruction have been combined with intracellular recordings (Turner and Schwartzkroin, 1980, 1983; Brown and Johnston, 1983; Durand *et al.*, 1983) to check and supplement the electrotonic modeling. In either case, only two of the many electrotonic parameters can be measured directly with electrophysiological techniques—whole cell input resistance (R_{IN}) and the cell's time constant (t_0 or τ). Even these basic building blocks for the calculation of electrotonic structure must be derived from electrophysiological measurements, and in this derivation lie some intrinsic problems of the investigation. Input resistance, calculated simply from Ohm's law, can be easily computed by injecting a known constant-current pulse intracellularly, and measuring the steady-state voltage change produced by the pulse. However, the resistance so obtained depends on the resting membrane potential of the neuron; an input resistance calculated at -70 mV can be quite different from that obtained at -50 mV (the anomalous rectification phenomenon—see below). Most investigators (Barnes and McNaughton, 1980; Turner and Schwartzkroin, 1980, 1983; T. H. Brown *et al.*, 1981; Johnston, 1981; Wong and Prince, 1981; Durand *et al.*, 1983) have obtained R_{IN} values by plotting an I/V curve, and using the slope of a linear portion of this curve as the appropriate R_{IN} parameter. Variability in these determinations depends on the quality of the intracellular recording (injured neurons and/or those with leaky membranes may give results different from "healthy" cells)(Durand *et al.*, 1983), the type and resistance of the electrode (low-resistance electrodes generally yield lower values than high-resistance electrodes), and the voltage range of the chosen linear I/V plot. Input resistance of the granule cell is generally highest, with an average value of 40–45 megohms; the CA3 cell, although by far the largest of the three major cell types, has an R_{IN} of about 35 megohms; the CA1 neuron appears most variable, with an average input resistance of 25–30 megohms. These values are an order of magnitude higher than the input resistances measured for spinal cord motoneurons (Barrett and Crill, 1974), but are comparable to those determined for neocortical neurons (Lux and Pollen, 1966; Connors *et al.*, 1982).

Cell or membrane time constant has proved to be a somewhat complicated parameter to measure. Assuming a single exponential decay of the charging (or discharge) curve resulting from injection of a current pulse intracellularly, one can define the membrane time constant as the time for membrane potential to reach $1 - 1/e$ of its peak voltage (Spencer and Kandel, 1961a). However, in practice, the charging curve cannot be exactly fit by a single exponential function. Rather, investigators have determined at least two constants; the longer one, termed t_0 is much longer than the second (t_1), and is generally given as the membrane time constant. Durand *et al.* (1983) have shown that the most accurate measure of these time constants is carried out with very short (0.5 msec) pulse injections, so that the active conductances of the cell membrane are not involved. The measurements made with the short pulse method are generally similar to those made from longer current pulse injections (50–100 msec). The longest time constant has been found in CA3 pyramidal neurons (average of 25 msec) followed by CA1 cells (about 15 msec), and the granule cells (about 11 msec); interneurons tend to have extremely short (for hippocampus) time constants. In general, these time constant values for hippocampal neurons are much longer than the time constants seen in motoneurons (Barrett and Crill, 1974).

The ratio between t_0 and t_1 has been used (based on arguments from the equivalent cylinder modeling theory) to calculate a measure, rho (ρ), which represents the ratio of the cell's dendritic and somatic conductances. When calculated using strictly electrophysiological data derived from time constant measurements, ρ's of 1.0–1.5 have been found for all cell types, with granule cells having the smallest ρ and the CA1 cells having the largest (T. H. Brown *et al.*, 1981; Johnston, 1981). However, when anatomical reconstructions are used to calculate the area of dendritic versus somatic membrane, and the ρ value then based on the ratio of dendritic membrane area to some membrane area, much larger ρ values are obtained (from 7.5 in granule cells to 16 in CA1 neurons) (Turner and Schwartzkroin, 1980). It is worth noting here that these two means for determining ρ, which produce such very different values, in fact do not measure the same thing. The small electrophysiologically derived ρ indicates that a large part of the cell is isopotential, including regions that would ordinarily be recognized (morphologically) as dendritic. Thus, voltage-clamping of these neurons should be relatively effective, with accurate clamp control of at least the proximal dendrites (Johnston and Brown, 1983). As determined with morphological data from HRP-injection reconstructions, however, the large ρ is primarily a statement of the relative preponderance of dendritic membrane in the hippocampal neurons; ρ in this sense is primarily an anatomical measure.

Perhaps the most descriptive electrotonic parameter is the electrotonic length (L) of hippocampal neurons. The L value for all hippocampal cell types is near 1. This small value indicates that these neurons are electrically rather short. Current injected in the distal synaptic region should have an appreciable effect on activity initiated at the soma, since a relatively large percentage of the injected current should actually reach the soma initial-segment region. The L value is arrived at rather differently, depending on whether it is strictly a product of equivalent cylinder calculations, or is based on the anatomical/electrophysiological reconstructions of the cell. Conceptually, the electrotonic length of a neuron has a somewhat different meaning, depending on the method of calculation. Using the equivalent cylinder model to determine L, the investigator must assume that dendritic branching follows the "three-halves power rule" (i.e., the diameter of a dendritic segment raised to the 3/2 power is equal to the sum of the diameters of its daughter dendrites, each raised to the 3/2 power, or $d^{3/2} = d_1{}^{3/2} + d_2{}^{3/2}$), and that all the dendritic branches terminate at the same "distance" from the soma. Studies using intracellular dye injections have shown that this first assumption is generally met by hippocampal cells (although not exactly), but that the second assumption is poorly satisfied in most of these cells. Thus, an L value of 1.0 determined with equivalent cylinder calculations suggests that all the dendrites end at an electrotonic distance of one length constant. A similar L of 1.0, using the anatomical reconstruction technique, says that the *average* dendritic L is 1; however, any given dendritic branch could terminate at other electrotonic distances. Individual dendrite L's of 0.5 to 2.0 were commonly found with the reconstruction technique (Turner and Schwartzkroin, 1980).

Despite these differences between equivalent cylinder modeling and cellular reconstruction methods, it is striking that all cell types in hippocampus have similar such short average L values (as compared, for instance, to motoneurons). It appears that despite the fact that these neurons are invested with rather elaborate dendritic trees (in order to provide surface area on which various synaptic inputs can be properly segregated?), the cell structure is designed so that even synapses occurring at distal locations can have significant electrical effects on somatic integration of inputs (Andersen *et al.*, 1980b). Almost paradoxically, the granule cells were generally found to have the largest L's although they appear to have the least elaborate dendritic trees. Granule cells were also found to best fit the equivalent cylinder model (i.e., with regard to dendritic branching), especially if a somatic "leak" conductance were incorporated into the model to account for the damage produced by electrode impalement (Durand *et al.*, 1983).

Since the equivalent cylinder model has led to electrotonic values generally similar to those found by methods incorporating anatomical reconstruction of the neuron, it seems that (despite its implicit simplifying assumptions) it provides a reasonable first approximation of hippocampal neuronal structure. However, the model is of little help in providing information about the cells' membrane capacitance and resistivity values. These values are needed to calculate many of the other electrotonic parameters, and are generally assumed, using values given in the literature for other cell membranes. Thus, assumption of a membrane capacitance (C_m) of 1 μF/cm^2 for all the cell types has led to calculation of membrane resistivity (R_m) of 3000–8000 ohms-cm^2 for the various hippocampal neurons. This assumed membrane capacitance value, however, is taken from cells whose structure and function are considerably different from the hippocampal neurons. Cellular reconstruction techniques allow investigators to make independent estimations of C_m and R_m. Such calculations have resulted in C_m's of 3–7 μF/cm^2 and in R_m's of 12,000–25,000 ohms-cm^2 (Turner and Schwartzkroin, 1980; Durand *et al.*, 1983). All such estimations of C_m and R_m, however, also assume that the character of the membrane is uniform throughout the cell. This necessary simplifying assumption represents a very unlikely situation.

The problem with such assumptions is particularly well illustrated by the results of incorporating dendritic spines into the model of hippocampal neurons (Turner and Schwartzkroin, 1983). Cell reconstruction techniques have made it possible to explicitly include dendritic spines in cell models. It is clear from looking at a picture of a hippocampal pyramidal cell or granule cell that: (1) the spines add a significant surface area (and therefore presumably a significant conductance) to the cell, and (2) most synapses are made onto spines, so the spines should intuitively play a major role in determining the effectiveness of synaptic input. The role of spines in modulating synaptic efficacy was modeled by Rall (1974), who showed theoretically that changes of the spine neck diameter and/or length could alter the ease with which synaptic current was transferred from dendritic synapse to soma. Spine distribution in the Turner and Schwartz-kroin (1983) modeling study was based on interspine distances as seen in Golgi preparations (Minkwitz, 1976), and spine dimensions were based on an average of those reported in the literature (Westrum and Blackstad, 1962) or directly measured in electron microscopic (EM) studies. The results of such electrotonic modeling were unexpected, for inclusion of spines only marginally changes the determined electrotonic parameters (less than 10% change from values determined without spines). Further, the model suggests that spines play only a minor role in modulating synaptic efficacy. This lack of effect is due to the extremely high cell input resistance "seen" at the base of the spine (where they attach to the dendrite). Thus, even with thin, narrow spine necks, the spine resistance was insignificant relative to the cell input resistance at its point of insertion; it is this resistance ratio that theoretically determines the power of the spine to control synaptic current flow. Although it is possible that the result of this modeling accurately assesses the role of spines in cell electrotonic function, it is perhaps more likely that the nature of the spine membrane (internal resistance, membrane capacitance, and resisitivity) has not been truly appreciated. If the spine differs significantly from the rest of the cell, the spine may well have special electrotonic significance.

3. Membrane Conductances and Action Potentials

Neuronal membrane conductances have been recognized as a primary factor determining cell behavior. Since Hodgkin and Huxley (1952) elucidated the conductances underlying the axon action potential in the squid, most of the studies of such conductances have been most successfully carried out in invertebrate preparations. Similar studies on *in situ* mammalian cortical neurons have been limited since control of the extracellular fluid ionic composition is impossible in conventional *in vivo* mammalian experiments. Introduction of the *in vitro* slice preparation to study mammalian cortical structures has allowed more exacting investigation of membrane conductances, which has revealed a complex set of channels in these neurons (Crill and Schwindt, 1983). In addition to hippocampus, the neocortex (Connors *et al.*, 1982; Stafstrom *et al.*, 1982), cerebellum (Llinás and Sugimori, 1980a,b), inferior olive (Llinás and Yarom, 1981a,b), and thalamus (Llinás and Jahnsen, 1982) have been well investigated. For the purposes of the present view, the membrane conductances will be discussed according to the major ionic species thought to be involved in neuronal activity.

3.1. Sodium (Na$^+$)

As is the case in most other neurons, there is one primary sodium conductance channel in hippocampal pyramidal neurons [however, see Stafstrom *et al.* (1982) for another sodium channel in neocortical cells]. It apparently has characteristics similar to those described by Hodgkin and Huxley (1952) for squid giant axon, and is responsible for the depolarizing phase of the cell's action potential. The sodium conductance (g_{Na}) channel is voltage-dependent and inactivates relatively rapidly. The precise kinetics of this channel have been poorly quantitated in hippocampal neurons for technical reasons; necessary voltage-clamp analysis has been limited to a single-electrode clamp procedure (because of the difficulty of impaling the same neuron with two separate electrodes), and these "time-sharing" clamps have had inadequate time resolution to carefully analyze the fast sodium channel. Qualitatively, g_{Na} appears to be at least partially "on" at resting potential and inactivates quickly with depolarizations of 20 mV or so. The voltage-dependent sodium channel is blocked by tetrodotoxin (TTX) added extracellulary to the bathing medium (Schwartzkroin and Slawsky, 1977); there is no evidence for a TTX-resistant sodium channel. Intracellular injection of the local anesthetic derivative QX 314 also blocks sodium channels (Connors and Prince, 1982); this intracellular treatment leads to an increase in cell input resistance and small-cell hyperpolarization, suggesting that there is a resting g_{Na}. Both TTX and QX 314 block the fast-rising action potentials thought to originate in the cell initial segment (IS) and soma regions (the "IS" and "soma" spikes). In addition, however, these treatments also block small-amplitude, fast-rising, all-or-none potentials variously termed "fast prepotentials," "d-spikes," "dendritic spikes," "electrotonic potentials," or "axon spikes" (Spencer and Kandel, 1961b; Schwartzkroin, 1975; Schwartzkroin and Prince, 1980b; MacVicar and Dudek, 1981). There is still considerable question about the localization of the voltage-dependent sodium channels responsible for the fast, action potential-like depolarizations.

Direct labeling of the sodium channels has not yet been satisfactorily accomplished for hippocampal pyramidal cells. Quantitative indications of Na^+ channel location and density can be derived from modeling studies (Traub and Llinás, 1979), in which channel parameters are experimentally adjusted in order to mimic the waveforms of experimentally recorded action potentials. Using this method, investigators have suggested that there is a high density of sodium channels at the IS and in the some membrane (as expected), and that there is also an appreciable g_{Na} in the pyramidal cell dendrites. According to one scheme, these dendritic channels are diffusely distributed at relatively low density throughout the dendritic tree. Another model suggests that there are dendritic "hot spots" of high sodium channel (TTX-sensitive) density, much as proposed by Spencer and Kandel (1961b) in their early intracellular studies of hippocampal neurons (*in vivo*).

That such sodium-mediated dendritic spikes are indeed generated in the pyramidal cell dendrites is supported by data from experiments in which intra-dendritic recordings were made (Wong *et al.*, 1979). In these penetrations, fast-rising TTX-sensitive potentials were observed to be larger in amplitude than the "d-spikes" recorded at the soma. These potentials were not electrotonically transmitted from the soma region, for they could still be observed when the dendrite was surgically disconnected from the soma (Benardo *et al.*, 1982). This procedure, however, did not rule out the possibility that these potentials were reflections of action potentials in electronically coupled neurons (MacVicar and Dudek, 1981). Dendritic localization of Na^+ channels capable of supporting regenerative spike generation is consistent with the observations that fast pre-potentials (fpp's) often are triggered by excitatory synaptic input and occur at the peak of EPSPs. However, this dendritic localization is inconsistent with the observation of antidromically elicited fpp's that are evoked by low-intensity alveus stimulation (considerably subthreshold for activation of IS or soma spikes in the pyramidal cells) (Schwartzkroin and Prince, 1980b). Similar potentials were observed by Eccles (1955) in motoneurons, and attributed to spikes in the axon (at a distant node of Ranvier) that did not invade the IS/soma region because of too large a "loading" effect. That such "m spikes" are also occurring in hippocampal neurons is indicated by the fact that fpp's elicited by antidromic stimulation can always be abolished by colliding the potential with an orthodromically traveling action potential (elicited by a short depolarizing current pulse injected into the cell soma) (Knowles *et al.*, 1982a). This interpretation of an antidromically invading axon spike also does not rule out the possibility that these fpp's are electronically coupled sodium potentials from other neurons.

3.2. Chloride (Cl⁻)

There is little evidence for a signficant chloride membrane channel that is not associated with a transmitter action. Blockade of chloride channels with drugs such as picrotoxin does not cause a change in cell input resistance. Recent studies have also indicated that there is little reason to suspect that an active chloride pump is involved in maintaining the proper chloride gradient across the cell membrane (Alger and Nicoll, 1983). Thus, the mechanism by which chloride is redistributed across the cell membrane has yet to be established.

3.3. Calcium (Ca²⁺)

Until relatively recently, there was little suspicion of a significant calcium conductance (g_{Ca}) in mammalian neurons other than at the presynaptic terminal. However, taking their example from investigations of inward calcium currents in a variety of invertebrate neurons, experimenters have found calcium channels to be rather common in cortical neurons, including the cerebellar Purkinje cell (Llinás and Sugimori, 1980a,b) and the hippocampal pyramidal cell (Schwartz-kroin and Slawsky, 1977; Wong and Prince, 1978; Wong and Schwartzkroin, 1982). The most significant hippocampal calcium conductance has been demonstrated in the CA3 neurons, where inward calcium current is thought to be responsible for much of the burst discharge so characteristic of these cells. The hippocampal g_{Ca} is voltage-dependent, with a relatively high activation threshold; i.e., the cell must be appreciably depolarized (to about -40 mV) to turn on the inward calcium current (Johnston *et al.*, 1980; Brown and Griffith, 1983b). A sufficiently high density of calcium channels to account for the generation of all-or-none calcium spikes has been demonstrated in hippocampal slice preparations; TTX treatment of the tissue blocks the lower-threshold sodium spikes, and allows the calcium spikes to be seen in isolation. Intracellular recordings from CA3 dendrites have shown these calcium spikes to be larger when recorded intradendritically, thus suggesting that the high density of calcium channels is primarily in the dendrites (Wong *et al.*, 1979; Benardo *et al.*, 1982). Modeling studies have confirmed that calcium spikes could be generated with a dendritic localization of g_{Ca} (Traub and Ilinás, 1979). It is unclear, however, whether any g_{Ca} exists in the soma membrane (however, see Benardo *et al.*, 1982). It is also uncertain whether calcium influx occurs as a graded process or primarily as a result of all-or-none calcium spikes. The common depolarizing afterpotential (DAP) (Kandel and Spencer, 1961; Fujita, 1975) in hippocampal neurons has been interpreted as a reflection of graded calcium entry (Wong and Prince, 1981), although alternative explanations of the DAP include its reflecting the slow charging of cell dendrites, perhaps by sodium influx. At least one form of the DAP, however, seems certainly attributable to calcium, since these potentials are blocked by such calcium antagonists as manganese (Mn^{2+}) and cadmium (Cd^{2+}). Wong and Prince (1981) have also shown that a summation of DAPs leads to the production of cell burst discharge.

The hippocampal calcium conductance has slow activation kinetics, and inactivates very slowly if at all (Brown and Griffith, 1983b). Thus, if calcium-activated repolarizing currents (see below) are blocked [e.g., with barium, tetraethylammonium (TEA), or 4-amino-pyridine (4-AP)], and the cell is depolarized above threshold for g_{Ca} activation, the cell will stay depolarized for prolonged periods (several seconds). Even with repolarizing currents intact, however, the calcium influx plays an important role in determining the discharge pattern of some hippocampal neurons. Brief depolarizations of CA3 cells trigger long-duration (10–30 msec) calcium spikes, which in turn serve as generators of sodium spike burst discharges (Wong and Prince, 1978; Wong and Schwartzkroin, 1982). Calcium spikes, and CA3 bursting, are abolished by calcium channel blockers (Mn^{2+}, Cd^{2+}), and potentiated by ions that flow through calcium channels more easily than the calcium ion itself (e.g., barium). The calcium ion chelator, EGTA, when injected into pyramidal neurons, also appears to potentiate calcium spike bursting (Schwartzkroin and Stafstrom, 1980).

Calcium and sodium inward currents (and outward potassium currents, see I_q below) in hippocampal neurons appear to account for one of the peculiarities of the cells' passive properties, the so-called "anomalous rectification" phenomenon (Hotson *et al.*, 1979). When hippocampal neurons are depolarized, the apparent input resistance of the cell increases; when the cells are hyperpolarized, the apparent resistance decreases. This phenomenon, which is particularly significant in the membrane range between resting potential and spiking threshold, does not represent a true change in membrane resistance (i.e., channels do not close with membrane depolarization); rather, the hyperpolarizing current pulses that are commonly used to measure input resistance cause a decrease in the number of channels that are open (compared to its original resting potential), and thus produce an apparently larger input resistance.

A second type of calcium channel, with low-threshold (i.e., when the cell is hyperpolarized) activation, has been described for other mammalian neurons (e.g., Llinás and Yarom, 1981a,b). Such a channel, which is inactivated at or near resting potential, and activated only after the cell has been hyperpolarized, has not yet been documented in hippocampal pyramidal neurons. However, many features of CA3 cell behavior are consistent with the existence of such channels in these cells. Two CA3 characteristics, in particular, suggest a low-threshold g_{Ca}: (1) postanodal depolarizations or spike discharge following hyperpolarizing current pulses or following IPSPs; and (2) spontaneous burst discharges only when the cell is relatively hyperpolarized, but single spike firing when the cell is slightly depolarized (inactivation of the low-threshold g_{Ca}). Thus, this newly demonstrated calcium conductance may also help determine hippocampal cell firing patterns.

3.4. Potassium (K$^+$)

The various potassium conductances (g_K) are unquestionably the most numerous and most complex of the ionic channels in hippocampal neurons. Virtually all the g_K's demonstrated in invertebrate neurons seem to be present also in these mammalian cortical cells. At least five such conductances can be distinguished using activation kinetics, thresholds, and pharmacological blocking agents. Most of the potassium conductances share the apparently hyperpolarizing, inhibitory role that follows from the fact that the potassium reversal potential is negative to the usual resting potential of pyramidal cells. However, the functional roles of these g_K's are varied, filling special needs.

3.4.1. Leak Conductance ($g_{K\ (leak)}$)

The resting potential of hippocampal neurons is determined primarily by the membrane's permeability (at rest) to potassium. These channels can be blocked by such agents as cesium (injected intracellularly) (Johnston *et al.*, 1980), and TEA (Schwartzkroin and Prince, 1980a; Brown and Griffith, 1983a); both these agents cause a large increase in the resting input resistance of the cell, presumably by blocking the leak conductance. Since there is apparently a significant leak of K$^+$ ions out of these cells, it seems necessary to postulate the existence of a tonically active potassium pump (sodium–potassium) that restores the proper distribution of ions. Indeed, when treated with pump inhibitors (e.g., ouabain), hippocampal neurons depolarize significantly (Segal, 1981a; Alger, 1984).

3.4.2. Delayed Rectifier ($g_{K\ (v)}$)

This potassium conductance is the "usual" fast, repolarizing conductance described by Hodgkin and Huxley (1952) and is involved in the hyperpolarizing phase of the action potential. However, it may turn off positive to the resting potential (Wong and Prince, 1981) leaving an apparent spike afterdepolarization that decays passively with the cell time constant. In hippocampal neurons, as in other neurons, this $g_{K\ (v)}$ appears to be voltage-sensitive. It is sensitive to the blocking agent TEA, which is extremely effective in causing a voltage-dependent broadening of the action potential (Schwartzkroin and Prince, 1980a). This repolarizing current seems particularly effective in interneurons that have extremely brief action potentials and large spike afterhyperpolarization; the interneurons are predictably very sensitive to TEA (Schwartzkroin and Mathers,

1978; Schwartzkroin and Prince, 1980a). Its primary role in hippocampal neurons appears to be associated with controlling the duration of the action potential and in contributing to spike afterhyperpolarizations (which in turn determines interspike trajectory and interval).

3.4.3. A-current ($g_{K\ (A)}$)

A fast potassium current, similar to the A-current, identified in invertebrate neurons, has also been revealed in hippocampal neurons (Gustafasson *et al.*, 1982). The A-current was uncovered in hippocampal slices treated with TTX (to block voltage-sensitive sodium channels) and Mn^{2+} (to block calcium channels). It was found to be "off" at cell resting potential, but quickly activated at levels just depolarized from rest (i.e., it is voltage-sensitive). Its kinetics are rapid (activation to peak in less than 15 msec, and rapid inactivation). It can be pharmacologically separated from the delayed rectifier, for $g_{K\ (A)}$ is blocked by low concentrations of 4-AP (0.1 mM) but is realtively insensitive to TEA and muscarine (see below). The functional role of this current is most likely to reduce the rate of cell firing at a given level of depolarization (i.e., contributes to firing adaptation).

3.4.4. M-current ($g_{K\ (M)}$)

The M-current is a potassium conductance that is activated at or near resting potential, which is blocked by cholinergic muscarinic agonists (Brown and Adams, 1980; Halliwell and Adams, 1982). In hippocampal neurons, this conductance is tonically activated at voltage levels near resting potential, thus contributing to determination of cell resting level. It is blocked by barium (1 mM) as well as muscarine (1 μm) at concentration levels that have no effects on other potassium conductances. Blockade of $g_{K\ (M)}$ produces an increase in cell input resistance and some cell depolarization. Thus, one of the primary actions of endogenous ACh is now thought to be via this depolarization mechanism (i.e., blockade of this potassium conductance) to produce a depolarizing modulatory effect. At least one form of the θ rhythm is undoubtedly mediated via the $g_{K(M)}$, for this θ is blocked by the muscarinic antagonist, atropine. The $g_{K\ (M)}$ is also responsible for some component of spike frequency adaptation (Madison and Nicoll, 1983).

3.4.5. Calcium-Dependent ($g_{K\ (Ca)}$)

The calcium-dependent potassium conductance has been one of the most widely studied currents in recent years (Alger and Nicoll, 1980a; Hotson and Prince, 1980; Schwartzkroin and Stafstrom, 1980; Hablitz, 1981; Nicoll and Alger, 1981; Brown and Griffith, 1983a), perhaps because the discovery of a significant calcium conductance in mammalian neurons has been such a surprise. The $g_{K\ (Ca)}$ is a relatively slow current, and thus can be easily analyzed, even with the slow (milliseconds) resolution of a single-electrode voltage clamp. The channels have a high conductance, and thus are also accessible to analysis by patch clamp techniques (Wong and Clark, 1983). This current is activated by the increase of free intracellular Ca^{2+}. Thus, this potassium conductance is normally abolished by blocking influx of calcium into the cell (e.g., with Mn^{2+}, Cd^{2+}, Co^{2+}). However, its calcium dependence can be more directly demonstrated by activating the $g_{K (Ca)}$ with injections of Ca^{2+} intracellularly, or by chelating intracellular Ca^{2+} with injections of EGTA. The former treatment results in a significant cell hyperpolarization with a reversal potential at the potassium reversal potential level; the latter treatment blocks the occurrence of calcium-activated hyperpolarizations such as follow repetitive spiking induced by depolarizing current injections. The $g_{K (Ca)}$ is also blocked by TEA and by barium. The calcium-dependent potassium conductance (1) is a major determinant of interspike interval ($g_{K (Ca)}$ triggered by calcium influx during spike APs); (2) serves to repolarize cells challenged by major depolarizing influences (such as would open the calcium channels); and (3) sets interburst interval in those neurons discharging in burst patterns. Effects of several drugs [e.g., alcohol (Carlen *et al.*, 1982), benzodiazepines (Carlen *et al.*, 1983)] and neurotransmitters [norepinephrine (Madison and Nicoll, 1982), dopamine (Benardo and Prince, 1982e)] have been attributed to this powerful stabilizing (hyperpolarizing) influence (see below).

3.4.6. Queer Current or Anomalous Rectifier ($g_{K (q)}$)

The "queer" current is a potassium conductance that has been so dubbed because its characteristics have been so difficult to examine (Adams and Halliwell, 1982; Halliwell and Adams, 1982). The role of this conductance has been difficult to elucidate, but investigators have suggested that it is involved in hippocampal anomalous rectification.

4. Local Circuitry and Cellular Interactions

4.1. Cell Types and Connections

The major cell types of hippocampus include the dentate granule cells and the pyramidal cells of Ammon's horn proper (Ramón y Cajal, 1911; Lorente de Nó, 1934). These are projection cells inasmuch as they send an axon out of the local area to make contact with neurons in other regions. The primary afferent input to each of the three major cell regions is excitatory (Andersen, 1975). Granule cells receive excitatory afferents from entorhinal cortex via the perforant pathway (Andersen *et al.*, 1966b,c; Lømo, 1971a). Electrophysiological laminar analysis, as well as morphological pathway tracing, has shown that perforant path fibers from lateral entorhinal cortex produce EPSPs on the distal third of the granule cell dendrite, and that fibers from medial entorhinal cortex produce EPSPs on the middle third of the dendritic tree (Blackstad, 1958; Hjorth-Simonsen and Jeune, 1972; Steward, 1976a; McNaughton and Barnes, 1977). McNaughton *et al.* (1981) have calculated that the unitary EPSP from medial perforant path is approximately 0.1 mV in amplitude (as recorded in the cell body). More distal EPSPs appear to be slower rising than the medial entorhinal

EPSP; this effect seems less a product of electronic decay than a real difference in the characteristics of lateral and medial entorhinal inputs (Abraham, 1982). Commissural afferents (from contralateral pyramidal cells) (Blackstad, 1956), associational fibers (from CA3–CA4 neurons) (Zimmer, 1971), and septal fibers (Rose *et al.*, 1976) synapse on proximal dendrites and produce excitatory effects (Steward *et al.*, 1977; Fantie and Goddard, 1982).

A similar afferent arrangement is seen in the pyramidal cell regions. The large CA3 pyramidal cells receive a potent excitatory input to their proximal dendrites from the granule cell mossy fibers (Andersen and Lømo, 1966; Yamamoto, 1972). This input is sufficiently large and proximal (electrotonically) that successful voltage clamp of the EPSP has recently been carried out (Brown and Johnston, 1983). The unitary EPSPs can be seen occurring spontaneously (Brown *et al.*, 1979). EPSP reversal potential has been found to be about 0 mV, with sodium implicated as the primary permeant ion associated with the large EPSP conductance increase. The CA3 neurons also receive excitatory commissural (Andersen and Lømo, 1966), entorhinal, and septal inputs, each to a specific portion of the dendritic tree. Finally, the smaller CA1 pyramidal cells are contacted by a primary excitatory input from Schaffer fibers (axon collaterals of CA3 pyramidal cells) (Andersen, 1960), as well as from commissural, septal (proximally) (Stanley *et al.*, 1979), and entorhinal (distally) inputs (Andersen and Lømo, 1966; Andersen *et al.*, 1966a, 1971b). While the entorhinal input to pyramidal cells of CA1 and CA3 synapse on the distal tips of their apical dendrites, the distal EPSPs are quite effective, as expected in a cell of relatively compact electrotonic structure (Andersen *et al.*, 1980b).

4.2. EPSPs and IPSPs

Synapses for all these excitatory afferents are made on pyramidal cell dendrites, particularly on spines (Hamlyn, 1963; Andersen *et al.*, 1966a). As such, the synaptic input may be further amplified by the intrinsic dendritic mechanisms typical of these neurons—dendritic spikes, and/or dendritic calcium depolarizations. The spine synapses all appear to be of the asymmetric type often associated with EPSPs (Gottlieb and Cowan, 1972).

Given the abundance of excitatory synapses, and the fact that all the major afferents produce EPSPs in the hippocampal projection cells, it is perhaps surprising that inhibitory potentials are the more powerful and ubiquitous features of hippocampal cell physiology (Kandel *et al.*, 1961; Spencer and Kandel, 1968; Purpura *et al.*, 1968). Inhibitory postsynaptic potentials occur spontaneously in pyramidal cells (Alger and Nicoll, 1980b; Brown and Johnston, 1980), and a summed IPSP is often the dominant cellular response to afferent stimulation. The initial excitatory event produced by the afferent volley is followed by a large IPSP that effectively limits the excitatory response to a single action potential, even in CA3 neurons that have intrinsic burst generation capabilities. This inhibition is thought to be mediated via inhibitory interneurons (Andersen *et al.*, 1964a,b, 1969). Initial models of inhibitory circuitry postulated a basket cell-like interneuron, located just basal to the pyramidal cell somata; this interneuron is excited by axon collaterals of pyramidal neurons, and in turn inhibits the pyramidal cell population. Such a recurrent or feedback inhibitory circuit has been confirmed in several studies: (1) Antidromic activation of pyramidal cells is followed by profound inhibition associated with an IPSP (Kandel *et al.*, 1961; Dunwiddie *et al.*, 1980). (2) Cell types have been characterized electrophysiologically with features distinct from the pyramidal cell, and consistent with the theoretical description of basket cell interneurons (Schwartzkroin and Mathers, 1978; Lee *et al.*, 1980; Fox and Ranck, 1981). (3) Electrophysiologically identified interneurons, intracellularly stained with HRP, have axons that give off collaterals within stratum pyramidale and make synaptic contact on pyramidal cell somata (Kunkel and Schwartzkroin, 1982). (4) Activation of pyramidal cells directly (intracellular depolarization) can produce excitation of interneurons, and direct activation of interneurons can produce inhibition of the pyramidal cell (Knowles and Schwartzkroin, 1981). The symmetric synapses thought to be responsible for this type of inhibition are localized primarily on the soma/initial segment region of the pyramidal cell (Gottlieb and Cowan, 1972; Schwartzkroin *et al.*, 1982; Somogyi *et al.*, 1983a), a site at which the IPSP has powerful control over cell action potential generation. The recurrent IPSP hyperpolarization initiated by antidromic stimulation is the result of a large increase in chloride conductance, with a reversal potential of approximately -70 mV (Spencer and Kandel, 1961c; Allen *et al.*, 1977; Eccles *et al.*, 1977; Dingledine and Langmoen, 1980; Alger and Nicoll, 1982a).

The hippocampal IPSP produced by orthodromic stimulation is very much more complex than the above picture of recurrent inhibition (Alger and Nicoll, 1982a; Schwartzkroin and Knowles, 1983). Several laboratories have shown that inhibition of pyramidal cells can be evoked with afferent stimulation subthreshold for triggering prior pyramidal cell activation (Alvarez-Leefmans, 1976; Lynch *et al.*, 1981). Recordings from interneurons have shown that these cells can be excited at short latency by very-low-intensity afferent stimulation (Schwartzkroin and Mathers, 1978). These findings are complemented by recent morphological demonstration of interneuron dendrites that reach into the afferent layers of hippocampus, and receive direct excitatory synapses from incoming afferents (Kunkel and Schwartzkroin, 1982; Frotscher and Zimmer, 1983). Thus, at least one class of identified inhibitory interneuron exerts a feed-forward inhibition onto the pyramidal cell. An IPSP of the feed-forward type has been demonstrated in electrophysiological studies. Orthodromic stimulation produces both an early chloride-mediated IPSP and a later, slow hyperpolarization (Fujita, 1979; Thalmann and Ayala, 1982; Alger and Nicoll, 1982a; Knowles *et al.*, 1982b; Alger, 1984). This second component appears to be generated on pyramidal cell dendrites (Leung, 1978), and due primarily to an increase in potassium conductance (Alger, 1984). The cells responsible for this IPSP component, and the sites of the relevant synapses, have not been determined.

4.3. Population Synchronization

Both the afferent EPSP pathways, and the local IPSP circuits, may potentially synchronize large populations of projection (pyramidal) cells. Excitatory EPSP contacts are made en passant, with a single afferent fiber affecting many target cells along its path (Andersen, 1975). The extrinsic excitatory pathways are in fact organized in "lamellae" of excitation (Andersen *et al.*, 1971b). Stimulation of an afferent input leads to excitation of not one but many cells that, when synchronously activated, generate large extracellular fields corresponding to EPSP activity (population EPSP) and action potential discharge (population spikes). Similarly, a single inhibitory interneuron affects large numbers of pyramidal cells since its axon ramifies for hundreds of micrometers (Lorente de Nó, 1934; Struble *et al.*, 1978; Kunkel and Schwartzkroin, 1982). In turn, the axon collaterals from many pyramidal neurons converge on a given interneuron. Thus, the interneuron–pyramidal cell interaction is one that can potentially recruit, in a phase-locked manner, a large population of neurons in rhythmic activity (Horowitz and Mates, 1975).

In addition to these major synaptic interactions, a number of other interactive pathways and mechanisms have been described in hippocampus. These include:

4.3.1. Electrotonic Coupling

Both morphological and electrophysiological evidence support the fact that electrotonic coupling exists among pyramidal cells and among granule cells. Dye coupling has been demonstrated with intracellular injections of Lucifer yellow (MacVicar and Dudek, 1980b; Andrew *et al.*, 1982; Knowles *et al.*, 1982a). In a high proportion (70–80%) of such injections, two or three neurons are subsequently found to be filled with the fluorescent dye. The pattern of dye coupling seen in hippocampus—two or three tightly related neurons—is rather different from coupling patterns in other CNS regions, where dye from a centrally injected neuron spreads out in a gradual "halo" to surrounding cells. Electrophysiological evidence for electrotonic coupling is less compelling. Knowles *et al.* (1982a) were unable to find convincing evidence of electrotonic coupling among CA1 pyramidal cells. However, using antidromic stimuli to trigger "short-latency depolarizations," Dudek and colleagues have been able to demonstrate coupling in a small percentage of cells; their indirect evidence of electronic coupling has been supported by simultaneous intracellular recordings of pairs of pyramidal cells and granule cells (MacVicar and Dudek, 1981, 1982; Taylor and Dudek, 1982a). Gap junctions have also been seen in freeze-fracture preparations of dentate and CA3 regions (Schmalbruch and Jahnsen, 1981; MacVicar and Dudek, 1982). Thus, electrotonic coupling certainly exists among some cells within the large population, but the degree of such connectivity and its functional significance are still unclear (Traub and Wong, 1981; Dudek *et al.*, 1983). Traub and Wong (1981) have suggested that electrotonic coupling could facilitate or disrupt synchronous discharge produced by chemical synapses, depending on the relative strength and timing of the chemical versus electrotonic connections.

4.3.2. Pyramidal Cell–Pyramidal Cell Excitatory Synapses

Chemical synapses between pyramidal cells have been inferred from observations of pyramidal cell-to-pyramidal cell EPSPs. It is not clear whether the connectivity between pyramidal cells is direct, or involves an excitatory interneuron (Andersen *et al.*, 1969; Lebovitz *et al.*, 1971). However, no such inter-neurons have been identified in hippocampus to account for recurrent excitation. In approximately 5% of CA3 pyramidal cell pairs, excitatory interactions have been found (MacVicar and Dudek, 1980a). This low degree of excitatory synaptic coupling appears to be sufficient to produce the recruitment of hyperexcitatory field activity typical of the CA3 region of hippocampus without requiring other excitatory and/or synchronizing influences (Traub and Wong, 1983a).

4.3.3. Ephaptic Interactions

Recent experiments have suggested that the large field potentials typical of hippocampus (probably resulting from the very regular dipole orientation of tightly packed projection neurons) are capable of influencing individual neuronal activity (Jefferys and Haas, 1982; Taylor and Dudek, 1982b; Turner *et al.*, 1983; Schwarzkroin, 1983a). Current flow associated with field potentials may discharge (or inhibit) neurons at the subliminal fringe of an active population. As such, the ephaptic mechanism could act to recruit additional neurons into an already active population. Although this function is poorly understood in the normal physiology of hippocampus, it appears that under traumatic conditions that affect membrane stability and cell input resistance (Purpura and Malliani, 1966), large cell populations may become synchronized ephaptically in the absence of any synaptic activity (Jefferys and Haas, 1982; Taylor and Dudek, 1982b).

4.3.4. Modulator Influences

A large number of neurotransmitter-like substances have been identified in hippocampus. These substances, discussed in the next section, may act to modulate the effects of transmitters at "primary" synapses or tonically control the level of cell excitability. ACh probably plays such a modulatory role (Alvarez-Leefmans and Gardner-Medwin, 1975; Benardo and Prince, 1981; Valentino and Dingledine, 1981; Krnjević and Ropert, 1981). Diffuse inputs into hippocampus from the raphe nuclei (serotonin) (Winson, 1980), locus coeruleus (norepinephrine) (Segal, 1982c; Dahl *et al.*, 1983), and ventral tegmental nuclei (dopamine) (Benardo and Prince, 1982e) have been identified but not yet studied in sufficient detail to explain their functional roles. Adenosine may also play a modulatory role (Lee and Schubert, 1982). Interneurons have been observed that react with antisera to cholecystokinin (CCK) (Handelmann *et al.*, 1981) and somatostatin (Feldman *et al.*, 1982; Kunkel *et al.*, 1983). These peptides may be colocalized with the primary inhibitory transmitter, GABA, and play some modulatory role during GABA inhibition (e.g., Vickery *et al.*, 1983). Similarly, dynorphin (an opiate substance) appears to be colocalized in mossy fiber terminals containing excitatory amino acid transmitters (McGinty *et al.*, 1983).

While our current picture of the basic simple synaptic organization of hippocampus has been confirmed by recent studies, there are additional layers of complexity still to be elucidated. It seems likely that several interneuron populations, with different functions, control the output of the projection neurons. Extrinsic afferents can modulate cell activity. Connectivity among cells, which form local circuits, is not so simple as originally postulated. Thus, there is a complex synaptic framework for processing data within the hippocampus.

5. Neurotransmitters

The relatively simple structure and well-defined circuitry of hippocampus have made it the subject of numerous studies concerning the identification and action of central neurotransmitters (Storm-Mathisen, 1977). These studies have been greatly facilitated by the development of the *in vitro* hippocampal slice preparation, coupled with the techniques of intracellular recording and microiontophoresis. A large number of transmitter candidates have been identified and studied. Some have received considerable attention, and are certain to have important functions in hippocampal physiology. These established transmitters include GABA, one or more glutamate-like substances, and ACh. Less well studied but clearly functional substances include serotonin (5HT) and norepinephrine (NE). The list of other agents now thought to have neuromodulatory roles on hippocampal neurons has grown to include histamine, adenosine, dopamine, and a variety of peptides. The functional roles of these putative neurotransmitters are not clearly understood. Even the conventional transmitters, GABA and ACh, apparently have complex functions.

In this section, we will review the evidence that these compounds act as neurotransmitters in hippocampus, using as guidelines a set of criteria that must be met for classification as a neurotransmitter: *presence* of the compound and/or its synthetic and metabolic enzymes, *release, synaptic mimicry, pharmacology of receptors,* and *termination of action.*

5.1. Acidic Amino Acids

A variety of experiments suggest that an acidic amino acid such as glutamate or aspartate is the primary excitatory neurotransmitter in the hippocampal formation. Both release and uptake of these amino acids have been described (Nadler *et al.,* 1977; Sandoval *et al.,* 1978; Wieraszko and Lynch, 1979). Iontophoretic application of these amino acids excites hippocampal neurons (Biscoe and Straughan, 1966), especially following dendritic application (Dudar, 1974; Schwartzkroin and Andersen, 1975). Finally, the reversal potentials for glutamate-evoked depolarizations and synaptically evoked EPSPs are similar (Hablitz and Langmoen, 1982).

The questions of which amino acid mediates synaptic excitation in which afferent pathway remains unanswered, primarily due to the complexities of several excitatory amino acid receptor subtypes and a paucity of receptor-selective antagonists (Watkins and Evans, 1981; Fagni *et al.,* 1983; Collingridge *et al.,* 1983a). Previous studies combining amino acid release and selective lesioning suggested glutamate as transmitter of the perforant path, aspartate and perhaps also glutamate as transmitter of CA3/CA4 associational and commissural fibers, and neither glutamate nor aspartate as transmitter of the mossy fibers (Nadler *et al.*, 1976, 1978). Generally, these proposals have been supported by recent electrophysiological and pharmacological studies (Crunelli *et al.*, 1983; Collingridge *et al.*, 1983b). Thus, the glutamate antagonist, glutamic acid diethyl ester, selectively antagonizes glutamate- and perforant path-evoked excitations, while α-aminoadipate selectively antagonizes excitations elicited by aspartate and commissural stimulation (Hicks and McLennan, 1979). Similarly, APB (2-amino-4-phosphonobutyric acid), which may antagonize both glutamate and aspartate, inhibits excitatory reponses at both perforant path and Schaffer collateral–commissural synapses, while APP (2-amino-3-phosphonopropionic acid), which may antagonize only aspartate, inhibits only Schaffer collateral–commissural synaptic responses (White *et al.*, 1979). Neither APB nor APP has any effect on mossy fiber-evoked EPSPs (White *et al.*, 1979; but see Yamamoto *et al.*, 1983).

More recently, excitatory amino acid receptors of the Schaffer-commissural system in hippocampus have been classified into four distinct subtypes, based on receptor sensitivities to a number of agonists and antagonists, and on receptor "desensitization" characteristics (Fagni *et al.*, 1983). This classification may prove useful in future studies in this area. Along these lines, L-glutamate and D,L-homocysteate, agonists at G_2 and G_1 (synaptic) receptors, respectively (Fagni *et al.*, 1983), elicit depolarizations due to a fast increase in conductance to sodium and potassium (Hablitz and Langmoen, 1982; Sawada *et al.*, 1982). Another glutamate agonist, NMA (*N*-methyl-D,L-aspartate), activates yet another receptor (Fagni *et al.*, 1983) to evoke a depolarization due to activation of a voltage-sensitive calcium conductance (Dingledine, 1983). The mechanism of action of the fourth receptor subtype, the so-called kainate receptor, has not been elucidated.

5.2. GABA

The major inhibitory neurotransmitter in the hippocampal formation is GABA. Biochemical studies have localized GABA and the enzyme responsible for its synthesis, glutamic acid decarboxylase (GAD), to virtually all regions and layers of the hippocampal formation. There appears, however, to be somewhat of a bimodal distribution such that GABA and GAD are concentrated in stratum pyramidale and stratum moleculare (Storm-Mathisen and Fonnum, 1971; Storm-Mathisen, 1972; Okada and Shimada, 1975). More recently, GAD has been localized immunohistochemically in a variety of nonpyramidal (interneuron) cell types throughout hippocampus and dentate gyrus (Ribak *et al.*, 1978; Seress and Ribak, 1983; Somogyi *et al.*, 1983b). Terminals containing GAD-like immunoreactivity have been shown by electron microscopy to make symmetric (presumably inhibitory) synaptic contacts with pyramidal and granule cell somata and their dendritic shafts (Ribak *et al.*, 1978), and with other interneurons (Kunkel and Schwartzkroin, 1982). In addition, the IS of the hippocampal pyramidal cell axon of some species receives a large number of symmetric synaptic contacts from one distinctive interneuronal type; almost all of these contacts are GAD-positive and therefore presumably GABAergic (Somogyi *et al.*, 1983b).

Multiple GABA receptors are present in the hippocampal formation. High- and low-affinity GABA receptor sites have been identified in receptor binding studies (Enna and Snyder, 1975; Beaumont *et al.*, 1978; Olsen *et al.*, 1981). In addition, a novel subtype of GABA receptor, the $GABA_B$ or baclofen-sensitive site, has been described (Hill and Bowery, 1981); this receptor has a high affinity for GABA and the GABA agonist baclofen but is not antagonized by classic GABA blockers such as bicuculline. Finally, Alger and Nicoll (1982b) have postulated the existence of "depolarizing" GABA receptors in the dendrites of CA1 pyramidal cells based on results of their electrophysiological and pharmacological studies. These receptors, which are extremely sensitive to bicuculline, may be "extrasynaptic" (D. A. Brown *et al.*, 1981).

IPSPs are a prominent feature of hippocampal neurons. The chemical mediator of recurrent inhibition appears to be GABA, both in hippocampus proper (Curtis *et al.*, 1979) and in dentate gyrus (Matthews *et al.*, 1981). GABA-evoked hyperpolarizations and recurrent IPSPs are antagonized by bicuculline (Curtis *et al.*, 1970; Alger and Nicoll, 1982a,b), and are mediated by an increased chloride conductance (Andersen *et al.*, 1964a; Ben-Ari *et al.*, 1981a; Alger and Nicoll, 1982a,b). The late feed-forward IPSP (Fujita, 1979; Alger and Nicoll, 1982a; Thalmann and Ayala, 1982) is typically associated with a minimal conductance change (as measured at the soma), is difficult to reverse with current injected at the soma, is resistant to blockade by bicuculline, and may be mediated by an increased conductance of K^+ rather than Cl^-. More recent studies suggest that the late IPSP may be mediated via an interaction of GABA with dendritic $GABA_B$ receptors; baclofen produces a hyperpolarization of hippocampal pyramidal cells that is resistant to bicuculline, reverses at about -85 mV, and is apparently due to an increased K^+ conductance (Newberry and Nicoll, 1983).

Yet another GABA-evoked response can be observed in the hippocampus. Application of GABA to the dendrites of pyramidal cells produces a depolarization rather than a hyperpolarization (Alger and Nicoll, 1979, 1982b; Andersen *et al.*, 1980a; Thalmann *et al.*, 1981; Djørup *et al.*, 1981; Mueller *et al.*, 1983). This dendritic depolarizing response reverses at about -40 mV, is associated with a decreased input resistance, appears to be mediated via an increased conductance to chloride and some cation(s), and is more sensitive to blockade by GABA antagonists than is the typical somatic hyperpolarizing response. The physiological significance of this response is yet to be determined; functional inhibition can result from the "shunting" effect (decreased input resistance), whereas "facilitation" may result from the voltage depolarization.

5.3. Acetylcholine

The septum is the source of a major input to virtually all areas of hippocampus (Raisman, 1966). Studies combining lesions with localization of the cholinergic enzymes acetylcholinesterase and choline acetyltransferase suggest that this pathway is cholinergic (Lewis *et al.*, 1967). Indeed, stimulation of the septum has been shown to promote the release of ACh in the hippocampus (Smith, 1974; Dudar, 1975). Radioligand binding studies have demonstrated the existence of both muscarinic (Kuhar and Yamamura, 1976; Kuhar *et al.*, 1981) and nicotinic (Marks and Collins, 1982) receptors in hippocampus.

Electrophysiological studies utilizing evoked field potentials suggest that septal input to the hippocampus is excitatory (Andersen *et al.*, 1961a,b; Krnjević and Ropert, 1982). Iontophoresis of ACh *in vivo* also elicits an excitatory response, manifested either as a slow increase in the spontaneous firing rate of single neurons recorded extracellularly (Biscoe and Straughan, 1966; Bland *et al.*, 1974), or as an enhancement of a fimbrial- or commissural-evoked field potential (Krnjević and Ropert, 1981).

Intracellular recording, primarily *in vitro* (but *in vivo* as well), has allowed a more detailed examination of the actions of ACh in hippocampus. The primary finding has been that ACh produces a slow postsynaptic depolarization associated with a moderate increase in input resistance (Benardo and Prince, 1981; Dodd *et al.*, 1981; Herrling, 1981; Segal, 1982a), probably due to closure of voltage-dependent K^+ channels (Dodd *et al.*, 1981; Benardo and Prince, 1982a,b). Halliwell and Adams (1982), using voltage clamp techniques, have demonstrated that the slow ACh-evoked depolarizing is due to a blockade of the M-current (I_M; Brown and Adams, 1980), an outward K^+ current that is slightly "on" on resting potential, is activated upon cell depolarization, and is inhibited by muscarinic agonists. A blockade of afterhyperpolarizations (AHPs) (i.e., inhibition of a calcium-activated potassium conductance) may also contribute somewhat to the slow cholinergic depolarization (Benardo and Prince, 1982a–c). Brown (1983) has proposed that the net effect of cholinergic inhibition of I_M (and $g_{K(Ca)}$) may not be depolarization and cell spiking *per se*, but rather a release of a general braking influence (through blockade of a tonic inhibitory potassium conductance), thus increasing neuronal excitability.

Investigators have also demonstrated a presynaptic action of ACh in hippocampus. Presynaptic inhibition, manifested as a reduction in the amplitude of the population spike, the extracellular field EPSP, and the intracellular EPSP, has been reported; this effect is especially pronounced when ACh is applied to synaptic regions in stratum radiatum (Yamamoto and Kawai, 1967; Hounsgaard, 1978, Valentino and Dingledine, 1981). Finally ACh has been reported to produce excitation in hippocampus via disinhibition (Ben-Ari *et al.*, 1981b; Haas, 1982). The mechanism by which ACh acts to produce disinhibition (i.e., suppression of firing of inhibitory neurons?, decrease GABA release?) is not known. The net effect of such an action, however, would be excitation of the postsynaptic pyramidal neuron. It may be that a cholinergic inhibition of the M-current in presynaptic terminals mediates both presynaptic inhibition and disinhibition; i.e., blockade of M-current produces terminal depolarization and so reduces release of both excitatory and inhibitory neurotransmitters.

Only a few investigators have examined the pharmacology of ACh-evoked effects in detail and with a variety of receptor-selective agonists and antagonists (Bird and Aghajanian, 1976; Benardo and Prince, 1982c). The results of these studies suggest that most, if not all, of the cholinergic responses in hippocampus are mediated by activation of muscarinic receptors. The role of nicotinic cholinergic receptors present in hippocampus (Marks and Collins, 1982) remains to be determined.

5.4. Norepinephrine

Noradrenergic afferents to hippocampus arise largely from the pontine nucleus locus coeruleus (LC); this pathway has been demonstrated histochemically by the Falck–Hillarp histofluorescence (Fuxe, 1965; Blackstad *et al.*, 1967), glyoxylic acid-induced histofluorescence (Lindvall and Bjorklund, 1974), immunofluorescence utilizing dopamine-β-hydroxylase as a marker (Swanson and Hartman, 1975), and autoradiographic tracing methods (Segal *et al.*, 1973; Jones and Moore, 1977). Norepinephrine (NE) is present in hippocampus at a concentration of about 0.5 μg/g (Moore, 1975). Biochemical studies, using radioligand binding, have demonstrated the existence of both α and β noradrenergic receptors in hippocampus (Crutcher and Davis, 1980; Palacios *et al.*, 1980; Young and Kuhar, 1980). The distribution of α receptors appears to correlate better with the local distribution of NE in hippocampus than does that of β receptors (Crutcher and Davis, 1980). Both α and β receptors appear to be linked to cyclic AMP-generating systems (Dolphin *et al.*, 1979; Daly *et al.*, 1981b; Segal *et al.*, 1981).

Local application of NE has been reported to alter pyramidal cell discharge *in vivo;* both decreases and increases in firing rate have been observed (Salmoiraghi and Stefanis, 1965; Biscoe and Straughan, 1966; Segal and Bloom, 1974a; Mueller *et al.*, 1982). Likewise, stimulation of LC has been shown to produce both decreases and increases in pyramidal cell firing (Segal and Bloom, 1974a,b). The actions of NE in hippocampus have also been examined with intracellular recording. Iontophoretic application of NE to cat hippocampal neurons *in vivo* evokes a hyperpolarization associated with a conductance decrease (Herrling, 1981). In addition, IPSP and EPSP amplitudes are decreased and increased, respectively. Application of NE *in vitro* also produces a hyperpolarization in most cases, although depolarizations are sometimes observed (Langmoen *et al.*, 1981; Segal, 1981a). The effect of NE on EPSPs is variable, where IPSPs are routinely depressed. The data of Langmoen *et al.* (1981) suggest that an increased chloride conductance and/or a blockade of anomalous rectification (Hotson *et al.*, 1979) underlies the NE-induced hyperpolarization. Segal (1981a) has proposed that because NE-evoked hyperpolarizations can be blocked by ouabain and low temperature, some of these responses are also mediated via an activation of a sodium/potassium pump. In a more recent study, Madison and Nicoll (1982) reported that NE produces a pronounced blockade of AHPs in pyramidal cells without interfering with calcium spikes. In these experiments, NE increased the number of action potentials evoked by glutamate or by a long (600 msec) depolarizing current pulse (blockade of accommodation); this response was observed even in the presence of an underlying NE-evoked hyperpolarization.

Analysis of the pharmacology of the NE actions in hippocampus is somewhat confusing. For example, Segal (1981a) reported that the β antagonist, sotalol, blocks NE-evoked hyperpolarizations, whereas Langmoen *et al.* (1981) observed only a partial antagonism of NE-induced hyperpolarizations by sotalol. A more extensive pharmacological analysis was performed by Madison and Nicoll (1982), with the finding that the noradrenergic blockade of AHPs—an *excitatory* rather than an *inhibitory* response—is mediated by β receptor activation. Pharmacological dissection of noradrenergic responses, using a variety of selective α and β agonists and antagonists, has been carried out at the field potential level by Mueller *et al.* (1981). In their *in vitro* studies, α receptors mediated inhibitory effects and β receptors mediated excitatory effects.

The primary action of NE may not be simply a membrane de- or hyperpolarization. Rather, membrane hyperpolarization may act in concert with the removal of an important inhibitory influence ($g_{K(Ca)}$) to increase the "signal-to-noise" ratio of input to the neuron, thereby making the neuron more responsive to certain synaptic signals and modulating its activity and excitability (Woodward *et al.*, 1979; Madison and Nicoll, 1982).

5.5. Serotonin

Spectrophotofluorometric analyses have demonstrated the presence of 5HT in the hippocampal formation (Wimer *et al.*, 1973; Moore and Halaris, 1975). An uptake system, presumably located in serotonergic nerve terminals and associated with termination of action of synaptically released 5HT, has also been demonstrated (Gage and Thompson, 1980). The 5HT fibers in hippocampus arise from the midbrain raphe nuclei, as demonstrated by a variety of techniques (Fuxe, 1965; Conrad *et al.*, 1974; Segal and Landis, 1974; Moore and Halaris, 1975; Azmitia and Segal, 1978; Steinbusch, 1981). Hippocampus contains a large number of 5HT receptors (Bennett and Snyder, 1976), with a relatively greater number of $5HT_1$ than $5HT_2$ receptors (Peroutka and Snyder, 1981). 5HT receptors have been shown to be coupled to adenylate cyclase (Barbaccia *et al.*, 1983).

Iontophoretic application of 5HT *in vivo* depresses the firing rate of hippocampal pyramidal neurons (Biscoe and Straughan, 1966; Segal, 1975). Stimulation of the dorsal and median raphe nuclei mimic the action of iontophoretically administered 5HT (Segal, 1975), suggesting that 5HT has a net inhibitory function in hippocampus.

The ionic basis for the 5HT-elicited inhibition has been examined *in vitro* with intracellular recording. 5HT produces a hyperpolarization of CA1 pyramidal neurons in slices from rats (Segal, 1980a) and guinea pigs (Jahnsen, 1980); a decrease in input resistance accompanies the hyperpolarization. Jahnsen (1980) has noted a decreased EPSP amplitude following 5HT administration. The 5HT response appears to be a direct postsynaptic action in that it is not affected by conditions that block synaptic transmission. In CA1 neurons, the hyperpolarization appears sensitive to changes in extracellular potassium (Segal, 1980a), and iontophoretic application of 5HT causes a measurable change in extracellular K^+ concentration (Segal and Gutnick, 1980). In some CA1 cells, a depolarization associated with an increase in input resistance has also been reported (Jahnsen, 1980); the ionic mechanisms for this effect may be a decrease in potassium and/or chloride conductances. There is some confusion about 5HT effects on CA3 neurons and granule cells. Segal (1981c) reported a potassium-sensitive hyperpolarization in granule cells, but a different mechanism of hyperpolarization in CA3 neurons. A chloride-mediated conductance increase was found by Assaf *et al.* (1981) in recordings from dentate neurons.

5.6. Dopamine

For many years it was thought that dopamine (DA) was present in the hippocampus only as a precursor of NE. More recently, however, several lines of evidence suggested the existence of a distinct dopaminergic projection to hippocampus. First, Hökfelt *et al.* (1974), using a modification of Falck–Hillarp histofluorescence technique, observed the presence of likely DA fibers in hippocampus. Second, based on an apparent lack of dopamine-β-hydroxylase, Swanson and Hartman (1975) suggested that many fibers previously thought to contain NE might actually contain DA. Third, studies examining the levels of DA and its metabolites after lesions and pharmacological manipulations have confirmed a DA projection from the substantia nigra and the ventral tegmental area (Scatton *et al.*, 1980; Ishikawa *et al.*, 1982). Finally, DA receptors (Bischoff *et al.*, 1979) and a DA-sensitive adenylate cyclase (Dolphin *et al.*, 1979) have been demonstrated in hippocampus.

Iontophoretic application of DA *in vivo* inhibits hippocampal pyramidal cell discharge (Biscoe and Straughan, 1966; Segal and Bloom, 1974a). Intracellular recording in CA1 neurons shows that DA (in micromolar concentrations) produces a slow hyperpolarization associated with a conductance increase (Benardo and Prince, 1982d,e). An augmentation of current-evoked AHPs is also observed. The effects of DA are mimicked by DA agonists (apomorphine and epinine) and blocked by DA antagonists (flupenthixol and chlorpromazine). The DA-evoked response appears to involve an increased K^+ conductance; the hyperpolarization reverses at about -85 mV, and persists when IPSPs are reversed by intracellular Cl^- injection. The DA effects are blocked by intracellular EGTA, suggesting a dependence on intracellular Ca^{2+}. Benardo and Prince (1982d,e) concluded that DA enhances a Ca^{2+}-dependent K^+ conductance by increasing the intracellular Ca^{2+} concentration through effects on some Ca^{2+} buffering mechanism; Ca^{2+} influx itself (Ca^{2+} spikes) was not monitored by these investigators. These findings suggest that DA not only has a general inhibitory effect in hippocampus, but also may be most effective in modulating bursting activity in these neurons.

5.7. Histamine

The hippocampal formation receives a putative histaminergic projection from the supramammillary region of the midbrain (Segal and Landis, 1974; Barbin *et al.*, 1976; Watanabe *et al.*, 1983). Histamine (HA) receptors are present in hippocampus and appear to be coupled to adenylate cyclase (Haas *et al.*, 1978; Schwartz *et al.*, 1980).

The majority of hippocampal pyramidal cells *in vivo* are inhibited by iontophoretically applied HA (Haas and Wolfe, 1977). This effect is blocked by metiamide, an H_2 antagonist, but not by mepyramine, an H_1 antagonist. An inhibitory action of HA has been demonstrated with intracellular recording *in vitro* as well (Haas, 1981). Histamine and impromidine, an H_2 agonist, evoke hyperpolarizations and minimal conductance changes (measured at the soma) in most CA1 pyramidal neurons and dentate granule cells. The hyperpolarizations persist in low calcium/high magnesium medium, and are not altered following intracellular chloride injection. Haas (1981) therefore proposed that HA activates a dendritic potassium conductance.

A few hippocampal pyramidal cells are depolarized by HA (Segal, 1980b, 1981b; Haas, 1981). These depolarizations are blocked by conditions that abolish synaptic transmission (low calcium/high magnesium medium, TTX), and so are thought to be mediated presynaptically (increased release of excitatory transmitter). The data of Segal (1981b) suggest that this presynaptic action of HA might be mediated via H_1 receptors.

5.8. Adenosine

Fairly compelling evidence has accumulated in the past few years indicating that adenosine functions as an inhibitory neurotransmitter in hippocampus. Iontophoretic application of adenosine or its related nucleotides was shown to depress the firing of single units recorded extracellularly (Kostopoulos and Phillis, 1977). This inhibitory action of adenosine was later confirmed utilizing the *in vitro* slice preparation (Schubert and Mitzdorf, 1979; Dunwiddie and Hoffer, 1980; Okada and Ozawa, 1980). Specifically, adenosine decreased population spike and field EPSP amplitudes in CA1 and CA3. As the presynaptic fiber potential was unchanged by adenosine, it was suggested that the inhibitory action of adenosine is due to presynaptic inhibition (e.g., inhibition of release of excitatory transmitter, as has been documented to occur in the periphery; see Fredholm and Hedqvist, 1980).

Intracellular analyses have demonstrated a postsynaptic adenosine action. Adenosine produces a hyperpolarization of hippocampal pyramidal neurons, perhaps due to an increased potassium conductance (Okada and Ozawa, 1980; Segal, 1982b). Siggins and Schubert (1981) observed that low concentrations of adenosine (5 μM) elicit a presynaptic inhibition (reduction of intracellularly recorded EPSP) without any effect on postsynaptic membrane potential, and that higher concentrations (10–20 μM) also evoke a postsynaptic hyperpolarization. Adenosine may depress inhibitory as well as excitatory transmission; adenosine decreases IPSP amplitude (Siggins and Schubert, 1981; Segal, 1982b) and reduces recurrent inhibition as measured by paired pulse stimulation (Lee and Schubert, 1982). Finally, Proctor and Dunwiddie (1983) have shown that adenosine inhibits calcium spikes in CA1 pyramidal neurons.

Hippocampus contains two subtypes of adenosine receptors, designated A_1 and A_2. The A_2 receptor has a high affinity (nM) for adenosine and related analogues, demonstrates stereospecificity, and mediates an inhibition of adenylate cyclase. In contrast, the A_2 receptor has a lower affinity (μM) for adenosine and adenosine analogues, has nearly equal affinities for *l*- and *d*-phenylisopropyladenosine, and activates adenylate cyclase (Daly *et al.*, 1981a; Snyder, 1981). The electrophysiological actions of adenosine in hippocampus appear to be mediated by A_1 receptors; the rank order of potency of a series of adenosine agonists for inhibition of the field EPSP correlates well with that for inhibition of A_1 receptor binding (Reddington *et al.*, 1982). In addition, the magnitude of adenosine-evoked depression of evoked activity correlates with the density of A_1 receptors as determined autoradiographically (Lee *et al.*, 1983a,b).

All of these receptor-mediated actions of adenosine are blocked by methylxanthines at concentrations below those needed to antagonize phosphodiesterase (Daly *et al.*, 1981a; Snyder, 1981). In addition, methylxanthines themselves increase hippocampal excitability *in vitro*, suggesting that endogenous adenosine exerts a tonic inhibitory influence on hippocampal neurons (Dunwiddie, 1980; Dunwiddie *et al.*, 1981). Adenosine may be released from pre- or postsynaptic elements (see Fredholm and Hedqvist, 1980); Lee *et al.* (1982) have demonstrated a presynaptic release of adenosine in hippocampus.

5.9. Peptides

5.9.1. Opiates

Early experiments demonstrated a low enkephalin content within hippocampus (Hong *et al.*, 1977). Subsequently, the dentate and regions CA3–CA4 were shown to contain about twice as much enkephalin as the other hippocampal regions (Hong and Schmid, 1981). Immunocytochemical studies have demonstrated enkephalin-like immunoreactivity in two separate projection systems, the mossy fibers (Gall *et al.*, 1981; Stengaard-Pedersen *et al.*, 1981), and the lateral entorhinal cortex input to stratum lacunosum–moleculare of Ammon's horn (Gall *et al.*, 1981). In addition, enkephalin-like immunoreactivity has been found within the somata of dentate granule cells, some pyramid-shaped cells in area CA1, and various scattered interneurons (Gall *et al.*, 1981). Finally, more recent immunocytochemical studies have demonstrated that the endogenous opiate found in the mossy fiber system is dynorphin rather than enkephalin (McGinty *et al.*, 1983).

Initial electrophysiological studies demonstrated an excitatory action of opioid peptides on hippocampal pyramidal cells (Nicoll *et al.*, 1977). Extracellular investigations *in vivo* and *in vitro* suggested that this excitation is due to disinhibition (Zieglgänsberger *et al.*, 1979; Dunwiddie *et al.*, 1980; Lee *et al.*, 1980; Corrigall and Linseman, 1980). More recent intracellular studies have supported this hypothesis; IPSPs, but not responses to locally applied GABA, are suppressed by opiate agonists (Nicoll *et al.*, 1980; Gähwiler, 1980; Robinson and Deadwyler, 1981; Masukawa and Prince, 1982). Some investigators have suggested that opioid peptides might suppress dendritic feed-forward inhibition more than somatic recurrent inhibition (Nicoll *et al.*, 1980; Dingledine, 1981). Finally, the excitatory action of the opioid peptides is abolished by conditions that block synaptic transmission (Gähwiler, 1980).

Other investigators, however, have presented evidence against the hypothesis of disinhibition. Haas and Ryall (1980) observed that enkephalins produce an increase in the amplitude and duration of EPSPs evoked in CA1 pyramidal cells by stratun radiatum stimulation; no changes in IPSPs were observed. Similarly, Lynch *et al.* (1981) did not see any changes in feedback or feed-forward inhibition during enkephalin administration. Presynaptic facilitation (Haas and

Ryall, 1980) and an enhanced "EPSP–spike coupling" (Lynch *et al.*, 1981) may therefore mediate at least part of the opiate-induced excitation in hippocampus.

Some of the confusion surrounding the actions of opiates in the hippocampal formation is due to the existence of multiple subtypes of opiate receptors (Chang *et al.*, 1979), as well as more than one possible endogenous ligand (e.g., metenkephalin and dynorphin). Gähwiler and Maurer (1981) attempted to clarify this issue by examining the actions of agonists selective for μ, δ, or κ receptors. These investigators found that cultured hippocampal neurons possess primarily μ receptors. More recently, Henriksen *et al.* (1983) observed that some CA3 pyramidal neurons are, in fact, inhibited rather than excited by κ agonists such as dynorphin. Since the mossy fiber projection to CA3 pyramidal cells is excitatory (and presumably mediated by an excitatory amino acid), the finding of an apparently inhibitory opioid peptide (dynorphin) in this system is somewhat surprising. Dynorphin may exist as a "cotransmitter" in mossy fibers (McGinty *et al.*, 1983), and function there primarily to modulate the efficacy of excitatory amino acid-mediated synaptic transmission.

5.9.2. Other Peptides

A number of other peptides may function as neurotransmitters in hippocampus. Excitatory actions have been described for vasopressin/oxytocin (Mühlethaler *et al.*, 1982, 1983), corticotropin-releasing factor (CRF; Aldenhoff *et al.*, 1982), vasoactive intestinal peptide (VIP; Dodd *et al.*, 1979), cholecystokinin (CCK) and related peptides (Dodd and Kelly, 1981), and angiotensin II (Haas *et al.*, 1980). Both excitatory and inhibitory actions have been observed following application of somatostatin (Dodd and Kelly, 1978; Olpe *et al.*, 1980; Pittman and Siggins, 1981; Mueller and Schwartzkroin, 1983). The precise role of these peptides in normal hippocampal physiology is unknown at present. Recent experiments demonstrating colocalization of peptides with other conventional transmitters (Lundberg and Hökfelt, 1983) suggest a "neuromodulatory" role.

6. Plasticity

Experiments in recent years have show that, contrary to long-held beliefs, the mammalian CNS is plastic, with potential for change based on the experience of the organism. Nowhere has this plasticity been shown more dramatically than in hippocampus and related structures. At the morphological level, this property of hippocampus can be seen in a variety of phenomena: (1) sprouting of afferent pathways, to occupy synaptic sites vacated following lesions of other inputs (Lynch and Cotman, 1975; Steward, 1976b; Cotman and Nadler, 1978); (2) successful transplantation of hippocampus with tissue and fiber growth in a foreign environment (e.g., *in oculo*) (Hoffer *et al.*, 1977; Taylor *et al.*, 1980); and (3) as a target for transplanted tissue such as septum or LC (Björklund and Stenevi, 1979; Lewis and Cotman, 1980; Kromer *et al.*, 1981). In all these situations, the plastic afferents establish electrophysiologically functional connections, in appropriate patterns, and maintain predetermined pharmacological specificity.

These exciting experiments, however, constitute only one aspect of hippocampal plasticity, and are somewhat peripheral to the focus of this chapter on cellular electrophysiology. A variety of forms of electrophysiological plasticity have also been described in hippocampus. In these latter studies, it has been conclusively demonstrated that the efficacy of a synapse or the probability of cell discharge under certain proscribed conditions can be modified, and is a function of the history of activity at that synapse (or at different but related synapses). The various forms of synaptic plasticity have been particularly exciting inasmuch as they are candidates for mechanisms underlying learning and/or memory processes (Swanson *et al.*, 1982).

6.1. Paired-Pulse Inhibition

The simplest cases of synaptic plasticity in hippocampus are the paired-pulse inhibition and facilitation effects (Lømo, 1971b; Steward *et al.*, 1976, 1977; McNaughton, 1980; Creager *et al.*, 1980; Buzsaki and Eidelberg, 1982; Low *et al.*, 1983). When a given afferent pathway is stimulated with two pulses in rapid succession (a "conditioning" and then a "test" pulse), the response to the second or "test" pulse varies as a function of interpulse interval and intensity of the conditioning stimulus. At short intervals (i.e., less than 30 or 40 msec), the test response is inhibited. This inhibition can be measured as a decreased amplitude of the population spike or decreased probability of firing of a single neuron. However, the inhibition is not dependent on discharge of pyramidal cell action potentials, since the same phenomenon can be observed in EPSP amplitude changes, with stimuli subthreshold for spike initiation. It is generally agreed that this paired-pulse inhibition is mediated by the recurrent and feed-forward IPSPs elicited by the first of the two stimuli. That the effect is not restricted to homosynaptic mechanisms is demonstrated by the fact that antidromic stimulation as the "conditioning" pulse can result in test response inhibition.

6.2. Paired-Pulse Facilitation

Not so well understood is the paired-pulse facilitation seen with "conditioning-test" stimuli to an orthodromic pathway. This effect is also not dependent on spike initiation by the conditioning pulse, and is specifically homosynaptic (Steward *et al.*, 1977). Paired-pulse facilitation results in an increase in field EPSP and population spike amplitude, and an increase in intracellularly recorded EPSP amplitude and EPSP rate of rise (Lømo, 1971b; Schwartzkroin, 1975; Yamamoto *et al.*, 1980; Racine and Milgram, 1983). Such changes are unaccompanied by alterations in the presynaptic volley potential, and are thus thought to be due to short-lasting changes at the synapse itself (McNaughton, 1982). For example, residual calcium in the presynaptic terminals could result in greater transmitter release in response to the second stimulus. Alternatively, postsynaptic mechanisms have been proposed (Low *et al.*, 1983), including alterations in EPSP–spike "coupling." The paired-pulse facilitation has been described with a time constant of 80–100 msec, but can often be seen superimposed on a slower depression effect (perhaps due to transmitter depletion).

"Frequency facilitation" is seen in the pyramidal cell regions of hippocampus during repetitive afferent stimulation at low to moderate frequency (e.g., 1 to 15 Hz) and intensity (Andersen and Lømo, 1967; Creager *et al.*, 1980). During such trains of stimuli, the amplitude of evoked population spikes increases (and the number of population spikes evoked by the stimulus increases) with each successive pulse, a reflection of increased synchrony and repetitive firing of individual neurons. Frequency facilitation may be, at least in part, an extension of paired-pulse facilitation (Racine and Milgram, 1983), resulting from temporal and spatial summation of synaptic inputs. Frequency facilitation, however, is more clearly a heterosynaptic effect, i.e., inputs other than the one receiving repetitive stimulations can evoke the enhanced response. In addition, although facilitation of both the EPSP and population spikes can occur at low stimulus frequencies, enhancement of the population spike (and probability of cell discharge) can be seen at higher stimulus frequencies when the population EPSP appears depressed. This latter feature has suggested that the mechanism underlying frequency facilitation may be a generalized increase in postsynaptic cell excitability—e.g., cell depolarization as a consequence of increased extracellular potassium concentration. Repetitive afferent stimulation at low frequency may, in some hippocampal systems, lead to short-term depression of evoked responses (Alger and Teyler, 1976; Teyler and Alger, 1976). This habituation-like effect is thought to reflect a postsynaptic alteration (Lynch *et al.*, 1977).

A large number of potentiation phenomena that outlast the potentiating stimulus have been described. Phenomenologically, these various "augmentation," "enhancement," and "potentiation" effects differ according to time course and the characteristics of the stimulus train needed to evoke them. One such effect is the facilitation resulting from brief stimulus trains (time constant of only 5–7 sec). It is thought to be due to an increase in neurotransmitter release, perhaps analogous to posttetanic potentiation (PTP) (McNaughton, 1982; Racine *et al.*, 1983). More intense stimulus trains result in longer-lasting effects, with time constants ranging from 70 sec to 5 days or more. A general postsynaptic depression has also been identified following repetitive stimulation, particularly at low frequencies (slower than 1 Hz). This effect is apparently heterosynaptic, since its demonstration is not linked to a particular input pathway (Alger and Teyler, 1976; Lynch *et al.*, 1977). The mechanisms underlying these longer-lasting changes are not clear, and, in fact, may be multiple.

6.4. Long-Term Potentiation

"Long-term potentiation" (LTP) has been intensively studied *in vitro* as well as *in vivo* (Bliss and Gardner-Medwin, 1973; Douglas and Goddard, 1975; Schwartzkroin and Wester, 1975; Alger and Teyler, 1976; Lynch *et al.*, 1977; Andersen *et al.*, 1977; 1980c; Dunwiddie and Lynch, 1978; Yamamoto and Chujo, 1978; Misgeld *et al.*, 1979; Baudry and Lynch, 1980; Eccles, 1983; Voronin, 1983). It corresponds to the "potentiation-2" effect of Racine and Milgram (1983) and "enhancement" of McNaughton (1982). Conventionally, it is produced by 1- to 10-sec stimulus trains of 15–400 Hz, which result in marked increases in population spike responses (250% facilitation), increased probability of cellular discharge to a given input, and decreased latency to population spike peak. The synaptic effects are less clear. Most authors report a consistent but smaller increase in extracellular EPSP response (50%), and an increased rate of rise of the population EPSP; intracellularly recorded EPSPs may increase slightly or show no change. These changes persist for hours in *in vitro* preparations, and for days *in vivo*. Two forms of LTP have been reported, based on the input–output relationships of: (1) the stimulus intensity (or fiber volley) to population EPSP amplitude (V–E potentiation), and (2) population EPSP amplitude to population spike amplitude (E–S potentiation) (Andersen *et al.*, 1980c).

The LTP effect is primarily homosynaptic, appearing to require a minimal number of coactive (and geographically neighboring) afferents (McNaughton *et al.*, 1978). Some authors have found that stimulation of a heterosynaptic path may, in some systems, serve to "depotentiate" an already potentiated synapse (Wilson *et al.*, 1981; Levy and Steward, 1983). Since no change in presynaptic volley or postsynaptic cell properties are usually detected as a result of LTP, most investigators believe that the underlying mechanism is synaptic. The hypothesis is supported by the observation that LTP requires calcium (indeed, it may be induced by high calcium levels) (Dunwiddie and Lynch, 1979; Wigström *et al.*, 1979; Turner *et al.*, 1982) and intact synaptic transmission (Dunwiddie *et al.*, 1978). Further, LTP is blocked by protein synthesis inhibitors (Stanton and Sarvey, 1983; Steward and Brassel, 1983). Among the hypotheses advanced to account for LTP are the following: (1) There is an increase in the afferent terminal volley or a recruitment of afferent terminal collaterals (Low and BeMent, 1980; Wigström and Gustafsson, 1981; (2) there is an increase in transmitter release (either increased quanta or increased quantal size) (McNaughton, 1982; Baxter and Brown, 1983); (3) afferent terminals are hyperpolarized, thus leading to larger-amplitude presynaptic depolarizations (Sastry, 1982); (4) the postsynaptic membrane becomes supersensitive to the afferents' transmitter by the "uncovering" of additional receptors (Baudry and Lynch, 1980); (5) there is a change in dendritic spine shape that results in more effective transfer of synaptic current (Fifkova and Van Harreveld, 1977); (6) there is a shift in a dendritic trigger zone so as to increase the efficiency of coupling between EPSP and action potential initiation (Wilson *et al.*, 1981; Low *et al.*, 1983); (7) field (ephaptic) effects depolarize neurons near threshold (Turner *et al.*, 1984); (8) inhibitory local circuit effects are decreased (Yamomoto and Chujo, 1978). There are supportive data for all these possibilities, but there is little consensus at present for which of these mechanisms might actually be critical. Even the question of whether the primary effect is pre- or postsynaptic is unresolved. It is hoped that some answers to the questions about mechanisms will provide important insights regarding mechanisms of short-term memory, a function widely ascribed to hippocampus.

6.5. Learning and Memory

The widely held belief that hippocampus is involved in memory/learning processes is based largely on lesion–behavior studies. However, early studies of unit activity during learning paradigms also implicated hippocampal neurons in the learning processes (Olds, 1972; Olds *et al.*, 1972). More recent work from a variety of laboratories shows hippocampal cell involvement in a number of behaviors. Ranck and associates (Ranck, 1973; Muller *et al.*, 1983) have shown that many hippocampal cells fire exclusively in well-determined spatial/behavioral situations, a finding that is consistent with the possible role of hippocampus as a spatial cognitive map (O'Keefe and Nadel, 1978). Hippocampal cell involvement in an auditory discrimination task has been demonstrated by Deadwyler *et al.* (1979), although the nature of the involvement remains somewhat puzzling. Thompson and collaborators have carried out extensive classical conditioning studies in which hippocampal pyramidal cells were shown to "learn" to discharge in response to a conditioning stimulus (Berger and Thompson, 1978; Thompson *et al.*, 1980). This involvement in classical conditioning has recently been shown to interact with long-term potentiation, suggesting that these phenomena may share common mechanisms (Barnes and McNaughton, 1983; Berger, 1983).

There is little question that the activity of hippocampal neurons can be altered as a function of the animals' experience, and therefore—by definition—participate in learning-like phenomena. It is unclear, however, where hippocampus "sits" in the chain of neuronal changes accompanying learning/memory. Many learning tasks, which show hippocampal cellular involvement, are unaffected by hippocampal lesions. Yet, plasticity is easily demonstrated in hippocampal neurons and many candidate cellular mechanisms can be investigated. Plasticity thus remains one of the intriguing characteristics of hippocampal neurons.

7. Epileptogenesis

Another salient and perhaps related feature of hippocampus is its tendency to produce epileptiform discharges, and its frequent involvement in complex partial seizures of the temporal lobe (Green, 1964; Engel *et al.*, 1982). Experimenters commonly find that even moderate mechanical distortion (e.g., from introducing a microelectrode into hippocampus) can initiate epileptiform events. The low seizure threshold of this limbic structure, and its natural propensity to produce afterdischarge and bursts of action potentials, are critical to hippocampal involvement in epileptogenesis. Some clues as to the mechanisms underlying this seizure susceptibility can be found in both the intrinsic cell properties and synaptic connectivity of hippocampus.

As described in Section 3, there are a variety of depolarizing membrane conductances that can, under special conditions, render hippocampal neurons hyperexcitable. These mechanisms are particularly pronounced in the CA2–CA3 pyramidal cell population (Wong and Traub, 19830, and give these cells certain "pacemaker"-like qualities (Hablitz and Johnston, 1981; Wong and Schwartz-kroin, 1982). Even under normal conditions, these pyramidal cells tend to fire in burst patterns, due to the large calcium conductance of the dendrites (and perhaps soma). Synaptic input does not normally trigger synchronous burst output, however, since the excitatory PSP is closely followed by a powerful IPSP that hyperpolarizes the cell membranes.

Both *in vivo* and *in vitro* slice studies have shown, however, that blockade of the IPSP inevitably leads to epileptiform burst activity (Dingledine and Gjerstad, 1980; Schwartzkroin and Prince, 1980b). Such agents as bicuculline, picrotoxin, and penicillin appear to be epileptogenic (Dichter and Spencer, 1969a,b; Schwartzkroin and Prince, 1977) to the extent that they block various components of the GABA receptor/chloride ionophore complex.

The question of whether epileptiform bursting, and particularly whether the paroxysmal depolarization shift (PDS), is due to intrinsic cellular properties or to synaptic effects (ie.g., a "giant" EPSP) has been widely debated and explicitly tested in hippocampus (Dichter and Spencer, 1969a; Schwartzkroin and Prince, 1978; Johnston and Brown, 1981). On the one hand, investigators have shown that epileptiform bursts appear similar to endogenously generated discharges especially in their calcium dependence (Wong and Prince, 1979). It has been hypothesized, therefore, that epileptiform activity results when disinhibition releases an intrinsic burst propensity; the large inward current carried by calcium (and sodium) is not offset by inhibitory influences, and cells stay depolarized for longer periods of time (Schwartzkroin and Wyler, 1980). On the other hand, investigators have shown that epileptiform bursting in hippocampus meets criteria for synaptically generated events, not for endogenously generated discharge (Johnston and Brown, 1981, 1984). It now seems clear that both intrinsic cellular and synaptic events contribute to epileptogenesis (Schwartzkroin, 1983b; Wong *et al.*, 1984). The current, unanswered question appears to be whether the bursting propensity of hippocampal pyramidal cells is *necessary* for the generation of its peculiar rhythmic, synchronized discharges.

A number of investigators have attempted to model mechanisms of hippocampal synchronization. Phasic hyperpolarizing mechanisms, such as the IPSP or the Ca^{2+}-dependent potassium-mediated AHP, are effective synchronizing agents. However, both of these potentials may be reduced by epileptogenic agents (e.g., bicuculline blocks GABA-mediated IPSPs and produces epileptiform activity; TEA blocks a variety of potassium conductances and leads to burst discharge—Schwartzkroin and Pedley, 1979). Thus, the synchronizing effects of these hyperpolarizations are not necessary for development of epileptiform activity. Traub and Wong (1981, 1983a) have combined information about CA3 pyramidal cell bursting properties and pathways of interaction to model epileptiform bursting in hippocampus (as a result of blocking GABA-mediated inhibition). This model, and subsequent experimental work by these investigators (Traub and Wong, 1983b; Wong and Traub, 1983), suggest that a small number of "pacemaker" neurons, with a few sufficiently powerful recurrent excitatory connections, can initiate synchronized bursting. A requirement of this model is that all cells in the population have at least a low frequency of excitatory connections with each other. In this model, the burst properties of the neurons serve as amplifiers for excitatory synaptic input, and AHPs help phase the rhythmicity of the network synchronicity. Although the intrinsic bursting properties of hippocampal neurons are not *essential* to the establishment of synchrony, these characteristics bestow upon hippocampus its uniquely low seizure threshold. Electrotonic and ephaptic interactions may also contribute to and/or modulate the development of hippocampal synchrony (Dudek *et al.*, 1983). The vast majority of work on hippocampal epileptogenicity has centered on interictal burst events, rather than on seizure. Control of hippocampal excitability, and reduc-

tion of bursting activity, is based on a number of intrinsic and circuitry mechanisms. As described briefly above, intrinsic cellular depolarizing and hyperpolarizing properties are normally set in a delicate balance. Similarly, excitatory
and inhibitory synaptic connections are normally balanced so as to restrict spread
of excitability.

Neurotransmitters are now identified that modulate cellular excitability, and
may be critical in the development of seizure activity. As discussed above, ACh
may increase general excitability by blocking the M-current (Benardo and Prince,
1982a). It contrast, DA depresses epileptiform cellular discharge through its
apparent action on intracellular calcium and calcium-dependent potassium conductances (Benardo and Prince, 1982e). Both anticonvulsant and proconvulsant
effects have been observed with NE; which effects are manifested apparently
depends on which receptor subpopulation is most strongly activated (Mueller
and Dunwiddie, 1983).

In the interictal hippocampal focus, a surround inhibitory field provides a
means of preventing seizure onset and spread (Dichter and Spencer, 1969a;
Traub, 1983). With the breakdown of protective mechanism, seizures are generated and recruit larger cell populations. Although the reasons for loss of
control are not clear, it is known that seizure onset is accompanied by a large
increase in extracellular potassium concentration and a substantial decrease in
extracellular calcium concentration (Fisher *et al.*, 1976: Krnjević *et al.*, 1980) (and
glial depolarization—Schwartzkroin and Prince, 1979). Such changes in extracellular environment may play a role in the transition from interictal to ictal
activity, and in the spread of epileptiform activity (Yaari *et al.*, 1983).

8. Conclusion

The study of hippocampal cell properties has been pursued in *in vitro* and
in vivo preparations, ranging from cell cultures to awake, behaving animals. It
is hoped that a better understanding of single-cell properties will lead to a better
understanding of what the hippocampus does, and how it does it. Toward this
end, single-cell properties are currently being investigated using modern patch
clamp techniques on isolated neuronal membrane (Numann *et al.*, 1982; Wong
and Clark, 1983). Characteristics of voltage- and transmitter-dependent channels
can be quantitatively described using such techniques. At the other end of the
spectrum, cellular involvement in a variety of learning situations is being studied.
This examination of cellular plasticity has been extended to animals in which
regenerative (following lesions and transplantations) growth has occurred. These
analyses of hippocampal neurons not only provide information about the hippocampus itself, but also serve as models for examination of other, more complex
cortical structures. The various membrane conductances and patterns of connectivity observed in hippocampal cells have been useful paradigms for analysis
of neocortical pyramidal cells. Recent *in vitro* studies of cortical neurons suggest
that, as in the CA2–CA3 hippocampal cells, there is a population of pacemaker-
like endogenous bursters that initiate epileptiform activity (Connors *et al.*, 1982;
Prince, 1983). Neocortical pyramidal cells have also been found to have a complex
distribution of conductances that can be voltage or transmitter modulated. Such

cellular properties may well be generalizable to a wide range of neurons. A detailed understanding of hippocampal cell properties has therefore been an important milestone toward better appreciation of the complexities of cortical neurons.

ACKNOWLEDGMENTS. We are grateful to the following people for their help and contributions to this review: F. Doolittle, J. Franck, M. Haglund, L. Reece, and J. Taube. Work in the authors' laboratory is supported by NIH Grants NS 00413, NS 15317, NS 18895, NS 17111, and NS 07012; and by NSF Grant BNS 82009906.

9. References

Abraham, W. C., 1982, Failure of cable theory to explain differences between medial and lateral perforant path evoked potentials, *Proc. Univ. Otago Med. Sch.* **60**:23–24

Adams, P. R., and Halliwell, J. V., 1982, A hyperpolarization-induced inward current in guinea pig hippocampal neurones, *J. Physiol. (London)* **324**:62P–63P.

Aldenhoff, J. B., Gruol, D. L., and Siggins, G. R., 1982, Corticotropin releasing factor (CRF) depolarizes and excites pyramidal neurons of the hippocampal slice preparation, *Soc. Neurosci. Abstr.* **8**:983.

Alger, B. E., 1984, Characteristics of a slow hyperpolarizing synaptic potential in rat hippocampal neurons, *J. Neurophysiol.* **52**:892–910.

Alger, B. E., and Nicoll, R. A., 1979, GABA-mediated biphasic inhibitory responses in hippocampus, *Nature* **281**:315–317.

Alger, B. E., and Nicoll, R. A., 1980a, Epileptiform burst hyperpolarization: Calcium-dependent potassium potential in hippocampal CA1 pyramidal cells, *Science* **210**:1122–1124.

Alger, B. E., and Nicoll, R. A., 1980b, Spontaneous inhibitory post-synaptic potentials in hippocampus: Mechanism for tonic inhibition, *Brain Res.* **200**:195–200.

Alger, B. E., and Nicoll, R. A., 1982a, Feed-forward dendritic inhibition in rat hippocampal pyramidal cells studied in vitro, *J. Physiol. (London)* **328**:105–123.

Alger, B. E., and Nicoll, R. A., 1982b, Pharmacological evidence for two kinds of GABA receptor on rat hippocampal pyramidal cells studied in vitro, *J. Physiol. (London)* **328**:125–141.

Alger, B. E., and Nicoll, R. A., 1983, Ammonia does not selectively block IPSPs in rat hippocampal pyramidal cells, *J. Neurophysiol.* **49**:1381–1391.

Alger, B. E., and Teyler, T. J., 1976, Long-term and short-term plasticity in CA1, CA3 and dentate regions of the rat hippocampal slice, *Brain Res.* **110**:463–480.

Allen, G. I., Eccles, J., Nicoll, R. A., Oshima, T., and Rubia, F. J., 1977, The ionic mechanisms concerned in generating the i.p.s.ps of hippocampal pyramidal cells, *Proc. R. Soc. London Ser. B* **198**:363–384.

Alvarez-Leefmans, F. J., 1976, Functional synaptic organization of inhibitory pathways in the dentate gyrus of the rabbit, *Exp. Brain Res. Suppl.* **1**:229–234.

Alvarez-Leefmans, F. J., and Gardner-Medwin, A. R., 1975, Influences of the septum on the hippocampal dentate area which are unaccompanied by field potentials, *J. Physiol. (London)* **249**:14P–16P.

Andersen, P., 1960, Interhippocampal impulses. II. Apical dendritic activation of CA1 neurones, *Acta Physiol. Scand.* **48**:178–208.

Andersen, P., 1975, Organization of hippocampal neurons and their interconnections, in: *The Hippocampus* 1 (R. L. Isaacson and K. H. Pribram, eds.), Plenum Press, New York, pp. 155–175.

Andersen, P., and Lømo, T., 1966, Mode of activation of hippocampal pyramidal cells by excitatory synapses on dendrites, *Exp. Brain Res.* **2**:247–260.

Andersen, P., and Lømo, T., 1967, Control of hippocampal output by afferent volley frequency, *Prog. Brain Res.* **27**:400–412.

Andersen, P., Bruland, H., and Kaada, B. R., 1961a, Activation of the dentate area by septal stimulation, *Acta Physiol. Scand.* **51**:17–28.

Andersen, P., Bruland, H., and Kaada, B. R., 1961b, Activation of the field CA1 of the hippocampus by septal stimulation, *Acta Physiol. Scand.* **51**:29–40.

Andersen, P., Eccles, J. C., and Løyning, Y., 1964a, Location of postsynaptic inhibitory synapses of hippocampal pyramids, *J. Neurophysiol.* **27**:592–607.

Andersen, P., Eccles, J. C., and Løyning, Y., 1964b, Pathway of postsynaptic inhibition in the hippocampus, *J. Neurophysiol.* **27**:608–619.

Andersen, P., Blackstad, T. W., and Lømo, T., 1966a, Location and identification of excitatory synapses on hippocampal pyramidal cells, *Exp. Brain Res.* **1**:236–248.

Andersen, P., Holmqvist, B., and Voorhoeve, P. E., 1966b, Entorhinal activation of dentate granule cells, *Acta Physiol. Scand.* **66**:448–460.

Andersen, P., Holmqvist, B., and Voorhoeve, P. E., 1966c, Excitatory synapses on hippocampal apical dendrites activated by entorhinal stimulation, *Acta Physiol. Scand.* **66**:461–472.

Andersen, P., Gross, G. N., Lømo, T., and Sveen, P., 1969, Participation of inhibitory and excitatory interneurones in the control of hippocampal cortical output, in: *The Interneuron* (M. A. B. Brazier, ed.), University of California Press, Los Angeles, pp 415–465.

Andersen, P., Bliss, T. V. P., and Skrede, K. K., 1971a, Unit analysis of hippocampal population spikes, *Exp. Brain Res.* **13**:208–221.

Andersen, P., Bliss, T. V. P., and Skrede, K. K., 1971b, Lamellar organization of hippocampal excitatory pathways, *Exp. Brain Res.* **13**:222–238.

Andersen, P., Bland, B. H., and Dudar, J. D., 1973, Organization of the hippocampal output, *Exp. Brain Res.* **17**:152–168.

Andersen, P., Sundberg, S. H., Sveen, O., and Wigström, H., 1977, Specific long-lasting potentiation of synaptic transmission in hippocampal slices, *Nature* **266**:736–737.

Andersen, P., Dingledine, R., Gjerstad, L., Langmoen, I. A., and Mosfeldt-Laursen, A., 1980a, Two different responses of hippocampal pyramidal cells to application of gamma-amino butyric acid, *J. Physiol. (London)* **305**:279–296.

Andersen, P., Silfvenius, H., Sundberg, S. H., and Sveen, O., 1980b, A comparison of distal and proximal dendritic synapses on CA1 pyramids in hippocampal slices in vitro, *J. Physiol. (London)* **307**:273–299.

Andersen, P., Sundberg, S. H., Sveen, O., Swann, J. W., and Wigström, H., 1980c, Possible mechanisms for long-lasting potentiation of synaptic transmission in hippocampal slices from guinea-pigs, *J. Physiol. (London)* **302**:463–482.

Andrew, R. D., Taylor, C. P., Snow, R. W., and Dudek, F. E., 1982, Coupling in rat hippocampal slices: Dye transfer between CA1 pyramidal cells, *Brain Res. Bull.* **8**:211–222.

Assaf, S. Y., Crunelli, V., and Kelly, J. S., 1981, Action of 5-hydroxytryptamine on granule cells in the rat hippocampal slice, *J. Physiol. (Paris)* **77**:377–380.

Azmitia, E. C., and Segal, M., 1978, An autoradiographic analysis of the differential ascending projections of the dorsal and median raphe nuclei in the rat, *J. Comp. Neurol.* **179**:641–668.

Barbaccia, M. L., Brunello, N., Chuang, D.-M., and Costa, E., 1983, Serotonin-elicited amplification of adenylate cyclase activity in hippocampal membranes from adult rat, *J. Neurochem.* **40**:1671–1679.

Barbin, G., Garbarg, M., Schwartz, J.-C., and Storm-Mathisen J., 1976, Histamine synthesizing afferents to the hippocampal region. *J. Neurochem.* **26**:259–263.

Barnes, C. A., and McNaughton, B. L., 1980, Physiological compensation for loss of afferent synapses in rat hippocampal granule cells during senescence, *J. Physiol. (London)* **309**:473–485.

Barnes, C. A., and McNaughton, B. L., 1983, Where is the cognitive map?, *Soc. Neurosci. Abstr.* **9**:649.

Barrett, J. N., and Crill, W. E., 1974, Specific membrane properties of cat motoneurons, *J. Physiol. (London)* **239**:301–324.

Baudry, M., and Lynch, G., 1980, Hypothesis regarding the cellular mechanisms responsible for long-term synaptic potentiation in the hippocampus, *Exp. Neurol.* **68**:202–204.

Baxter, D., and Brown, T. H., 1983, Quantal analysis of long-term synaptic potentiation, *Soc. Neurosci. Abstr.* **9**:103.

Beaumont, K., Chilton, W. S., Yamamura, H. I., and Enna, S. J., 1978, Muscimol binding in rat brain: Association with GABA receptors, *Brain Res.* **148**:153–162.

Benardo, L. S., and Prince, D. A., 1981, Acetylcholine induced modulation of hippocampal pyramidal neurons, *Brain Res.* **211**:227–234.

Benardo, L. S., and Prince, D. A., 1982a, Cholinergic excitation of mammalian hippocampal pyramidal cells, *Brain Res.* **249**:315–331.

Benardo, L. S., and Prince, D. A., 1982b, Ionic mechanisms of cholinergic excitation in mammalian hippocampal pyramidal cells, *Brain Res.* **249:**333–344.

Benardo, L. S., and Prince, D. A., 1982c, Cholinergic pharmacology of mammalian hippocampal pyramidal cells, *Neuroscience* **7:**1703–1712.

Benardo, L. S., and Prince, D. A., 1982d, Dopamine modulates a Ca^{++}-activated potassium conductance in mammalian hippocampal pyramidal cells, *Nature* **297:**76–79.

Benardo, L. S., and Prince, D. A., 1982e, Dopamine action on hippocampal pyramidal cells, *J. Neurosci.* **2:**415–423.

Benardo, L. S., Masukawa, L. M., and Prince, D. A., 1982, Electrophysiology of isolated hippocampal pyramidal dendrites, *J. Neurosci.* **2:**1614–1622.

Ben-Ari, Y., Krnjević, K., Reiffenstein, R. J., and Reinhardt, W., 1981a, Inhibitory conductance changes and action of gamma-aminobutyrate in rat hippocampus, *Neuroscience* **6:**2445–2463.

Ben-Ari, Y., Krnjević, K., Reinhardt, W., and Ropert, N., 1981b, Intracellular observations on the disinhibitory action of acetylcholine in the hippocampus, *Neuroscience* **6:**2475–2484.

Bennett, J. P., Jr., and Snyder, S. H., 1976, Serotonin and lysergic acid diethylamide binding in rat brain membranes: Relationship to postsynaptic serotonin receptors, *Mol. Pharmacol.* **12:373–389.**

Berger, T., 1983, Long term potentiation of hippocampal synaptic transmission accelerates behavioral learning, Paper presented at the First Biennial Symposium on Neural Mechanisms of Conditioning, Marine Biological Laboratory, Woods Hole, Mass.

Berger, T. W., and Thompson, R F., 1978, Neuronal plasticity in the limbic system during classical conditioning of the rabbit nictitating membrane response. I. The hippocampus, *Brain Res.* **145:**323–346.

Bird, S. J., and Aghajanian, G. K., 1976, The cholinergic pharmacology of hippocampal pyramidal cells: A microiontophoretic study, *Neuropharmacology* **151:**273–282.

Bischoff, S., Scatton, B., and Korf, J., 1979, Dopamine metabolism, spiperone binding and adenylate cyclase activity in the adult rat hippocampus after ingrowth of dopaminergic neurones from embryonic implants, *Brain Res.* **179:**77–84.

Biscoe, T. J., and Straughan, D. W., 1966, Microelectrophoretic studies of neurones in the cat hippocampus, *J. Physiol. (London)* **183:**341–359.

Björklund, A., and Stenevi, U., 1979, Regeneration of monoaminergic and cholinergic neurons in the mammalian central nervous system, *Physiol. Rev.* **59:**62–100.

Blackstad, T. W., 1956, Commissural connections of the hippocampal region in the rat with special reference to their mode of termination, *J Comp. Neurol.* **105:**417–538.

Blackstad, T. W., 1958, On the termination of some afferents to the hippocampus and fascia dentata, *Acta Anat.* **35:**202–214.

Blackstad, T. W., Fuxe, K., and Hökfelt, T., 1967, Noradrenaline nerve terminals in the hippocampal region of the rat and the guinea pig, *Z. Zellforsch.* **7:**463–473.

Bland, B. H., Kostopoulos, G. K., and Phillis J. W., 1974, Acetylcholine sensitivity of hippocampal formation neurons, *Can. J. Physiol. Pharmacol.* **52:**966–971.

Bland, B. H., Andersen, P., and Ganes, T., 1975, Two generators of hippocampal theta activity in rabbits, *Brain Res.* **94:**199–218.

Bliss, T. V. P., and Gardner-Medwin, A. R., 1973, Long-lasting potentiation of synaptic transmission in the dentate area of the unanesthetized rabbit following stimulation of the perforant path, *J. Physiol. (London)* **232:**357–374.

Brown, D. A., 1983, Slow cholinergic excitation—a mechanism for increasing neuronal excitability, *Trends Neurosci.* **6:**302–307.

Brown, D. A., and Adams, P. R., 1980, Muscarinic suppression of a novel voltage-sensitive K^+ current in a vertebrate neurone, *Nature* **283:**673–676.

Brown, D. A., and Griffith, W. H., 1983a, Calcium-activated outward current in voltage-clamped hippocampal neurones of the guinea-pig, *J. Physiol. (London)* **337:**287–301.

Brown, D. A., and Griffith, W. H., 1983b, Persistent slow inward calcium current in voltage-clamped hippocampal neurones of the guinea pig, *J. Physiol. (London)* **337:**303–320.

Brown, D. A., Higgins, A. J., Marsh, S., and Smart, T. G., 1981, Actions of GABA on mammalian neurons, axons, and nerve terminals, in: *Amino Acid Neurotransmitters* (F. V. DeFeudis and P. Mandel, eds.), Raven Press, New York, pp. 321–326.

Brown, T. H., and Johnston, D., 1980, Two classes of miniature synaptic potentials in CA3 hippocampal neurons, *Soc. Neurosci. Abstr.* **6:**10.

Brown, T. H., and Johnston, D., 1983, Voltage-clamp analysis of mossy fiber synaptic input to hippocampal neurons, *J. Neurophysiol.* **50:**487–507.

Brown, T. H., Wong, R .K. S., and Prince, D. A., 1979, Spontaneous miniature synaptic potentials in hippocampal neurons, *Brain Res.* **177:**194–199.

Brown, T. H., Fricke, R. A., and Perkel, D. H., 1981, Passive electrical constants in three classes of hippocampal neurons, *J. Neurophysiol.* **46:**812–827.

Buzsaki, G., and Eidelberg, E., 1982, Convergence of associational and commissural pathways on CA1 pyramidal cells of the rat hippocampus, *Brain Res.* **237:**283–295.

Carlen, P. L., Gurevich, N., and Durand, D., 1982, Ethanol in low doses augments calcium-mediated mechanisms measured intracellularly in hippocampal neurons, *Science* **215:**306–309.

Carlen, P. L., Gurevich, N., and Pole, P., 1983, Low-dose benzodiazepine neuronal inhibition: Enhanced Ca^{++}-mediated K^+ conductance, *Brain Res.* **271:**358–364.

Chang, K. J., Cooper, B R., Hazum, E., and Cuatrecasas, P., 1979, Multiple opiate receptors: Different regional distribution in the brain and differential binding of opiates and opioid peptides, *Mol. Pharmacol.* **16:**91–104.

Collingridge, G. L., Kehl, S. J., and McLennan, H., 1983a, The antagonism of amino acid-induced excitations of rat hippocampal CA1 neurones in vitro, *J. Physiol. (London)* **334:**19–31.

Collingridge, G. L., Kehl, S. J., and McLennan, H., 1983b, Excitatory amino acids in synaptic transmission in the Schaffer collateral–commissural pathway of the rat hippocampus, *J. Physiol. (London)* **334:**33–46.

Connors, B. W., and Prince, D. A., 1982, Effects of local anesthetic QX-314 on the membrane properties of hippocampal pyramidal neurons, *J. Pharmacol. Exp. Ther.* **200:**476–481.

Connors, B. W., Gutnick, M. J., and Prince, D. A., 1982, Electrophysiological properties of neocortical neurons in vitro, *J. Neurophysiol.* **48:**1302–1320.

Conrad, L. C. A., Leonard, C. M., and Pfaff, D W., 1974, Connections of the median and dorsal raphe nuclei in the rat: An autoradiographic and degeneration study, *J. Comp. Neurol.* **156:**179–206.

Corrigall, W. A., and Linseman, M. A., 1980, A specific effect of morphine on evoked activity in the rat hippocampal slice, *Brain Res.* **192:**227–238.

Cotman, C. W., and Nadler, J. V., 1978, Reactive synaptogenesis in the hippocampus, in: *Neuronal Plasticity* (C. W. Cotman, ed.), Raven Press, New York, pp. 227–271.

Creager, R., Dunwiddie, T., and Lynch, G., 1980, Paired-pulse and frequency facilitation in the CA1 region of the in vitro rat hippocampus, *J. Physiol. (London)* **299:**409–424.

Crill, W. E., and Schwindt, P. C., 1983, Active currents in mammalian central neurons, *Trends Neurosci.* **6:**236–240.

Crunelli, V., Forda, S., and Kelly, J. S., 1983, Blockade of amino acid-induced depolarizations and inhibition of excitatory post-synaptic potentials in rat dentate gyrus, *J. Physiol. (London)* **341:**627–640.

Crutcher, K. A., and Davis, J. N., 1980, Hippocampal alpha- and beta-adrenergic receptors: Comparisons of ^{3}H-dihydroalprenolol and ^{3}H-WB 4101 binding with noradrenergic innervation in the rat, *Brain Res.* **182:**107–117.

Curtis, D. R., Felix, D., and McLennan, H., 1970, GABA and hippocampal inhibition, *Br. J. Pharmacol.* **40:**881–883.

Dahl, D., Bailey, W. H., and Winson, J., 1983, Effect of norepinephrine depletion of hippocampus on neuronal transmission from perforant pathway through dentate gyrus, *J. Neurophysiol.* **49:**123–133.

Daly, J. W., Bruns, R. F., and Snyder, S. H., 1981a, Adenosine receptors in the central nervous system: Relationship to the central actions of methylxanthines, *Life Sci.* **28:**2083–2097.

Daly, J. W., Padgett, W., Creveling, C. R., Cantacuzene, D., and Kirk, K. L., 1981b, Cyclic AMP-generating systems: Regional differences in activation by adrenergic receptors in rat brain, *J. Neurosci.* **1:**49–59.

Deadwyler, S. A., West, M., and Lynch, G., 1979, Activity of dentate granule cells during learning: Differentiation of perforant path input, *Brain Res.* **169:**29–43.

Dichter, M., and Spencer, W. A., 1969a, Penicillin-induced interictal discharges from the cat hippocampus. I. Characteristics and topographical features, *J. Neurophysiol.* **32:**649–662.

Dichter, M., and Spencer, W. A., 1969b, Penicillin-induced interictal discharges from the cat hippocampus. II. Mechanisms underlying origin and restriction, *J. Neurophysiol.* **32:**663–687.

Dingledine, R., 1981, Possible mechanisms of enkephalin action on hippocampal CA1 pyramidal neurons, *J. Neurosci.* **1:**1022–1035.

Dingledine, R., 1983, N-methyl aspartate activates voltage-dependent calcium conductance in rat hippocampal pyramidal cells, *J. Physiol. (London)* **343**:385–405.

Dingledine, R., and Gjerstad, L., 1980, Reduced inhibition during epileptiform activity in the in vitro hippocampal slice, *J. Physiol. (London)* **305**:297–313.

Dingledine, R., and Langmoen, I. A., 1980, Conductance changes and inhibitory actions of hippocampal recurrent IPSPs, *Brain Res.* **185**:277–287.

Djørup, A., Jahnsen, H., and Mosfeldt-Laursen, A., 1981, The dendritic response to GABA in CA1 of the hippocampal slice, *Brain Res.* **219**:196–201.

Dodd, J., and Kelly, J. S., 1978, In somatostatin an excitatory transmitter in the hippocampus?, *Nature* **273**:674–675.

Dodd, J., and Kelly, J. S., 1981, The actions of cholecystokinin and related peptides on pyramidal neurones of the mammalian hippocampus, *Brain Res.* **205**:337–350.

Dodd, J., Kelly, J. S., and Said, S. I., 1979, Excitation of CA1 neurones of the rat hippocampus by the octacosapeptide, vasoactive intestinal polypeptide (VIP), *Br. J. Pharmacol.* **66**:125P.

Dodd, J., Dingledine, R., and Kelly, J. S., 1981, The excitatory action of acetylcholine on hippocampal neurones of the guinea pig and rat maintained in vitro, *Brain Res.* **207**:109–127.

Dolphin, A., Hamont,, M., and Bockaert, J., 1979, The resolution of dopamine and beta-1 and beta-2 adrenergic-sensitive adenylate cyclase activities in homogenates of cat cerebellum, hippocampus, and cerebral cortex, *Brain Res.* **179**:305–317.

Douglas, R. J., 1975, The development of hippocampal function: Implications for theory and for therapy, in: *The Hippocampus*, Vol. 2 (R. L. Isaacson and K. H. Pribram, eds.), Plenum Press, New York, pp. 327–361.

Douglas, R. M., and Goddard, G. V., 1975, Long-term potentiation of the perforant path–granule cell synapse in the rat hippocampus, *Brain Res.* **86**:205–215.

Dudar, J. D., 1974, In vitro excitation of hippocampal pyramidal cell dendrites by glutamic acid, *Neuropharmacology* **13**:1083–1089.

Dudar, J. D., 1975, The effect of septal nuclei stimulation on the release of acetylcholine from the rabbit hippocampus, *Brain Res.* **83**:123–133.

Dudek, F. E., Andrew, R. D., MacVicar, B. A., Snow, R. W., and Taylor, C. P., 1983, Recent evidence for and possible significance of gap junctions and electrotonic synapses in the mammalian brain, in: *Basic Mechanisms of Neuronal Hyperexcitability* (H. H. Jasper and N. M. Van Gelder, eds.), Liss, New York, pp. 31–73.

Dunwiddie, T. V., 1980, Endogenously released adenosine regulates excitability in the in vitro hippocampus, *Epilepsia* **21**:541–548.

Dunwiddie, T. V., and Hoffer, B. J., 1980, Adenine nucleotides and synaptic transmission in the in vitro rat hippocampus, *Br. J. Pharmacol.* **69**:59–68.

Dunwiddie, T., and Lynch, G., 1978, Long-term potentiation and depression of synaptic responses in the rat hippocampus: Localization and frequency dependency, *J. Physiol. (London)* **276**:353–367.

Dunwiddie, T., and Lynch, G., 1979, The relationship between extracellular calcium concentrations and the induction of hippocampal long-term potentiation, *Brain Res.* **169**:103–110.

Dunwiddie, T., Madison, D., and Lynch, G., 1978, Synaptic transmission is required for long-term potentiation, *Brain Res.* **150**:413–417.

Dunwiddie, T., Mueller, A., Palmer, M., Stewart, J., and Hoffer, B., 1980, Electrophysiological interactions of enkephalins with neuronal circuitry in the rat hippocampus. I. Effects on pyramidal cell activity, *Brain Res.* **184**:311–330.

Dunwiddie, T. V., Hoffer, B. J., and Fredholm, B. B., 1981, Alkylxanthines elevate hippocampal excitability: Evidence for a role of endogenous adenosine, *Naunyn-Schmiedebergs Arch. Pharmacol.* **316**:326–330.

Durand, D., Carlen, P. L., Gurevich, N., Ho, A., and Kunov, H., 1983, Electrotonic parameters of rat dentate granule cells measured using short current pulses and HRP staining, *J. Neurophysiol.* **50**:1080–1097.

Eccles, J. C., 1955, The central action of antidromic impulses in motor nerve fibres, *Pfluegers Arch. Gesamte Physiol. Menschen Tiere* **260**:385–415.

Eccles, J. C., 1983, Calcium in long-term potentiation as a model for memory, *Neuroscience* **10**:1071–1081.

Eccles, J. C., Nicoll, R. A., Oshima, T., and Rubia, F. J., 1977, The anionic permeability of the inhibitory postsynaptic membrane of hippocampal pyramidal cells, *Proc. R. Soc. London Ser. B* **198**:315–361.

Engel, J., Jr., Kuhl, D. E., Phelps, M. E., and Crandall, P. H., 1982, Comparative localization of epileptic foci in partial epilepsy by PCT and EEG, *Ann. Neurol.* **12:**529–537.

Enna, S. J., and Snyder, S. H., 1975, Properties of gamma-aminobutyric acid (GABA) binding in rat brain synaptic membrane fractions, *Brain Res.* **100:**81–97.

Fagni, L., Baudry, M., and Lynch, G., 1983, Classification and properties of acidic amino acid receptors in hippocampus. I. Electrophysiological studies of an apparent desensitization and interactions with drugs which block transmission, *J. Neurosci.* **3:**1538–1546.

Fantie, B. D., and Goddard, G. V., 1982, Septal modulation of the population spike in the fascia dentata produced by perforant path stimulation in the rat, *Brain Res.* **252:**227–237.

Feldman, S. C., Dreyfus, C. F., and Lichtenstein, E. S., 1982, Somatostatin neurons in the rodent hippocampus: An in vitro and in vivo immunocytochemical study, *Neurosci. Lett.* **33:**29–34.

Fifkova, E., and Van Harreveld, A., 1977, Long-lasting morphological changes in dendritic spines of dentate granular cells following stimulation of the entorhinal area, *J. Neurocytol.* **6:**211–230.

Fisher, R. S., Pedley, T. A., Moody, W. J., Jr., and Prince, D. A., 1976, The role of extracellular potassium in hippocampal epilepsy, *Arch. Neurol.* **33:**76–83.

Fox, S. E., and Ranck, J. B., Jr., 1981, Electrophysiological characteristics of hippocampal complex-spike cells and theta cells, *Exp. Brain Res.* **41:**399–410.

Fredholm, B. B., and Hedqvist, P., 1980, Modulation of neurotransmission by purine nucleotides and nucleosides, *Biochem. Pharmacol.* **29:**1635–1643.

Frotscher, M., and Zimmer, J., 1983, Commissural fibers terminate on non-pyramidal neurons in the guinea pig hippocampus—A combined Golgi/EM degeneration study, *Brain Res.* **265:**289–293.

Fujita, Y., 1975, Two types of depolarizing after-potentials in hippocampal pyramidal cells of rabbits, *Brain Res.* **94:**435–446.

Fujita, Y., 1979, Evidence for the existence of inhibitory postsynaptic potentials in dendrites and their functional significance in hippocampal pyramidal cells of adult rabbits, *Brain Res.* **175:**59–69.

Fuxe, K., 1965, Evidence for the existence of monoamine neurons in the central nervous system. IV. The distribution of monoamine terminals in the central nervous system, *Acta Physiol. Scand. Suppl.* **247:**37–85.

Gaffan, D., 1974, Recognition impaired and association intact in the memory of monkeys after transection of the fornix, *J. Comp. Physiol. Psychol.* **86:**1100–1109.

Gage, F. H., and Thompson, R. G., 1980, Differential distribution of norepinephrine and serotonin along the dorsal–ventral axis of the hippocampal formation, *Brain Res. Bull.* **5:**771–773.

Gähwiler, B. H., 1980, Excitatory action of opioid peptides and opiates on cultured hippocampal pyramidal cells, *Brain Res.* **194:**193–203.

Gähwiler, B. H., and Maurer, R., 1981, Involvement of mu-receptors in the opioid-induced generation of bursting discharges in hippocampal pyramidal cells, *Regul. Peptides* **2:**91–96.

Gall, C., Brecha, N., Karten, H. J., and Chang, K. J., 1981, Localization of enkephalin-like immunoreactivity to identified axonal and neuronal populations of the rat hippocampus, *J. Comp. Neurol.* **198:**335–350.

Gottlieb, D. I., and Cowan, W. M., 1972, On the distribution of axon terminals containing spheroidal and flattened synaptic vesicles in the hippocampus and dentate gyrus of the rat and cat, *Z. Zellforsch.* **129:**413–429.

Green, J. D., 1964, The hippocampus, *Physiol. Rev.* **44:**561–608.

Green, J.D., and Petsche, H., 1961, Hippocampal electrical activity. IV. Abnormal electrical activity, *Electroencephalogr. Clin. Neurophysiol.* **13:**868–879.

Green, J. D., Maxwell, D. S., Schindler, W. J., and Stumpf, C., 1960, Rabbit EEG "theta" rhythm: Its anatomical source and relation to activity in single neurons, *J. Neurophysiol.* **23:**403–420.

Gustafsson, B., Galvan, M., Grafe, P., and Wigström, H., 1982, A transient outward current in a mammalian central neurone blocked by 4-aminopyridine, *Nature* **299:**252–254.

Haas, H. L., 1981, Histamine hyperpolarizes hippocampal neurones in vitro, *Neurosci. Lett.* **22:**75–78.

Haas, H. L., 1982, Cholinergic disinhibition in hippocampal slices of the rat, *Brain Res.* **233:**200–204.

Haas, H. L., and Ryall, R. W., 1980, Is excitation by enkephalins of hippocampal neurones in the rat due to presynaptic facilitation or to disinhibition?, *J. Physiol.* (*London*) **308:**315–330.

Haas, H. L., and Wolf, P., 1977, Central actions of histamine: Microelectrophoretic studies, *Brain Res.* **122:**269–294.

Haas, H. L., Wolf, P., Palacios, J. M., Garbarg, M., Barbin, G., and Schwartz, J.-C., 1978, Hypersensitivity to histamine in the guinea pig brain: Microiontophoretic and biochemical studies, *Brain Res.* **156:**275–291.

Haas, H. L., Felix, D., Celio, M. R., and Inagami, T., 1980, Angiotensin II in the hippocampus: A histochemical and electrophysiological study, *Experientia* **36:**1394–1395.

Hablitz, J. J., 1981, Altered burst responses in hippocampal CA3 neurons injected with EGTA, *Exp. Brain Res.* **42:**483–485.

Hablitz, J. J., and Johnston, D., 1981, Endogenous nature of spontaneous bursting in hippocampal pyramidal neurons, *Cell. Mol. Neurobiol.* **1:**325–334.

Hablitz, J. J., and Langmoen, I. A., 1982, Excitation of hippocampal pyramidal cells by glutamate in the guinea pig and rat, *J. Physiol. (London)* **325:**317–331.

Halliwell, J. V., and Adams, P. R., 1982, Voltage-clamp analysis of muscarinic excitation in hippocampal neurons, *Brain Res.* **250:**71–92.

Hamlyn, L. H., 1963, An electron microscope study of pyramidal neurons in the Ammon's horn of the rabbit, *J. Anat.* **97:**189–201.

Handelmann, G. E., Meyer, D. K., Beinfeld, M. C., and Oertel, W. H., 1981, CCK-containing terminals in the hippocampus and derived from intrinsic neurons: An immunohistochemical and radioimmunological study, *Brain Res.* **224:**180–184.

Henriksen, S. J., Chouvet, G., and Bloom, F., 1983, Differential responses of hippocampal neurons to endogenous opioid peptides, and opiate alkaloids suggest multiple opiate receptors, *Soc. Neurosci. Abstr.* **9:**1130.

Herrling, P L., 1981, The membrane potential of cat hippocampal neurons recorded in vivo displays four different reaction-mechanisms to iontophoretically applied transmitter agonists, *Brain Res.* **212:**331–343.

Hicks, T. P., and McLennan, H., 1979, Amino acids and the synaptic pharmacology of granule cells in the dentate gyrus of the rat, *Can. J. Physiol. Pharmacol.* **57:**973–978.

Hill, D. R., and Bowery, N. G., 1981, ^{3}H-baclofen and ^{3}H-GABA bind to bicuculline-insensitive $GABA_B$ sites in rat brain, *Nature* **290:**149–152.

Hjorth-Simonsen, A., and Jeune, B., 1972, Origin and termination of the hippocampal perforant path in the rat studied by silver impregnation, *J. Comp. Neurol.* **144:**215–232.

Hodgkin, A. L., and Huxley, A. F., 1952, A quantitative description of membrane current and its application to conduction and excitation in nerve, *J. Physiol. (London)* **117:**500–544.

Hoffer, B. J., Seiger, Å., Taylor, D., Olson, L., and Freedman, R., 1977, Seizures and related epileptiform activity in hippocampus transplanted to the anterior chamber of the eye, *Exp. Neurol.* **54:**233–250.

Hökfelt, T., Ljungdahl, Á., Fuxe, K., and Johansson, O., 1974, Dopamine nerve terminals in the rat limbic cortex: Aspects of the dopamine hypothesis of schizophrenia, *Science* **184:**177–179.

Hong, J.-S., and Schmid, R., 1981, Intrahippocampal distribution of Met^5-enkephalin, *Brain Res.* **205:**415–418.

Hong, J.-S., Yang, H. Y., Fratta, W., and Costa, E., 1977, Determination of methionine-enkephalin in discrete regions of rat brain, *Brain Res.* **134:**383–386.

Horowitz, J. M., and Mates, J. W B., 1975, Signal dispersion within a hippocampal neural network, *Comput. Biol. Med.* **5:**283–296.

Hotson, J. R., and Prince, D. A., 1980, A calcium activated hyperpolarization follows repetitive firing in hippocampal neurons, *J. Neurophysiol.* **43:**409–419.

Hotson, J. R., Prince, D. A., and Schwartzkroin, P. A., 1979, Anomalous inward rectification in hippocampal neurons, *J. Neurophysiol.* **42:**889–895.

Hounsgaard, J., 1978, Presynaptic inhibitory action of acetylcholine in area CA1 of the hippocampus, *Exp. Neurol.* **62:**787–797.

Isaacson, R. L., and Pribram, K. H. (eds.), 1975, *The Hippocampus,* Vols. 1 and 2, Raven Press, New York.

Ishikawa, K., Ott, T., and McGaugh, J. L., 1982, Evidence for dopamine as a transmitter in dorsal hippocampus, *Brain Res.* **232:**222–226.

Jahnsen, H., 1980, The action of 5-hydroxytryptamine on neuronal membranes and synaptic transmission in area CA1 of the hippocampus in vitro, *Brain Res.* **197:**83–94.

Jefferys, J. G. R., and Haas, H L., 1982, Synchronized bursting of CA1 hippocampal pyramidal cells in the absence of synaptic transmission, *Nature* **300:**448–450.

Johnston, D., 1981, Passive cable properties of hippocampal CA3 pyramidal neurons, *Cell. Mol. Neurobiol.* **1:**41–55.

Johnston, D., and Brown, T. H., 1981, Giant synaptic potential hypothesis for epileptiform activity, *Science* **211**:294–297.

Johnston, D., and Brown, T. H., 1983, Interpretation of voltage-clamp measurements in hippocampal neurons, *J. Neurophysiol.* **50**:464–486.

Johnston, D., and Brown, T. H., 1984, Mechanisms of neuronal burst generation, in: *Electrophysiology of Epilepsy* (P. A. Schwartzkroin and H. V. Hweal, eds.), Academic Press, New York, pp. 277–301.

Johnston, D., Hablitz, J. J., and Wilson, W. A., 1980, Voltage clamp discloses slow inward current in hippocampal burst-firing neurones, *Nature* **286**:391–393.

Jones, B. E., and Moore, R. Y., 1977, Ascending projections of the locus coeruleus in the rat. II. Autoradiographic study, *Brain Res.* **127**:23–53.

Kandel, E. R., and Spencer, W. A., 1961, Electrophysiology of hippocampal neurons. II. After-potentials and repetitive firing, *J. Neurophysiol.* **24**:243–259.

Kandel, E. R., Spencer, W. A., and Brinley, F. J., Jr., 1961, Electrophysiology of hippocampal neurons. I. Sequential invasion and synaptic organization, *J. Neurophysiol.* **24**:225–242.

Knowles, W. D., and Schwartzkroin, P. A., 1981, Local circuit synaptic interactions in hippocampal brain slices, *J. Neurosci.* **1**:318–322.

Knowles, W. D., Funch, P. G., and Schwartzkroin, P. A., 1982a, Electrotonic and dye coupling in hippocampal CA1 pyramidal cells in vitro, *Neuroscience* **7**:1713–1722.

Knowles, W. D., Schwartzkroin, P. A, and Schneiderman, J. H., 1982b, Three types of hyperpolarizations in hippocampal CA3 neurons, *Soc. Neurosci. Abstr.* **8**:412.

Kostopoulos, G. K., and Phillis, J. W., 1977, Purinergic depression of neurons in different areas of the rat brain, *Exp. Neurol.* **55**:791–824.

Kramis, R., Vanderwolf, C. H., and Bland, B. H., 1975, Two types of hippocampal rhythmical slow activity in both the rabbit and the rat: Relations to behavior and effects of atropine, diethylether, urethane, and pentobarbital, *Exp. Neurol.* **49**:58–85.

Krnjević, K., and Ropert, N., 1981, Septo-hippocampal pathway modulates hippocampal activity by a cholinergic mechanism, *Can. J. Physiol. Pharmacol.* **59**:911–914.

Krnjević, K., and Ropert, N., 1982, Electrophysiological and pharmacological characteristics of facilitation of hippocampal population spikes by stimulation of the medial septum, *Neuroscience* **7**:2165–2183.

Krnjević, K., Morris, M. E., and Reiffenstein, R. J., 1980, Changes in extracellular Ca^{++} and K^+ activity accompanying hippocampal discharges, *Can. J. Physiol. Pharmacol.* **58**:579–583.

Kromer, L. F., Björklund, A., and Stenevi, U., 1981, Regeneration of the septohippocampal pathway in adult rats is promoted by utilizing embryonic hippocampal implants as bridges, *Brain Res.* **210**:173–200.

Kuhar, M. J., and Yamamura, H. I., 1976, Localization of cholinergic muscarinic receptors in rat brain by light microscopic radioautography, *Brain Res.* **110**:229–243.

Kuhar, M. J., Taylor, N., Wamsley, J. K., Hulme, E. C., and Birdsall, N. J. M., 1981, Muscarinic cholinergic receptor localization in brain by electron microscopic autoradiography, *Brain Res.* **216**:1–9.

Kunkel, D. D., and Schwartzkroin, P. A., 1982, Interneuron morphology in the CA1 region of rabbit hippocampus, *Soc. Neurosci. Abstr.* **8**:216.

Kunkel, D. D., Schwartzkroin, P. A., and Hendrickson, A. E., 1983, Immunocytochemistry of somatostatin in CA1 of rabbit hippocampus, *Soc. Neurosci. Abstr.* **9**:218.

Langmoen, I. A., Segal, M., and Andersen, P., 1981, Mechanisms of norepinephrine actions on hippocampal pyramidal cells in vitro, *Brain Res.* **208**:349–362.

Lebovitz, R. M., Dichter, M., and Spencer, W. A., 1971, Recurrent excitation in the CA3 region of cat hippocampus, *Int. J. Neurosci.* **2**:99–108.

Lee, H. K., Dunwiddie, T., and Hoffer, B., 1980, Electrophysiological interactions of enkephalins with neuronal circuitry in the rat hippocampus. II. Effects on interneuron excitability, *Brain Res.* **184**:331–342.

Lee, K., and Schubert, P., 1982, Modulation of an inhibitory circuit by adenosine and AMP in the hippocampus, *Brain Res.* **246**:311–314.

Lee, K., Schubert, P., Gribkoff, V., Sherman, B., and Lynch, G., 1982, A combined in vivo/in vitro study of the presynaptic release of adenosine derivatives in the hippocampus, *J. Neurochem.* **38**:80–83.

Lee, K. S., Reddington, M., Schubert, P., and Kreutzberg, G., 1983a, Regulation of the strength of adenosine modulation in the hippocampus by a differential distribution of the density of A_1 receptors, *Brain Res.* **260**:156–159.

Lee, K. S., Schubert, P., Reddington, M., and Kreutzberg, G. W., 1983b, Adenosine receptor density and the depression of evoked neuronal activity in the rat hippocampus in vitro, *Neurosci. Lett.* **37**:81–85.

Leung, L. S., 1978, Hippocampal CA1 region—Demonstration of antidromic dendritic spike and dendritic inhibition, *Brain Res.* **158**:219–222.

Levy, W. B., and Steward, O., 1983, Temporal contiguity requirements for long-term associative potentiation/depression in the hippocampus, *Neuroscience* **8**:791–797.

Lewis, E. R., and Cotman, C. W., 1980, Mechanisms of septal lamination in the developing hippocampus revealed by outgrowth of fibers from septal implants. I. Positional and temporal factors, *Brain Res.* **196**:307–330.

Lewis, P. R., Shute, C. C. D., and Silver, A., 1967, Confirmation from choline acetylase analyses of a massive cholinergic innervation to the rat hippocampus, *J. Physiol. (London)* **191**:215–224.

Lieb, J. P., Engel, J. E., Jr., Gevins, A., and Crandall, P. H., 1981, Surface and deep EEG correlates of surgical outcome in temporal lobe epilepsy, *Epilepsia* **22**:515–538.

Lindvall, O., and Björklund, A., 1974, The organization of the ascending catecholamine neuron system in the rat brain as revealed by the glyoxylic acid fluorescence method, *Acta Physiol. Scand.* **412**:1–48.

Llinás, R., and Jahnsen, H., 1982, Electrophysiology of mammalian thalamic neurones in vitro, *Nature* **297**:406–408.

Llinás, R., and Sugimori, M., 1980a, Electrophysiological properties of in vitro Purkinje cell somata in mammalian cerebellar slices, *J. Physiol. (London)* **305**:171–195.

Llinás, R., and Sugimori, M., 1980b, Electrophysiological properties of in vitro Purkinje cell dendrites in mammalian cerebellar slices, *J. Physiol. (London)* **305**:197–213.

Llinás, R., and Yarom, Y., 1981a, Electrophysiology of mammalian inferior olivary neurones in vitro: Different types of voltage-dependent ionic conductances, *J. Physiol. (London)* **315**:549–567.

Llinś, R., and Yarom, Y., 1981b, Properties and distribution of ionic conductances generating electroresponsiveness of mammalian inferior olivary neurones in vitro, *J. Physiol. (London)* **315**:569–584.

Lømo, T., 1971a, Patterns of activation in a monosynaptic cortical pathway: The perforant path input to the dentate area of the hippocampal formation, *Exp. Brain Res.* **12**:18–45.

Lømo, T., 1971b, Potentiation of monosynaptic EPSPs in the perforant path–dentate granule cell synapse, *Exp. Brain Res.* **12**:46–63.

Lorente de Nó, R., 1934, Studies on the structure of the cerebral cortex II. Continuation of the study of the ammonic system, *J. Psychol. Neurol.* **46**:113–177.

Low, W. C., and BeMent, S. L., 1980, Enhancement of afferent fiber activity in hippocampal slices, *Brain Res.* **198**:472–477.

Low, W. C., BeMent, S. L., and Whitehorn, D., 1983, Field-potential evidence for extrasynaptic alterations in the hippocampal CA1 pyramidal cell population during paired-pulse potentiation, *Exp. Neurol.* **80**:9–22.

Lundberg, J. M., and Hökfelt, T., 1983, Coexistence of peptides and classical neurotransmitters, *Trends Neurosci.* **6**:325–333.

Lux, H. D., and Pollen, D. A., 1966, Electrical constants of neurons in the motor cortex of the cat, *J. Neurophysiol.* **29**:207–220.

Lynch, G., and Cotman, C. W., 1975, The hippocampus as a model for studying anatomical plasticity in the adult brain, in: *The Hippocampus*, Vol. 1 (R. L. Isaacson and K. H. Pribram, eds.), Plenum Press, New York, pp. 123–154.

Lynch, G. S., Dunwiddie, T., and Gribkoff, V., 1977, Heterosynaptic depression: A postsynaptic correlate of long-term potentiation, *Nature* **266**:737–739.

Lynch, G. S., Jensen, R. A., McGaugh, J. L., Davila, K., and Oliver, M. W., 1981, Effects of enkephalin, morphine, and naloxone on the electrical activity of the in vitro hippocampal slice preparation, *Exp. Neurol.* **71**:527–540.

McGinty, J. F., Henriksen, S. J., Goldstein, A., Terenius, L., and Bloom, F. E., 1983, Dynorphin is contained within hippocampal mossy fibers: Immunochemical alterations after kainic acid administration and colchicine-induced neurotoxicity, *Proc. Natl. Acad. Sci. USA* **80**:589–593.

McNaughton, B. L., 1980, Evidence for two physiologically distinct perforant pathways to the fascia dentata, *Brain Res.* **199**:1–19.

McNaughton, B. L., 1982, Long-term synaptic enhancement and short-term potentiation in rat fascia dentata act through different mechanisms, *J. Physiol. (London)* **324**:249–262.

McNaughton, B. L., and Barnes, C. A., 1977, Physiological identification and analysis of dentate granule cell responses to stimulation of the medial and lateral perforant pathways in the rat, *J. Comp. Neurol.* **175**:439–454.

McNaughton, B. L., Douglas, R. M., and Goddard, G. V., 1978, Synaptic enhancement in fascia dentata: Cooperativity among coactive afferents, *Brain Res.* **157**:277–293.

McNaughton, B. L., Barnes, C. A., and Andersen, P., 1981, Synaptic efficacy and EPSP summation in granule cells of rat fascia dentata studied in vitro, *J. Neurophysiol.* **46**:952–966.

MacVicar, B. A., and Dudek, F. E., 1980a, Local synaptic circuits in rat hippocampus: Interaction between pyramidal cells, *Brain Res.* **184**:220–223.

MacVicar, B. A., and Dudek, F. E., 1980b, Dye-coupling between CA3 pyramidal cells in slices of rat hippocampus, *Brain Res.* **196**:494–497.

MacVicar, B. A., and Dudek, F. E., 1981, Electrotonic coupling between pyramidal cells: A direct demonstration in rat hippocampal slices, *Science* **213**:782–785.

MacVicar, B. A., and Dudek, F. E., 1982, Electrotonic coupling between granule cells of rat dentate gyrus: Physiological and anatomical evidence, *J. Neurophysiol.* **47**:579–592.

Madison, D. V., and Nicoll, R. A., 1982, Noradrenalin blocks accommodation of pyramidal cell discharge in the hippocampus, *Nature* **299**:636–638.

Madison, D. V., and Nicoll, R. A., 1983, Adaptation of action potential frequency in hippocampal pyramidal cells is regulated by calcium-activated potassium conductance and M-current, *Soc. Neurosci. Abstr.* **9**:601.

Marks, M. J., and Collins, A. C., 1982, Characterization of nicotine binding in mouse brain and comparison with the binding of alpha-bungarotoxin and quinuclidinyl benzilate, *Mol. Pharmacol.* **22**:554–564.

Masukawa, L. M., and Prince, D. A., 1982, Enkephalin inhibition of inhibitory input to CA1 and CA3 pyramidal neurons in the hippocampus, *Brain Res.* **249**:271–280.

Matthews, W. D., McCafferty, G. P., and Setler, P. E., 1981, An electrophysiological model of GABA-mediated neurotransmission, *Neuropharmacology* **20**:561–565.

Minkwitz, H.-G., 1976, Zur Entwicklung der Neuronenstruktur des Hippocampus wahrend der Pra- and Postnatalen Ontogenese der Albinoratte. III. Mitteilung: Morphometrische Erfassung der Ontogenetischen Veranderungen in Dendriten Struktur und Spine Besatz an Pyramiden-Neuronen (CA1) des Hippocampus, *J. Hirnforsch.* **17**:255–275.

Misgeld, U., Sarvey, J. M., and Klee, M. R., 1979, Heterosynaptic postactivation potentiation in hippocampal CA3 neurons: Long-term changes of the postsynaptic potential, *Exp. Brain Res.* **37**:217–229.

Moore, R. Y., 1975, Monoamine neurons innervating the hippocampal formation and septum: Organization and response to injury, in: *The Hippocampus*, Vol. 1 (R. L. Isaacson and K.H. Pribram, eds.), Plenum Press, New York, pp. 215–237.

Moore, R. Y., and Halaris, A. E., 1975, Hippocampal innervation by serotonin neurons of the midbrain raphe in the rat, *J. Comp. Neurol.* **164**:171–184.

Mueller, A. L., and Dunwiddie, T. V., 1983, Anticonvulsant and proconvulsant actions of alpha- and beta-noradrenergic agonists on epileptiform activity in rat hippocampus in vitro, *Epilepsia* **24**:57–64.

Mueller, A. L., and Schwartzkroin, P. A., 1983, Electrophysiological actions of somatostatin (SRIF) in rabbit hippocampus studied in vitro, *Soc. Neurosci. Abstr.* **9**:219.

Mueller, A. L., Hoffer, B. J., and Dunwiddie, T. V., 1981, Noradrenergic responses in rat hippocampus: Evidence for mediation by α and β receptors in the in vitro slice, *Brain Res.* **214**:113–126.

Mueller, A. L., Palmer, M. R., Hoffer, B. J., and Dunwiddie, T. V., 1982, Hippocampal noradrenergic responses in vivo and in vitro: Characterization of alpha and beta components, *Naunyn-Schmiedebergs Arch. Pharmacol.* **318**:259–266.

Mueller, A. L., Chesnut, R. M., and Schwartzkroin, P. A., 1983, Actions of GABA in developing rabbit hippocampus: An in vitro study, *Neurosci. Lett.* **39**:193–198.

Mühlethaler, M., Dreifuss, J. J., and Gähwiler, B. H., 1982, Vasopressin excites hippocampal neurones, *Nature* **296**:749–751.

Mühlethaler, M., Sawyer, W. H., Manning, M. M., and Dreifuss, J. J., 1983, Characterization of a uterine-type oxytocin receptor in the rat hippocampus, *Proc. Natl. Acad. Sci. USA* **80:**6713–6717.

Muller, R. U., Kubie, J. L., and Ranck, J. B., Jr., 1983, High resolution mapping of the "spatial" fields of hippocampal neurons in the freely moving rat, *Soc. Neurosci. Abstr.* **9:**646.

Nadler, J. V., Vaca, K. W., White, W. F., Lynch, G. S., and Cotman, C. W., 1976, Aspartate and glutamate as possible transmitters of excitatory hippocampal afferents, *Nature* **260:**538–540.

Nadler, J. V., White, W. F., Vaca, K. W., Redburn, D. A., and Cotman, C. W., 1977, Characterization of putative amino acid transmitter release from slices of rat dentate gyrus, *J. Neurochem.* **29:**279–290.

Nadler, J. V., White, W. F., Vaca, K. W., Perry, B. W., and Cotman, C. W., 1978, Biochemical correlates of transmission mediated by glutamate and aspartate, *J. Neurochem.* **31:**147–155.

Newberry, N. R., and Nicoll, R. A., 1983, Direct inhibitory action of baclofen on hippocampal pyramidal cells, *Soc. Neurosci. Abstr.* **9:**457.

Nicoll, R. A., and Alger, B. E., 1981, Synaptic excitation may activate a calcium-dependent potassium conductance in hippocampal pyramidal cell, *Science* **212:**957–959.

Nicoll, R. A., Siggins, G. R., Ling, N., Bloom, F. E., and Guillemen, R., 1977, Neuronal actions of endorphins and enkephalins among brain regions: A comparative microiontophoretic study, *Proc. Natl. Acad. Sci. USA* **74:**2584–2588.

Nicoll, R. A., Alger, B. E., and Jahr, C. E., 1980, Enkephalin blocks inhibitory pathways in the vertebrate CNS, *Nature* **287:**22–25.

Numann, R., Wong, R. K. S., and Clark, R., 1982, Electrophysiology of single dissociated cortical neurons, *Soc. Neurosci. Abstr.* **8:**413.

Okada, Y., and Ozawa, S., 1980, Inhibitory action of adenosine on synaptic transmission in the hippocampus of the guinea pig in vitro, *Eur. J. Pharmacol.* **68:**483–492.

Okada, Y., and Shimada, C., 1975, Distribution of γ-aminobutyric acid (GABA) and glutamate decarboxylase (GAD) activity in the guinea pig hippocampus—Microassay method for the determination of GAD activity, *Brain Res.* **98:**202–206.

O'Keefe, J., and Nadel, L., 1978, *The Hippocampus as a Cognitive Map*, Oxford University Press, London.

Olds, J., 1972, Learning and the hippocampus, *Rev. Can. Bio. Suppl.* **31:**215–238.

Olds, J., Disterhoft, J. F., Segal, M., Kornblith, C. L., and Hirsh, R., 1972, Learning centers of rat brain mapped by measuring latencies of conditioned unit responses, *J. Neurophysiol.* **35:**202–219.

Olpe, H.-R., Balcar, V. J., Bittiger, H., Rink, H., and Sieber, P., 1980, Central actions of somatostatin, *Eur. J. Pharmacol.* **63:**127–133.

Olsen, R. W., Bergman, M O., VanNess, P. C., Lummis, S. C, Watkins, A. E., Napias, C., and Greenlee, D. V., 1981, Gamma-aminobutyric acid receptor binding in mammalian brain: Heterogeneity of binding sites, *Mol. Pharmacol.* **19:**217–227.

Olton, D. S., Becker, J. T., and Handelmann, G. E., 1979, Hippocampus, space, and memory, *Behav. Brain Sci.* **2:**313–365.

Palacios, J. M., DeHaven, R. N., and Kuhar M. J., 1980, Localization of beta-adrenergic receptors in rat brain by light microscopic autoradiography, *Fed. Proc.* **39:**593.

Peroutka, S. J., and Snyder, S. H., 1981, Two distinct serotonin receptors: Regional variations in receptor binding in mammalian brain, *Brain Res.* **208:**339–347.

Petsche, H., Stumpf, C., and Gogolak, G., 1962, The significance of the rabbit's septum as a relay station between midbrain and hippocampus. I. The control of hippocampus arousal activity by septum cells, *Electroencephalogr. Clin. Neurophysiol.* **14:**201–211.

Pittman, Q. J., and Siggins, G. R., 1981, Somatostatin hyperpolarized hippocampal pyramidal cells in vitro, *Brain Res.* **221:**402–408.

Prince, D. A., 1983, Ionic mechanisms in cortical and hippocampal epileptogenesis, in: *Basic Mechanisms of Neuronal Hyperexcitability* (H. H. Jasper and N. VanGelder, eds.), Liss, New York, pp. 217–243.

Proctor, W. R., and Dunwiddie, T. V., 1983, Adenosine inhibits calcium spikes in hippocampal pyramidal neurons in vitro, *Neurosci. Lett.* **35:**197–201.

Purpura, D. P., and Malliani, A., 1966, Spike generation and propagation initiated in dendrites by transhippocampal polarization, *Brain Res.* **1:**403–406.

Purpura, D. P., Prelevic, S., and Santini, M., 1968, Hyperpolarizing increase in membrane conductance in hippocampal neurons, *Brain Res.* **7:**310–312.

Racine, R. J., and Milgram, N. W., 1983, Short-term potentiation phenomena in the rat limbic forebrain, *Brain Res.* **260**:201–216.

Racine, R. J., Milgram, N. W., and Hafncr, S., 1983, Long-term potentiation phenomena in the rat limbic forebrain, *Brain Res.* **260**:217–231.

Raisman, G., 1966, The connexions of the septum, *Brain* **89**:317–348.

Rall, W., 1969, Time constants and electrotonic length constants of membrane cylinders and neurons, *Biophys. J.* **9**:1483–1508.

Rall, W., 1974, Dendritic spines, synaptic potency and neuronal plasticity, in: *Cellular Mechanisms Subserving Changes in Neuronal Activity* (C. D. Woody, K. A. Brown, T. J. Crow, and J. D. Knispe, eds.), Brain Information Service, UCLA, Los Angeles, pp. 13–21.

Rall, W., 1977, Core conductor theory and cable properties of neurons, in: *Handbook of Physiology, The Nervous System*, Section I(E. R. Kandel, ed.), Williams & Wilkins, Baltimore, pp. 39–98.

Rall, W., and Rinzel, J., 1973, Branch input resistance and steady attenuation for input to one branch of a dendritic neuron model, *Biophys. J.* **13**:648–688.

Ramón y Cajal, S., 1911, *Histologie du systemé nerveux de l'Homme et des Vertébrés*, Maloine, Paris.

Ranck, J. B., Jr., 1973, Studies on single neurons in dorsal hippocampal formation and septum in unrestrained rats. Part 1. Behavioral correlates and firing repertoires, *Exp. Neurol.* **41**:461–534.

Reddington, M., Lee, K., and Schubert, P., 1982, An A_1-adenosine receptor characterized by ^{3}H-cyclohexyladenosine binding, moderates the depression of evoked potentials in a rat hippocampal slice preparation, *Neurosci. Lett.* **28**:275–279.

Ribak, C. E., Vaughn, J. E., and Saito, K., 1978, Immunocytochemical localization of glutamic acid decarboxylase in neuronal somata following colchicine inhibition of axonal transport, *Brain Res.* **140**:315–332.

Robinson, J. H., and Deadwyler, S. A., 1981, Intracellular correlates of morphine excitation in the hippocampal slice preparation, *Brain Res.* **224**:375–387.

Rose, A. M., Hattori, T., and Fibiger, H. C., 1976, Analysis of the septo-hippocampal pathway by light and electron microscopic autoradiography, *Brain Res.* **108**:170–174.

Salmoiraghi, G. C., and Stefanis, C. N., 1965, Patterns of central neuron responses to suspected transmitters, *Arch. Ital. Biol.* **103**:705–724.

Sandoval, M. E., Horch, P., and Cotman, C. W., 1978, Evaluation of glutamate as a hippocampal neurotransmitter: Glutamate uptake and release from synaptosomes, *Brain Res.* **142**:285–299.

Sastry, B. R., 1982, Presynaptic change associated with long-term potentiation in hippocampus, *Life Sci.* **30**:2003–2008.

Sawada, S., Takada, S., and Yamamoto, C., 1982, Excitatory actions of homocysteic acid on hippocampal neurons, *Brain Res.* **238**:282–285.

Scatton, B., Simon, H., Le Moal, M., and Bischoff, S., 1980, Origin of dopaminergic innervation of the rat hippocampal formation, *Neurosci. Lett.* **18**:125–131.

Schmalbruch, H., and Jahnsen, H., 1981, Gap junctions on CA3 pyramidal cells of guinea pig hippocampus shown by freeze fracture, *Brain Res.* **217**:175–178.

Schubert, P., and Mitzdorf, U., 1979, Analysis and quantitative evaluation of the depressive effect of adenosine on evoked potentials in hippocampal slices, *Brain Res.* **172**:186–190.

Schwartz, J.-C., Barbin, G., Duchemin, A. M., Garbarg, M., Palacios, J. M., Quach, T. T., and Rose, C., 1980, Histamine receptors in brain: Characterization by binding studies and biochemical effects, in: *Receptors for Neurotransmitters and Peptide Hormones* (G. Pepeu, M. J. Kuhar, and S. J. Enna, eds.), Raven Press, New York, pp. 169–182.

Schwartzkroin, P. A., 1975, Characteristics of CA1 neurons recorded intracellularly in the hippocampal in vitro slice preparation, *Brain Res.* **85**:423–436.

Schwartzkroin, P. A., 1983a, Mechanisms of cell synchronization in epileptiform activity, *Trends Neurosci.* **6**:157–160.

Schwartzkroin, P. A., 1983b, Local circuit considerations and intrinsic neuronal properties involved in hyperexcitability and cell synchronization, in *Basic Mechanisms of Neuronal Hyperexcitability* (N. VanGelder and H. H. Jasper, eds.), Liss, New York, pp. 75–108.

Schwartzkroin, P. A., and Andersen, P., 1975, Glutamic acid sensitivity of dendrites in hippocampal slices in vitro, in: *Physiology and Pathology of Dendrites* (G. Kreutzberg, cd.), Raven Press, New York, pp. 45–51.

Schwartzkroin, P. A., and Knowles, W. D., 1983, Local interactions in the hippocampus, *Trends Neurosci.* **6**:88–92.

Schwartzkroin, P. A., and Mathers, L. H., 1978, Physiological and morphological identification of a nonpyramidal hippocampal cell type, *Brain Res.* **157:**1–10.

Schwartzkroin, P. A., and Pedley, T. A., 1979, Slow depolarizing potentials in "epileptic" neurons, *Epilepsia* **20:**267–277.

Schwartzkroin, P. A., and Prince, D. A., 1977, Penicillin-induced epileptiform activity in the hippocampal in vitro preparation, *Ann. Neurol.* **1:**463–469.

Schwartzkroin, P. A., and Prince, D. A., 1978, Cellular and field potential properties of epileptogenic hippocampal slices, *Brain Res.* **147:**117–130.

Schwartzkroin, P. A., and Prince D. A., 1979, Recordings from presumed glial cells in the hippocampal slice, *Brain Res.* **161:**533–538.

Schwartzkroin, P. A., and Prince, D. A., 1980a, Effects of TEA on hippocampal neurons, *Brain Res.* **185:**169–181.

Schwartzkroin, P. A., and Prince, D. A., 1980b, Changes in excitatory and inhibitory synaptic potentials leading to epileptogenic activity, *Brain Res.* **183:**61–76.

Schwartzkroin, P. A., and Slawsky, M., 1977, Probable calcium spike in hippocampal neurons, *Brain Res.* **135:**157–161.

Schwartzkroin, P. A., and Stafstrom, C. E., 1980, Effects of EGTA on the calcium-activated afterhyperpolarization in hippocampal CA3 pyramidal cells, *Science* **210:**1125–1126.

Schwartzkroin, P. A., and Wester, K., 1975, Long-term facilitation of a synaptic potential following tetanization in the in vitro hippocampal slice, *Brain Res.* **89:**107–119.

Schwartzkroin, P. A., and Wyler, A. R., 1980, Mechanisms underlying epileptiform burst discharge, *Ann. Neurol.* **7:**95–107.

Schwartzkroin, P. A., Kunkel, D. D., and Mathers, L. H., 1982, Development of rabbit hippocampus: Anatomy, *Dev. Brain Res.* **2:**453–468.

Scoville, W. B., and Milner, B., 1957, Loss of recent memory after bilateral hippocampal lesions, *J. Neurol. Neurosurg. Psychiatry* **20:**11–21.

Segal, M., 1975, Physiological and pharmacological evidence for a serotonergic projection to the hippocampus, *Brain Res.* **94:**115–131.

Segal, M., 1980a, The action of serotonin in the rat hippocampal slice preparation, *J. Physiol. (London)* **303:**423–439.

Segal, M., 1980b, Histamine produces a Ca^{+2}-sensitive depolarization of hippocampal pyramidal cells in vitro, *Neurosci. Lett.* **19:**67–71.

Segal, M., 1981a, The action of norepinephrine in the rat hippocampus: Intracellular studies in the slice preparation, *Brain Res.* **206:**107–128.

Segal, M., 1981b, Histamine modulates reactivity of hippocampal CA3 neurons to afferent stimulation in vitro, *Brain Res.* **213:**443–448.

Segal, M., 1981c, Regional differences in neuronal responses to 5-HT: Intracellular studies in hippocampal slices, *J. Physiol. (Paris)* **77:**373–375.

Segal, M., 1982a, Multiple actions of acetylcholine at a muscarinic receptor studied in the rat hippocampal slice, *Brain Res.* **246:**77–87.

Segal, M., 1982b, Intracellular analysis of a postsynaptic action of adenosine in the rat hippocampus, *Eur. J. Pharmacol.* **79:**193–199.

Segal, M., 1982c, Norepinephrine modulates reactivity of hippocampal cells to chemical stimulation in vitro, *Exp Neurol.* **77:**86–93.

Segal, M., and Bloom, F. E., 1974a, The action of norepinephrine in the rat hippocampus. I. Iontophoretic studies, *Brain Res.* **72:**79–97.

Segal, M., and Bloom, F. E., 1974b, The action of norepinephrine in the rat hippocampus. II. Activation of the input pathway, *Brain Res.* **72:**99–114.

Segal, M., and Gutnick, M. J., 1980, Effects of serotonin on extracellular potassium concentration in the rat hippocampal slice, *Brain Res.* **195:**389–401.

Segal, M., and Landis, S., 1974, Afferents to the hippocampus of the rat studied with the method of retrograde transport of horseradish peroxidase, *Brain Res.* **78:**1–15.

Segal, M, Pickel, V., and Bloom, F. E., 1973, The projections of the nucleus locus coeruleus: An autoradiographic study, *Life Sci.* **13:**817–821.

Segal, M., Greenberger, V., and Hofstein, R., 1981, Cyclic AMP-generating systems in rat hippocampal slices, *Brain Res.* **213:**351–364.

Seifert, W., 1983, *Neurobiology of the Hippocampus*, Academic Press, New York.

Seress, L., and Ribak, C. E., 1983, GABAergic cells in the dentate gyrus appear to be local circuit and projection neurons, *Exp. Brain Res.* **50**:173–182.

Siggins, G .R., and Schubert, P., 1981, Adenosine depression of hippocampal neurons in vitro: An intracellular study of dose-dependent actions on synaptic and membrane potentials, *Neurosci. Lett.* **23**:55–60.

Smith, C. M., 1974, Acetylcholine release from the cholinergic septo-hippocampal pathway, *Life Sci.* **14**:2159–2166.

Snyder, S. H., 1981, Adenosine receptors and the actions of methylxanthines, *Trends Neurosci.* **4**:242–244.

Somogyi, P., Nunzi, M. G., Gorio, A., and Smith, A. D., 1983a, A new type of specific interneuron in the monkey hippocampus forming synapses exclusively with the axon initial segments of pyramidal cells, *Brain Res.* **259**:137–142.

Somogyi, P., Smith, A. D., Nunzi, M. G., Gorio, A., Takagi, H., and Wu, J. Y., 1983b, Glutamate decarboxylase immunoreactivity in the hippocampus of the cat: Distribution of immunoreactive synaptic terminals with special reference to the axon initial segment of pyramidal neurons, *J. Neurosci.* **3**:1450–1468.

Spencer, W. A., and Kandel, E. R., 1961a, Electrophysiology of hippocampal neurons. III. Firing level and time constant, *J. Neurophysiol.* **24**:260–271.

Spencer, W. A., and Kandel, E. R., 1961b, Electrophysiology of hippocampal neurons. IV. Fast prepotentials, *J. Neurophysiol.* **24**:272–285.

Spencer, W. A., and Kandel, E. R., 1961c, Hippocampal neuron responses to selective activation of recurrent collaterals of hippocampofugal axons, *Exp. Neurol.* **4**:149–161.

Spencer, W. A., and Kandel, E. R., 1968, Cellular and integrative properties of the hippocampal pyramidal cell and the comparative electrophysiology of cortical neuron, *Int. J. Neurol.* **6**:266–296.

Squire, L. R., 1982, The neuropsychology of human memory, *Annu. Rev. Neurosci.* **5**:241–273.

Stafstrom, C. E., Schwindt, P. C., and Crill, W. E., 1982, Negative slope conductance due to a persistent subthreshold sodium current in cat neocortical neurons in vitro, *Brain Res.* **236**:221–226.

Stanley, J. C., DeFrance, J. F., and Marchand, J. F., 1979, Tetanic and posttetanic potentiation in the septohippocampal pathway, *Exp. Neurol.* **64**:445–451.

Stanton, P. K., and Sarvey, J. M., 1983, Blockade of long-term potentiation in rat hippocampal CA1 region by the protein synthesis inhibitors emetine and cycloheximide, *Soc. Neurosci. Abstr.* **9**:678.

Steinbusch, H. W. M., 1981, Distribution of serotonin-immunoreactivity in the central nervous system of the rat—cell bodies and terminals, *Neuroscience* **6**:557–618.

Stengaard-Pedersen, K., Fredens, K., and Larsson, L.-I., 1981, Enkephalin and zinc in the hippocampal mossy fiber system, *Brain Res.* **212**:230–233.

Steward, O., 1976a, Topographic organization of the projections from the entorhinal area to the hippocampal formation of the rat, *J. Comp. Neurol.* **167**:285–314.

Steward, O., 1976b, Reinnervation of dentate gyrus by homologous afferents following entorhinal cortical lesions in adult rats, *Science* **194**:426–428.

Steward, O., and Brassel, S., 1983, Intrahippocampal injections of cycloheximide reversibly block long term potentiation, *Soc. Neurosci. Abstr.* **9**:860.

Steward, O., White, W. F., Cotman, C. W., and Lynch, G., 1976, Potentiation of excitatory synaptic transmission in the normal and in the reinnervated dentate gyrus of the rat, *Exp. Brain Res.* **26**:423–441.

Steward, O., White, W. F., and Cotman, C. W., 1977, Potentiation of the excitatory synaptic action of commissural, associational and entorhinal afferents to dentate granule cells, *Brain Res.* **134**:551–560.

Storm-Mathisen, J., 1972, Glutamate decarboxylase in the rat hippocampal region after lesions of the afferent fibre systems: Evidence that enzyme is localized in intrinsic neurons, *Brain Res.* **40**:215–235.

Storm-Mathisen, J., 1977, Localization of transmitter candidates in the brain: The hippocampal formation as a model, *Prog. Neurobiol.* **8**:119–181.

Storm-Mathisen, J., and Fonnum, F., 1971, Quantitative histochemistry of glutamate decarboxylase in rat hippocampal region, *J. Neurochem.* **18**:1105–1111.

Struble, R. B., Desmond, N. L., and Levy, W. B., 1978, Anatomical evidence for interlamellar inhibition in the fascia dentata, *Brain Res.* **152**:580–585.

Swanson, L. W., and Hartman, B. K., 1975, The central adrenergic system: An immunofluorescence study of the location of cell bodies and their efferent connections in the rat utilizing dopamine-beta-hydroxylase as a marker, *J. Comp. Neurol.* **163:**467–506.

Swanson, L. W., Teyler, T. J., and Thompson, R. F. (eds.), 1982, Hippocampal long-term potentiation: Mechanisms and implications for memory, *Neurosci. Res. Progr. Bull.* **20.**

Taylor, C. P., and Dudek, F. E., 1982a, A physiological test for electrotonic coupling between CA1 pyramidal cells in rat hippocampal slices, *Brain Res.* **235:**351–357.

Taylor, C. P., and Dudek, E. E., 1982b, Synchronous neural afterdischarges in rat hippocampal slices without active chemical synapses, *Science* **218:**810–812.

Taylor, D., Freedman, R., Seiger, Å., Olson, L., and Hoffer, B., 1980, Conditions for adrenergic hyperinnervation in hippocampus. II. Electrophysiological evidence from intraocular double grafts, *Exp. Brain Res.* **39:**289–299.

Teyler, T. J., and Alger, B. E., 1976, Monosynaptic habituation in the vertebrate forebrain: The dentate gyrus examined in vitro, *Brain Res.* **115:**413–425.

Thalmann, R. H., and Ayala, G. F., 1982, A late increase in potassium conductance follows synaptic stimulation of granule neurons of the dentate gyrus, *Neurosci. Lett.* **29:**243–248.

Thalmann, R. H., Peck, E. J., and Ayala, G. F., 1981, Biphasic response of hippocampal pyramidal neurons to GABA, *Neurosci. Lett.* **21:**319–324.

Thompson, R. F., Berger, T. W., Berry, S. D., Hoehler, F.K., Kettner, R. E., and Weisz, D. J., 1980, Hippocampal substrate of classical conditioning, *Physiol. Psychol.* **8:**262–279.

Traub, R. D., 1983, Cellular mechanisms underlying the inhibitory surround of penicillin epileptogenic foci, *Brain Res.* **261:**277–284.

Traub, R. D., and Llinás, R., 1979, Hippocampal pyramidal cells: Significance of dendritic ionic conductances for neuronal function and epileptogenesis, *J. Neurophysiol.* **42:**476–496.

Traub, R. D., and Wong, R. K. S., 1981, Penicillin-induced epileptiform activity in the hippocampal slice: A model of synchronization of CA3 pyramidal cell bursting, *Neuroscience* **6:**223–230.

Traub, R. D., and Wong, R. K. S., 1983a, Synaptic mechanisms underlying interictal spike initiation in a hippocampal network, *Neurology* **33:**257–266.

Traub, R. D., and Wong, R. K. S., 1983b, Synchronized burst discharge in disinhibited hippocampal slice. II. Model of cellular mechanism, *J. Neurophysiol.* **49:**459–471.

Turner, D. A., and Schwartzkroin, P. A., 1980, Steady-state electrotonic analysis of intracellularly stained hippocampal neurons, *J. Neurophysiol.* **44:**184–199.

Turner, D. A., and Schwartzkroin, P. A., 1983, Electrical characteristics of dendrites and dendritic spines in intracellularly stained CA3 and dentate hippocampal neurons, *J. Neurosci.* **3:**2381–2394.

Turner, R. W., Baimbridge, K. G., and Miller, J. J., 1982, Calcium-induced long-term potentiation in the hippocampus, *Neuroscience* **7:**1411–1416.

Turner, R. W., Richardson, T. L., and Miller, J. J., 1983, Role of ephaptic interactions in paired pulse and frequency potentiation of hippocampal field potentials, *Soc. Neurosci. Abstr.* **9:**733.

Turner, R. W., Richardson, T.L., and Miller J. J., 1984, Ephaptic interactions contribute to paired pulse and frequency potentiation of hippocampal field potentials, *Exp. Brain Res.* **59:**567–570.

Valentino, R. J., and Dingledine, R., 1981, Presynaptic inhibitory effect of acetylcholine in the hippocampus, *J. Neurosci.* **1:**784–792.

Vanderwolf, C. H., Kramis, R., Gillespie, L. A., and Bland, B. H., 1975, Hippocampal slow activity and neocortical low voltage fast activity: Relations to behavior, in: *The Hippocampus*, Vol. 2 (R. L. Isaacson and K. H. Pribram, eds.), Plenum Press, New York, pp. 101–128.

Vickery, B. G., Schmechel, D. E., and Haring, J. H., 1983, Study of GABAergic non-pyramidal neurons in plexiform layers and deep white matter of rat hippocampus, *Soc. Neurosci. Abstr.* **9:**408.

Voronin, L. L., 1983, Long-term potentiation in the hippocampus. *Neuroscience* **10:**1051–1069.

Watanabe, T., Taguchi, Y., Hayashi, H., Tanaka, J., Shiosaka, S., Tohyama, M., Kubota, H., Terano, Y., and Wada, H., 1983, Evidence for the presence of a histaminergic neuron system in the rat brain: An immunohistochemical analysis, *Neurosci. Lett.* **39:**249–254.

Watkins, J C., and Evans, R. H., 1981, Excitatory amino acid transmitters, *Annu. Rev. Pharmacol. Toxicol.* **21:**165–204.

Westrum, L. E., and Blackstad, T. W., 1962, An electron microscopic study of the stratum radiatum of the rat hippocampus (regio superior, CA1) with particular emphasis on synaptology, *J. Comp. Neurol.* **119:**281–309.

White, W. F., Nadler, J. V., and Cotman, C. W., 1979, The effect of acidic amino acid antagonists on synaptic transmission in the hippocampal formation in vitro, *Brain Res.* **164:**177–194.

Wieraszko, A., and Lynch, G., 1979, Stimulation-dependent release of possible transmitter substances from hippocampal slices studied with localized perfusion, *Brain Res.* **160**:372–376.

Wigström, H., and Gustafsson, B., 1981, Increased excitability of hippocampal unmyelinated fibres following conditioning stimulation, *Brain Res.* **229**:507–513.

Wigström, H., Swann, J. W., and Andersen, P., 1979, Calcium dependency of synaptic long-lasting potentiation in the hippocampal slice, *Acta Physiol. Scand.* **105**:126–128.

Wilson, R. C., Levy, W. B., and Steward, O., 1981, Changes in translation of synaptic excitation to dentate granule cell discharge accompanying long-term potentiation. II. An evaluation of mechanisms utilizing dentate gyrus dually innervated by surviving ipsilateral and sprouted crossed temporodentate inputs, *J. Neurophysiol.* **46**:339–355.

Wimer, R. E., Norman, R., and Eleftheriou, B. E., 1973, Serotonin levels in hippocampus: Striking variations associated with mouse strain and treatment, *Brain Res.* **63**:397–401.

Winson, J., 1974, Patterns of hippocampal theta rhythm in the freely moving rat, *Electroencephalogr. Clin. Neurophysiol.* **36**:291–301.

Winson, J., 1980, Raphe influences on neuronal transmission from perforant pathway through dentate gyrus, *J. Neurophysiol.* **44**:937–950.

Wong, R. K. S., and Clark, R. B., 1983, Single K^+ channel currents from hippocampal pyramidal cells of adult guinea pig, *Soc. Neurosci. Abstr.* **9**:602.

Wong, R. K. S., and Prince, D. A., 1978, Participation of calcium spikes during intrinsic burst firing in hippocampal neurons, *Brain Res.* **159**:385–390.

Wong, R. K. S., and Prince, D. A., 1979, Dendritic mechanisms underlying penicillin-induced epileptiform activity, *Science* **204**:1228–1231.

Wong, R. K. S., and Prince, D. A., 1981, Afterpotential generation in hippocampal pyramidal cells, *J. Neurophysiol.* **45**:86–97.

Wong, R. K. S., and Schwartzkroin, P. A., 1982, Pacemaker neurons in the mammalian brain: Mechanisms and function, in: *Cellular Pacemakers, Mechanisms of Pacemaker Generation*, Vol. 1 (D. O. Carpenter, ed.), Wiley, New York, pp. 237–254.

Wong, R. K. S., and Traub, R. D., 1983, Synchronized burst discharge in disinhibited hippocampal slice. I. Initiation in CA2–CA3 region, *J. Neurophysiol.* **49**:442–458.

Wong, R. K. S., Prince, D. A., and Basbaum, A. I., 1979, Intradendritic recordings from hippocampal neurons, *Proc. Natl. Acad. Sci. USA* **76**:986–990.

Wong, R. K. S., Traub, R. D., and Miles, R., 1984, Epileptogenic mechanisms as revealed by studies of the hippocampal slice, in: *Electrophysiology of Epilepsy* (P. A. Schwartzkroin and H. V. Wheal, eds.), Academic Press, New York, pp. 253–275.

Woodward, D. J., Moises, H. C., Waterhouse, B. D., Hoffer, B. J., and Freedman, R., 1979, Modulatory actions of norepinephrine in the central nervous system, *Fed. Proc.* **38**:2109–2116.

Yaari, Y., Konnerth, A., and Heinemann, U., 1983, Spontaneous epileptiform activity of CA1 hippocampal neurons in low extracellular calcium solutions, *Exp. Brain Res.* **51**:153–156.

Yamamoto, C., 1972, Activation of hippocampal neurons by mossy fiber stimulation in thin brain sections in vitro, *Exp. Brain Res.* **14**:423–435.

Yamamoto, C., and Chujo, T., 1978, Long-term potentiation in thin hippocampal sections studied by intracellular and extracellular recordings, *Exp. Neurol.* **58**:242–250.

Yamamoto, C., and Kawai, N., 1967, Presynaptic action of acetylcholine in thin sections from the guinea pig dentate gyrus in vitro, *Exp. Neurol.* **19**:176–187.

Yamamoto, C., Matsumoto, K., and Takagi, M., 1980, Potentiation of excitatory postsynaptic potentials during and after repetitive stimulation in thin hippocampal sections, *Exp. Brain Res.* **38**:469–477.

Yamamoto, C., Sawada, S., and Takada, S., 1983, Suppressing action of 2-amino-4-phosphonobutyric acid on mossy fiber-induced excitation in the guinea pig hippocampus, *Exp. Brain Res.* **51**:128–134.

Young, W. S., and Kuhar, M. J., 1980, Noradrenergic alpha-1 and alpha-2 receptors: Light microscopic autoradiographic localization, *Fed. Proc.* **39**:593.

Zieglgänsberger, W., French, E., Siggins, G., and Bloom, F., 1979, Opioid peptides may excite hippocampal pyramidal neurons by inhibiting adjacent inhibitory interneurons, *Science* **205**:415–417.

Zimmer, J., 1971, Ipsilateral afferents to the commissural zone of the fascia dentata demonstrated in decommissurated rats by silver impregnation, *J. Comp. Neurol.* **142**:393–416.

9

The Hippocampal
Formation of the
Primate Brain
A Review of Some Comparative Aspects of
Cytoarchitecture and Connections

DOUGLAS L. ROSENE and GARY W. VAN HOESEN

1. Introduction

The long-standing interest of neuroscientists in the hippocampal formation has occurred from the perspective of two rather different points of view. On the one hand, the comparatively simple cytoarchitecture of the hippocampal formation and the laminar segregation of its extrinsic and intrinsic afferents make it an interesting and relatively simple model system for experimental manipulation and investigation. Chapter 8 in this volume, by Schwartzkroin and Mueller, is a thoughtful review of how effective the hippocampus has been as a model system for neurophysiological studies using the *in vitro* slice preparation. Other investigations have utilized the hippocampal formation to study the effects of genetic defects in neuronal development (e.g., Nowakowski and Davis, 1985),

A key to the abbreviations used in the illustrations is given in Section 10, pp. 448–450.

DOUGLAS L. ROSENE • Department of Anatomy, Boston University School of Medicine, Boston, Massachusetts 02118.   GARY W. VAN HOESEN • Departments of Anatomy and Neurology, University of Iowa College of Medicine, Iowa City, Iowa 52242.

345

collateral sprouting induced by deafferentation (e.g., Lynch *et al.*, 1972; Cotman and Nadler, 1978), or intracerebral transplantation (e.g., Frotscher and Zimmer, 1986). While most of the studies that use the hippocampal formation as a model system have focused on the rodent, the other major interest in the hippocampal formation has grown out of a variety of clinical and experimental data derived from humans and nonhuman primates. These latter investigations have focused on the disruption of certain aspects of the memory process produced by hippocampal lesions as first described in human neurosurgical patients (Scoville and Milner, 1957; Penfield and Milner, 1958) and subsequently investigated in nonhuman primates (e.g., Moss *et al.*, 1981). These studies have engendered the view that the hippocampus is an important, if not essential, component of the neural systems responsible for normal learning and memory, especially the anterograde episodic and contextual aspects of memory. In human patients with hippocampal lesions the generic aspects of memory are largely preserved, i.e., a car is still a car, a dog is still a dog, etc., but learning and remembering whose car it might be or whose dog it is are impossible.

The present chapter is motivated largely by this latter point of view and concentrates on the structure of the primate hippocampal formation and features of its anatomical organization that may reflect its role in higher cognitive processes in primates. In this regard there are several themes that occur throughout the following discussion. One is the notion that the mammalian hippocampal formation is *not* a phylogenetically static structure as its rather consistent cytoarchitecture might suggest. A corollary of this is that the primate hippocampal formation *is* a progressive structure that has developed in concert with the expanding primate neocortex. An additional theme is that the primate hippocampal formation is likely to have structural features and connections that have no homologue in rats, rabbits, guinea pigs, or other nonprimates in which the hippocampal formation has been investigated. Hence, drawing inferences about either structural or functional aspects of the hippocampal formation of a primate such as the monkey or man based on our knowledge of the structure and function of the hippocampal formation in the guinea pig or rat may be quite misleading.

Because the ultimate focus of our interest in the hippocampal formation is its function in man, this review will focus on investigations conducted in nonhuman primates and our own work in the rhesus monkey. While the monkey is much closer phylogenetically to man than any other readily available laboratory animal, the phylogenetic distance between monkey and man is still enormous, with divergence from a common ancestor estimated to have occurred somewhere between 27 and 33 million years ago. In contrast, divergence between chimpanzee and man occurred between 6 and 8 million years ago (Templeton, 1983; Sibley and Ahlquist, 1984). Hence, inferences from studies of the monkey hippocampal formation to man may also be misleading and are certain to be incomplete. Nevertheless, it is our contention that current understanding of some of the unique anatomical features of the monkey hippocampal formation, the distinctive ways in which it is similar to that of man, and the ways in which it differs from that of nonprimates all clearly lead to important insights into the likely organization of the human hippocampus, the range of potential additional changes likely to be observed in the human hippocampus, and hence the potential role of the human hippocampus in learning and memory.

In considering the diverse applications of nomenclature in studies of the hippocampal formation, it is useful to consider the distinctly inglorious origin and early history of this anatomical term. As described below and illustrated in Fig. 1, the term *hippocampus* originated as a descriptor of the convoluted structure observed grossly in the floor of the lateral ventricle of the human brain. In his review of hippocampal etymology, Lewis (1923) states:

> The flight of fancy which led Arantius, in 1587, to introduce the term *hippocampus* is recorded in what is perhaps the worst anatomical description extant. It has left its readers in doubt whether the elevations of cerebral substance were being compared with fish or beast, and no one could be sure which end was the head. Accordingly the familiar term for which Arantius is responsible is commonly misused and seldom understood. . . .

Lewis also provides a translation of Arantius's original description of the convolutions he apparently observed in the floor of the inferior horn of the lateral ventricle:

> At the base of these ventricles, which face inward toward the median line, an elevation of white substances rises up and, as it were, grows there. This is raised up from the inferior surface like an appendage, and is continuous with psalloid body, or lyra. In its length it extends toward the anterior parts and the front of the brain, and is provided with a flexuous figure of varying thickness. This recalls the image of a Hippocampus, that is, of a little sea-horse. Rather, perhaps it suggests the form of a white silk-worm, embracing at that point the beginning of the spinal marrow. . . . Of this structure the part constituting the head is nearest to the ventricle known as the third, but the body, bent back and passing over into the tail, is drawn forward toward the anterior parts. So, for the purpose of distinguishing the ventricles above, it has been found convenient to refer to them as the ventricles of the Hippocampus, or of the silk-worm.

In retrospect, it seems likely that Arantius was describing the convoluted bulge of the hippocampal formation as it lies in the floor of the inferior horn of the lateral ventricle of the human brain as shown in Fig. 1. As Gertz *et al.* (1972) have demonstrated, the rostral or uncal end of the hippocampus shows from one to five convolutions, the "flexuous figure" of Arantius, which conjured up in his mind the "flexuous" appearance of the Mediterranean sea horse, the hippocampus. Unfortunately, Arantius did not provide an illustration of the hippocampus to clarify which end was the head or which end was closer to the third ventricle.

According to Lewis (1923), the term *hippocampus* apparently caught the attention of early anatomists and it subsequently appeared in numerous anatomical descriptions. The following account, again according to Lewis, outlines the early history of studies describing the hippocampus and the various names applied to it. Apparently the first clear illustration of the hippocampus was not published until 1729 by Duveroni, almost 150 years after Arantius's original description. Perhaps because of this, the acceptance of the term was not universal as Winslow, in 1732 (before publication of Duveroni's figure), described the structure in the floor of the inferior horn of the lateral ventricle as a "ram's horn" and in 1742 Garengeot described these ram's horns as "the horns of Ammon," an Egyptian God often depicted with horns. In addition, Diemer-

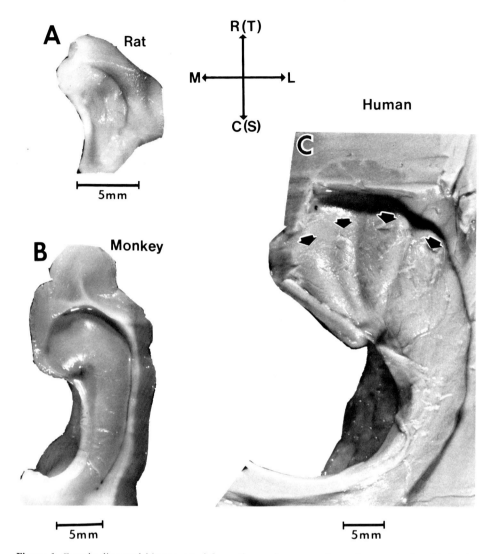

Figure 1. Grossly dissected hippocampal formation as it appears from the ventricular side in the rat (A), monkey (B), and man (C). Note that the caudal (C) end of the primate hippocampal formation corresponds to the septal (S) end of the rat hippocampal formation. However, in the rat, the septal end of the hippocampal formation is located rostrally rather than caudally. In the primate the temporal (T) end of the hippocampal formation is located at the rostral end of the inferior horn of the lateral ventricle. In C, the bold arrows mark the convolutions of the human hippocampus.

broeck in 1672 described the same structure as the "pedes hippocampi" or feet of the hippocampus. The descriptions accompanying both of these new terms, *pes hippocampi* and *Ammon's horn*, were no clearer and were probably even less justified as descriptors of the hippocampus than Arantius's original. Nevertheless, these competing terms also caught the attention of early anatomists as synonyms for this unusual part of the cortex.

While the term *hippocampus* has become the accepted name for this bulge in the floor of the inferior horn of the lateral ventricle (*Nomina Anatomica*, 1983), all three terms have survived and have been applied to the anatomy of the hippocampal formation in a variety of ways. Thus, the term *hippocampus* is generally used to cover both the dentate gyrus and all the pyramidal subfields except the subiculum unless it is qualified as *hippocampus proper*, referring only to the pyramidal subfields exclusive of the subiculum. The term *Ammon's horn* (*Cornu Ammonis*) refers to all the pyramidal subfields except the subiculum (e.g., Lorente de Nó, 1934) and is thus equivalent to *hippocampus proper*. The term *pes hippocampi* is used to designate the convoluted anterior part of the hippocampus as it appears grossly in the floor of the ventricle (e.g., Cassell and Brown, 1984) and hence may include the underlying dentate gyrus and subiculum as well as the ammonic subfields since all are present in the grossly visible "pes hippocampi." In this regard it is useful to remember that the original usage of the term *hippocampus* designated the entire grossly visible and convoluted structure that displayed the convolutions of the sea horse and it was certainly not limited to any particular cytoarchitectonic subdivisions. Thus, the modern limitation of the term *hippocampus* or the so-called "hippocampus proper" to only the part composed of a tightly packed, narrow layer of pyramidal neurons constitutes another variation on the original usage.

Modern usage has restricted the term *hippocampus* to regions characterized by the narrowest bands of pyramidal cells that Ramón y Cajal referred to as the regio inferior and regio superior and Lorente de Nó (1934) divided into four subfields of the Cornu Ammonis: CA1, CA2, CA3, and CA4. These areas are also designated the *hippocampus proper* in recognition of the fact that this usage of the term *hippocampus* excludes the dentate gyrus and subiculum, both of which are clearly part of the grossly defined hippocampus in the inferior horn of the lateral ventricle and share the simple three-layered cytoarchitecture of allocortex (Filimonoff, 1947). As described by Stephan and Andy (1970), this hippocampal allocortex is more specifically designated the archicortex in distinction to the allocortical olfactory areas, which are designated as paleocortex. Because of the original usage of the name *hippocampus* and the similarity of these archicortical regions, the term *hippocampal formation* (HF) will be used in this review to designate all of the allocortex (archicortex) within the curled bulge of the grossly defined hippocampus: the dentate gyrus (DG) or fascia dentata, the hippocampus proper [corresponding to the CA1–CA4 subfields of Lorente de Nó (1934) or the regio inferior and regio superior of Ramón y Cajal (1968)], and the subiculum (including the prosubiculum). These basic architectonic subdivisions were originally based upon the identification of unique cell types in Golgi impregnations. However, with the description of these cell types in mind, careful examination of well-prepared Nissl-stained sections allows these subfields to be readily identified. These basic subfields are indicated on the coronal section through the hippocampal formation of the monkey shown in Fig. 2A where the approximate borders between different subfields are indicated by arrows. As shown in the corresponding line drawing in Fig. 2B, the exact borders between many of the subfields are oblique rather than perpendicular to the pyramidal cell layers. These oblique borders are the result of the horizontally shifted overlap of the cell types that characterize each of these different subfields, and complicate

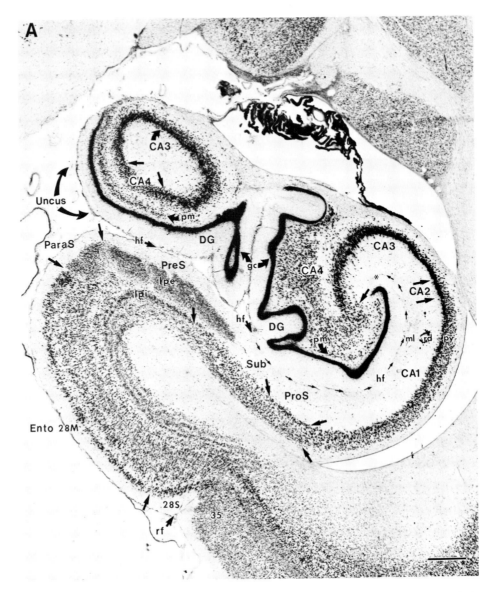

Figure 2. Architectonic subdivisions of the hippocampal formation of the rhesus monkey. In A the approximate boundaries of the subfields are indicated by the sharp arrows. However, these boundaries are usually not orthologonal to the pyramidal cell layer. Instead, as shown by the corresponding line drawing in B, the transition from one cytoarchitectonic subdivision to another is usually characterized by a horizontally shifted overlap of the cell types characteristic of both subdivisions. This horizontally shifted overlap results in the oblique borders illustrated in B. Bar = 0.5 mm.

the identification of each subfield in Nissl sections and probably contribute to frequent differences in identification in different studies. The details of these cytoarchitecture designations and a comparison of their features in rat, monkey, man are described in more detail in Section 4.

Four unifying features support the usefulness of the common classification

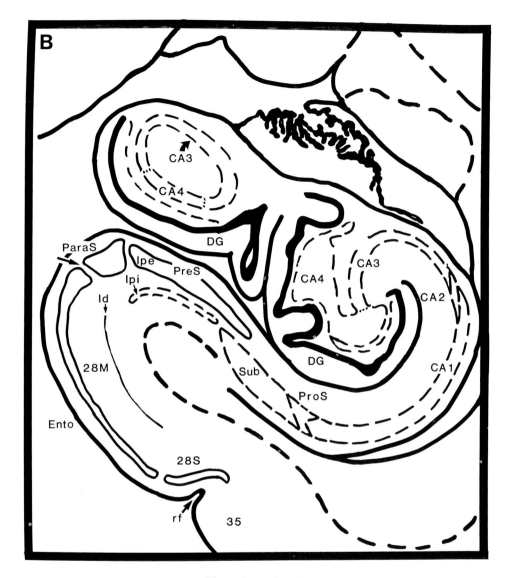

Figure 2. *(continued)*

of these distinct areas under the term *hippocampal formation*. First, all of these areas are the simplest type of cortex, allocortex, and are comprised of only three cortical layers: (1) a superficial plexiform layer of dendrites, axons, glia, and a few scattered neurons, (2) a deeper prominent cellular layer composed of predominantly one cell type, granule cells in the dentate gyrus and pyramidal cells in the hippocampus proper and the subiculum, (3) an underlying polymorph layer of dendrites and axons and scattered polymorphic neurons. An example of this allocortex from the CA1 subfield of the monkey is illustrated in Fig. 3. Second, all of these areas receive their major source of direct afferent input from the adjacent periallocortical entorhinal areas and input terminates in the more superficial part of the molecular layer. Third, these areas are tightly linked together by a serial set of intrinsic connections beginning in the dentate gyrus and terminating in the subiculum at the transition with the adjacent periallo-cortex of the presubiculum. Fourth, all of these subdivisions display a laminar organization of both extrinsic and intrinsic afferents that is highly segregated with little overlap. On all of these counts the adjacent periallocortical areas such

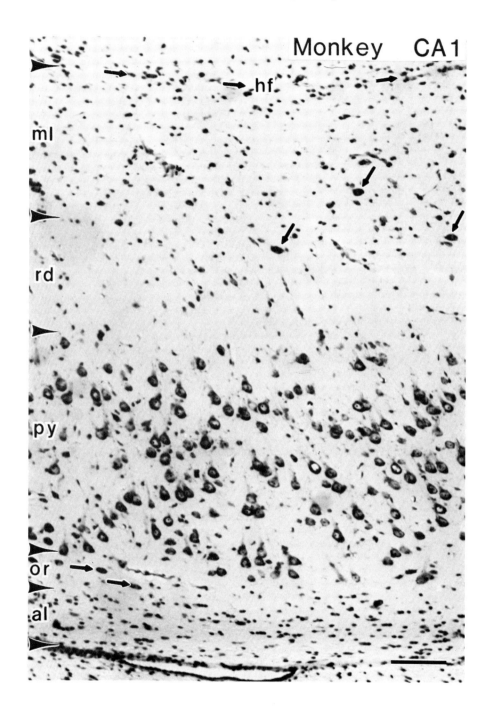

as the presubiculum, parasubiculum, and entorhinal area, which some authors include in the term *hippocampal formation,* constitute distinctly different morphological entities. Thus, in this discussion the term *hippocampal formation* will be used to designate all of the three-layered archicortex of the medial temporal lobe: the dentate gyrus (fascia dentata), the so-called hippocampus proper, and the subiculum. In this usage the term *hippocampal formation* corresponds closely with the original use of the term *hippocampus* and also has the virtue of being limited to one type of cortex.

3. Phylogenetic Considerations

While the basic cytoarchitecture of the hippocampal formation is remarkably constant in mammalian phylogeny and allows ready identification of the homologous structures in different species, it is also clear, as illustrated in Fig. 4, that there are striking differences between hippocampal formation cytoarchitecture of the rat and the monkey or man as well as clear differences between monkey and man. In light of these differences in hippocampal morphology, it is important to consider them in the context of evolution and phylogeny. One issue is whether any differences in hippocampal morphology represent phylogenetically "new and progressive" changes that are structural correlates of progressive elaboration of hippocampal function, or whether they may represent "regressive" alterations that are structural correlates of decreased or vestigial hippocampal function. Of course, one must also consider whether these differences in morphological appearance could be simple epiphenomena that have no significance for hippocampal function. To the extent that one can answer this type of question with either of the first two alternatives and determine the relationship between any two species such as monkey and man, then one can formulate both morphological and functional predictions about the hippocampal formation of man based upon experimental observations in the monkey.

Addressing these questions requires a brief consideration of some of the nomenclature used to classify the hippocampal formation. As described above, the hippocampal formation is composed of a simple three-layered allocortex and along with the allocortical olfactory cortex, the periallocortical entorhinal and cingulate cortices and the amygdaloid and septal nuclei comprise the phylogenetically oldest structures of the mammalian telencephalon (White, 1965).

Figure 3. Photomicrograph of the CA1 subfield of the monkey hippocampal formation taken from a 10-μm paraffin section stained with thionin. It serves to illustrate the main characteristics of three-layered allocortex. Superficially beneath the obliterated hippocampal fissure (hf) there is a plexiform layer, which in CA1 is further subdivided into a superficial stratum moleculare (ml) that has many glia and a deeper stratum radiatum (rd) that has fewer glia. There are a few scattered neurons (arrows) in this plexiform layer, particularly at the border of the stratum moleculare and stratum radiatum. The second layer is the stratum pyramidale (py) or pyramidal cell layer, which is composed primarily of medium-size pyramidal cells that, unlike in the rat, are loosely packed. The third layer is the stratum oriens (or) or polymorphic layer, which is composed of scattered polymorphic neurons (arrows) that are often fusiform-shaped in the CA1 region. Bar = 100 μm.

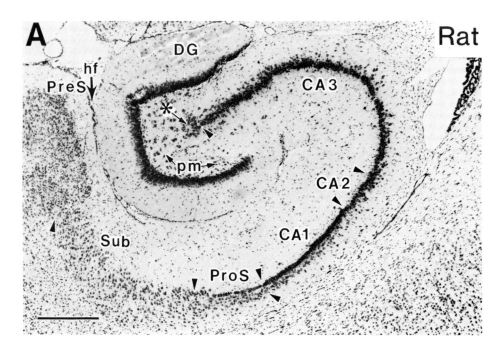

Figure 4. Nissl-stained coronal sections through the hippocampal formation of the rat (A), monkey (B), and man (C) with the approximate boundaries of the corresponding cytoarchitectonic subdivisions marked by arrowheads. The asterisk in A marks the small cluster of hilar neurons that may correspond to the CA4 subfields of monkey and man. Note that while there is striking similarity in the overall arrangement of the hippocampal formation in all three species, this similarity decreases as one proceeds from the dentate gyrus (DG) through the CA subfields toward the subiculum. Furthermore, it is also clear that the CA1 and subicular subfields occupy a proportionally larger part of the hippocampal formation as one proceeds from rat to monkey to man. The section in A is a 10-μm-thick, paraffin-embedded horizontal section through the middle part of the ventral hippocampal formation of the rat. The sections in B and C are both celloidin-embedded coronal sections through the main body of the hippocampal formation. The section in B is 30 μm thick and that in C is 50 μm thick. Bars = 0.5 mm (A, B), 1 mm (C).

Based upon the observation of comparative neuroanatomists that the telencephalon of many primitive vertebrates is dominated by afferents from the olfactory system, many past and even a few current conceptualizations of the phylogenetic development of the telencephalon emphasize its possible development from a primordial olfactory brain and often label these structures the "rhinencephalon," i.e., the "nose-brain." Since there is ample behavioral, physiological, and morphological evidence that the olfactory system in primates and especially in man has either regressed or at least failed to develop along with the neocortex, classification of the hippocampal formation as part of the rhinencephalon often leads to the impression that it too has regressed. However, many investigators (e.g., Brodal, 1947; Pribram and Kruger, 1954; Pribram, 1961) have pointed out that in mammalian brains in general and primate brains in particular, *direct* olfactory bulb input is largely limited to the anterior olfactory nucleus, primary olfactory cortex (prepyriform cortex), olfactory tubercle (anterior perforated

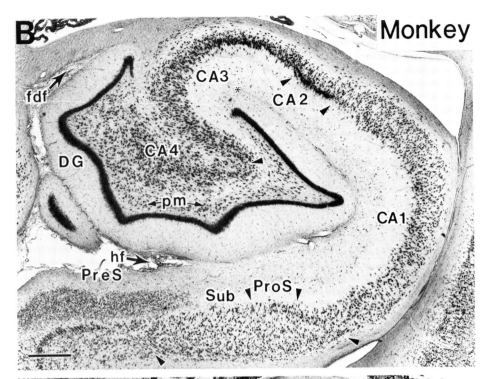

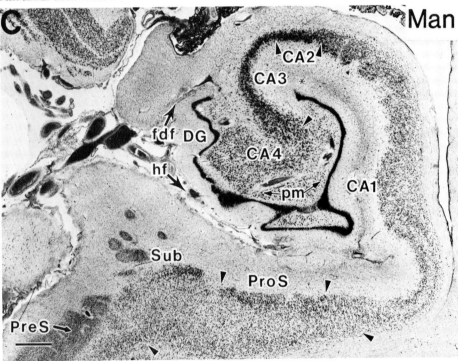

Figure 4. (*continued*)

substance), and corticomedial amygdala and is not even a predominant *indirect* input to most of the other structures often included in the "rhinencephalon" such as the hippocampal formation, entorhinal cortex, cingulate cortex, septal area, and the basolateral amygdala. For this and a variety of other morphological and developmental reasons (e.g., see White, 1965), the term *rhinencephalon* should be limited to the olfactory bulb, anterior olfactory nuclei, olfactory tubercle, primary olfactory cortex (paleocortex or prepyriform or piriform cortex), and perhaps the corticomedial amygdala, while the remainder of the phylogenetically older structures of the telencephalon that border the interventricular foramen are best designated the "limbic lobe" or the "limbic system" when the subcortical structures with which they are directly connected are included.

This separation of the olfactory and the limbic systems serves to emphasize the independence in function of these two systems but does not free the primate hippocampal formation from guilt by association with a vestigial or regressive olfactory system from which it presumably developed. This presumptive olfactory origin can be questioned on a number of grounds. First, in an interesting comparative study of the olfactory and limbic systems, Riss *et al.* (1969) put forth the alternate hypothesis that the original limbic system structures of the telencephalon, the archicortex, and the preoptic and septal areas may predate the development of the olfactory system. Some of the evidence for this is that the nervus terminalis, a cranial nerve that is thought to be sensitive to the internal chemical milieu and that projects to the septal and preoptic areas, is present in amphioxus, a vertebrate that lacks an olfactory system. According to this view, the olfactory nerve developed from the limbic system, i.e., differentiated from the nervus terminalis as the "nerve of the limbic system" sensitive to the external chemical milieu. A second and related point is the observation (White, 1965) that in a major developmental abnormality, the arhinencephalic monster, when the telencephalic vesicle fails to divide the telencephalon medium (septal and preoptic areas), is absent and the olfactory structures (bulb and nerves) also fail to develop even though the limbic cortices develop as a ring surrounding the interventricular foramen. White (1965) points out that this may indicate the structures of the limbic cortical ring originated before the olfactory structures, which may have developed from the telencephalon medium. Finally, the olfactory cortex differs from the limbic cortices such as the hippocampus as well as from the rest of the telencephalon in failing to develop from a cortical plate. From this perspective the hippocampal formation could be looked upon as the original association cortex of the telencephalon and may have continued to evolve in concert with the expanding neocortex, independent of evolutionary changes in the olfactory system.

In any discussion of "phylogenetic" differences between extant species, it is important to keep in mind that no two living species are direct phylogenetic descendants of each other or of any other living species and that the brains of their predecessors, including the last common ancestor, are not available for study. Consequently, statements about interspecies differences in homologous structures such as the hippocampal formation are not based upon true phylogenetic data derived from examining a genealogical series of related organisms. Instead, inferences about phylogenetic relationships must be made on the basis of other criteria and a variety of assumptions that should be made explicit (e.g., Campbell, 1982). First, identification of something labeled the "hippocampal formation" in several species is a claim of homology that is based simply upon morphological similarity and cannot logically exclude the possibility that evolutionary pressures have led to the convergent or parallel evolution of two different structures into a structure with a high degree of morphological similarity. If this were the case, a wide variety of distinct differences in both morphological detail and function would be expected. While it would still be of interest to understand the possible contribution of the observed morphological differences to differential function, this would have no significance for the phylogeny of a given area. An example of this type of convergent or parallel evolution is the "cruciate" sulcus of cats and dogs, which the study of endocasts of predecessors has shown to be absent in the common ancestor of both species (Radinsky, 1969). Second, even if morphological similarity is sufficient to identify homologous structures, comparisons of the development of any given structure between two extant species where one is thought to be "higher" on the phylogenetic scale may reflect only selective evolutionary pressures that were unique to one of the two species rather than a "progressive" aspect of the "higher" phylogenetic species.

With the foregoing caveats in mind, there are several lines of evidence suggesting that the hippocampal formation is not a regressive or vestigial structure but has undergone a "progressive" development in the course of primate phylogeny. One indication of this progression is the cytological elaboration of the ammonic and subicular subfield that occurs in primate phylogeny and is fully described in Section 4 and illustrated in Figs. 4–6. A second line of evidence is the elaboration of corticocortical connections between the hippocampal formation and the cerebral cortex that occurs in primates and is described in Section 6. A third line of evidence derives from comparative studies of the size (volume) of the hippocampal formation in a series of insectivores, prosimians, and simians by Stephan and Andy (1970). Because interspecies comparisons of the proportional volumes (ratios) of two structures within the brain cannot determine which structure may have enlarged and comparisons of absolute volumes of brain structures are confounded by the fact that larger animals have larger brains, Stephan and Andy (1970) applied the allometric method to make interspecies comparisons of the volume of homologous limbic system structures. For example, even though the hippocampus of primates is much larger than in the rat, this information alone provides no clue as to whether the hippocampal formation has progressed, regressed, or remained static in terms of its contribution to CNS function. Conversely, the hippocampal formation in the rat makes up a larger relative volume of the telencephalon than it does in primates but this does not necessarily indicate that it has regressed in primates. Instead, this change in relative volume could result if both the hippocampal formation and the neocortex were expanding in size and function with the neocortex expanding more rapidly.

Rather than compare absolute volumes or relative CNS volumes, the allometric method takes the volume of the structure relative to the body weight of the organism. An underlying assumption of this method is that it takes a larger brain (more neurons) to control a larger body and if a brain structure increased in volume as predicted by increased body weight in larger organisms, this would reflect the status quo, i.e., no change in the functional potential of the structure. Thus, if a 1-kg rat grew to the 70-kg size of the average human, one would expect the brain to grow and the allometric method predicts the expected volume of the different CNS structures such as the hippocampal formation or the neo-cortex in the 70-kg rat. Structures that were larger than the predicted value would have "progressed" and would have increased functional potential while structures that were smaller than predicted would have "regressed" and would have decreased functional potential. Blumberg (1984) has provided an excellent discussion of the general principles of the allometric method as it applies to a variety of different organ systems and structural features and how it may be useful for studying hominid evolution from fossils of probable ancestors. While scaling to body weight is a common comparative approach for those studying the evolution of the brain, it is not without its own problems and limitations. Many of these problems relative to the evolution of the primate brain are dis-cussed by Radinsky (1982) and Martin (1982). However, one obvious problem worth noting is that in any given species, evolutionary pressures in a particular environment may select for an increase or decrease in body size independent of the effects upon brain size.

Using this allometric approach, Stephan and Andy (1970) measured the volumes of a variety of allocortical forebrain structures in 22 insectivores (e.g., basal or primitive insectivores such as the hedgehog and progressive insectivores such as moles and otter shrews), 20 prosimians (e.g., the tree shrew and galago), and 21 simians (e.g., the rhesus monkey, chimp, and man). Since the insectivores as a group are thought to be among the most primitive mammals and are presumed to have a common ancestor with primates, Stephan and Andy (1970) used the basal insectivores as the extant species most representative of this last common ancestor. On this basis they have used the allometric method to predict the volume of brain structures for simians and prosimians (of a given weight) predicted by the relationship of brain volume and body weight in the basal insectivores as a group. For various allocortical structures, they calculated "pro-gression indices" as the ratio of the observed volume to the predicted volumes. With this index, numbers greater than 1 indicate a "progressive" enlargement exceeding that which could be attributed to changes in body size alone while indices less than 1 indicate a "regressive" decrease in size relative to that predicted by body weight. Stephan and Andy (1970) utilized these allometric data from extant species to construct "an ascending primate scale" that they propose reflects phylogenetic development of the brain. Such conclusions about a phylogenetic scale may be overstated since convergent and/or divergent evolutionary pressures over millions of years have probably acted independently upon most of these species to alter individual brain structures and other body features. However, the comparative measurements provided by Stephan and Andy are useful in identifying those brain structures that are *likely* to have undergone a progressive enlargement that *may* be reflected in increased functional potential.

The application of this method to questions of evolutionary change in limbic system structures such as the hippocampal formation is best illustrated by looking at the olfactory system, which conventional wisdom holds has functionally regressed in primate phylogeny, and the neocortex, which has clearly progressed. Stephan and Andy reported that the olfactory bulb accounts for 17.6% of the volume of the telencephalon in basal insectivores, 2.9% in prosimians, and 0.2% in simians. For the neocortex, volume measurements demonstrate that it accounts for 22.0% of the volume of the telencephalon in basal insectivores, 71.5% in prosimians, and 87.6% in simians. Because of this dramatic change in neocortex, it may be that the olfactory system has not regressed but has only failed to progress at the same rate as the neocortex and consequently occupies progressively less of the volume of the telencephalon. The allometric analysis of Stephan and Andy yields progression indices for the olfactory bulb of progressive insectivores that range from about 0.4 (a relative allometric decrease) to 1.5 (a relative allometric increase) with a median of about 1. However, the indices for the prosimians range from about 1.2 to 0.1 with the median around 0.6 and the indices for simians range from about 0.2 to 0.02 with a median of about 0.1. In fact, the lowest value in this group is 0.02 for man and indicates that the volume of the human olfactory bulb is only about 2% of that predicted for a basal insectivore of the same size. These progression indices support the idea that there may have been an actual (not a relative) diminution of the olfactory bulb in prosimians and an even greater regression in simians corresponding with the decrease in the functional significance of this system.

The importance of these data lies in consideration of whether or not phylogenetically ancient structures of the limbic system such as the hippocampal formation have undergone a similar regression in relative size. On the other hand, if the hippocampal formation has instead progressed in relative size (even if overshadowed by the development of the neocortex), then one would expect that there may be a corresponding progressive elaboration of function and perhaps of morphological features. For the hippocampal formation the volume measurements of Stephan and Andy (1970) demonstrate that the hippocampal formation accounts for 14.3% of the volume of the telencephalon in basal insectivores, 7.0% in prosimians, and 2.6% in simians, i.e., the same pattern as the olfactory bulb. However, the allometric method demonstrates an average progression index of 2.3 for the hippocampal formation in prosimians and simians with most of the values falling between 1.5 and 3.0. For the simians the largest progression index is 4.2 for the human hippocampal formation and the smallest is about 1.3 for the gorilla with the other simians (e.g., monkeys, chimps) falling in between. This outcome serves to illustrate the difficulty of interpreting these data in any given instance since on functional grounds it seems likely that a great ape like the gorilla should have a progression index closer to that of man than the monkey. In this particular case, one cannot determine whether the surprisingly small value for the hippocampal formation of the gorilla is due to selective evolutionary pressures producing less progression in size (and presumably function) or whether the small value is a result of evolutionary pressures selecting for an atypical increase in body weight. Intuition argues for the latter explanation but there appears to be no definitive way to prove this. In any case, the value of this comparative approach is that it suggests that structures with progression indices greater than 1 are likely to have undergone progressive phylogenetic development that may be reflected both morphologically and functionally. An underlying theme of this chapter is that the hippocampal formation of both monkey and man is not a regressive structure, nor is it simply an enlarged version of the hippocampal formation of the rat. Rather, the hippocampal formation is a structure that has undergone a progressive development in primate phylogeny that is reflected in many levels of its morphological organization (cytoarchitectonics, histochemistry, connectivity) and suggests a functional progression as well. The relative change in the size of the hippocampal formation in rat, monkey, and man is illustrated in Fig. 1 (gross dissections) and Fig. 4 (coronal sections).

4. Comparative Cytoarchitectonics

The following section is a comparative discussion of the cytoarchitecture of the hippocampal formation in three different species: rat, monkey, and man. These three were not chosen because there is any presumption that they comprise a phylogenetic series or progression. The rat is important because it has been the species utilized in a majority of published papers on the anatomy, physiology, and behavioral function of the hippocampal formation. The human hippocampus is included for two reasons. First, it is the primary motivation behind most studies of the hippocampal formation. Second, despite cursory similarities the human hippocampus is strikingly different from that of the rat. The monkey hippocampus is the focus of this section because it is the closest species to the human where it is practical to conduct a full range of neurobiological investigations. Hence, its similarities and differences from the human hippocampal formation are important to circumscribe potential extrapolations from monkey to man. Furthermore, the similarities and differences between the hippocampal formation of the monkey and the rat are important in attempting to understand observed differences in the experimental observations in these two species.

As shown in Fig. 4, the basic appearance of a Nissl-stained coronal section through the hippocampal formation of each of these three species is indeed similar. The major cytoarchitectonic subdivisions of each of these three species are labeled and there is no mistaking the fact that these appear to be homologous structures. On the other hand, closer inspection of each of these cytoarchitectonic subfields reveals striking differences that apparently increase as one proceeds from the proximal dentate gyrus through the ammonic subfields (CA4–CA1) to the most distal subiculum, adjacent to presubiculum. Figures 5 and 6 illustrate the comparative appearance in these three species of four cytoarchitectonic subdivisions of the hippocampal formation: the dentate gyrus (DG), CA3 subfield, CA1 subfield, and subiculum (Sub). One obvious conclusion of this comparison is the relatively stable cytoarchitectonic appearance of the dentate gyrus (Fig. 5A–C). The only major alteration is the more dispersed appearance of the prominent polymorphic neurons (pm) underlying the granule cell layer in the human dentate gyrus and the thinner molecular layer of the rat. In the CA3 subfield the most striking difference is the increasing dispersion of the large pyramidal cells of the stratum pyramidale (py) as one goes from rat to monkey to man (Fig. 5D–F). This is even more evident in the stratum pyramidale of the CA1 subfield in monkey and man where, at first glance, one might not accept this as the subfield homologous to the CA1 of the rat (Fig. 6A–C). Finally, the subiculum in the money and man also shows a dramatic increase in dispersion of neurons in the pyramidal cell layer (Fig. 6D–F). This also allows the increasing heterogeneity of cell types in the subiculum compared to the other subfields to be readily observed. In the discussion that follows, these and three other cytoarchitectonic subdivisions of the monkey hippocampal formation will be described in detail and compared to the corresponding areas in the rat and human brain. In addition to cytoarchitectonic criteria, our subdivision of the hippocampal formation into a total of seven areas is based upon histochemical data as well as data from experimental studies of connectivity. Some of the histochemical and connectional data are mentioned below but the details appear in Sections 5 and 6, respectively.

4.1. Longitudinal Levels of the Hippocampal Formation

In understanding the primate hippocampal formation, one of the most important points to consider is the longitudinal topography. In the rat a large part of the hippocampal formation is found dorsal to the thalamus and its rostral tip almost reaches the foramen of Monro just behind the septal area. The caudal tip of the hippocampal formation extends ventrally to reach the base of the brain just caudal and dorsal to the amygdala. Thus, the rostral-to-caudal longitudinal axis of the rat hippocampal formation is often described as the septotemporal axis. In the monkey and man the entire hippocampal formation is located in the temporal lobe and the most "rostral" part of the hippocampal formation begins rostromedially in the uncus of the medial temporal lobe. Caudally, the hippocampal formation extends into the atrium of the lateral ventricle where the efferent fibers of the fornix ascend around the posterolateral aspect of the thalamus and attach to the inferior aspect of the splenium of the corpus callosum. They continue rostrally beneath the callosum as the fornix to enter the parenchyma at the foramen of Monro. In equating different longitudinal levels of the primate hippocampal formation to the rat hippocampal formation, the septal or rostral end of the dorsal hippocampus of the rat is equivalent to the splenial or caudal end of the primate hippocampal formation. Similarly, the temporal end of the rat hippocampal formation is equivalent to the most *rostral* tip of the primate hippocampal formation where it reaches the medial surface of the temporal lobe as part of the uncus. These relationships can be appreciated in Fig. 1 where the gross hippocampi of the three species are aligned in parallel.

In all three species the hippocampal formation is curved in the dorsoventral plane but in both monkey and man there is also a pronounced medial flexure into the uncus. This dorsoventral curvature and particularly the medial flexure produces considerable variation in the appearance of the hippocampal formation when cut in coronal sections because of tangential cuts through many of the rostral subfields. The effect of this curvature is illustrated for the monkey hippocampal formation in Fig. 7. The entire longitudinal axis of the primate hip-

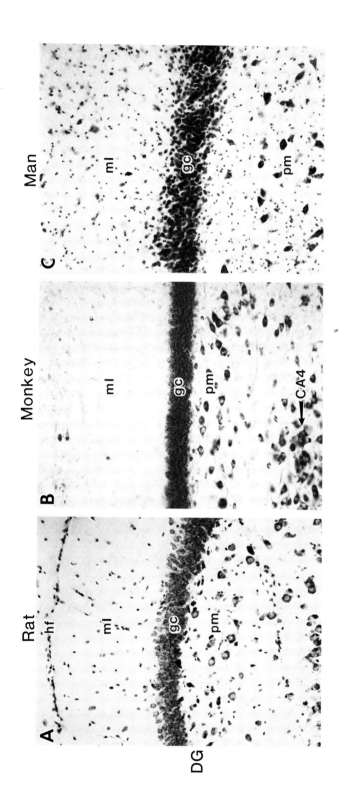

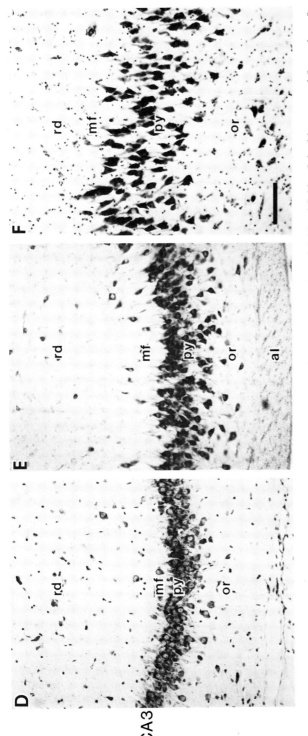

Figure 5. Photomicrographs taken at the same magnification through the dentate gyrus (DG) and CA3 subfields of the hippocampal formation of the rat, monkey, and man. Note that the appearance of the dentate gyrus is relatively constant in the three species but that there is clear dispersion of the pyramidal cell layer in the CA3 subfield. The photomicrographs of the rat hippocampal formation were taken from the same 10-μ-thick, paraffin-embedded horizontal section shown in Fig. 4A; those of the monkey were taken from the same 30-μm-thick, celloidin-embedded coronal section shown in Fig. 4B; but those of the human were taken from the 30-μm-thick, celloidin-embedded coronal section shown in Fig. 8B. Bar = 100 μm.

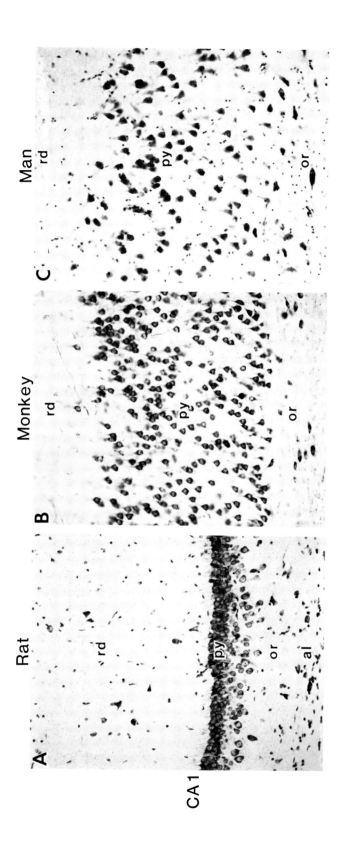

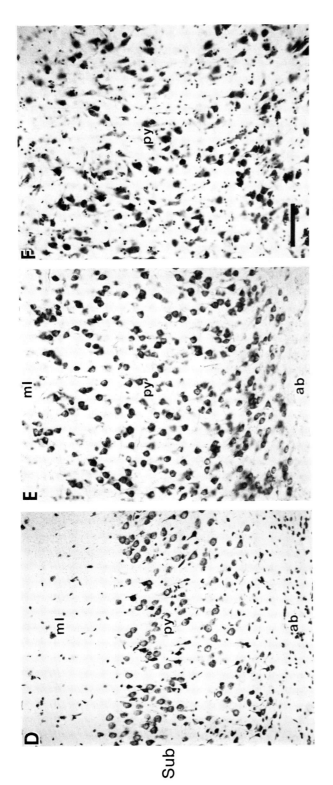

Figure 6. Photomicrographs taken through the subiculum and CA1 subfields of the hippocampal formation of the rat, monkey, and man at the same magnification and from the same sections used for Fig. 5. Note the striking increase in the dispersion and thickness of the pyramidal cell layer of the CA1 subfield of monkey and man compared to the rat, and the further exaggeration of this trend in the subiculum. Bar = 100 μm.

pocampal formation is indicated on the dissected specimen shown in the center of Fig. 7. The accompanying photomicrographs are thionin-stained coronal sections taken through four different anterior–posterior coronal levels. Their approximate planes of section are indicated on the dissection. Section A is taken through the most *anterior* end of the hippocampal formation, which we have designated the genu since, as indicated by the arrows on the dissection, it is at the genu where the main body of the hippocampal formation bends first medially and then even slightly caudally to reach the surface of the brain in the uncus. The most rostral or temporal end of the longitudinal axis of the hippocampal formation is shown in Fig. 7B and this level is labeled the uncus and will be referred to as the uncal hippocampus. It corresponds topographically with the temporal end of the rat hippocampus. However, it is important to note that this *rostral* end of the longitudinal axis of the monkey hippocampus is not found in the most anterior section. Thus, at the anterior level of the genu where the section in Fig. 7A was taken, neither the dentate gyrus nor subfield CA4 is present, but in the more caudal section shown in Fig. 7B both are present and the continuity of the dentate gyrus (DG) from the medial surface of the uncal hippocampus laterally into the anterior part of the main body of the hippocampal formation can be seen. It is in the main body of the hippocampal formation where its basic configuration can be recognized. While the uncal hippocampus constitutes one longitudinal level of the hippocampal formation, the main body of the hippocampal formation can be further subdivided into three additional levels: an anterior body (B), a mid body (C), and a posterior body (D). The posterior body is contiguous with the inferior and lateral pulvinar nuclei and constitutes approximately the caudal third of the main body. The mid body is contiguous with the lateral geniculate nucleus and constitutes the middle third of the main body. The anterior body (B) is contiguous with both the optic tract and the uncal hippocampus and constitutes the rostral third of the main body. While the genu of the hippocampal formation is a distinct morphological entity and useful for descriptive purposes, it does not constitute an additional complete level of the longitudinal axis of the hippocampal formation because the CA1 and subicular subfields observed there actually belong to the more caudally located dentate gyrus and CA3 subfields of the uncus (B). Hence, the uncus and genu together comprise the fourth level of the monkey hippocampal formation. Some of the relationships of the uncus, genu, and anterior body can also be appreciated in the series of horizontal and sagittal sections shown in Figs. 14 and 15, respectively.

Three levels of the hippocampal formation of the monkey (uncus, genu, and anterior body) correspond to the so-called "pes hippocampi" of human neuroanatomical and neuropathological literature (Gertz *et al.*, 1972; Cassell and Brown, 1984). In the primate brain, mechanical forces of the expansion of both the temporal lobe and the hippocampal formation presumably produce both the medial flexure and, in the human, the infolding of the rostral hippocampal formation as it is compressed along its longitudinal axis (Stephan, 1963). This infolding results in the appearance of one to five convolutions in the "pes hippocampi" of the human brain (Gertz *et al.*, 1972). These convolutions are indicated by arrows on the dissected human hippocampus shown in Fig. 1 and on

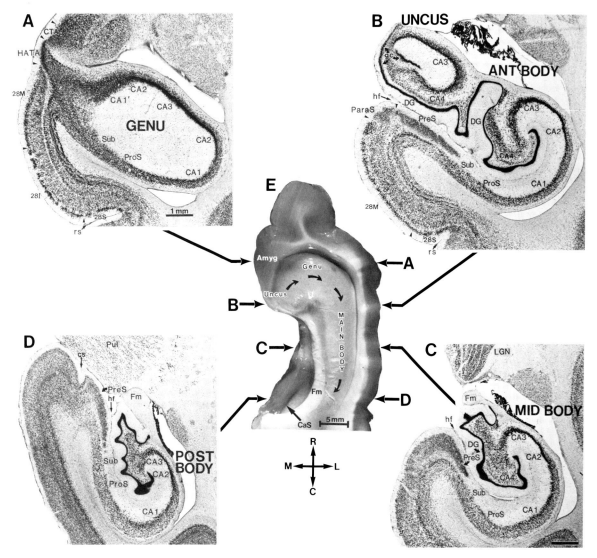

Figure 7. Coronal sections through four locations along the longitudinal axis of the monkey hippocampal formation. The medial flexure of the longitudinal axis is indicated on the gross dorsal (superior) view of the hippocampal formation (E) as it is seen in the floor of the inferior horn of the lateral ventricle in the right hemisphere. The approximate plane of section for the coronal sections in A–D are indicated on E by the arrows. The section in A is taken through the genu, the most rostral part of the medial flexure, and illustrates the absence of the dentate gyrus (which turns medially further caudal) as well as the insertion of the hippocampal–amygdaloid transition area (HATA) between the medial entorhinal cortex (28M) and the cortical–amygdaloid tran-sition area (CTA) and the rest of the amygdala dorsally. The section in B illustrates the continuity of the dentate gyrus as it rotates medially on the caudal aspect of the flexure to reach the medial surface of the hemisphere on the uncus. Note that only the dentate gyrus and the CA4 and CA3 subfields are present in the uncus while laterally in the an-terior body all the hippocampal subfields now have their usual appearance. The sections in C and D illustrate the typical arrangement and appearance of the subdivisions of the monkey hippocampal formation as one proceeds cau-dally through the middle level of the main body (C) to the posterior third of the longitudinal axis beneath the pulvinar (D). Bar = 1.0 mm.

the coronal section through the genu (pes) shown in Fig. 8A. Similar convolutions probably produced the "flexuous" appearance first noted by Arantius in 1587 (Lewis, 1923) and, like the increase in sulci and gyri of the primate neocortex, probably reflect the phylogenetic increase in the size of the primate hippocampal formation, i.e., the progression of Stephan and Andy (1970). The coronal section through the genu (pes hippocampi) of the human brain shown in Fig. 8A reveals four convolutions and an underlying cytoarchitectonic arrangement quite similar

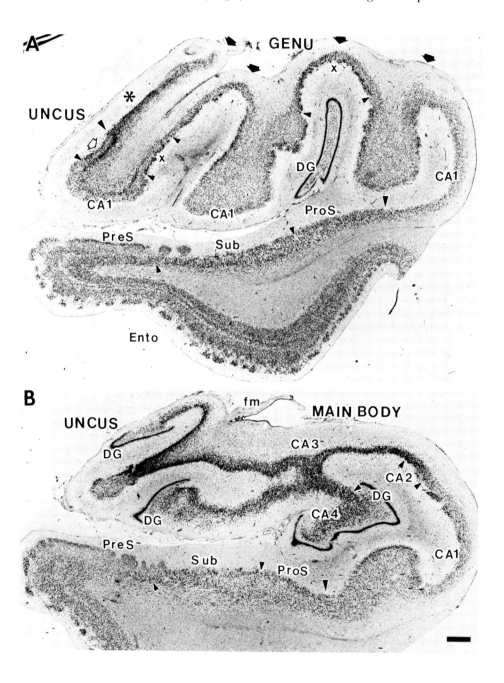

to that of the monkey genu (Fig. 7A) where oblique or tangential sections obscure the normal appearance of the different subfields. Similarly, a more caudal section through the uncus and main body of the human hippocampus reveals an arrangement of subfields quite similar to the monkey with the main body showing the characteristic arrangements of all the subfields.

Clearly the appearance, in coronal sections, of the genu and uncal levels of the primate hippocampal formation is unique due to the curvature of the hippocampus. However, understanding these rostral (temporal) levels of the hippocampal formation is also complicated by the appearance of several unique or atypical dorsomedial subfields that clearly are part of the uncal hippocampus. We have designated these subfields CA1′ and the hippocampal–amygdaloid transition area (HATA). These subfields are located dorsomedially at the level of the genu (Fig. 7A) and as illustrated in Fig. 9 are topographically (in relation to the CA3 and CA2 subfields) in the same positions as the ventrally located CA1 and subicular subfields. However, where the subiculum is continuous with layer VI of the presubiculum (Fig. 7A) and/or the entorhinal cortex (Fig. 7B), the HATA is at points contiguous with the cortical–amygdaloid transition area (CTA) of the amygdala (Fig. 9A) and/or layer VI of the entorhinal cortex (Fig. 7A). Some of the unique cytoarchitectonic, histochemical, and connectional characteristics that set these rostromedial subfields apart from the remainder of the monkey hippocampal formation and have led us to apply these particular unique labels are discussed more fully in Sections 5 and 6.

However, the common presentation of the primate hippocampal formation is derived from sections through the main body of the hippocampal formation. As illustrated in Fig. 7B–D, the cytoarchitecture of the main body of the hippocampal formation appears to be relatively constant throughout all three rostrocaudal levels of the main body. While the absolute size and relative proportions of the hippocampal subfields display some rostrocaudal variation, principally due to the posterodorsal curvature up toward the splenium, topographically there is a good correspondence of these subfields with the typical picture of the

---

Figure 8. Two 30-μm-thick, celloidin-embedded coronal sections through the rostral part of the human hippocampal formation. The section in A was taken through the rostral part of the genu and four of the convolutions that characterize this level (the "pes hippocampi") are indicated by bold arrows. The subfields are indicated as in previous illustrations, with three exceptions. Medially where the hippocampal formation reaches the medial surface of the hemisphere (the rostral part of the human uncus) there are two subfields present that cannot be unequivocally identified. On the basis of topographic position, relative cell size, and relative cell packing density, it seems likely that the region marked with the asterisk corresponds to the HATA of the monkey (Figs. 7A and 9A) while the region marked with the open arrow corresponds to the CA1′ subfield of the monkey (Figs. 7A and 9). The regions marked with the "x" are tangential cuts through the CA2 and CA1 subfields, which result in an extensive and patchy overlap. While this illustrates the topographic similarity of this level to the equivalent level of the monkey hippocampal formation (Fig. 7A), it also demonstrates the much greater complexity produced by the more pronounced flexure and medial compression of the human hippocampal formation. The section in B was taken from the same block, at the back of the medial flexure, behind the convolutions. It illustrates the appearance of the uncal hippocampus (the caudal part of the human uncus) as well as the rostral end of the main body of the hippocampal formation. This illustrates the topographic similarity of this level to the equivalent level of the monkey hippocampal formation shown in Figs. 2A and 7B. Bar = 1.0 mm.

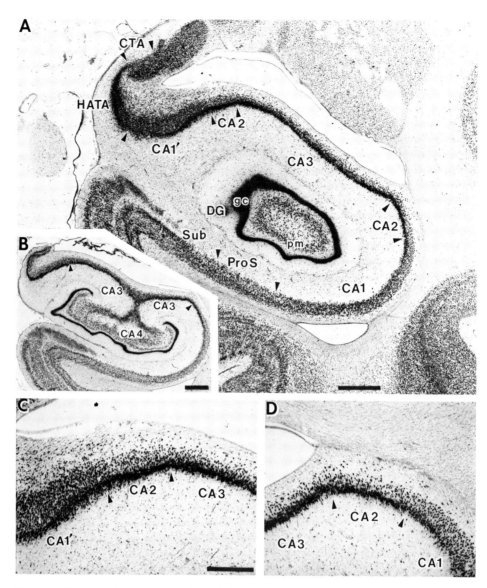

Figure 9. The section in A was taken through the middle of the genu of the hippocampal formation of the rhesus monkey and illustrates the dorsomedial continuation of the CA2 subfield and its continuity with subfield CA1′ and the HATA. The inset in B shows a section slightly caudal to A and illustrates the point at which the CA3 subfield emerges from the hilus of the dentate gyrus as these subfields turn medially. In C and D higher-power photomicrographs taken from the section shown in A demonstrate the difference between the transition from the CA2 subfield to the dorsomedial CA1′ subfield (C) and the transition from the CA2 subfield to the ventrolateral CA1 subfield. Bars = 1.0 mm (A, B), 0.5 mm (C, D).

hippocampal formation of the rat (Fig. 4A) as well as with similar levels of the human (Figs. 4C and 8B). The principal features of each of these subfields through the main body of the hippocampal formation are described below and this is followed by a discussion of the subfields present in the uncal hippocampal formation.

4.2. Cytoarchitecture of the Main Body of the Hippocampal Formation

The dentate gyrus: The dentate gyrus, also referred to as the fascia dentata, is the most medial gray of the monkey hippocampal formation. It is characterized by a single densely packed layer of small "granule" cells (Fig. 5) that form medial, central, and lateral blades in the monkey (Fig. 4B). This small gyrus is separated by the fimbriodentate fissure from the fibers of fimbria dorsally. Ventrally and then laterally, it is separated from the subiculum, CA1, CA2, and part of the CA3 subfield by the partially obliterated hippocampal fissure (Figs. 2A and 4B), the fundus of which reaches almost to the end of the lateral blade of the dentate gyrus. Since the choroid plexus, which seals off the inferior horn of the lateral ventricle, attaches to the fimbria, the medial part of the dentate gyrus is located outside the ventricle and is covered with pia. Unlike other sulci or fissures, the hippocampal fissure is "obliterated" over most of its extent as the afferent fibers from the entorhinal cortex pass directly across the fissure between the molecular layer of the underlying subiculum and the molecular layer of the dentate gyrus. While the location of the fissure is clearly marked by penetrating blood vessels, the normal layer of pia is incomplete at best and usually undetectable in the deepest part of the fissure. The granule cells have an apical tuft of dendrites that forms a distinct superficial molecular layer that is usually divided into "thirds" on the basis of unique afferent inputs and histochemical characteristics. The region deep to the granule cell layer is referred to as the hilus of the dentate gyrus and encloses two distinct groups of cells. The first group is found immediately below the granule cell layer and is a discontinuous layer of polymorphic neurons, which constitutes the third layer of the dentate gyrus allocortex. As illustrated in Fig. 10, this polymorphic layer forms a distinct band in man and monkey but it consists of dispersed neurons in the rat. At least some of these polymorphic neurons send their axons to the inner third of the molecular layer as the dentate gyrus association pathway (e.g., Swanson *et al.*, 1978). In the monkey, the second group of neurons lies deep to the polymorphic layer, is often separated from it by a relatively cell-free zone, and consists of a relatively compact group of polymorphic neurons that appear to correspond to the CA4 subfield of modified ammonic pyramids of Lorente de Nó (1934).

The CA4 subfield: Amaral (1978), on the basis of a Golgi study of the hilar region of 28-day-old rats, has argued that all the neurons of the dentate gyrus hilus are polymorphic cells that represent the convergence of the polymorphic layers of the dentate gyrus and the CA3 subfield of the hippocampus proper. Lorente de Nó (1934) designated these neurons as a CA4 subfield of modified Ammon's horn pyramids. On the basis of his Golgi study and other reports that indicated the hilar neurons were dominated by afferent input from the dentate gyrus, Amaral argued that the CA4 terminology of Lorente de Nó be discarded. As shown in Fig. 10A, the polymorphic neurons of the hilus of the rat dentate gyrus do appear to be homogeneously dispersed except for a small cluster of neurons (asterisk in Figs. 10A and 4A) near the tip of the pyramidal cell layer of the CA3 subfield. However, the hilar neurons in the monkey and man clearly form two distinct groups, a polymorphic layer and a prominent CA4 cluster (Figs. 4B,C and 10B,C). In addition, our observations in the monkey indicate that only the polymorphic neurons give rise to the dentate gyrus association and

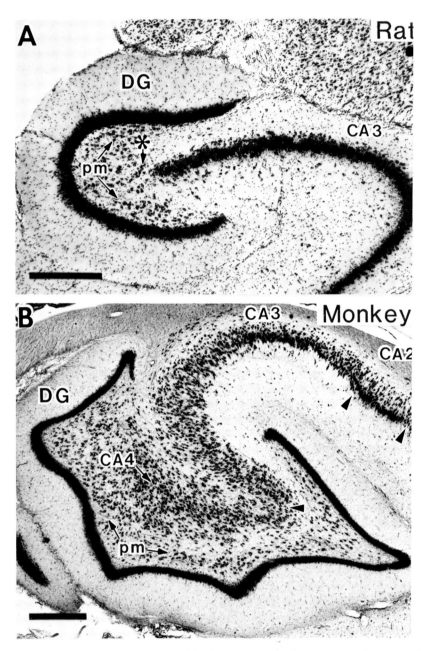

Figure 10. Photomicrographs of the hilus of the dentate gyrus in the rat (A), monkey (B), and man (C). In B the clear distinction between the polymorphic layer of the dentate gyrus and the diffuse CA4 subfield is quite evident in the hippocampal formation of the monkey and this same distinction is also evident for the human hippocampal formation in C. However, in the rat two distinct populations of neurons are not evident in the hilus although in many sections there is a small cluster of neurons at the tip of the internal blade of the CA3 subfield (marked by the asterisk here and for a different section in Fig. 4A) which may be the equivalent of the CA4 subfield of primates. Bars = 0.1 mm (A), 0.5 mm (B), 1.0 mm (C).

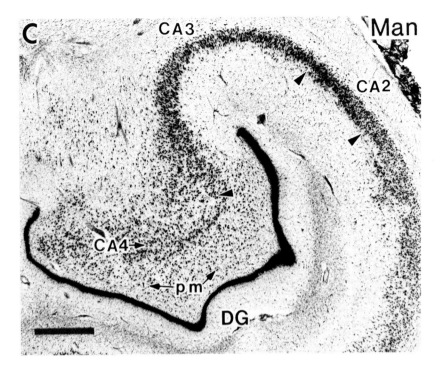

Figure 10. (*continued*)

commissural projections while the CA4 neurons project out of the hippocampal formation to the septal area. Consequently, we have retained the CA4 designation for the primate hippocampal formation. However, on the basis of the Nissl stain appearance of the hilar region in the rat (Figs. 4A and 10A), it seems likely that Amaral's (1978) designation of the hilar cells as part of the dentate gyrus may be correct with the possible exception of the small clusters marked by the asterisk, which could be the homologue of the neurons we apply the CA4 designation to in the primate. In any case, the CA4 subfield in the monkey is clearly distinct from the polymorphic layer of the dentate gyrus and has some histochemical and connectional characteristics in common with the CA3 subfield as described below. This region of the hippocampal formation requires a detailed analysis with the Golgi stain much like that done in the rat (Amaral, 1978).

The CA3 subfield: This is the archetypical pyramidal cell subfield of the hippocampal formation and is characterized by a narrow layer of densely packed and intensely chromophilic pyramidal neurons (Figs. 10 and 5). This layer begins adjacent to the cluster of CA4 neurons within the hilus of the dentate gyrus and curves laterally and then ventrally around the lateral blade of the dentate gyrus granule cells and the fundus of the obliterated hippocampal fissure (Figs. 2A, 4B, and 10B). The apical dendrites of these pyramidal cells extend superficially toward the pia of the hippocampal fissure where the plexiform layer that they constitute is classically divided into three distinct layers. Proximal to the pyramidal cell layer, approximately the inner fifth of this plexiform layer is occupied by the "mossy fibers" that originate from the granule cells of the dentate gyrus. In Nissl-stained sections this layer can often be discerned as a clear area and is classically designated the stratum lucidum. As illustrated in Fig. 11, in the monkey the stratum lucidum also stands out as an AChE-poor zone and in the Timm's stain clearly corresponds to the distribution of the zinc-rich mossy fibers, so we simply label it the mossy fiber layer (mf). Immediately above the mossy fiber layer is the stratum radiatum, which occupies the next two-fifths of the plexiform layer and corresponds to the zone of termination of the Schaffer collaterals of the CA3 pyramidal cells. It is both AChE-positive and stains intensely with Timm's stain (Fig. 11). Finally, the outer two-fifths of this plexiform layer has been designated as the stratum lacunosum and stratum moleculare. For convenience, we refer to this as simply the stratum moleculare or molecular layer and it corresponds to the zone of termination of extrinsic afferents from the entorhinal cortex (Van Hoesen and Pandya, 1975). This most superficial layer is lightly stained in both AChE and Timm's preparations as shown in Fig. 11.

The CA2 subfield: Like the CA4 subfield, there has been some controversy over whether or not this is a distinct subfield. According to Lorente de Nó (1934), the pyramidal cell layer of the CA2 subfield is characterized by the presence of large, intensely chromophilic pyramidal neurons that are similar in most respects to the CA3 pyramids except that they do not receive a "mossy fiber" input from the dentate gyrus onto "thorns" on their apical dendrites. According to this criterion, there would be no mossy fiber layer (stratum lucidum) in the CA2 subfield and this can be readily observed in carefully prepared Nissl sections (Figs. 10B and 11B) as well as in material prepared with the AChE (Fig. 11A) or Timm's (Fig. 11C) procedures. A close inspection of Fig. 10B reveals CA3-like pyramids continuing superficially beyond the end of the mossy fiber layer into the CA2 subfield (eventually overlapping some CA1-type pyramids). This relationship is confirmed for the monkey in Fig. 11 where the AChE-free and Timm's positive mossy fiber layer terminate while the CA3-like pyramids continue. As described in subsequent sections, studies of connectivity also confirm the limitation of the mossy fiber projection to the CA3 subfield and demonstrate some unique afferent inputs to the CA2 subfield.

However, for reasons that are not entirely clear, Amaral and his collaborators (Amaral and Cowan, 1980; Veazy *et al.*, 1982; Amaral *et al.*, 1984; Bakst and Amaral, 1984) generally disregard the CA terminology of Lorente de Nó (1934) and include the CA2 subfield with the CA3 subfield as the "regio inferior" of Ramón y Cajal. In explaining this terminology, Bakst and Amaral (1984, p. 349) state that they define regio inferior as "characterized by large pyramidal cells which are innervated by the axons of the granule cells, the so-called mossy fibers . . ." and that they consider a transition zone that corresponds to the CA2 zone of Lorente de Nó "to be part of regio inferior. . . ." Yet they go on to explain that this "transition zone . . . is characterized by fairly large, darkly staining cells which do not receive mossy fiber input." Not only is this a contradiction of their definition of regio inferior but it exactly corresponds to Lorente de Nó's definition of the CA2 subfield. It is also interesting that in an earlier study (Veazy *et al.*, 1982) these investigators reported a supramammillary projection to the monkey hippocampal formation that was exclusively confined to the region corresponding to the CA2 subfield of Lorente de Nó (1934). They state that this

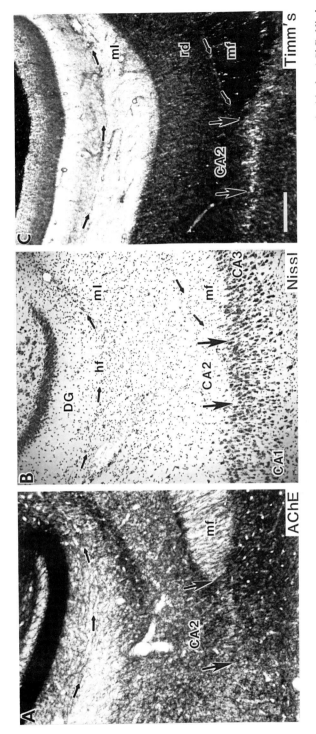

Figure 11. Photomicrographs taken from three sections of the CA2 region of the monkey hippocampal formation processed with the AChE, Nissl, and Timm's procedures. These sections demonstrate that the mossy fiber layer (stratum lucidum) of the CA3 subfield, which is heavily stained by Timm's method (C), is relatively AChE-free (A), and ends at the border with the CA2 subfield even though large chromophilic CA3-like neurons continue superficially in CA2 as far as the CA1 border (B). Bar = 200 μm.

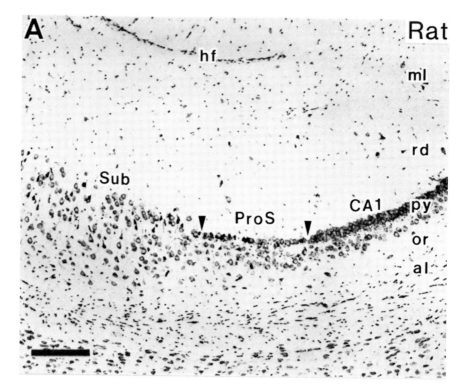

Figure 12. Appearance of the prosubicular subfield of the hippocampal formation of the rat (Fig. 4A), monkey (Fig. 4B), and man (Fig. 8B). In B the prosubiculum of the monkey is characterized primarily by the presence of clusters of tightly packed small neurons that occur both superficially and deeper in the pyramidal cell layer. In addition, the CA1–prosubicular border is also characterized by three other features. First, it can be noted that the stratum radiatum can be identified by the absence of glia and that it extends only a short distance over the pyramidal layer of the prosubiculum. Second, the distinctive and uniform pyramids of the CA1 stratum pyramidale are replaced by a heterogeneous population of neurons. Third, the stratum oriens ends beneath the pyramidal cell layer of the prosubiculum. While all of these features also characterize the prosubiculum of the rat and man, in the rat (A) this subfield is not well developed and these features are much less evident. While the prosubiculum of the human hippocampal formation (C) is very well developed and displays these same features, they are somewhat obscured by the increased dispersion of neurons in the human prosubiculum as well as the adjacent CA1 and subiculum. Bars = 200 μ (A, B), 0.5 mm (C).

projection "seems to exclude the terminal zone occupied by the mossy fibers." Aside from this issue, use of the regio inferior designation for the CA3 and CA2 subfields in the monkey is at best confusing since the CA3 and CA2 subfields are, at all levels, *superior* to the CA1 (regio superior) subfield! Without belaboring this point further, we have followed the terminology of Lorente de Nó (1934) to acknowledge the clear distinction of the CA2 subfield from the adjacent CA3 and CA1 subfields and to avoid the confusing designation of the superiorly placed CA3 and CA2 subfields as a regio inferior.

The CA1 subfield: The CA1 subfield in primates (monkey and man) is quite distinct from that in the rat shown in Fig. 4. A higher-magnification comparison of these subfields in Fig. 6A–C demonstrates that the CA1 subfield of the rat is

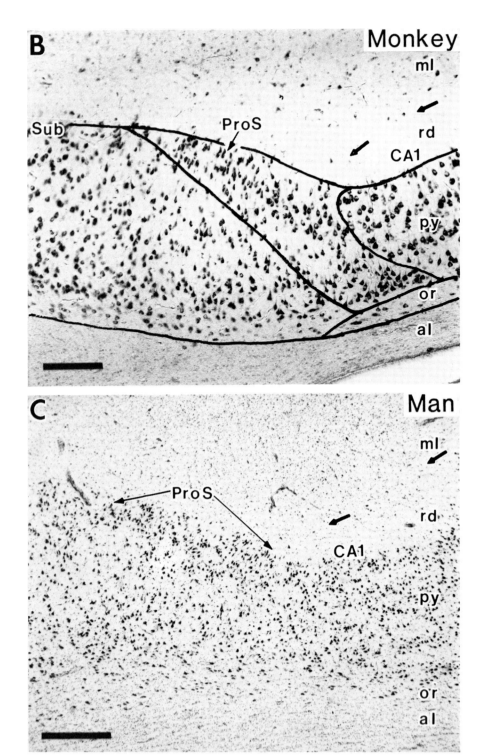

Figure 12. (*continued*)

composed of a thin, tightly packed layer of neurons that are clearly smaller than the pyramids of the CA3 subfield, but in both monkey and man the pyramidal cell layer of CA1 is much wider and less densely packed than CA3 and is composed of neurons that are nearly as large as the CA3 neurons. In fact, except for its topographic position between the CA2–3 subfields and subiculum–prosubiculum, the CA1 subfield of the primate hippocampal formation bears such little resemblance to the more widely recognized CA1 layer of the rat that it is often mistaken for the more similar subiculum (e.g., Fig. 18-10, Carpenter, 1976; but corrected in Fig. 18-12 of Carpenter and Sutin, 1983). At its border with the CA2 subfield, the CA1 pyramidal cells first appear beneath the more chromophilic CA2 neurons, which gradually thin and end superficially (Figs. 2 and 4B). This horizontally shifted overlap of adjoining subfields is a common feature of most of the cytoarchitectonic transitions in the hippocampal formation and also in the adjacent presubiculum and other periarchicortices. However, it is important to note that we do not consider the presence of a horizontal overlap of two adjacent fields sufficient cause to designate the area of overlap as a distinct cytoarchitectonic region. Thus, the CA2 field is identified because of the unique morphology and connections of the CA2 pyramidal cells and not simply as an area where CA3 pyramidal cells overlap with adjacent CA1 pyramids.

The prosubiculum: Lorente de Nó (1934) identified a small cytoarchitectonic zone located between the subiculum and the CA1 subfield as the prosubiculum. His designation of the prosubiculum was based upon a number of criteria, one of which was the observation that the border of the prosubiculum and the CA1 subfield is the point at which the Schaffer collaterals of the stratum radiatum end. In addition, based upon Golgi studies he concluded that the superficial part of stratum pyramidale in the prosubiculum was composed of small modified ammonic pyramids. While Lorente de Nó (1934) states that the dendritic aborization of these modified prosubicular pyramids differs from CA1 pyramids due to the lack of a stratum radiatum, his drawings of Golgi-impregnated sections from the mouse (Figs. 11 and 13 of Lorente de Nó, 1934) and monkey (Fig. 30 of Lorente de Nó, 1934) indicate that the most striking feature of these superficial pyramids is that they are relatively small. In fact, this is an extremely distinctive feature of the prosubiculum; and allows this area to be explicitly identified in Nissl-stained material as shown in Fig. 12 for the rat, monkey, and man. In all three species the prosubiculum is most clearly identified by the cluster of superficial small pyramids that begin at the tip of the stratum radiatum. However, these small pyramids, which we use to define the prosubiculum, do not continue throughout all three of the prosubicular subfields identified by Lorente de Nó. Thus, our delineation of the prosubiculum includes all of prosubiculum C of Lorente de Nó and a part of his prosubiculum B but the remainder of prosubiculum B and all of his prosubiculum A are included in the subiculum. In addition to the absence of superficial small pyramids from these latter areas, we identify them as part of the subiculum principally because of the presence of large subicular pyramids that project to the mammillary bodies. While both the termination of stratum radiatum and the appearance of the small pyramids in clusters in the superficial part of stratum pyramidale are the most salient features of the prosubiculum in a Nissl stain, an interesting additional correlate is the

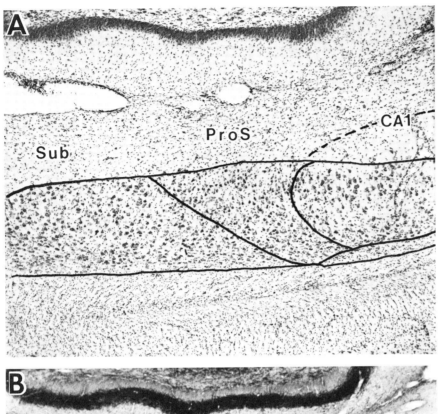

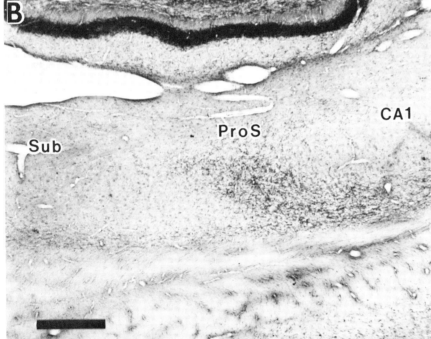

Figure 13. Prosubiculum shown at higher power in two adjacent sections from a rhesus monkey. The section in B was processed for the demonstration of AChE and shows a good correspondence of AChE reaction product with the pyramidal cell layer of the prosubiculum. Bar = 0.5 mm.

disappearance of stratum oriens at the distal border of CA1. Our observations also demonstrate that the prosubiculum as defined by these criteria is characterized by the presence of an AChE-dense zone that corresponds almost exactly with the cytoarchitectonic limits of the prosubiculum as shown in Fig. 13. This characteristic as well as some unique connections of the prosubiculum are discussed in more detail in Sections 5 and 6.

Despite these explicit criteria, the usefulness of designating the prosubiculum as a distinct subfield has not been universally accepted. For example, Bakst and Amaral (1984) despite noting the increased density of AChE staining in this region assert that this area should simply be considered a transition zone between CA1 and the subiculum and suggest that the small cells may be a superficial excursion of the stratum oriens. Despite the absence of the stratum oriens from the subicular subfields, this latter suggestion seems unlikely in view of the morphological differences between the polymorphic neurons of the stratum oriens and the small superficial pyramids of the prosubiculum (e.g., Lorente de Nó, 1934). In our view the prosubiculum does not constitute a transitional zone between the subiculum and the CA1 subfield because it does not display an intermingling of or even intermediate histochemical or morphological features of these two areas. Instead, it has its own unique and independent features. Consequently, there seems to be little value in either adopting a new designation (i.e., CA1–subiculum transition) or ignoring Lorente de Nó's designation of this area as the prosubiculum.

The subiculum: The architecture of the subiculum in the monkey, rat, and man is quite distinctive as shown in Figs. 4 and 6D–F. However, in all three species it is characterized by the appearance of large pyramid-shaped neurons that begin beneath the distal extremity of the small prosubicular pyramids. As a result, the border with the prosubiculum is characterized by typical horizontally shifted overlap of the characteristic cell type. The layer of subicular pyramids widens and continues distally to another overlapping border below the superficial layer of small pyramidal neurons in the lamina principalis externa of the presubiculum. In Nissl-stained material from the rat, monkey, and man (Fig. 6D–F), the subicular pyramids are much larger than the ammonic pyramids of the CA1 subfield and much larger than the small pyramids of the prosubiculum. In addition, in place of a stratum oriens there is a deep layer of somewhat smaller and more densely packed pyramids that gives way to fusiform neurons adjacent to the underlying white matter of the angular bundle. These deep layers increase in relative thickness and density of cells as one proceeds distally from the prosubiculum to the presubiculum. Compared with the prosubiculum or CA1 subfields, the subiculum is clearly a more complex but nevertheless three-layered allocortex.

4.3. Cytoarchitecture of the Uncal Hippocampal Formation

General considerations: As illustrated in Fig. 7, the uncal part of the primate hippocampal formation is the most rostral tip of its longitudinal axis. Due to the medial flexure this is also the most medial part and the point where the hippocampal formation emerges from the inferior horn of the lateral ventricle to appear on the medial surface of the hemisphere. While these topographic relationships are important for localization along the longitudinal axis, as Stephan (1963) has noted, the medial flexure that forms the genu and the uncus in the primate brain may be a result of the mechanical forces exerted on the hippocampal formation by the expanding temporal lobe neocortex. Similarly, the convolutions that characterize uncal and genual levels of the human hippocampal formation (Figs. 1 and 8) may be the result of longitudinal compression of the expanding hippocampal formation. What makes the uncal hippocampus important are the unique architectonic, histochemical, and connectional features of several of the uncal subfields. While Lorente de Nó (1934) argued that all of the subfields were constant along the longitudinal aspect of the hippocampus, others have noted a variety of differences. For instance, McLardy (1963) described a number of unique cell and fiber characteristics of the uncal hippocampus and concluded that this part of the hippocampal formation was relatively primitive in comparison with the main body. While it is often difficult to determine whether there is more heuristic value in splitting things apart on the basis of differences or lumping things together on the basis of common features, several characteristics of some of the subfields of the uncal hippocampal formation are so unique that they must be considered unique entities.

The uncal dentate gyrus, CA4, CA3, and CA2 subfields: The dentate gyrus and the three hippocampal subfields intimately related to it (CA4–2) turn medially across the posterior part of the genu to reach the medial surface of the caudal uncus as shown in Figs. 7 and 9 for the monkey and Fig. 8 for man. The related CA1, and subicular subfields also turn medially around a larger radius so that they occupy the lateral and then rostral parts of the genu but never reach the uncus. Thus, in the uncal hippocampus only the dentate gyrus and the CA4, CA3, and slightly more anteriorly located CA2 subfields are present (Figs. 2A and 7B). While this explanation for the absence of some subfields in the uncus is not immediately obvious, it appears that the medial flexure begins as the fundus of the hippocampal fissure turns medially and slightly dorsally (in the coronal plane) until the fissure reaches the medial surface of the hemisphere in the caudal aspect of the uncus. This can be appreciated by examining in order Figs. 7B, 9B, 9A and then comparing these coronal sections with the horizontal sections of Fig. 14B,C. Thus, the lateral blade of the dentate gyrus swings medially just caudal to the medial excurion of the fundus of the hippocampal fissure so that the lateral blade of the dentate gyrus emerges on the surface of the uncus (Figs. 2A and 7B). In contrast, the CA1 subfield located lateral to the fundus of the hippocampal fissure is forced to follow a larger radius of curvature that carries it rostral to the hippocampal fissure (Fig. 14A,B) before turning medially. Assuming that along the longitudinal axis of the hippocampal formation each individual subfield has an "equivalent" length so that each millimeter of CA3 subfield has a corresponding millimeter of dentate gyrus medially and CA1 subfield laterally, then since all the subfields begin caudally at approximately the same point beneath the splenium, when the medial flexure occurs rostrally, the subfields located lateral and ventral to the fundus of the hippocampal fissure (CA1, prosubiculum, and subiculum) must bend around a larger radius than

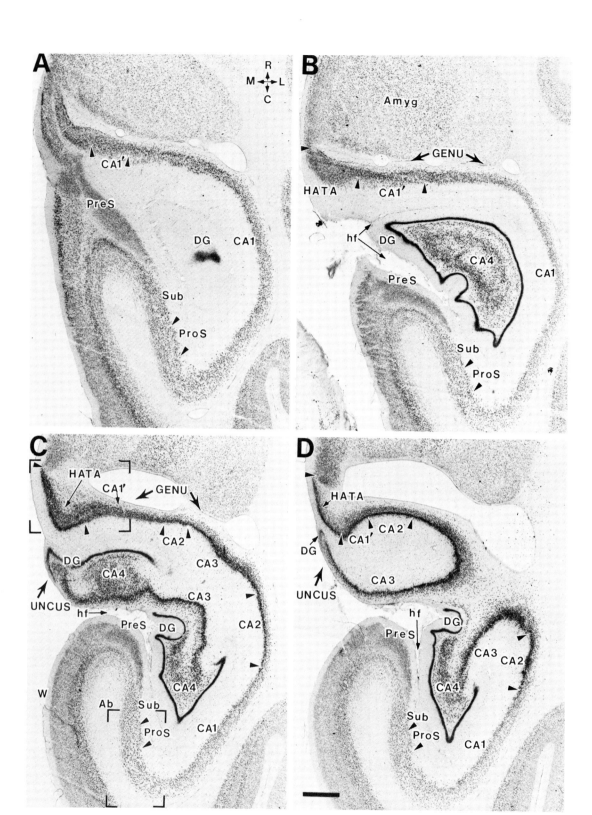

the subfields located medial and dorsal to the fundus. Hence, the equivalent lengths of these ventral and lateral subfields will not extend as far medially and the equivalent segments will not be found in the same coronal plane.

While histochemical and connectional features that distinguish the uncal dentate gyrus and CA4, CA3, and CA2 subfields from the same subfields of the main body are described in Sections 5 and 6, there are only minor cytoarchitectonic differences in these fields at different longitudinal levels. As shown in Fig. 7B, the lateral-to-medial continuity of the dentate gyrus can be observed as well as the superior location of the CA3 and CA2 subfields. This is best shown in Fig. 9B where the dorsal emergence of the CA2 subfield from within the hilus of the medially extended dentate gyrus can be observed. Further rostrally (Figs. 9A and 7A) toward the front of the genu, the CA3 subfield is present superiorly and is flanked both medially and laterally by the CA2 subfield. As shown in Fig. 9A, the lateral CA2 subfield is bordered laterally by the archetypical CA1 subfield. The serial progression through the prosubiculum and subiculum to the presubiculum of the periarchicortex is also evident. However, Fig. 9A also demonstrates that the medial progression from the medial CA2 subfield toward the uncus is not typical as one proceeds through two cytoarchitectonically distinct subfields, CA1′ and HATA. These two subfields are dorsomedially adjacent to the most rostral part of CA2 and rostrally they reach the medial surface of the uncus between the entorhinal cortex (ventrally) and the CTA dorsally as shown in Fig. 9A (also Fig. 7A a bit farther rostrally). Because of the unique features of these two areas, they deserve a more complete discussion.

The dorsomedial CA1′ subfield: In the most anteromedial part of the genu, subfield CA2 is readily distinguished by its densely chromophilic neurons and the absence of the dentate gyrus mossy fibers and the corresponding stratum lucidum. At levels anterior to Fig. 7A, it is clear that this medial CA2 subfield is continuous with the lateral CA2 subfield and simply constitutes the dorsomedial curvature of the CA2 subfield slightly rostral to CA3. However, throughout the genu the medial border of this dorsomedial CA2 subfield abuts a subfield that topographically should correspond to the CA1 subfield but architectonically is quite different as shown in Figs. 9C,D and 14–16. Nevertheless, this subfield shares some of the characteristics of the CA1 subfield so we have retained the CA1 designation but acknowledge the many differences by referring to it as CA1′.

As shown in Fig. 9A,C,D, the CA1′ subfield is composed of neurons that are smaller and much more densely packed than those of the ventrolateral CA1 subfield. Cytoarchitectonically, this region is composed of pyramid-shaped neurons and we have verified this in our Golgi-stained preparations from this area (Ekstein and Rosene, unpublished observations). Additional perspectives on the topographic position of the CA1′ subfield are presented in Figs. 14 and 15,

Figure 14. Four horizontal sections through the uncus, genu, and anterior body of the hippocampal formation of the rhesus monkey. The section in A is most dorsal and subsequent sections are taken progressively farther ventral in the temporal lobe. The continuity of CA1 with the prosubiculum ventrally and caudally and CA1′ dorsomedially is illustrated in A–C and the appearance of the sharp border of the HATA with the amygdala dorsally is shown in B–D. Bar = 1.0 mm.

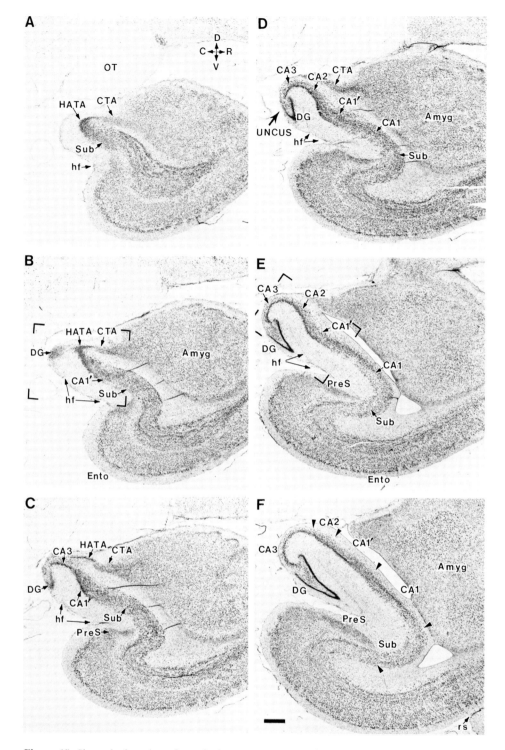

Figure 15. Six sagittal sections through the uncus, genu, and anterior body of the hippocampal formation of the rhesus monkey, the section in A being the most medial and F the most lateral. Like Fig. 14, these sections illustrate the appearance and location of the HATA and CA1′ subfields in the dorsomedial hippocampal formation. Bar = 1.0 mm.

which are, respectively, series of horizontal and sagittal sections that include the uncus, genu, and anterior body of the hippocampal formation. As shown in Fig. 14A,B, in the most rostral part of the genu the CA1 subfield is continuous with the CA1′ subfield, which separates typical CA1 from the HATA. However, the more ventral horizontal section shown in Fig. 14C illustrates the separation of the CA1′ from the CA1 subfield by the CA2 and CA3 subfields similar to that observed in the coronal section of Fig. 9A. In the sagittal sections in Fig. 15, which begin in the HATA of the uncus and progress laterally into the genu, these same topographic relationships appear with the CA1′ subfield inserted between the CA2 and CA1 subfields (Fig. 15E,F) and between the HATA dorsally and the subiculum ventrally (Fig. 15B). Despite the continuity and the topographic similarity of the CA1′ subfield to CA1, these illustrations and the higher-magnification comparisons taken from them and shown in Fig. 16 clearly demonstrate the unique appearance and location of the CA1′ subfield. In Fig. 8A a corresponding area of the human hippocampal formation has been marked with

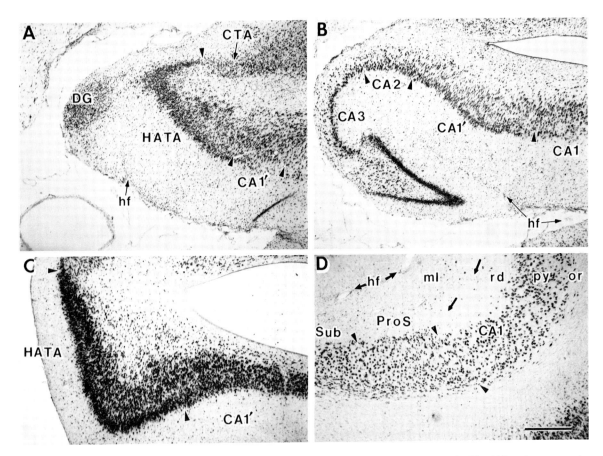

Figure 16. The sections in A and B are higher-power photomicrographs of the sections shown in Fig. 15B and 15E, respectively, and illustrate the appearance of the HATA and CA1′ subfields. The photomicrographs in C and D were taken from the section shown in Fig. 14C and compare the CA1′–HATA transition dorsomedially with the CA1–prosubicular transition ventrolaterally. Bar = 0.5 mm.

an open arrow. Some of the unique histochemical and connectional features of this area are presented in subsequent sections.

The dorsomedial HATA: As one proceeds medially from CA1′ there is a further decrease in cell size and an increase in packing density as the pyramidal cell layer turns dorsally and becomes interposed between the entorhinal cortex and the CTA (Figs 7A, 9A, 14A–D, 15A,B). In addition, both stratum radiatum and stratum oriens, which are present in the CA1′ subfield, stop at the transition to the HATA. Because of this unique topographic position, the unique cytoarchitecture of this area, and the fact that these neurons appear to have connections that are very different from any of the other hippocampal subfields, we have designated this area the HATA. While it is topographically in the position of the subiculum and prosubiculum and at the level shown in Figs. 7A and 15A is continuous with the subiculum, as shown in Fig. 16, the neurons in the HATA are much smaller and much more densely packed than neurons in the subiculum, prosubiculum, CA1 or CA1′ subfields. In common with the subiculum, our retrograde labeling experiments have shown that neurons in the HATA project through the fornix to the mammillary complex but anterograde labeling experiments demonstrate that these fibers terminate in the tuberomammillary nucleus rather than in the medial or lateral mammillary nuclei where all other subicular neurons terminate (Ekstein and Rosene, 1987). We have also observed that neurons in the HATA are *not* labeled following an HRP injection into the anterior thalamic nucleus, which labels all levels of the subiculum. It is important to note that this area does *not* correspond to the area Price (1981) has designated the amygdalohippocampal area. This latter area apparently corresponds to what we designate the CTA as well as the adjacent posterior part of the cortical amygdaloid nucleus [see Saunders and Rosene (1987) for additional illustrations]. In addition, our HATA is entirely on the "hippocampal" side of the area Price labels the amygdalohippocampal area. In Fig. 8A a potentially homologous region in the uncal hippocampus of the human hippocampal formation is designated with an asterisk. While much more needs to be learned about the HATA, it is clearly a part of the hippocampal formation in its location, histochemical characteristics, and connections but is so distinct from all the other hippocampal subfields that a separate designation is necessary. However, it is likely that as we discover more about this unique area, another more meaningful designation may be needed.

The ventrolateral CA1, prosubiculum, and subiculum: As illustrated in Fig. 7B and confirmed by our histochemical observations and studies of connectivity, the CA1, prosubiculum, and subiculum that are present beneath the uncal hippocampus, are actually subfields related to the dentate gyrus, CA4, CA3, and CA2 subfields of the anterior body. The subicular and CA1 subfields related to the uncal hippocampus are located more rostrally in the genu (Fig. 7C). In this regard the connections and architecture of these subfields at both levels (Fig. 7A,B) are typical of the entire main body of the hippocampal formation.

The subfields and layers of the monkey hippocampal formation: A summary of the location of all the subfields and their laminar subdivisions is presented in Fig. 17. This illustration was taken from a section through the back of the genu where all the subfields represented in the uncus, genu, and main body of the monkey hippocampal formation are present. This level is just slightly posterior to the level shown in Fig. 9B.

5.   Neurohistochemistry

The data on neurohistochemistry presented in this section will be limited to those aspects that clarify some of the more interesting cytoarchitectonic issues discussed in the preceding section. Furthermore, these descriptions are based upon triplets of adjacent sections of both rat and rhesus monkey hippocampus prepared respectively with Timm's stain for heavy metals, the AChE histochemical procedure, and the thionin stain. In some cases a few Timm's and AChE sections were counterstained with thionin as well. This material was processed according to a combined perfusion protocol that also allows simultaneous demonstration of HRP, AChE, and Timm's reactions in the same brain (Moss and Rosene, 1984). The focus of this discussion will be on the monkey hippocampal formation but occasional reference will be made to our own observations on the human hippocampal formation as well as to published reports on all three species. The discussion of comparative densities of AChE reaction product is based in part upon quantitative assessment of both normal densities and densities after fornix transection. For the specifics of these quantitative assessments the reader

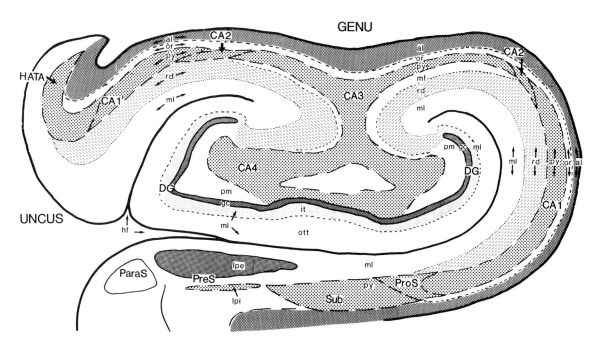

Figure 17. Drawing, from a section through the monkey hippocampal formation at a level similar to that of the section shown in Fig. 9B, illustrating the location of all the hippocampal subfields and laminae discussed identified in the rhesus monkey hippocampal formation.

is referred to Moss and Rosene (1987) and Moss *et al.* (1987). Like the preceding section, this will be organized according to architectonic zone and topographic level within the hippocampal formation.

5.1. The Main Body of the Hippocampal Formation

As described above, in terms of the general topography of architectonic fields, the main body of the primate hippocampal formation is most similar to the rat hippocampal formation. Typical AChE staining patterns for the rat, monkey, and man and Timm's staining patterns for the rat and monkey are illustrated in Fig. 18. While the basic pattern of staining in these different species is similar, there are also a number of interesting differences.

In the dentate gyrus of the rat, the molecular layer shows three distinct bands of Timm's staining (e.g., Haug, 1973). These bands (Fig. 19D) each occupy approximately one-third of the width of the molecular layer and hence have been designated the inner third (proximal to the granule cell layer), the middle third, and the outer third (abutting the hippocampal fissure). Each of these Timm's stained bands appears to correspond to a unique band of afferent termination. The inner third corresponds to the zone of termination of the commissural and association pathways that originate from neurons in the hilus of the dentate gyrus (e.g., Swanson *et al.*, 1978). The lightly stained middle third of the molecular layer corresponds to the zone of termination of afferents arising from the medial subdivision of the entorhinal cortex while the darker staining outer third corresponds to the zone of termination of afferents from the lateral subdivision of the entorhinal cortex (e.g., Steward, 1976). In the monkey, Timm's stain always demonstrates a dense and distinct inner third but the distinction between the middle and outer thirds is more difficult to demonstrate and there is often a vague "transition zone" (asterisk in Figs. 19E and 20C) between the two. It is interesting to speculate that this transition zone may be a result of the large subdivision of entorhinal cortex designated 28I by Van Hoesen and Pandya (1975), which is intermediate in its cytoarchitectonic characteristics and perhaps its connections between the lateral and medial subdivisions of the entorhinal cortex.

In AChE-reacted sections there is also a differential pattern of reaction product within the molecular layer of the dentate gyrus but this does not correspond particularly well with the divisions established with Timm's stain as a comparison of Fig. 19A and D demonstrates. Thus, as indicated in Fig. 19A, in AChE preparations of the rat hippocampal formation the inner third of the dentate gyrus molecular layer is divided into an AChE-dense zone immediately proximal to the granule cell layer and a relatively AChE-free zone more distally. Since in the rat the AChE staining in the proximal part of the inner third is abolished by lesions of the septal area where cholinergic input to the hippocampal formation originates (e.g., Mellgren and Srebro, 1973), this zone of the dentate gyrus has also been referred to as the "septal–commissural" zone (e.g., Mosko *et al.*, 1973). However, many investigations of septal projections to the hippocampal formation of the rat have failed to demonstrate any distinct termination

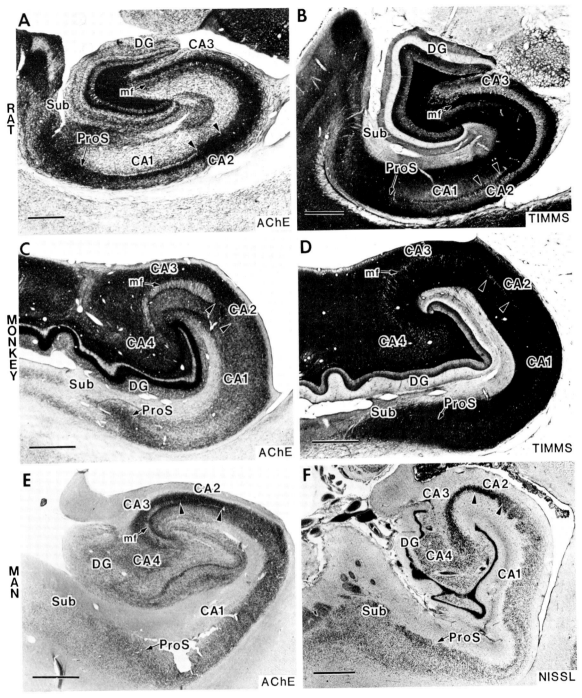

Figure 18. (*Left*) Sections through the hippocampal formation of the rat (A), monkey (C), and man (E) prepared with AChE; (*right*) matched sections prepared with Timm's procedure (B, D) or the thionin stain (F). These sections demonstrate the specific histochemical characteristics associated with specific subdivisions of the hippocampal formation. Bars = 0.5 mm (A, B), 1.0 mm (C, D), 2.0 mm (E, F).

corresponding to this AChE-rich zone (e.g., Swanson and Cowan, 1979) and despite some reports of selective septal projections to this area (Mosko *et al.*, 1973; Crutcher *et al.*, 1981) the bulk of the evidence suggests that in the rat, the AChE-dense zone does not receive a correspondingly dense projection from the septal area even though there is a slight increase in the density of anterograde label over the superficial part of the granule cell layer (e.g., Milner *et al.*, 1983).

In the dentate gyrus of the monkey, the picture of AChE staining is quite different from that in the rat. As shown in Fig. 19B, the entire inner third of the molecular layer is filled with dense AChE reaction production. Unlike the rat, in the monkey this AChE-dense zone corresponds almost precisely with the dense Timm's stained inner third as illustrated in Fig. 20. In addition, like the rat, the inner third of the molecular layer in the monkey is the zone of termination for the dentate gyrus association system (see below). While this increased AChE-dense zone might suggest an expansion and/or increased density of the septohippocampal projection to the monkey dentate gyrus, two observations argue strongly against this. First, in the monkey we have observed that transections of the fornix that disconnect septal and/or basal forebrain cholinergic input to the hippocampal formation result in only minor loss of AChE reaction product in this layer even though, like the rat, there is dramatic depletion throughout the hippocampal formation (Moss *et al.*, 1987). Second, we have observed that injections of radiolabeled amino acids into the medial septal nucleus or other cholinergic nuclei of the basal forebrain in monkeys do not result in a distribution of anterograde label corresponding to this AChE-dense inner third. Instead, anterograde label is distributed uniformly throughout the inner third of the molecular layer with only a slight increase in density in the superficial part of the granule cell layer. This correspondence of the association zone and the AChE-dense zone raises the possibility that some aspect of the intrinsic association system may be cholinesterase-positive or even cholinergic. The presence of AChE-positive neurons in the hilus of the dentate gyrus is well known (e.g., Lewis and Shute, 1967) but it is not known if these are the same neurons that give rise to the dentate gyrus association system and even if they are, there are no reports that these neurons contain ChAT, the definitive marker of cholinergic neurons. Since AChE may be present postsynaptically in neurons that are only cholinoceptive, presynaptically in association with noncholinergic projections, and may well have some noncholinergic functions (Greenfield, 1984), the significance of the expansion of the AChE-dense zone in the monkey as well as the preservation of AChE reaction product after fornix transection is unclear.

The relationship of the two principal afferents and both these histochemical stains in the dentate gyrus of the rat and the monkey is summarized in Fig. 21. Quantitative measurements of the areas occupied by these different systems were made from coronal sections through the mid body of hippocampal formation of the monkey and horizontal sections through the middle level of the ventral hippocampal formation of the rat. The histochemical reactions were prepared from adjacent frozen sections while the association and entorhinal afferents were demonstrated using the anterograde transport of amino acids and paraffin embedding methods. In both the monkey and rat the relative distributions of the entorhinal and association afferents are quite close and Timm's stain also

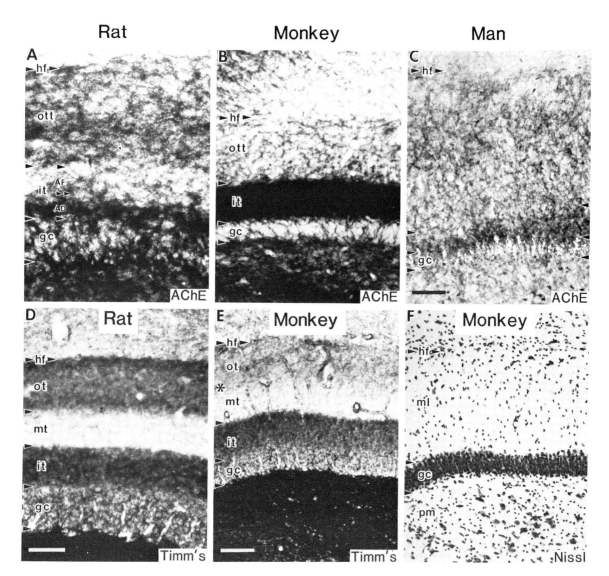

Figure 19. Appearance of the dentate gyrus of the rat (A), monkey (B), and man (C) in tissues reacted for the demonstration of AChE (*top*) and corresponding appearance (*bottom*) of the dentate gyrus in tissue prepared with Timm's stain for heavy metals, except that the section in F is a thionin-stained section of monkey hippocampus matching B and E. The asterisk in E marks the vague transition between the lightly staining middle third and the denser staining outer third of the molecular layer of the dentate gyrus of the monkey hippocampal formation. In comparing the AChE patterns note that in A the inner third (it) of the molecular layer of the dentate gyrus of the rat is divided into an AChE dense zone (AD) and a slightly larger AChE free (AF) zone. However in B the inner third (it) of the monkey dentate gyrus is completely AChE dense while in C the human dentate gyrus shows an AChE dense zone that, like the rat, does not occupy the entire inner third but like the monkey there is no AChE free zone. Bars = 200 μm (C), 50 μm (D, also applies to A), 100 μm (E, also applies to B and F).

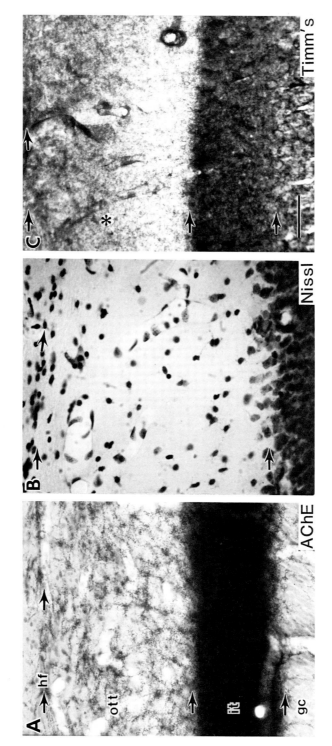

Figure 20. Comparison of high-power photomicrographs of the dentate gyrus of the rhesus monkey prepared with the AChE, Nissl, or Timm's procedures. Note the close correspondence between the AChE-dense inner third of the molecular layer (A) and Timm's stained inner third (C). In C the asterisk marks the gradual transition between the denser outer third and the less dense inner third. Bar = 50 μm.

shows a good correspondence. It is only in AChE material that the differences described above became apparent. In any case, these observations raise the possibility that in the monkey, in comparison to the rat, there may be something quite different in some functional aspects of the cholinergic innervation of the dentate gyrus and/or its interaction with the dentate gyrus association system.

In an attempt to determine if the dentate gyrus of the human displays AChE staining patterns similar to the monkey, we have prepared some sections of human hippocampus. As shown in Fig. 18E the overall AChE distribution in the human hippocampal formation is more similar to the monkey (Fig. 18C) than the rat (Fig. 18A). However, the AChE staining picture of the dentate gyrus of the human differs from both the rat and the monkey. As shown in Fig. 19C the AChE-dense band proximal to the granule cell layer appears to occupy only about 10 to 15% of the molecular layer in the human, a value similar to the 13% observed in the rat but quite different from the 30% seen in the monkey (see Fig. 21). In addition, AChE in the remainder of the molecular layer is more uniformly distributed and of higher intensity relative to the dense supragranular zone than in either the monkey or the rat and there is no distinctive AChE-free zone superficial to the AChE-dense zone as there is in the rat. Whether the AChE-dense supragranular zone in the human dentate gyrus is coextensive with the "inner third" as defined by Timm's stain or with the termination zone of the dentate gyrus association system as it is in the monkey or occupies only a part of these zones as it does in the rat is not known. If it is coextensive with the association zone in the human, this would indicate that zone of the entorhinal afferent termination may occupy proportionally more of the molecular layer in the human than it does in either the rat or monkey. While this narrow zone of AChE-dense reaction product in the inner third and more diffuse distribution in the remainder of the molecular layer in the human dentate gyrus is consistent across several brains, it is possible that the apparent reduction in the width of the inner third and increase in the outer two-thirds (relative to the monkey) is a function of postmortem changes in AChE activity or distribution. In any case, the significance of this AChE-dense zone in both primates and rodents remains to be determined.

While the distribution of AChE reaction product in the inner third of the molecular layer of the dentate gyrus in the rat and monkey and its preservation after fornix transection in the monkey but not the rat constitute a striking difference between these two species, a comparison of both AChE distribution and Timm's staining patterns in the other hippocampal subfields reveals at least as many additional species differences as there are similarities. Furthermore, when there are differences between the rat and monkey, examination of the human hippocampal formation generally reveals a pattern more similar to that of the monkey rather than the rat.

For example, in both the rat and monkey there is dense AChE reaction product in the hilus of the dentate gyrus (including both the dentate gyrus polymorphic layer and the CA4 subfield) and in stratum oriens and stratum pyramidale of the CA3 and CA2 subfields as shown in Fig. 18A,C (for the monkey see also Bakst and Amaral, 1984; Moss and Rosene, 1987). However, in the monkey, but not the rat, there is a decrease in AChE density in the polymorphic layer immediately beneath the granule cells and then two denser bands in the

RAT   MONKEY

TIMMS

A

←— hf —→

ml

40%   40%

30%   29%

30%   31%

←— gc —→

ENTO

B

←— hf —→

ml

70%   67%

30%   33%

←— gc —→

ASSOC

←— hf —→

C

ml

72%   68%

28%   32%

←— gc —→

ACHE

←— hf —→

D

ml

72%   70%

15%

13%   30%

←— gc —→

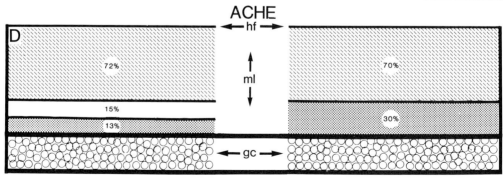

CA4 region of the hilus. While these differential patterns are not evident in the hilus in the rat (perhaps reflecting the relative areas of the polymorphic layer and the CA4 subfield described above), a similar pattern that appears to correspond to the polymorphic and CA4 zones is also seen in the human hippocampal formation (Fig. 18E,F).

In the comparable sections prepared with Timm's stain (Fig. 18B,D), it can be observed that the hilus of the dentate gyrus in the rat is stained intensely and relatively uniformly whereas in the monkey the hilus is stained most intensely in the polymorphic zone and less intensely in the CA4 zone (although this is not readily apparent in Fig. 18D). While comparable Timm's stained material for the human hippocampal formation is not available, the published report of Timm's staining of endogenous metal sulfides in the human hippocampal formation (Cassell and Brown, 1984) appears to demonstrate this same differential in the hilus of the dentate gyrus.

In the CA3 subfield of the rat, there is dense AChE reaction product in the stratum lucidum, which is occupied primarily by the granule cell mossy fibers (Fig. 18A). In contrast, in the monkey the mossy fiber zone (stratum lucidum) is most notable for its very low level of AChE reaction product as shown in Figs. 11A and 18C. In addition, more superficially in the CA3 and CA2 subfields of the monkey, the stratum radiatum has significant AChE reaction product and the stratum moleculare has both a very dense AChE-positive zone adjacent to the stratum radiatum and a less dense zone adjacent to the hippocampal fissure. In the rat, the stratum radiatum has relatively little AChE and the stratum moleculare does not show the two distinct bands of reaction product. In the human hippocampal formation the distribution of AChE in the CA3 and CA2 subfields is most similar to that seen in the monkey with dense AChE reaction product in the stratum oriens and stratum pyramidale, relatively little AChE reaction product in the mossy fiber layer, less dense reaction product in the stratum radiatum, and some evidence of two bands of reaction product in the molecular layer. The feature most common to all three species is the homogeneously dense reaction product seen in the stratum oriens and stratum moleculare of the CA2 subfield.

Similarly, Timm's stain of the CA3 and CA2 subfields presents a very similar picture in the rat and monkey where the densely staining mossy fiber projection occupies the hilus of the dentate gyrus and stratum lucidum of CA3. In both species, Timm's mossy fiber staining ends abruptly at the CA3–CA2 border and serves to differentiate the CA2 subfield from CA3 even in Nissl stains where the stratum lucidum can usually be identified. This observation agrees with the earlier report of Otsuka *et al.* (1976) in the monkey. It has been confirmed in the human brain by Cassell and Brown (1984) who reported that even without

←

Figure 21. Comparison of the proportion of the dentate gyrus molecular layer in the monkey and the rat determined by four different techniques: (A) Timm's stain for heavy metals, (B) anterograde labeling with amino acids of the entorhinal afferents to the dentate gyrus, (C) anterograde labeling with amino acids of the dentate gyrus association pathway, (D) the AChE histochemical procedure. Note the good correspondence between species of all these measures except the AChE procedure.

sulfide perfusion, Timm's stain could demonstrate the mossy fiber projection through the stratum lucidum of the CA3 subfield. All these reports agree that the mossy fiber staining stops abruptly at the CA2–CA3 border. The Timm's pattern in the remainder of the CA3 and CA2 subfields is identical in the monkey and rat with dense staining occupying the stratum radiatum but little or no staining of the stratum moleculare (Fig. 18B,D).

In both the rat and monkey there is generally less AChE reaction product in the CA1 subfield than in the comparable layers of the CA3 and CA2 subfields. Like these areas the stratum oriens and stratum pyramidale of the CA1 subfield have the greatest AChE density in both the rat and monkey. However, in the superficial layers there is a striking difference between these two species. In the monkey there is significant AChE reaction product in the stratum radiatum where it is comparable in density to that in the stratum oriens and stratum pyramidale (Fig. 18C) but the density in the stratum radiatum decreases as one proceeds from the border with the CA2 subfield toward the prosubiculum. In contrast, the stratum moleculare in the monkey is virtually free of AChE reaction product. In the rat the pattern of AChE reaction product in these two layers is exactly reversed with the stratum radiatum relatively free of reaction product while there is significant reaction product in most of the stratum moleculare. A comparison of the AChE pattern in the human reveals that it follows the pattern of the monkey with uniformly dense reaction product in this stratum oriens, stratum pyramidale, and stratum radiatum and that the density of this reaction product decreases near the prosubiculum (Fig. 18E). Similarly, the stratum moleculare of the human hippocampal formation is almost free of AChE reaction product.

In Timm's stain, both the rat and the monkey show a prominent band of staining in the CA1 subfield that is coextensive with the stratum oriens, stratum pyramidale, and stratum radiatum of the CA1 subfield and the stratum moleculare is relatively unstained in both species as shown in Fig. 18B,D. To the extent that Timm's staining reflects the location of different afferents (Haug, 1973), this similarity suggests that most features of the principal afferents to these layers (the Schaffer collateral system and entorhinal perforant path) may be phylogenetically stable or at least comparable in the rat and monkey. There are no data available in the human on this issue.

In the rat both the subiculum and the small prosubicular subfields show dense AChE reaction product throughout all layers. This AChE staining is most dense in the prosubiculum and lightest at the border with the presubiculum (Fig. 18A). The distribution of AChE reaction product in the monkey is similar in the prosubiculum where there is denser reaction product throughout all layers than in the adjacent CA1 subfield. However, in contrast to the rat, the subiculum is nearly free of AChE reaction product except for a narrow band in the deep part of the stratum pyramidale (Fig. 18 A versus C). In the human hippocampal formation, AChE reaction product appears to follow the same pattern as the monkey with denser AChE reaction product distinguishing the prosubiculum from both CA1 and the subiculum (Fig. 18C). In this regard the area that we have classified as the prosubiculum in the rat, monkey, and man on the basis of the small superficial pyramids (Fig. 12) appears to be characterized as well by increased AChE reaction product in all three species (e.g., Fig. 13). However, in the monkey and man this AChE pattern also differentiates the prosubiculum from the subiculum but this distinction does not appear to hold for the rat. The significance of the AChE-free subiculum of the primate is unclear but may reflect a further differentiation of these two subicular subfields in primates.

Like the distribution of the AChE reaction product in the prosubiculum and subiculum, Timm's stain also differentiates the monkey from the rat. In the rat there is a distinct increase in Timm's staining in the stratum pyramidale of the prosubiculum and then a slight decrease in the subiculum (Fig. 18D). However, in the monkey, Timm's staining pattern does not change appreciably in the stratum pyramidale of the prosubiculum and subiculum from the stratum pyramidale of CA1.

To the extent that the AChE histochemical reaction and Timm's stain for heavy metals assess cholinergic innervation and general afferent organization, respectively, the data reviewed above suggest that the histochemical organization of most subfields of the hippocampal formation of the monkey and man are quite similar but that there are a number of features that distinguish both from the hippocampal formation of the rat.

5.2. The Uncus and Genu of the Hippocampal Formation

The foregoing descriptions of AChE and Timm's staining patterns apply to the entire main body of the monkey hippocampal formation. Figure 22 presents adjacent sections through the mid part of the main body of the monkey hippocampal formation prepared with AChE, Nissl, and Timm's procedures. The Nissl section (Fig. 22B) presents the comparable cytoarchitectonic delineation of the various subfields as described in Section 4 for comparison with the histochemical features described in Section 5.1. In Figs. 23 and 24, similar sets of adjacent sections from the same case are presented at the level of the anterior body and uncus (Fig. 23) and the genu (Fig. 24). Comparison of the genu and uncus (Figs. 24 and 23) with the anterior body and mid body (Figs. 23 and 22) indicates that the histochemical features of the main body generally apply to the uncus and genu of the monkey hippocampal formation. However, there are a few exceptions to this as well as some unique features that are important to note.

With regard to AChE staining it is clear that the entire dentate gyrus as well as the CA4, CA3, and CA2 subfields of the uncus and genu show much greater AChE density than similar subfields of the anterior or mid body even though the relative staining patterns within each subfield are similar (Figs. 22–24). This corresponds to a similar distribution in the rat where AChE density is greater in the ventral hippocampus, as well as in the guinea pig (Geneser-Jensen, 1972). The CA1, prosubiculum, subiculum at all levels show similar AChE staining patterns. However, at the level of the genu, the two unique subfields, CA1′ and the HATA, each have a distinct pattern. In the CA1′ subfield the density of AChE reaction product is greater than in the CA1 subfield, even in the same section (Fig. 24). However, the distribution of AChE reaction product in CA1′ is similar to CA1 with relatively dense staining in the stratum oriens, stratum pyramidale, and stratum radiatum but little AChE reaction product in the stratum moleculare. In the HATA there is a decrease in AChE staining relative to

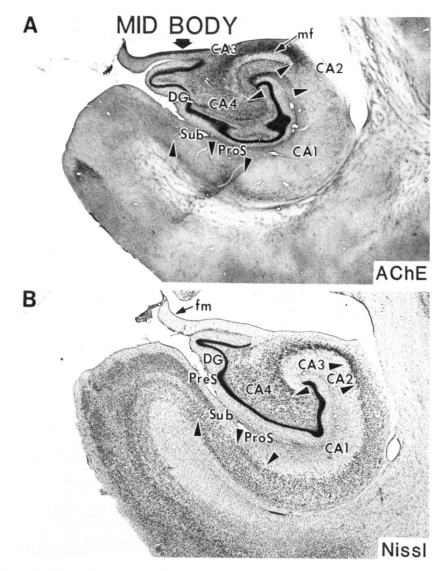

Figure 22. Three adjacent 40-µm-thick frozen sections through the middle level of the main body of the hippocampal formation of the rhesus monkey prepared according to AChE, Nissl, or Timm's procedures. Bar = 1.0 mm.

the adjacent CA1' subfield but a modest density of AChE reaction product is found throughout the stratum pyramidale while the molecular layer is free of reaction product. These features serve to distinguish the HATA from the pro-subiculum and subiculum since in the prosubiculum AChE increases relative to the adjacent CA1 subfield while in the subiculum AChE reaction product is relatively absent from the stratum pyramidale.

The basic Timm's staining pattern for these different levels appears to be very stable for all of the typical cytoarchitectonically defined subfields. As shown in Fig. 24, the mossy fiber layer clearly distinguishes the medial and lateral parts

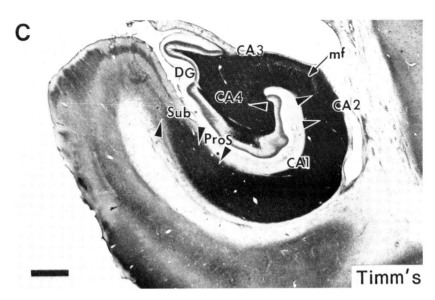

Figure 22. *(continued)*

of the CA2 subfield from the intervening CA3 subfield in the genu. In the uncus, the Timm's staining pattern also serves to confirm the cytoarchitectonic observations that only the dentate gyrus, CA4, and CA3 are generally present. Interestingly, while the Timm's pattern in these uncal subfields is normal, the overall density is clearly reduced relative to the main body, even in the same section (e.g., Fig. 23). However, the most interesting features of Timm's stain occur in the CA1′ and HATA. As shown in Fig. 24, the dense Timm's staining of the stratum radiatum but the light staining of the stratum moleculare that characterize the CA3, CA2, and CA1 subfields continue into CA1′ but the density dramatically decreases. This is the opposite of the change in AChE staining. In the HATA, Timm's pattern is even more unique since the stratum pyramidale is unstained while the stratum moleculare is densely stained. In both regards this is exactly the opposite of the pattern in all of the other ammonic and subicular subfields and clearly distinguishes the HATA as a unique subfield.

In summary, the histochemical characteristics of the uncus and genu of the hippocampal formation serve to confirm the identification of the HATA and CA1′ as unique subfields. Furthermore, when taken together the obvious increased density of AChE and decreased density of Timm's staining suggest that there may be unique reciprocal changes in the cholinergic and other afferent innervation of the uncus and genu.

6. Connectivity

The connectivity of the hippocampal formation has been a focus of intense investigation by neuroscientists for most of the past 40 years, and Blackstad's (1956) early work was one of the first to use the then new suppressive silver

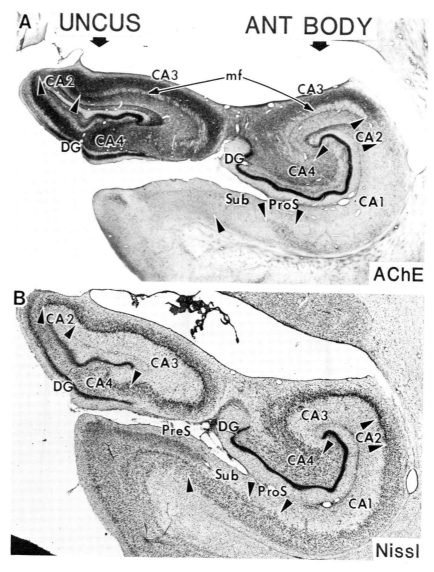

Figure 23. Three adjacent 40-μm-thick frozen sections through the uncus and anterior level of the main body of the hippocampal formation of the rhesus monkey prepared according to AChE, Nissl, or Timm's procedures. They are from the same case as Fig. 22. Bar = 1.0 mm.

impregnation methods. As a result, there is a wealth of information on this topic, especially from the many investigations using axoplasmic transport tracer techniques in the rat where a majority of these studies have been conducted. This literature is so extensive that no attempt will be made to review all these studies. Instead, this section will focus on those aspects of hippocampal connectivity that are common to both the rat and monkey but especially those that are unique to the monkey. Before proceeding with this discussion, two issues should be considered regarding the interpretation of axoplasmic transport data. The sensitivity

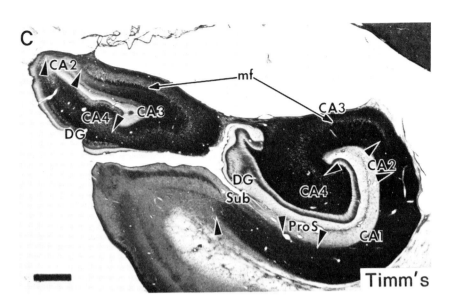

Figure 23. *(continued)*

of these axoplasmic transport methods has provided exquisite confirmation of many aspects of hippocampal connectivity that were subject to dispute or confusion when only methods utilizing normal material or lesion-induced degeneration were available. On the other hand, these new methods have also resulted in a number of isolated reports that describe aspects of hippocampal connectivity that do not fit into our conventional thinking about the hippocampal formation. While some of these reports may represent new and unique aspects of hippocampal connectivity that should change the way we think about the hippocampal formation, others may represent examples of the "effective injection site" problem or "excessive sensitivity."

The issue of excessive sensitivity is in essence an issue of how to interpret a "few" retrogradely labeled neurons or "light" anterograde label. With techniques as sensitive as current axoplasmic flow methods, these "minor" connections can appear quite convincing. Deciding whether these should be reported as a minor connection or dismissed as an anomaly is often dependent upon how well they fit into current theories. While it is certainly reasonable to simply describe and illustrate all of the evidence generated by these techniques, once these "light" connections are part of the literature they tend to strengthen with age even though the minor connection may in fact have little functional significance. To illustrate this point, one can imagine that during the course of neonatal development some neurons form connections that simply reflect the recapitulation by ontogeny of phylogenetically obsolete connections. It is now clear that one of the basic mechanisms critical to the development of the brain is the death of "excess" neurons or the dying back of "excess" axonal connections (e.g., Reh and Kalil, 1982; Finlay and Slattery, 1983). According to this scenario, these "misplaced" neurons and/or their axons normally die back during development. However, if only a few of these neurons and/or axons survive as "aberrant" or

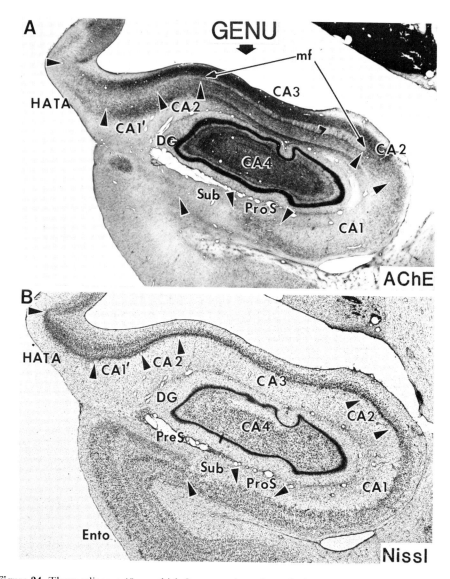

Figure 24. Three adjacent 40-μm-thick frozen sections through the genu of the hippocampal formation of the rhesus monkey prepared according to AChE, Nissl, or Timm's procedures. They are from the same case as Figs. 22 and 23. Bar = 1.0 mm.

"anomalous" remnants of former connectivity, it is not only possible but likely that these will be detected by the careful use of axoplasmic transport techniques. For example, many of us have observed a few neurons retrogradely labeled with HRP in completely unexpected loci. In this case, even if the axon that carried the HRP retrograde tracer were an aberrant or vestigial reflection of a former connection, the HRP filling may be intense. If the skeptical but careful investigator excludes all of the potential technical problems as possible explanations, then this small number of consistently labeled neurons may be reported as a

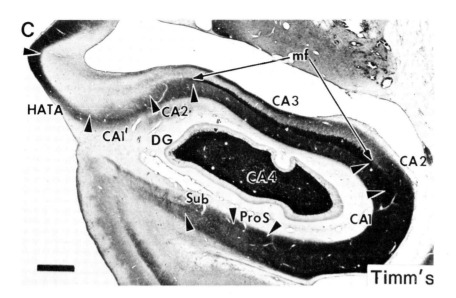

Figure 24. *(continued)*

new connection simply because the HRP technique is so sensitive and the appearance of a few labeled neurons so striking.

A similar problem arises in the interpretation of the exact locus of the tracer injection site from which effective uptake and axoplasmic transport occurred. In essence, the problem of the effective injection site is a function of two unavoidable aspects of the axoplasmic transport technique. The first problem results from the fact that tracer uptake and axoplasmic transport are dynamic processes that require time: from hours to days. Because of this temporal requirement, injection sites of any tracer are always examined at a time interval after the injection when sufficient uptake and transport have occurred. Yet because this is a dynamic process, the injection site at the end of the interval will never fully reflect its state (e.g., size, concentration gradients) during the uptake and transport process. Hence, uptake and transport may readily have occurred in an area that at the time of sacrifice shows little or no evidence of a tracer injection. The second problem results from the fact that the tracer within the injection is distributed across a concentration gradient and that neural elements (e.g., cell bodies, axons) located at different points within the graded injection site may either concentrate transported tracer into a few neurons or axons or dilute it among a larger population. Thus, if a few distant neurons all have axonal arborizations that cover the entire injection site, they are likely to take up and retrogradely transport large amounts of tracer, intensely labeling this small population of neurons. On the other hand, if a small population of neurons all have axons that arborize only in a very small part of the same injection site, they may not take up and transport sufficient tracer to appear retrogradely labeled. The important message of the foregoing discussion for the following review of hippocampal connectivity is that one must be very skeptical in single-tracer studies of unusual positive results, especially "minor" connections, and take special care not to draw far-reaching conclusions from negative results.

With these caveats in mind, the details of hippocampal connectivity will be considered in four separate sections: extrinsic afferent input, intrinsic connections, commissural connections, and extrinsic efferent output. Each of these different systems is exceedingly complex and this complexity grows steadily as new studies are published. However, the number of available studies that have focused upon the monkey hippocampal formation are few. Nevertheless, there do appear to be a number of unifying principles around which each of these systems of connections is organized. For hippocampal extrinsic afferents most major inputs terminate in specific laminae that are sharply defined and delimited from other inputs. Intrinsic hippocampal connections show a similar specificity in their termination but are organized as a serial relay through the different architectonic zones leading from the dentate gyrus through the ammonic subfields and into the subiculum. Overlap of major extrinsic or intrinsic afferents is the exception rather than the rule. The extrinsic hippocampal efferents appear to be organized as a set of parallel connections. Thus, hippocampal projections to the septal area are organized as a set of parallel connections from both the ammonic and the subicular subfields while the diencephalic connections originate as parallel connections from two subdivisions of the subiculum and the cortical efferents originate as parallel connections from both the subiculum and the CA1 subfield.

6.1. Extrinsic Afferents

In the monkey, like the rat, the principal afferent input to all parts of the hippocampal formation originates in the adjacent entorhinal cortex (Hjorth-Simonsen, 1972; Hjorth-Simonsen and Jeune, 1972; Van Hoesen and Pandya, 1975; Steward, 1976), and terminates in the outer two-thirds of the molecular layer of the dentate gyrus and throughout the entire molecular layer (stratum lacusom-moleculare) of the ammonic subfields. In the monkey and rat there is an additional dimension of vertical organization of this termination in the molecular layer of the dentate gyrus and the CA3 subfield while there is a horizontal organization in the molecular layer of the CA1 subfield. This organization has been carefully described by Steward (1976) for the rat and generally corresponds with that described in the monkey by Van Hoesen and Pandya (1975). In the rat, Steward demonstrated that afferents originating in the medial entorhinal area terminate in the middle third of the molecular layer of the dentate gyrus and the deeper half of the molecular layer of the CA3 subfield while those originating from the lateral entorhinal area terminate in the outer third of the molecular layer of the dentate gyrus and the outer half of the CA3 molecular layer. However, entorhinal afferents to the molecular layer of the CA1 and subicular subfields are differentiated along a horizontal dimension so that afferents originating from the medial entorhinal cortex terminate near the CA3 end of the CA1 molecular layer while those from the lateral entorhinal cortex terminate near the subicular end of the CA1 molecular layer. An additional feature of the entorhinal afferent input to the rat hippocampal formation is the "lamellar" organization of this afferent system as reported by Hjorth-Simonsen and Jeune (1972) and Wyss (1981). According to this notion (Andersen *et al.*, 1971), the longitudinal extent of the hippocampal formation is composed of a series of identical and adjacent lamellae each consisting of a short segment of intrinsically connected hippocampal subfields that receive afferent input from a topographically limited part of the entorhinal cortex. This organization has also been confirmed in the rat by studies utilizing injections of the retrograde tracer HRP into the hippocampal formation, which demonstrated that the entorhinal afferents to the hippocampus originate in a topographic pattern, primarily from neurons in layers II and III (Ruth *et al.*, 1982; Steward and Scoville, 1976). Finally, apparently following the principle that the more lateral (subicular) parts of the hippocampal formation receive afferent input from the more lateral parts of the entorhinal cortex, we have also demonstrated that the perirhinal cortex in the lateral bank of the rhinal sulcus projects to the molecular layer of the subiculum (Kosel *et al.*, 1983).

In comparing these observations in the rat with the organization of entorhinal afferents in the monkey a number of prominent differences deserve comment. First, while the afferent input from the lateral and medial entorhinal cortices follows the same principles of laminar termination as the rat, there is little indication that the entorhinal input to different longitudinal levels of the hippocampal formation is organized according to a lamellar plan (Van Hoesen and Pandya, 1975). Instead, entorhinal projections to the hippocampal formation, even from small injections limited to part of one subdivision, cover over half of the longitudinal axis. Another feature of the temporal lobe afferent input to the monkey hippocampal formation is that in addition to the perirhinal input, cortical afferents to the molecular layer of the subiculum originate in the proisocortex and even the neocortex (areas TH and TF) of the posterior parahippocampal gyrus (Van Hoesen *et al.*, 1979) while there was no evidence for cortical inputs beyond the perirhinal area in the rat (Kosel *et al.*, 1983). Additional neocortical inputs to the monkey hippocampal formation have also been reported to originate from the frontal lobe (Leichnetz and Astruc, 1975) and from area TE of the temporal lobe (Schwerdtfeger, 1979) but we have been unable to confirm these in our own material. In any case, since it is not possible to identify temporal lobe cortical areas in the rat that are likely to be homologous to areas TF and TH of the posterior parahippocampal gyrus and there is no evidence of cortical inputs beyond the perirhinal area in the rat, it is likely that this parahippocampal input constitutes a true species difference that may reflect the increased neocortical connectivity of the primate hippocampal formation.

On the basis of retrograde tracing experiments, Amaral and Cowan (1980) reported that subcortical afferents to the monkey hippocampal formation were quite similar to those observed in the rat. They reported retrogradely labeled neurons in the brain stem (locus coeruleus, midline raphe, reticular formation), the diencephalon (supramammillary nucleus, lateral hypothalamic area), the basal forebrain (medial septal nucleus, diagonal band, and nucleus basalis), and the amygdala (anterior amygdaloid area and basolateral nucleus). With the exception of the amygdala and locus coeruleus, these results confirm a similar HRP study in the squirrel monkey by DeVito (1980). While these subcortical afferents generally correspond to those reported in the rat using the retrograde transport of HRP, only a few of these afferents have been demonstrated by anterograde techniques in the rat and even fewer in the monkey. Consequently, with a few exceptions, very little is known of the exact termination pattern of these subcortical afferents within the monkey hippocampal formation. While the good correspondence of retrograde labeling in the rat and monkey suggests that subcortical afferents may be phylogenetically conservative, surprisingly there are a few clear differences when the anterograde termination of these subcortical connections is determined.

Thus, one very interesting projection that has been demonstrated in the monkey (Veazy *et al.*, 1982) arises from the supramammillary nucleus in the hypothalamus. In the dentate gyrus the distribution of anterograde label was quite similar to that observed in the rat (Wyss *et al.*, 1979) with a very narrow band of label overlying the superficial part of the granule cell layer and the adjacent supragranular part of the molecular layer. Surprisingly, Veazy *et al.*, (1982) reported that unlike the rat, the supramammillary projection also terminated in the stratum pyramidale and stratum radiatum of the hippocampus proper immediately distal to the termination of the mossy fibers in the CA3 subfield. Veazy *et al.* (1982) describe this area as the CA3–CA1 (regio inferior–regio superior) transition zone but, as mentioned above, recognize that this corresponds to subfield CA2 of Lorente de Nó (1934). The specificity of this supramammillary projection as well as the unique cytoarchitecture of the CA2 pyramids and lack of mossy fiber termination clearly supports the identification of a CA2 subfield at least in primates. While the termination of the supramammillary projection in the dentate gyrus is similar to that reported in the rat (Wyss *et al.*, 1979), recent reports in the rat have failed to demonstrate a supramammillary projection to the CA2 subfield (Haglund *et al.*, 1984), suggesting that this subcortical projection may be unique to the monkey. Despite our warning about the cautious approach to negative results, the projection to the CA2 subfield in the monkey and its absence in the rat may reflect a phylogenetic difference in subcortical diencephalic input to the primate hippocampal formation.

Other subcortical hippocampal afferents arise from the amygdaloid complex. In the rat and cat, Krettek and Price (1977) have reported that these afferents arise principally from the basolateral nucleus and terminate in the pyramidal layer and proximal part of the molecular layer of the subiculum. On the basis of HRP injections into the monkey hippocampal formation, Amaral and Cowan (1980) reported retrogradely labeled neurons in the basolateral nucleus of the amygdala. In our own material, using both HRP and different fluorescent retrograde tracers, we have confirmed the presence of retrogradely labeled neurons in the laterobasal nucleus but have also observed that the majority of retrogradely labeled neurons in the amygdala are located in the mediobasal, cortical, and accessory basal nuclei (Saunders *et al.*, 1987). Furthermore, on the basis of injections of radiolabeled amino acids into the amygdala, we have demonstrated that projections from the laterobasal and mediobasal nuclei terminate in the pyramidal and molecular layers of the subiculum and prosubiculum, a pattern similar to that reported for the basolateral nucleus of the rat and cat by Krettek and Price (1977) except that in the monkey the projection is shifted toward the prosubiculum. In the cat and rat, Krettek and Price reported that the amygdaloid afferents did not terminate throughout the entire longitudinal extent of the hippocampal formation but were limited to the ventral subiculum but in the monkey this amygdaloid projection extends throughout the entire longitudinal extent of the hippocampal formation. An additional unique observation in the monkey is that the projection arising from the accessory basal nucleus and adjacent cortical nucleus terminates in the molecular layer of the CA3 and CA2 subfields as well as in the subiculum–prosubiculum. As illustrated in Fig. 25, this unique projection is especially strong in the uncus, genu, and anterior body but also extends throughout the entire extent of the hippocampal formation (Saunders *et al.*, 1987). This amygdaloid input to the CA3 and CA2 subfields is another example of an aspect of the hippocampal formation that appears to be unique to the monkey and is of particular interest since it appears to arise mainly from the accessory basal nucleus, an amygdaloid nucleus that is unique in its development in the primate brain and may not have an exact homologue in the rat or cat (Price, 1981).

Another major subcortical afferent to the hippocampal formation arises from the magnocellular nuclei of the basal forebrain [Divac, 1975; Mesulam, *et al.*, 1983: the medial septal nucleus (MS), the vertical nucleus of the diagonal band (VDB), the horizontal nucleus of the diagonal band (HDB), and the nucleus basalis (NB)]. In the rat this afferent system has been referred to as the septohippocampal system and is generally regarded as a cholinergic system although Amaral and Kurz (1985) have recently demonstrated that a significant proportion of the hippocampal projection neurons are probably not cholinergic. The termination of the septohippocampal system has been inferred on the basis of the distribution of AChE reaction product in the hippocampal formation since AChE activity in the hippocampal formation of the rat is almost totally abolished by transection of the fornix (Lewis and Shute, 1967) or lesions of the septal area (Mellgren and Srebro, 1973). However, it has become clear that the system is considerably more complicated since in the rat this afferent system originates from both the medial septal nucleus and the nucleus of the vertical limb of the diagonal band and perhaps (depending upon one's application of this nomenclature) from the horizontal nucleus of the diagonal band and from the nucleus basalis (see Lynch *et al.*, 1978; Amaral and Kurz, 1985) although there are far fewer hippocampal projection neurons in these more lateral subdivisions of the basal forebrain. However, there have been two major problems in our understanding of this afferent system that are still only partially resolved. First, studies utilizing anterograde tracing techniques to demonstrate the hippocampal projections of these basal forebrain areas (principally the septal area) have not consistently reported distributions of anterograde label that correspond with the distribution of AChE (degeneration: Mosko *et al.*, 1973; autoradiography: Rose and Shubert, 1977; Lynch *et al.*, 1978; Swanson and Cowan, 1979; Milner *et al.*, 1983; anterograde HPR: Crutcher *et al.*, 1981). The most prominent example of this problem is the AChE-dense supragranular zone in the inner third of the molecular layer of the dentate gyrus where fornix lesions abolish AChE staining in the rat (but not the monkey) while anterograde tracing experiments are

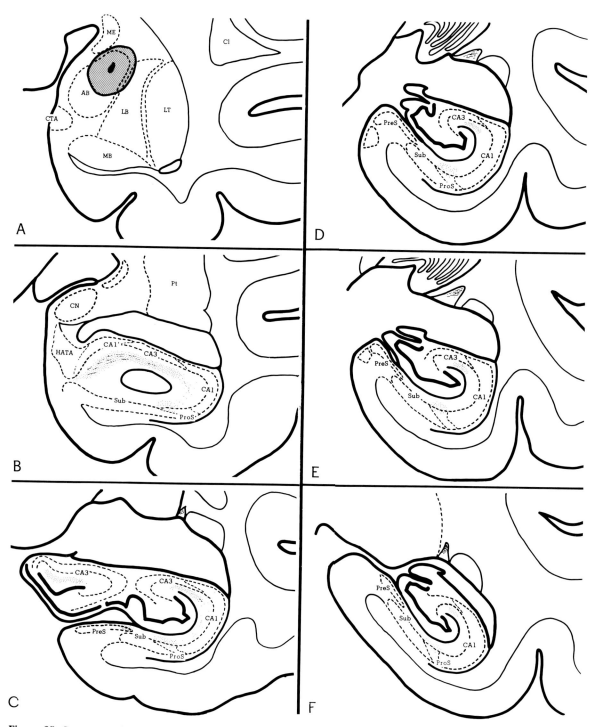

Figure 25. Summary of the results of an injection of radiolabeled amino acids (A) centered in the accessory basal nucleus of the amygdala of the rhesus monkey. As shown in B and C this injection produced label over the molecular layer of the CA3, CA2, and CA1′ subfields in the uncus, genu, and anterior body as well as the prosubiculum of the genu and anterior body. The prosubicular and CA3 label also continued back through the entire longitudinal axis of the hippocampal formation (D–F). Modified from Saunders *et al.* (1987).

divided as to whether or not there is a basal forebrain projection to this area. If AChE reaction product exactly marked the cholinergic septohippocampal projection, one might expect the anterograde tracing experiments to demonstrate termination in more areas than AChE reaction product is distributed since numerous studies (e.g., Amaral and Kurz, 1985) have demonstrated that there are a substantial number of noncholinergic hippocampal projection neurons in the basal forebrain. But to the contrary, the distribution of AChE reaction product is more extensive than patterns of anterograde label. One possible explanation of this is that there may be additional sources of AChE reaction product such as another extrinsic cholinergic input and/or an intrinsic source such as AChE- or ChAT-positive neurons (Milner *et al.*, 1983; Frotscher and Leranth, 1985). From all of these studies a few conclusions can be drawn. First, most studies agree that there is a strong projection from the medial septal nucleus and/or diagonal band to the hilus of the dentate gyrus, to stratum oriens of the CA3 and CA2 subfields and to the molecular and pyramidal layers of the subiculum. Second, these studies also agree that there is a less intense projection to the entire molecular layer of the dentate gyrus and ammonic subfields, to stratum radiatum of the CA3 subfield, and to stratum oriens of the CA1 subfield.

While there are no recent published studies of the anterograde projections from the basal forebrain to the hippocampal formation in the monkey, our own unpublished observations reveal similar anomalies. Thus, in the dentate gyrus the entire inner third of the molecular layer shows dense AChE reaction product but injections of radiolabeled amino acids throughout the basal forebrain have failed to demonstrate any specific evidence of greater terminal label in this layer than in the rest of the molecular layer of the dentate gyrus. Overall the pattern of termination in the monkey hippocampal formation is similar to that reported in the rat with the densest anterograde label in the hilus of the dentate gyrus and stratum oriens of the CA3 and CA2 subfields. In addition, there is significant uniformly distributed label in the molecular layer of the dentate gyrus and the stratum pyramidale and stratum radiatum of the CA3 and CA2 subfields. There is also label in the same parts of the CA1 subfield but it is reduced relative to CA3 and CA2. In the subicular subfields there was significant label in the stratum moleculare and stratum pyramidale of the prosubiculum but very little evidence of any projection to the subiculum. In addition, we have observed two other features of this termination pattern. First, regardless of the locus of injection or the site of termination, anterograde label is always most dense at the uncal level of the hippocampal formation and decreases at more posterior levels. Second, medial injections that are centered in the medial septum and medial part of the nucleus of the vertical limb of the diagonal band label the dentate gyrus and ammonic subfields most intensely while injections in the lateral part of the diagonal band and/or nucleus basalis produce dense label over the prosubiculum and CA1 subfield. While these two general trends correspond with similar organization described in the rat hippocampal formation by Milner *et al.* (1983), judging by published illustrations and our own material both tendencies are much more extreme in the monkey hippocampal formation.

While afferents to the hippocampal formation from the thalamus and various brain-stem monoaminergic nuclei have been demonstrated in the monkey only with retrograde transport techniques (e.g., Amaral and Cowan, 1980) in the rat their termination in the hippocampal formation has been demonstrated with anterograde transport techniques (Herkenham, 1978; Azmitia and Segal, 1978) or histofluorescence techniques (Loy *et al.*, 1980). Of these projections the most interesting is the thalamic projection from the nucleus reuniens. While all of the other brain-stem projections terminate relatively diffusely in the hippocampal formation, in the rat (Herkenham, 1978) this projection terminates in a sharp band limited to the stratum moleculare of both the subiculum (including the prosubiculum) and the CA1 subfield of the ventral hippocampal formation of the rat. If a similar thalamic afferent input exists in the monkey, it would overlap extensively with afferent input from the entorhinal cortex, perirhinal cortex, posterior parahippocampal cortices, and the amygdaloid complex that terminate in the stratum moleculare of the subiculum, prosubiculum, and CA1 subfields of the monkey. If this projection is not found in the monkey (and the paucity of retrogradely labeled thalamic neurons resulting from hippocampal HRP injections suggests this might be the case), then it could be that the region dominated by diencephalic input in the rat is completely dominated by telencephalic input in the monkey.

In summary, the principal extrinsic cortical afferent inputs to the hippocampal formation terminate in the molecular layer of all subfields. Furthermore, as one proceeds from the molecular layer (outer two-thirds) of the dentate gyrus (the most medial allocortex), laterally through the molecular layer of the ammonic subfields to the molecular layer of the prosubiculum and subiculum, this cortical input originates successively from the periallocortical entorhinal area, the proisocortical perirhinal cortex (area 35), and the proisocortex and neocortex (areas TH and TF) of the posterior parahippocampal gyrus. In the dentate gyrus and ammonic subfields the only other major extrinsic inputs to the molecular layers arise from the amygdala (accessory basal projection to the CA3 and CA2 subfields) and the less prominent basal forebrain input to the molecular layer of both the dentate gyrus and the CA3 and CA2 subfields. For the molecular layer of the CA1 subfield, only the possible thalamic input described above appears to be a potential additional extrinsic afferent. The basal forebrain input to the stratum moleculare of the prosubiculum and subiculum appears to overlap with amygdaloid input to these layers as well as with the proisocortical and neocortical inputs from the posterior parahippocampal gyrus to the molecular layer of these subfields. Thus, all of the areas of predominant extrinsic afferent termination are characterized by a convergence of at least several subcortical afferents with the major cortical afferents.

In addition to these inputs to zones apparently dominated by extrinsic afferent input, there are also some important extrinsic afferents that terminate in areas dominated by major intrinsic afferent systems (see below). Thus, the basal forebrain projection to the hilus of the dentate gyrus, and to the stratum oriens, stratum pyramidale, and stratum radiatum of the ammonic subfields appears to constitute the major extrinsic afferent input to these areas but this input overlaps extensively with major intrinsic afferent systems described in the following section (mossy fibers to the hilus of the dentate gyrus and Schaffer collateral projections to the stratum oriens, pyramidale, and radiatum of the CA3, CA2, and CA1 subfields). The basal forebrain and amygdaloid projections to the stratum pyramidale and the proximal part of the molecular layer of the prosubiculum and subiculum overlap with the major intrinsic projection of the CA1 subfield to these same areas. The supramammillary projection to the supragranular part of the inner third of the dentate gyrus molecular layer is the only specific extrinsic afferent input to any part of the inner third and it overlaps with the intrinsic dentate gyrus association pathway (see below). The supramammillary projection to the CA2 subfield overlaps with the intrinsic Schaffer collateral system.

6.2. Intrinsic Afferents and Efferents

One of the most striking features of the hippocampal formation is the highly ordered and serially arranged chain of intrinsic connections that link adjacent cytoarchitectonically defined subfields. In the following section the extensive studies of the intrinsic projection systems in the rat will first be described and then compared with our own observations in the monkey (Rosene and Van Hoesen, 1977). While our observations in the monkey were only described briefly in that short report, the discussion below also relies upon and describes some subsequent observations that have all confirmed the basic features of our original description.

There are at least two intrinsic projections that arise from the dentate gyrus: the mossy fiber system and the dentate gyrus association pathway. The mossy fibers are the zinc-rich efferents of the granule cells of the dentate gyrus and these have been shown by a number of techniques (silver degeneration: Blackstad *et al.*, 1970; Hjorth-Simonsen, 1973; Timm's stain degeneration: Haug *et al.*, 1971; autoradiography: Swanson *et al.*, 1978; anterograde HRP: West *et al.*, 1982) to project to the dentate gyrus polymorphic layer and/or the CA4 subfield as well as the classic projection through the stratum pyramidale and stratum lucidum of the CA3 subfield. Ultrastructural studies of Timm's stained normal material (Haug, 1967) or hippocampal slices injected intracellulary with HRP (Claiborne *et al.*, 1986) have confirmed that these granule cell axons give rise to axons and collaterals that form en passage mossy fiber synapses in the dentate gyrus hilar region and the CA4 and CA3 subfields of the rat. These large mossy fiber boutons make multiple synaptic contacts with invaginating spines. The boutons range from 1 or 2 μm in size on mossy fiber collaterals in the hilus (Claiborne *et al.*, 1986) to 5 μm in size on the principal mossy fibers in the CA3 subfield where the enlarged invaginating spines of the CA3 pyramids are referred to as thorns (Laatsch and Cowan, 1966; Amaral and Dent, 1981). This projection can be demonstrated in normal material by application of Timm's stain for heavy metals, which densely stains these axons (Haug, 1973), and this is illustrated for the rat and monkey in Figs. 18 and 24. In both species the distal end of the mossy fiber projection exactly defines the end of the CA3 subfield and the beginning of the CA2 subfield where the large chromophilic neurons similar to the CA3 pyramidal cells lack mossy fiber input. These relationships are illustrated for the monkey CA2 subfield in Fig. 11 and can be compared with the rat in Fig. 18. This same relationship has been confirmed in the human by Cassell and Brown (1984) using Timm's stain in unperfused tissue. Studies in the rat (Swanson *et al.*, 1978) and our own observations in the monkey indicate that this projection is organized in a topographic lamellar fashion so that one limited segment of the dentate gyrus sends its mossy fibers to only a limited segment of the dentate gyrus hilus, CA4 and CA3 subfields. As illustrated in Fig. 26, an injection of radiolabeled amino acids that involves the dentate gyrus (Fig. 26D) produces label in a narrow band of rostrally directed fibers as shown in Fig. 26C,D.

The hilar cells of the dentate gyrus and/or the CA4 subfield give rise to a dentate gyrus association pathway that terminates within the inner third of the molecular layer of the dentate gyrus. In the rat this system has been demonstrated with many different techniques (silver degeneration: Hjorth-Simonsen, 1973; silver degeneration and HRP: Laurberg, 1979; autoradiography: Swanson *et al.*, 1978) and in contrast to the limited lamellar topography of the mossy fiber projection this system appears to act as a longitudinal association pathway since it extends for a considerable distance along the longitudinal axis of the hippocampal formation. The origin of this system in the hilus of the dentate gyrus has also been confirmed in the rabbit by Berger *et al.* (1981). Our own observations in the monkey confirm the presence of this dentate gyrus association pathway, and its termination in the inner third of the molecular layer of the dentate gyrus following an injection of radiolabeled amino acids into the CA4 subfield and hilus of the dentate gyrus as illustrated in Fig. 27. We have also observed its extensive spread throughout the longitudinal axis of the hippocampal formation where it appears to extend in a caudal direction all the way to the posterior body (Fig. 27F) following an injection into the uncal hippocampus (Fig. 27C). As shown in Fig. 26, when only the hilus of the dentate gyrus is included in an injection at the level of the mid body of the hippocampal formation, the dentate gyrus association pathway is also labeled as far caudal as the posterior body (Fig. 26F) but rostrally does not reach the uncus (Fig. 26B). This suggests that this longitudinal pathway is polarized and has a longer extent in the caudal direction.

The CA3 subfield gives rise to an intrinsic projection that appears to correspond to the so-called Schaffer collateral system of classical Golgi impregnation studies (e.g., Lorente de Nó, 1934). According to these studies, CA3 and possibly CA2 pyramidal neurons send their main axon into the fimbria–fornix but give off an axon collateral that ascends into the stratum radiatum and then courses laterally through the stratum radiatum of the CA1 subfield where it contacts the proximal part of the apical dendrites of the CA1 pyramidal cells. In the rat, experimental studies using a variety of techniques (silver degeneration: Hjorth-

Figure 26. Summary of the results of an injection of radiolabeled amino acids (D) centered in the CA1 subfield that also spread into the granule cell and polymorphic layers of the dentate gyrus. The relatively limited and rostrally directed mossy fiber projection arising from the involvement of the granule cell layer courses forward in C–A while the weak but distinct labeling of the dentate gyrus association system arising from the polymorphic layer of the hilus is present from the most rostral level (A) to the most caudal level (F) of the dentate gyrus. The major projection system revealed by this injection is the ammonic subicular projection, which, like the mossy filter projection, is rostrally directed and relatively limited in its longitudinal spread as shown in C and B where the CA1 projection to layer V of the entorhinal cortex is also demonstrated.

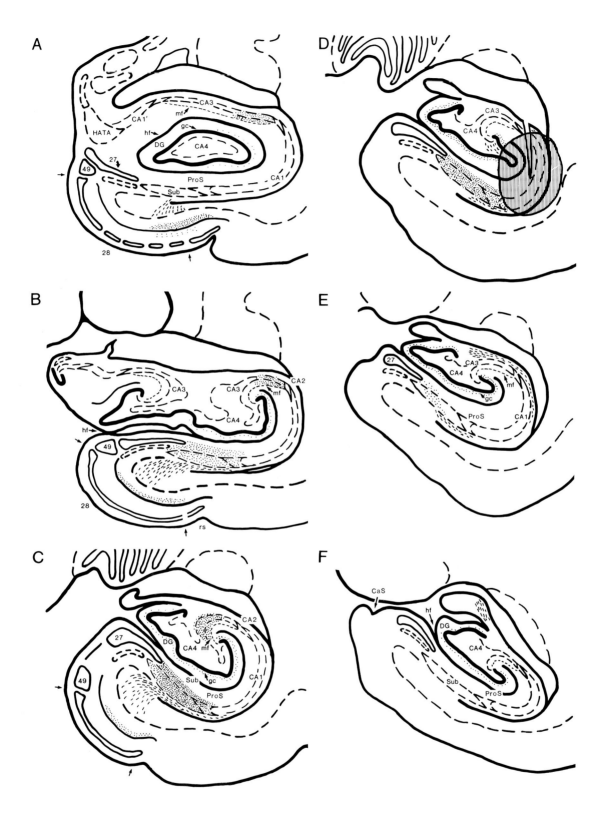

Simonsen, 1973; silver degeneration and HRP: Laurberg, 1979; autoradiography: Swanson *et al.*, 1978) have demonstrated that the Schaffer collateral projection originates in the CA3 subfield and terminates in the stratum radiatum and to a lesser extent in the stratum oriens of the CA3, CA2, and CA1 subfields. These studies have also demonstrated that this projection is not organized in a lamellar fashion but shows a considerable degree of divergence along the longitudinal axis of the hippocampal formation. Using intracellular injection of HRP, Finch *et al.* (1983) have demonstrated that at least some of the CA3 pyramids in the rat do indeed send an axon into the fimbria and collaterals into the Schaffer collateral system that reaches into the CA1 subfield and shows considerable divergence. Lorente de Nó (1934) proposed that the CA2 subfield gave rise to a "longitudinal association" projection that did not cover the entire stratum radiatum of the adjacent CA1 subfield but instead was limited to the stratum radiatum in and around the borders of the CA2 subfield where it extended a considerable distance along the longitudinal axis. In the monkey we have not been able to identify a longitudinal projection separate from the Schaffer collateral system.

While these studies in the rat agree on the origin in CA3 and termination in CA3, CA2, and CA1 of this Schaffer collateral projection, Swanson *et al.* (1978) reported two additional features of this system that are at variance with most other published reports. First, they report that injections of radiolabeled amino acids into the CA3 subfield label the Schaffer collateral system as well as a projection beyond the CA1 subfield into the subiculum and even the presubiculum. Second, these authors also report an identical projection system arising from CA4 and/or hilus of the dentate gyrus. To date, there is no convincing experimental confirmation in rats of either the CA4 origin of the Schaffer collateral system or its extension into the subiculum. In the monkey our own observations confirm the existence of a Schaffer collateral system that originates in the CA3 subfield and terminates in the CA3, CA2, and CA1 subfields as shown in Fig. 27A. In order of intensity, this projection terminates most heavily in the stratum radiatum, stratum pyramidale and stratum oriens of the CA1, CA2, and CA3 subfields as illustrated in Fig. 29A. Furthermore, our observations agree with those in the rat in demonstrating a large longitudinal extent for this system that is caudally directed like the dentate gyrus association system but is more limited in its longitudinal extent, especially from the uncus. In addition, our observations fail to demonstrate either a CA4 origin or a subicular termination for this system as described by Swanson *et al.* (1978). On the other hand, we do observe a weak projection to the prosubiculum, a subfield not recognized by any of the rat studies.

Figure 27. Summary of the results of an injection of radiolabeled amino acids into the uncal level of the hippocampal formation (C), which completely labeled the dentate gyrus, CA4 and CA3 subfields, and also spread into the underlying lamina principalis externa of the presubiculum. As shown in A and B, the Schaffer collateral system was labeled but only at the level of the genu and anterior body (A–C) while the dentate gyrus association pathway in the inner third of the dentate gyrus molecular layer was labeled throughout the entire longitudinal extent of the hippocampal formation. The label over layer III of the entorhinal cortex was caused by the spread of the injection into the presubiculum.

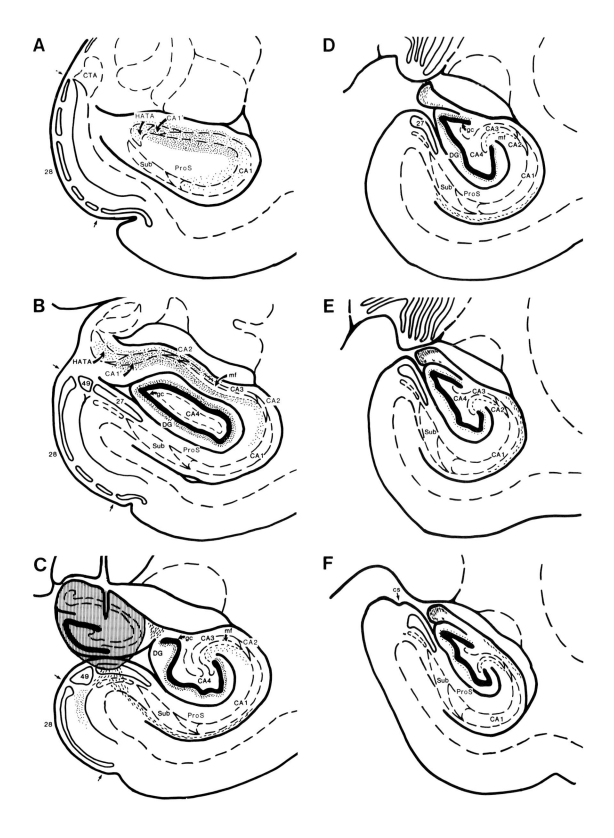

The final link in this serial chain of intrinsic connections originates in the CA1 subfield, which sends a strong intrinsic projection to the deep half of the stratum moleculare and throughout the stratum pyramidale of the subiculum. In the rat this projection has been demonstrated by Hjorth-Simonsen (1973) using silver degeneration methods and by Swanson *et al.* (1978) using the autoradiographic method. Both studies agree that the projection arises from the CA1 subfield and terminates in the pyramidal cell layer and in the deeper half of the molecular layer of the subiculum. Hjorth-Simonsen (1973) emphasizes that the projection is stronger at the distal (presubicular) end of the subiculum while Swanson *et al.* (1978) emphasize that the termination is heaviest in the deep part of the molecular layer. Both studies also have reported that this projection, like the mossy fiber system but in contrast to the Schaffer collateral or dentate gyrus association systems, is topographically organized in a lamellar fashion with only limited spread along the longitudinal axis of the hippocampal formation. Our observations in the monkey essentially agree with these results. As illustrated in Fig. 26, following an injection of radiolabeled amino acids into the CA1 subfield there is dense label over the subiculum that extends for a short distance rostrally. Unlike the rat this ammonic–subicular projection appears to terminate equally in the pyramidal and deep molecular layers as well as throughout the entire lateral to medial extent of the subiculum. On the other hand, in the monkey, the CA1 subfield appears to send only a weak projection to the prosubiculum where there is also a weak Schaffer collateral projection. Despite a few reports (Berger *et al.*, 1980; Kohler, 1985) to the contrary, the subiculum appears to have no strong intrinsic projections but instead, together with the prosubiculum, gives rise to the most complex and extensive set of extrinsic projections of all the hippocampal subfields [see Rosene and Van Hoesen (1977) and below].

In summary, in both the rat and monkey there are four distinct and prominent intrinsic connectional systems in the hippocampal formation: the dentate gyrus association system, the mossy fiber system, the Schaffer collateral system, and the ammonic–subicular system. Despite the many differences in the cytoarchitecture and histochemistry of the hippocampal formation in these two species, these intrinsic association systems are remarkably similar in their organization. This fact suggests that these intrinsic systems may be among the most phylogenetically stable aspects of the organization of the hippocampal formation, perhaps reflecting their functional importance and the stability of that function as a basic aspect of hippocampal organization. The serial chain from entorhinal afferent input through the dentate gyrus mossy fiber pathway, the CA3 Schaffer collateral system, and the CA1 ammonic–subicular system to the subiculum is summarized in Fig. 28.

Of these four intrinsic systems, the mossy fiber system and the ammonic–subicular system are topographically organized as narrow lamellar projection systems with no significant longitudinal spread. As such, they serve merely to link adjacent subfields in the serial chain of connections leading from the dentate gyrus to the subiculum. The other two intrinsic association systems, the dentate gyrus association system and the Schaffer collateral system, while topographically organized have a broad distribution along the longitudinal axis of the hippocampal formation. This difference between the lamellar and the longitudinal pathways has been confirmed electrophysiologically in the rat (Rawlins and Green, 1977). The dentate gyrus association system is unique in its limitation to one subfield, the dentate gyrus. However, it originates from a different set of neurons than the granule cell mossy fiber projection to the CA3 subfield but it is in a position to receive mossy fiber input and hence may provide both feedback to and extensive longitudinal integration of the granule cell output. While the Schaffer collateral system serves as a longitudinal association pathway within the CA3 subfield and along the CA2 and CA1 subfields as well, it also serves as a serial link from the CA3 subfield to the CA2 and CA1 subfields (and perhaps from the CA2 subfield to the CA1 subfield). At the very least, the serial link and longitudinal projections clearly originate from intermingled CA3 pyramidal cells and there is evidence that the same neuron may subserve both functions (Rawlins and Green, 1977). The functional significance of these orthogonally arranged but intertwined longitudinal and serial association systems is not obvious but it is important to note that there is no longitudinal association system within the subicular subfields, the final common pathway for most hippocampal extrinsic projections (Rosene and Van Hoesen, 1977).

6.3. Commissural Afferents and Efferents

In the rat, the vast majority of studies on the commissural connections of the hippocampal formation have concluded that the two longitudinally distributed systems, the dentate gyrus association pathway and the Schaffer collateral system, both have a contralateral projection that largely mirrors their ipsilateral distribution (Gottlieb and Cowan, 1973; Hjorth-Simonsen and Laurberg, 1977; Fricke and Cowan, 1978; Laurberg, 1979). On the other hand, the two topographically limited lamellar systems, the mossy fiber system and the ammonic–subicular system, have no crossed component in the rat or any other species investigated thus far (Swanson *et al.,* 1978; notwithstanding the contrary report of CA1 commissural projections by Voneida *et al.,* 1981). In one sense this pattern of commissural connectivity makes perfect sense since those ipsilateral systems organized to provide ipsilateral longitudinal integration are *a priori* the most likely to participate in and share the commissural integration and the topographically isolated lamellar systems seem *a priori* to remain isolated from the influences of commissural input.

The details of the origin, course, and termination of these commissural systems have been extensively studied in the rat but these details are largely unimportant for understanding the commissural connections of the primate brain because the most striking feature of the monkey hippocampal formation is the complete lack of commissural connections from all but the most anterior (uncal) levels of the hippocampal formation (Amaral *et al.,* 1984; Demeter *et al.,* 1985). While a crossed Schaffer collateral system and a crossed dentate gyrus association system similar to those observed in the rat are clearly demonstrated from injections of radio labeled amino acids (Fig. 29) or HRP into the uncal hippocampal formation, they rapidly diminish in strength as one proceeds cau-

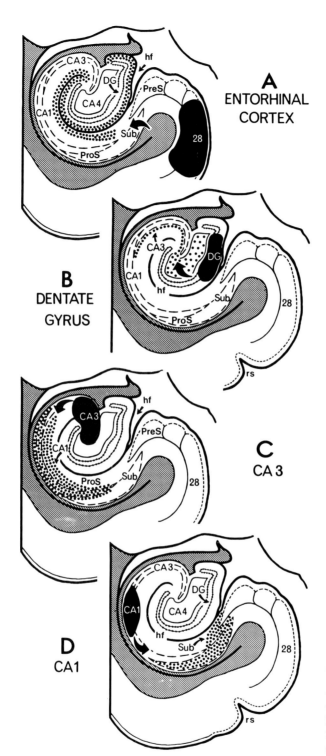

Figure 28. Summary of the serial chain of intrinsic connections that relay extrinsic afferent input (A: from the entorhinal cortex) from the dentate gyrus through the mossy fiber projection of the granule cells to the, CA3 subfield (B) where the Schaffer collateral system projects to the CA1 and prosubicular subfields (C) that in turn project to the subiculum (D) where the greatest diversity of hippocampal efferents originate. From Rosene and Van Hoesen (1977).

dally along the longitudinal axis of the hippocampal formation and do not extend caudally beyond the anterior body of the hippocampal formation. Furthermore, similar injections into the mid body or posterior body of the hippocampal formation fail to demonstrate any commissural connections whatsoever. In addition to these two hippocampal commissural systems, in the rat there is also a crossed projection from the entorhinal area to the opposite hippocampal formation, the so-called crossed temporoammonic system (Steward, 1976), which also mirrors the ipsilateral entorhinal projections. Amaral *et al.* (1984) describe a similar but insubstantial projection in the cynomolgus monkey while our own observations have failed to demonstrate this in the rhesus monkey. In any case, both studies demonstrate that compared to the rat (and other nonprimate mammals) the commissural connections of the monkey hippocampal formation are dramatically reduced and restricted in their distribution. This stands in sharp contrast to the relative similarities in both afferent inputs and intrinsic connections described above and appears to constitute a major species difference. The significance of this difference is unclear but it may reflect a growing functional linkage between the hippocampal formation and the increasingly lateralized cerebral cortex of primates. In the monkey some evidence of functional lateralization of the cerebral cortex has been reported (e.g., Hamilton, 1983) and in the human, Milner (1970) has reported that unilateral temporal lobe damage involving the hippocampal formation produces memory defects that reflect the lateralization of hemispheric function. Consequently, it is possible that the absence of hippocampal commissural connections reflects the advancing lateralization of cortical function in the monkey and the critical role that the hippocampal formation plays in cortical function in primates.

6.4. Extrinsic Efferents

The extrinsic connections of the hippocampal formation have been a focus of intense interest almost since it was first demonstrated by Gudden in 1881 that the fibers in the fornix that projected to the mammillary bodies originated from the hippocampal formation. While subsequent experimental studies using degeneration methods in rats (e.g., Raisman *et al.*, 1966) and monkeys (Simpson, 1952) identified various parts of the ammonic subfields as the origin of these fibers, more recent axoplasmic transport studies have demonstrated that these actually originate in the subicular subfields (Swanson and Cowan, 1975, 1977; Meibach and Siegel, 1975, 1977b). These same studies have also demonstrated that projections to the septal area originate in both the subiculum and the ammonic subfields. Our own studies in the monkey confirm these observations (Rosene and Van Hoesen, 1977; Ekstein and Rosene, 1987). As illustrated in Fig. 30 following an injection of HRP into the mammillary bodies of the monkey, retrogradely labeled neurons in the hippocampal formation are restricted to the subiculum. However, as shown in Fig. 31, after an HRP injection into the basal forebrain that included the ventral part of the septal area as well as the diagonal band nuclei, retrogradely labeled neurons were found in all the ammonic subfields as well as the subiculum.

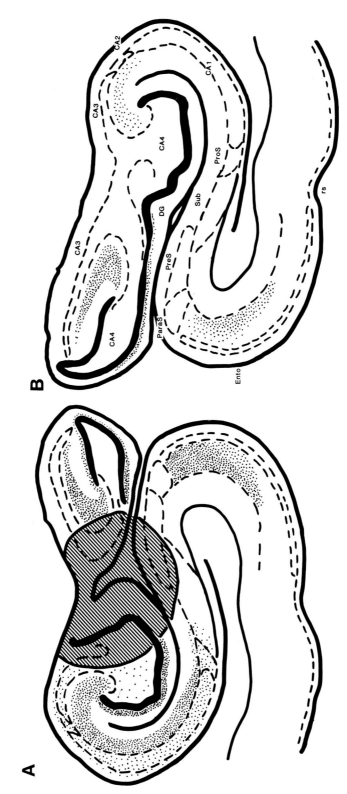

Figure 29. Summary of the results of an injection of radiolabeled amino acids (A) centered in the dentate gyrus, CA4 and CA3 subfields of the caudal genu, lateral part of the uncal hippocampus, and medial part of the anterior body. As shown in A the intrinsic Schaffer collateral system and dentate gyrus association system are both labeled. Like Fig. 27, the labeling over layer III of the entorhinal cortex is a result of spread of the injection ventrally into the presubiculum. The mirror-image contralateral projections cross the midline in the ventral hippocampal commissure and as shown in B are relatively strong in the uncal hippocampus and progressively diminish in the anterior body. No hippocampal commissural projections are observed caudal to the level illustrated in B. The contralateral projection to layer III of the entorhinal cortex originates in the presubiculum and crosses the midline in the dorsal hippocampal commissure.

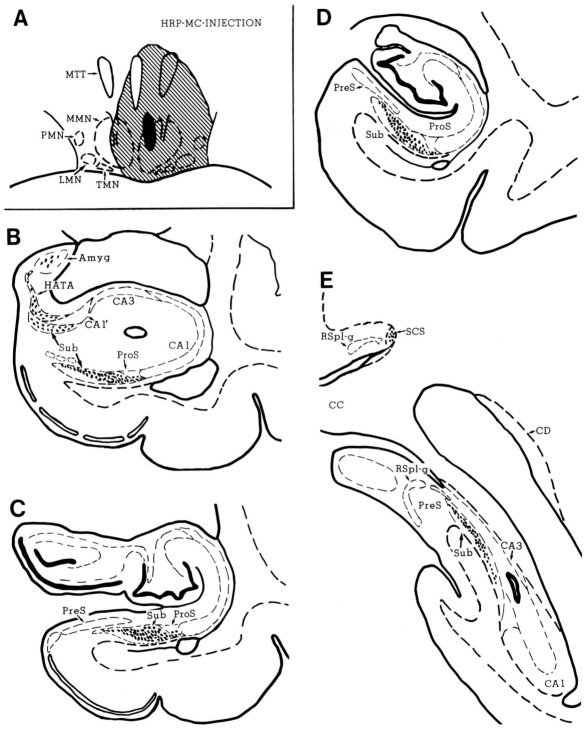

Figure 30. Summary of the results of an injection of HRP centered in the medial mammillary nucleus of the rhesus monkey (A). As shown in B–E, retrogradely labeled neurons were found in the subiculum throughout all levels of the hippocampal formation as well as in the HATA rostrally (B) and the supracallosal subiculum caudally (E). No retrogradely labeled neurons were found in any other subfields of the hippocampal formation following this injection. From Ekstein and Rosene (1987).

While these observations correspond to those reported in the rat, our studies of the origin of the mammillary body projection have also demonstrated two additional sources of the fornix projection to the mammillary bodies (Ekstein and Rosene, 1987): the supracallosal continuation of the subiculum into the cingulate gyrus (Fig. 30, B4; and Fig. 31) and the rostrally located HATA (Fig. 30, B1). Both observations have also been confirmed by anterograde transport of radiolabeled amino acids (Ekstein and Rosene, 1987). As summarized in Fig. 32, these anterograde observations demonstrate that the projections to the medial mammillary nucleus from the subiculum and supracallosal subiculum are topographically organized while the projection from the HATA terminates exclusively in the tuberomammillary nucleus. An additional observation is that the

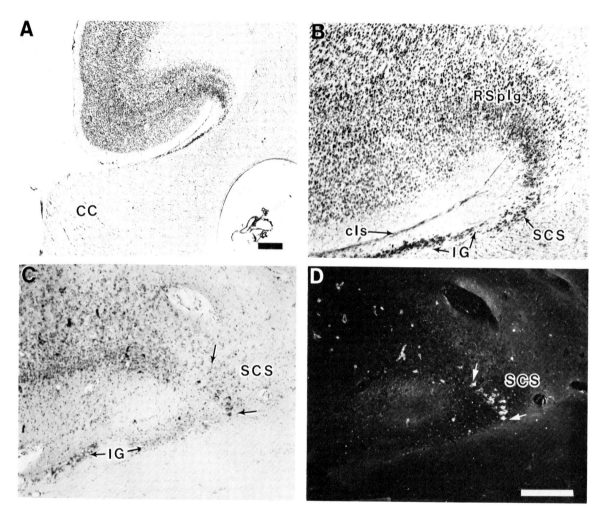

Figure 31. The location and cytoarchitectonic appearance of the supracallosal subiculum of the rhesus monkey are shown in A and B. The location of retrogradely labeled neurons following the HRP injection into the mammillary bodies illustrated in Fig. 30 is demonstrated in brightfield (C) and darkfield (D) photomicrographs of the section illustrated in Fig. 30E Bar = 1.0 mm (A), 200 μm (C, applies to A and D as well).

lateral extension of the subiculum beneath the presubiculum gives rise to a projection that terminates in the lateral mammillary nucleus (Ekstein and Rosene, 1987, and Fig. 32B). This appears to correspond to the observations of Edinger *et al.* (1979) in the rabbit and Krayniak *et al.* (1979) in the squirrel monkey except that these investigators identify these neurons as the deep cells of the presubiculum.

The anterior thalamic nuclei are the other principal diencephalic site of termination of postcommissural fornix projections from the hippocampal formation. As described above, studies in the rat by Swanson and Cowan (1977) and Meibach and Siegel (1977b) have demonstrated that these thalamic projections originate from the subicular subfields and not from the ammonic subfields of the hippocampal formation. This has been confirmed in the squirrel monkey (Krayniak *et al.*, 1979) and the cynomolgus monkey (Aggleton *et al.*, 1986) as well as by our own observation in the rhesus monkey that an injection of HRP into the anterior thalamic nuclei labeled neurons only in the subiculum. In agreement with Aggleton *et al.* (1986), we have also observed that the anterior thalamic projections from the subiculum originate in the deepest quarter of the stratum pyramidale of the subiculum and appear to have little overlap with the more superficial cells that give rise to the mammillary projection, suggesting that these projections arise from two distinct populations. However, the resolution

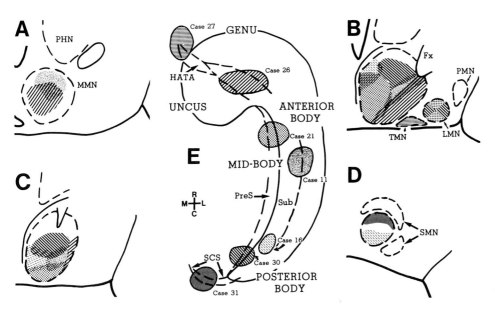

Figure 32. Summary of the location of injections of radiolabeled amino acids into the HATA, the subiculum, and the supracallosal subiculum along the longitudinal axis of the hippocampal formation of the rhesus monkey. The topographic distribution of anterograde label in the medial mammillary nucleus following injections along the longitudinal extent of the subiculum is summarized in A–D. Furthermore, while the supracallosal subiculum also projects topographically to the medial mammillary nucleus (D), as shown in B only medially placed subicular injections produced label over the lateral mammillary nucleus and the injection into the HATA produced label only over the tuberomammillary nucleus. Modified from Ekstein and Rosene (1987).

of this issue as well as the question of whether or not there are any neurons that project to both the thalamus and the mammillary body awaits appropriate double-labeling experiments with fluorescent retrograde tracers. In addition, Aggleton *et al.* (1986) also reported nonfornix projections from the subiculum to the laterodorsal and medial pulvinar nuclei. However, our own observations following injections of radiolabeled amino acids into all subfields of the hippocampal formation indicate that the laterodorsal projection originates from the presubiculum while the medial pulvinar projection arises from the cortex of the posterior parahippocampal gyrus that lies immediately beneath the subiculum. Nevertheless, there is general agreement in both the rat and the monkey that the ammonic subfields appear to project only as far as the septal area and only the subiculum projects beyond the septal area to the diencephalon.

As described in both the monkey (Siegel *et al.*, 1975; Krayniak *et al.*, 1979) and the rat (Swanson and Cowan, 1977; Meibach and Siegel, 1977a), the projection from the CA1, CA2, and CA3 subfields to the septal area originates from the pyramidal cells of these fields. There is disagreement, however, on whether septal projections originate from the CA4 subfield and/or the hilus of the dentate gyrus with Swanson and Cowan (1977) reporting no anterograde evidence for a projection when injections were limited to the hilus of the dentate gyrus of the rat. However, retrograde studies in the squirrel monkey (Krayniak *et al.*, 1979) and the rat (Chronister and DeFrance, 1979) both illustrated retrogradely labeled neurons in the hilus of the dentate gyrus that were clearly not part of the CA3 subfield following HRP injections into the septal area. Our own studies in the rhesus monkey have also demonstrated retrograde labeling in CA4 and/or hilar polymorphic neurons (Fig. 33). Thus, there is some reason to believe that either nonpyramidal cells of the polymorphic layer of the dentate gyrus and/or the "modified" pyramids of the CA4 subfield project to the septal area. These nonpyramidal projection neurons are of particular interest since several investigators have observed septal projections from other nonpyramidal cells in the stratum oriens and stratum radiatum of the CA3, CA2, and CA1 subfields of the rat (Chronister and DeFrance, 1979; Alonso and Kohler, 1982).

In the monkey we have observed similar nonpyramidal projection neurons in the stratum oriens of the ammonic subfields labeled following HRP injections into the septal area of the monkey as shown in Fig. 33. These labeled neurons were fusiform in shape and, like other nonpyramidal cells in the hippocampal formation, are usually thought to be local circuit neurons that project only within the hippocampal formation. To investigate this further we have examined our cases with HRP injections confined to the hippocampal formation and as shown in Fig. 34 have observed similar fusiform-shaped neurons retrogradely labeled in the stratum oriens caudal to the injection site. This observation suggests that these fusiform neurons have a rostrally directed intrinsic projection within the

Figure 33. Summary of the results of an injection of HRP (A) into the ventral part of the septal nucleus, the vertical limb of the diagonal band, the the rostral part of the preoptic area. As shown in B–F, at one level or another retrogradely labeled neurons were observed in all subfields of the hippocampal formation: CA4—D and E; CA3—B and C; CA1—B–D; Sub—B–F. In addition, retrogradely labeled fusiform-shaped neurons (arrows) were observed in the stratum oriens of the CA3, CA2, and CA1 subfields over the entire length of the hippocampal formation.

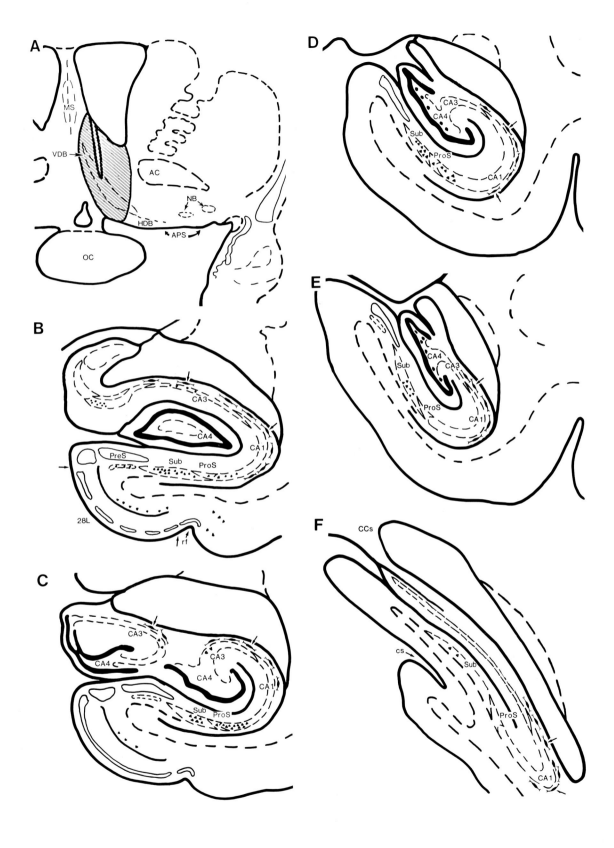

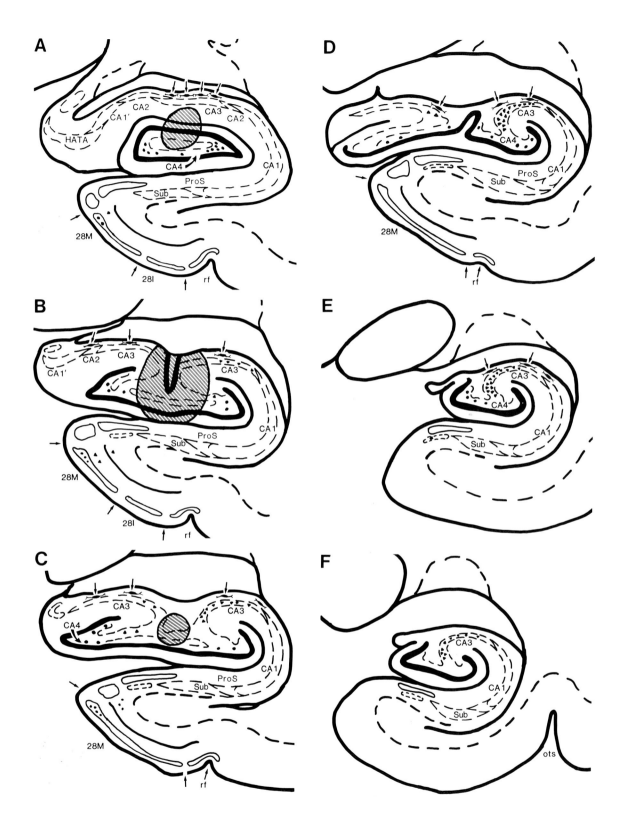

hippocampal formation. In our material these retrogradely labeled fusiform neurons of the stratum oriens correspond to the fusiform-shaped neurons of the stratum oriens that are evident in both Nissl-stained material as well as Golgi preparations. Examples of these fusiform neurons in both Golgi and Nissl material are shown in Fig. 35 as well as a typical CA1 pyramidal neuron and a fusiform-shaped neuron that was retrogradely labeled after the basal forebrain HRP injection shown in Fig. 33. In our Golgi preparations, the principal dendrites of these fusiform neurons extend transversely in the stratum oriens for at least several millimeters and side branches extend at least into the stratum pyramidale. While we have been unable to trace the axon of these Golgi-impregnated fusiform neurons, the existence of both intrinsic and extrinsic projections from similar-shaped neurons raises the possibility that individual fusiform neurons may have both a local axon collateral and a subcortically projecting axon. The resolution of this issue of collateralization awaits appropriate double-label experiments with fluorescent retrograde tracers.

In addition to these subcortical projections that travel in the fornix, the hippocampal formation also projects rostrally through the subcortical white matter of the temporal lobe to the amygdaloid complex in both the rat (Ottersen, 1982) and the monkey (Rosene and Van Hoesen, 1977; Saunders *et al.*, 1987). On the basis of the retrograde transport from HRP injections into the amygdala of the rat, Ottersen (1982) demonstrated that these projections originate from both the subiculum and the temporal part of the CA1 subfield and appear to project widely within the amygdala although no anterograde evidence was presented. We have examined this issue more closely in the monkey utilizing both anterograde and retrograde methods (Saunders *et al.*, 1987) and have confirmed that projections to the amygdaloid complex originate from both the subiculum and the CA1 subfield but our observations indicate that in the monkey the prosubiculum is the main source of hippocampal efferent projections to the amygdala. As shown in Fig. 36, an injection of radiolabeled amino acids centered in the prosubiculum produces strong anterograde label over the cortical and mediobasal nuclei and modest label over the laterobasal nucleus. A more rostral injection involving the CA1′ subfield (not illustrated) produced label over these same areas but in addition produced label over the accessory basal nucleus. While Ottersen (1982) reported retrograde labeling in both the subiculum and CA1 after HRP injections into the lateral amygdaloid nucleus of the rat, we found no evidence of this projection in the monkey. In the monkey, injections of retrograde tracers into the amygdala confirmed that most labeled cells from an accessory basal injection were observed in CA1′ while injections in the medial basal and cortical nuclei retrogradely labeled the prosubiculum (Saunders *et al.*, 1987).

Figure 34. Summary of the results of an injection of HRP into the dentate gyrus, CA4 and CA3 subfields of the genu of the hippocampal formation in the rhesus monkey. As expected, CA3, CA4, and polymorphic neurons of the dentate gyrus were retrogradely labeled throughout the entire longitudinal extent of the hippocampal formation. In addition, fusiform-shaped neurons (arrows) were retrogradely labeled in the stratum oriens of the CA3, CA2, and CA1 subfields from the genu all the way back to the mid body of the hippocampal formation, suggesting that these fusiform neurons may participate in some intrinsic connections.

From these studies it is apparent that the subiculum gives rise to more diverse extrinsic projections than the ammonic subfields and that the subicular subfields of the monkey have a more extensive and complex subcortical projection than the subiculum of the rat. While subcortical connectivity has been the focus of most studies of the hippocampal formation, it is clear that there are also direct projections from the hippocampal formation to the cerebral cortex (e.g., Hjorth-Simonsen, 1971; Rosene and Van Hoesen, 1977; Swanson and Cowan, 1977). In this regard it is of interest that the majority of these cortical projections appear to originate from the subiculum and/or prosubiculum while the others originate from the adjacent CA1 subfield and that both the extent and the diversity of these projections also seem to be greater in the monkey than the rat.

Thus, in the monkey we described hippocampal efferents that originate in

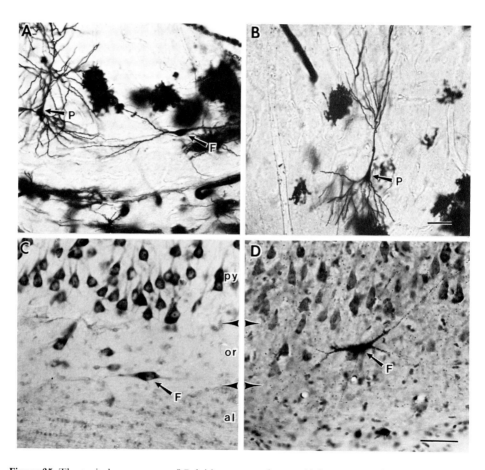

Figure 35. The typical appearance of Golgi-impregnated pyramidal neurons (P) in the CA1 subfield of the monkey hippocampal formation is shown in A and B as well as the appearance of a Golgi-impregnated fusiform-shaped neuron (F) of the stratum oriens in A. The appearance of these fusiform neurons in a Nissl (thionin)-stained section is shown in C as well as the appearance of a fusiform neuron retrogradely labeled with HRP after the injection into the basal forebrain illustrated in Fig. 33. (B also applies to A and D to C.) Bars = 50 μm.

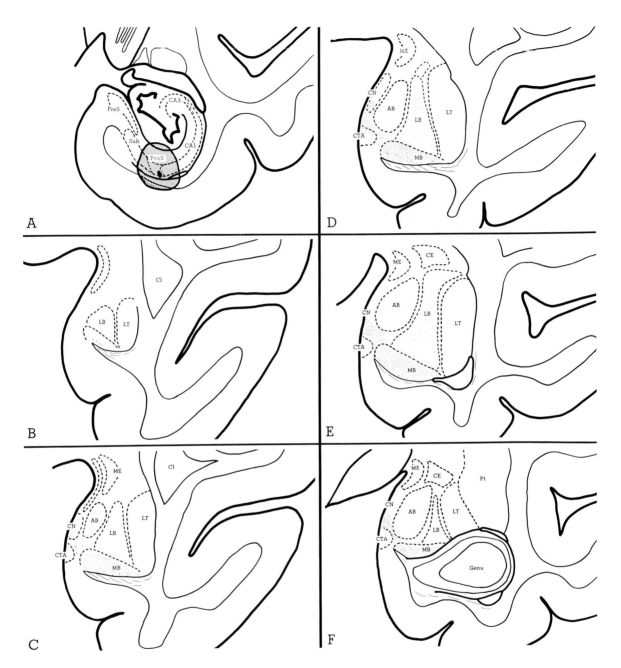

Figure 36. Summary of the results of an injection of radiolabeled amino acids (A) centered in the prosubiculum of the hippocampal formation of the rhesus monkey. This injection produced anterogradely transported label over the medial basal and cortical nuclei of the amygdala as well as very light labeling over the lateral basal nucleus. The origin of these projections in the prosubiculum was confirmed by placing injections of fluorescent retrograde tracers into the amygdala. (Modified from Saunders *et al.*, 1986).

the subiculum and project to a diversity of areas in the cerebral cortex. As illustrated in Fig. 37, these projections reached the entorhinal cortex, the perirhinal cortex, the proisocortex of the temporal pole, a proisocortical part of the posterior parahippocampal gyrus, the retrosplenial cortex of the posterior cingulate gyrus, the medial frontal and anterior cingulate cortex adjacent to the genu and rostrum of the corpus callosum, and the medial part of the orbitofrontal cortex (Rosene and Van Hoesen, 1977). Studies in the rat have also reported some cortical connections that appear to be homologous to those in the monkey. For example, Hjorth-Simonsen (1971) and later Swanson and Cowan

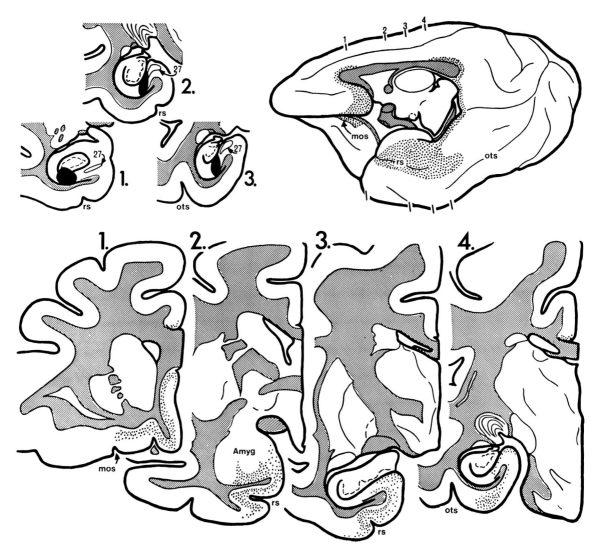

Figure 37. Summary of the diverse cortical projections of the subiculum of the hippocampal formation of the monkey. These include the medial frontal and orbital frontal cortices, the amygdala, the entorhinal cortex, the posterior parahippocampal gyrus, and the retrosplenial cortex. (Modified from Rosene and Van Hoesen, 1977).

(1977) described a projection from the CA3 subfield to the entorhinal cortex but in a subsequent report (Swanson *et al.*, 1978) these authors reported that a projection to the entorhinal cortex originated from the CA1 subfield and did not mention a CA3 projection. Swanson *et al.* (1978) also described a projection from CA3 to the cingulate cortex, from both CA1 and the subiculum to the perirhinal cortex and from the subiculum to the medial frontal cortex. In a later study, Swanson (1981) also reported a projection to the medial frontal cortex that originated from the same CA1 pyramidal cells that project to the entorhinal area. Additional studies in the rat (Meibach and Siegel, 1977b) and the guinea pig (Sorensen and Shipley, 1979; Sorensen, 1980) have demonstrated that the hippocampal projection to the cingulate cortex originates in the subiculum and terminates in the retrosplenial area and the projection to the entorhinal cortex originates in the subiculum as well as the CA1 subfields. However, there has been no evidence confirming the descriptions of cortical projections from the CA3 subfield and our own observations in the monkey have not demonstrated these projections.

While we originally emphasized the subiculum as the origin of cortical projections in the monkey (Rosene and Van Hoesen, 1977) all of our initial subicular injections also involved the prosubiculum and several of them also involved a part of the adjacent CA1 subfield. In our subsequent investigations using both anterograde and retrograde tracers, it is clear that many of these cortical projections originate in the prosubiculum and that there are also extensive cortical projections from limited parts of CA1. Thus, we have demonstrated that projections to layer 5 of the entorhinal cortex originate in both the subiculum and subfield CA1 (Saunders and Rosene, 1987) although as shown in Fig. 38 these two projections have somewhat different patterns of termination in different subdivisions of the entorhinal cortex. While detailed studies of other hippocampal cortical projections are still in progress,they demonstrate that the subiculum and/or prosubiculum give rise to at least part of all the cortical projections illustrated in Fig. 37 and that parts of the CA1 subfield also contribute to the medial frontal, entorhinal, and temporal neocortical projections. On the other hand, the retrosplenial projection originates solely from the subiculum. Finally, Goldman-Rakic *et al.* (1984) have recently reported that neurons in the subiculum were retrogradely labeled after large injections into the dorsolateral prefrontal cortex of the rhesus monkey, leading further support to the importance of the subiculum as the final common pathway for hippocampal output and its central role as an output from the hippocampal formation to the cerebral cortex.

6.5. Summary and Conclusions

The origin of some of the efferent connections of the monkey hippocampal formation are summarized in Fig. 39. The layers and subfields correspond to those illustrated in Fig. 17 and are based upon the section shown in Fig. 9B. For simplicity, the extrinsic afferents and the commissural projections present at this level as well as the projections of the HATA and CA1′ subfields have been omitted. Nevertheless, this illustrates the pattern of serial intrinsic connections as well as the origin of both subcortical and cortical projections. On the basis of this summary, the foregoing review, and our own studies and unpublished observations in the monkey, several principles of the organization of hippocampal connections can be derived, particularly with regard to intrinsic, commissural, and extrinsic projections.

First, like the rat, the major afferent inputs to the monkey hippocampal formation originate from the periallocortex of the entorhinal area and distribute to the molecular layer of all subfields. However, in the monkey there is also a significant afferent input that originates from proisocortical and even neocortical areas in the posterior parahippocampal gyrus and terminates in the molecular layer of the subiculum, the prosubiculum, and adjacent CA1 subfields where other telencephalix afferents from the amygdala and basal forebrain also ter-

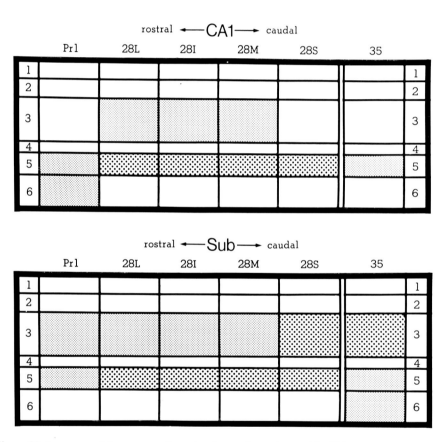

Figure 38. Summary of the pattern of termination we have observed in different layers of different subdivisions of the entorhinal cortex following injections of radiolabeled amino acids into different rostrocaudal levels of CA1 or the subiculum. Relatively light projections are indicated by the fine stippling and heavy projections by the coarse stippling. While there is a similar rostrocaudal topography in the projections from both of these subfields to the different subdivisions of the entorhinal and perirhinal cortices as well as a general correspondence in the layers and subdivisions where we observe termination, it is clear that the projection from the subiculum is more extensive. (Modified from Saunders and Rosene, 1987).

minate. Second, the serial chain of intrinsic connections begins in the most medially placed allocortical subfield, the dentate gyrus (which only receives extrinsic cortical afferents from the entorhinal area). This serial chain of intrinsic connections proceeds laterally (toward the neocortex) through successive ammonic subfields (CA3, CA2, CA1) to the last allocortical subfield, the subiculum. Third, the dentate gyrus, where this chain originates, only has intrinsic projections within the hippocampal formation but except for the subiculum, each successive subfield gives rise to increasingly complex extrinsic efferent projections as well as intrinsic projections that are part of the serial chain leading to the subiculum. Fourth, despite a few reports to the contrary (Berger *et al.*, 1980; Kohler, 1985), the subiculum appears to have no strong intrinsic projections but instead gives rise to the most complex and extensive set of extrinsic projections of all the hippocampal subfields. Fifth, commissural connections in the monkey are limited to the rostral third of the hippocampal formation (uncal hippocampus and part of the anterior body) so that a large part of the monkey hippocampal formation may be available for participation in highly lateralized functions of

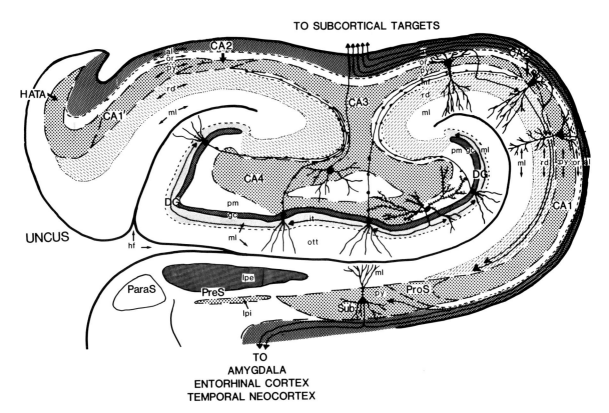

Figure 39. Summary of the origin of intrinsic and extrinsic projections from different subfields of the hippocampal formation. For convenience the projections of the HATA and CA1′ subfields as well as the commissural connections of this level are omitted. Furthermore, when an area gives rise to both intrinsic and extrinsic projections, they are illustrated as collateral projections of the same neuron although they may instead arise from different populations of neurons in the same subfield.

the neocortex. However, where the commissural connections are present in the monkey hippocampal formation, they mirror an ipsilateral intrinsic pathway. Finally, on top of this serial chain of intrinsic projections there are also several longitudinally arranged intrinsic connections that serve to provide a longitudinal integration of the activity of these different subfields.

7. Fiber Tracts of the Hippocampal Formation

The major connections of the hippocampal formation travel in several distinct fiber pathways both within the hippocampal formation and extrinsic to it. The principal fiber pathways are illustrated at four longitudinal levels of the monkey hippocampal formation in Fig. 40. Most of these fiber pathways carry both efferents and afferents although usually one or the other predominates.

7.1. The Alveus

The alveus is the name given to the white matter that lies deep to the pyramidal cell layers of the hippocampal formation and is exposed in the floor of the inferior horn of the lateral ventricle as illustrated in Fig. 40A–D. Axons of the hippocampal output neurons as well as some afferents travel in the alveus either to or from the fimbria or to or from the angular bundle. In the monkey the alveus is composed of heavily myelinated fibers most of which travel an oblique course moving along the longitudinal axis of the hippocampal formation as they travel superiorly or inferiorly around the circumference of the hippocampal formation. Axons destined to terminate within the hippocampal formation generally do not travel in the alveus.

7.2. The Fimbria

Many extrinsic projection fibers from the subiculum, prosubiculum, and CA subfields enter the alveus (Fig. 39) and travel superiorly and posteriorly onto the dorsal aspect of the hippocampal formation where they coalesce to form the white matter bundle known as the fimbria (Fig. 40A–D). This name means "fringe" and the appropriateness of this designation is obvious from Fig. 7E where this white matter bundle first appears at the posterior aspect of the genu, between the uncal hippocampus and the anterior body. As shown in Fig. 40A, in the more anterior levels of the genu only the alveus is present. However, fibers from the uncal hippocampus travel laterally and those from the anterior body travel medially where they join at the back of the genu to form the fimbria. It is at this point that the choroid plexus attaches to the free or distal tip of the fimbria and joins it to the inferior surface of the thalamus, forming the medial wall of the inferior horn of the lateral ventricle. This "choroidal" tip of the fimbria can be conveniently referred to as the distal tip in contrast to the part that is adherent to the dentate gyrus, which constitutes the proximal end of the fimbria. At this rostral origin of the fimbria, fibers from the uncus lie most medial in its distal tip while fibers from the genu and then the anterior body lie at respectively more lateral or proximal positions. Fibers that originate at more caudal levels of the main body of the hippocampus travel through the alveus to the fimbria where they occupy its most lateral part (see Ekstein and Rosene, 1987) and as a result of this lamellar addition of fibers, the size of the fimbria increases dramatically as one proceeds posteriorly (e.g., Fig. 40C versus D). Throughout its course the fimbria is separated from the dentate gyrus by the fimbrio dentate fissure (Fig. 40B). While it has been traditionally thought that the fimbria was composed entirely of efferent fibers of the hippocampal formation, as described more fully below, the fimbria also contains fibers originating from the septal area and other subcortical loci as well as commissural afferents and efferents of the uncal hippocampus and other commissural fibers that originate in the presubiculum, entorhinal cortex, and even the adjacent proisocortical and neocortical subfields of the posterior parahippocampal gyrus (Demeter *et al.*, 1985).

7.3. The Fornix

As shown in Fig. 7E at the level of the calcarine sulcus, the posterior body of the hippocampal formation thins and turns medially as it ends just beneath the splenium of the corpus callosum (Fig. 40D). While the hippocampal formation continues dorsally around the splenium as a small supracallosal hippocampal continuation, the induseum griseum, the fibers of the fimbria remain in a subcallosal position where the *proximal* part of the fimbria becomes attached to the inferior surface of the corpus callosum. The distal tip of the fimbria remains fixed anteriorly where it is attached by the choroid plexus to the thalamus. As these fimbria fibers separate from the hippocampal formation and ascend around the lateral aspect of the pulvinar, they become the posterior column of the fornix as shown in Figs. 40D and 41F. The term *fornix* means vault or arch and describes the course of the fornix from its inferior position in the temporal lobe beneath the thalamus up around the pulvinar and over the top of the thalamus to the foramen of Monro anteriorly. Because of the way the proximal part of the fornix ascends and moves medially to reach the inferior surface of the splenium, the distal tip of the fimbria, which was located medial to the proximal end of the fimbria in the inferior horn of the lateral ventricle, comes to lie laterally in the body of the lateral ventricle. Nevertheless, if one considers the part of the fornix attached to the corpus callosum as the proximal end and the "choroidal" tip the distal end, then these terms describe the location of the same fibers in both the fimbria and the fornix, only the medial–lateral orientation has reversed.

7.4. The Dorsal Fornix

In the rodent a midline projection pathway from the temporal parts of the hippocampal formation has been identified and designated the "dorsal fornix."

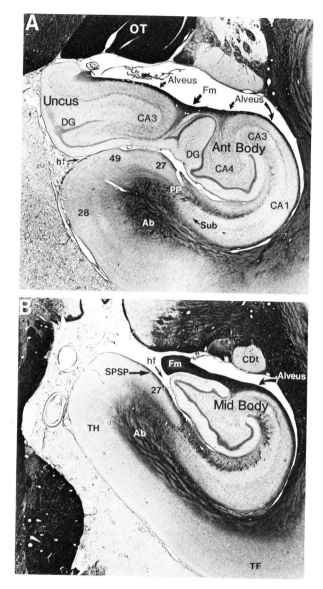

Figure 40. Myelin-stained frozen sections through the hippocampal formation of the rhesus monkey. These sections were taken at four levels along the longitudinal axis of the hippocampal formation and are indicated as 1A, 1B, 1C, and 1D on Fig. 42. The section in D illustrates the most caudal aspect of the posterior body of the hippocampal formation where it ascends in the atrium of the lateral ventricle toward the splenium where the fimbria attaches to the ventral surface and then separates from the hippocampal formation to continue forward as the fornix. The increasing thickness of the fimbria as well as the superficial presubicular pathway (SPSP) can be followed as one proceeds from rostral (B) to caudal (D) levels. Bar = 1.0 mm. Modified from Demeter *et al.*, 1985.

Throughout most of its subcallosal course it is separated by the dorsal hippocampal formation from the more laterally placed fimbria. It joins with the fimbria to form a unified fornix just in back of the septal area where the dorsal hippocampal formation has ended. As discussed more fully elsewhere (Ekstein and Rosene, 1987), the term *dorsal fornix* has been applied inconsistently in the pri-

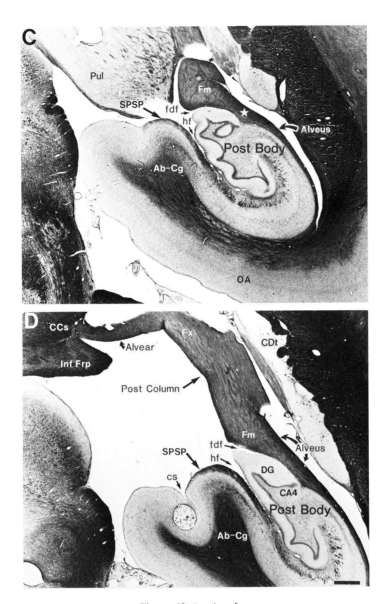

Figure 40. (*continued*)

mate to a variety of fiber bundles (McLardy, 1955; Poletti and Creswell, 1977) but has generally been applied to fibers that run in part of their course *dorsal* to the corpus callosum and that do not in any way correspond to the dorsal fornix as described in the rat. Our investigation of the fornix labeling following injections of radiolabeled amino acids into all levels of the subiculum (Ekstein and Rosene, 1987) as well as our observations on the course of fiber projections from radiolabeled amino acid injections in the ammonic subfields indicate that in the monkey there is no evidence of a distinct midline projection pathway that would be homologous with the dorsal fornix of the rat (e.g., Wyss *et al.*, 1980). It seems likely on topographic grounds that the dorsal fornix of the rat is produced by the separation of some projection fibers of the alveus from those in the fimbria by the presence of a dorsal (infracallosal) hippocampal formation in the rodent. In this sense the dorsal fornix of the rodent might be more appropriately designated as a dorsal or midline alveus since it carries fibers that would run in the alveus of the monkey hippocampal formation but would join the fimbria at the splenium to form a single distinct fornix beneath the corpus callosum.

7.5. The Callosal Perforating Fibers of the Fornix

In primates the term *dorsal fornix* has variously been applied to any fornix fibers that were thought to originate or travel dorsal to the corpus callosum. While various investigators (e.g., McLardy, 1955; Poletti and Creswell, 1977) have thought that these fibers originated in either the temporal or the cingulate cortex, we have recently identified the origin, course, and distribution of some similar fibers (Ekstein and Rosene, 1987). However, to avoid confusion with the dorsal fornix of the rat as well as to provide a more accurate designation, we have described these fibers as callosal perforating fornix fibers. These fibers originate in neurons of the supracallosal subiculum (Fig. 30E) medial to the induseum griseum in the posterior cingulate gyrus. Axons of these neurons travel anteriorly and ventromedially *through* the corpus callosum to join the midline or most proximal part of the fornix just posterior to the septum. These fibers then continue as part of the postcommissural fornix to terminate in the medial mammillary nucleus along with fibers from the subiculum of the hippocampal formation. Hence, despite their unique origin, these callosal perforating fornix fibers constitute a part of the fornix in every sense of other fibers of hippocampal origin.

7.6. The Angular Bundle and Perforant or Temporoammonic Pathway

The angular bundle was the term applied by Ramón y Cajal to the white matter that lies deep to both the subicular subfield of the hippocampal formation and the laterally adjacent entorhinal cortex (Fig. 40A–D). The fibers that comprise the angular bundle were thought to be afferents to the hippocampal formation originating from the entorhinal cortex and entering the hippocampal formation by perforating through the pyramidal cell layer of the subiculum before distributing in the molecular layer of all hippocampal subfields. Because

Figure 41. Myelin-stained frozen sections through the fornix and hippocampal commissures of the rhesus monkey. These sections were taken at eight levels of the fornix as indicated by levels 2A–2H on Fig. 42. Note that posteriorly the alvear part of the fimbria–fornix system is closely applied to the inferior limb of the forceps major (Inf Frp) of the corpus callosum (F–H). The three subdivisions of the hippocampal commissural system—the ventral hippocampal commissure (VHC), the hippocampal decussation (HD), and the dorsal hippocampal commissure (DHC)—are indicated as discrete bundles, they are continuous, one with another, and there is some overlap of crossing fibers in the different parts at their respective borders. Nevertheless, each of these carries a distinct set of crossing fibers. Bar = 1.0 mm. Modified from Demeter *et al.* (1985).

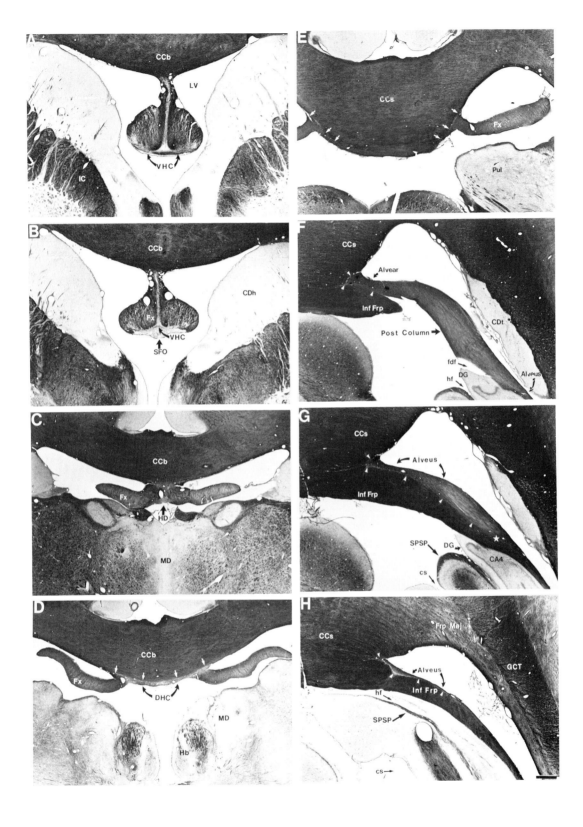

of their course through the subiculum, these afferent fibers from the angular bundle are often referred to as the perforant pathway. Although one might argue that this term should be restricted to the point of perforation only, it has come to be applied to the entire entorhinal projection to the hippocampal formation. Similarly, the term *temporoammonic pathway* has also been applied to the entire projection system even though the term might suggest that it refers only to fibers terminating in the ammonic or CA1–CA4 subfields of the hippocampal formation. In addition, it is now clear that in both rodents and primates, efferent fibers from the hippocampal formation enter the angular bundle from the alveus and travel for variable distances within the angular bundle before terminating in the entorhinal, perirhinal (Saunders and Rosene, 1987), and posterior parahippocampal cortices (Rosene and Van Hoesen, 1977). It is also clear that at posterior levels the angular bundle is in continuity with fibers from the cingulum bundle, which will reach the presubiculum (Pandya *et al.*, 1981). Furthermore, at these caudal levels the angular bundle also contains fibers from the posterior parahippocampal gyrus that project directly to the subiculum, prosubiculum, and adjacent part of the CA1 subfield (Van Hoesen *et al.*, 1979). In order to eliminate ambiguity and more accurately reflect the appropriate connectivity, it is suggested that the term *temporoammonic pathway* be avoided and the term *perforant pathway* be restricted to those afferent fibers that actually perforate the subiculum en route to the hippocampal formation. Following past usage, it seems reasonable to apply the term *angular bundle* to the white matter beneath the subiculum at both the level of the entorhinal and posterior parahippocampal cortices except posteriorly at the level of the calcarine sulcus where its continuity with the cingulum is apparent.

7.7. Superficial Presubicular Pathway

As shown in Fig. 40D, the molecular layer overlying the presubiculum at the level of the posterior body of the hippocampal formation is heavily myelinated. A similar myelination has been reported in the human brain by McLardy (1974) who, on the basis of both normal and pathological material, proposed that the fibers in this layer constituted a nonperforant presubicular pathway that, like the perforant pathway, carried afferents into the hippocampal formation. He proposed that these afferents originated in the posterior cingulate cortex. However, our experimental observations in monkeys indicate that this fiber bundle is a superficial efferent pathway composed of fibers that originate in the subiculum and prosubiculum and course through the molecular layer of the presubiculum to reach the molecular layer of the retrosplenial cortex. Vogt (1976) has demonstrated that beneath the splenium of the corpus callosum in the rostral lip of the calcarine sulcus, the presubiculum is continuous with the granular retrosplenial cortex (area 29) and Rosene and Van Hoesen (1977) described nonfornix projections in the monkey that terminated in the retrosplenial area. In fact, it is clear that these subicular efferents travel superficially in the molecular layer of the presubiculum to the retrosplenial cortex where they terminate in the granular layer. We are not certain if there are additional myelinated fibers in this layer or whether the subicular fibers terminate en passage in the presubiculum. In the latter case, this fiber pathway would, at least in part, constitute an additional cortical projection from the subiculum. Nevertheless, it is clear that a significant proportion of the myelinated fibers in the superficial layer of the presubiculum are extrinsic hippocampal efferents. Hence, despite McLardy's original description, these fibers do not strictly constitute a nonperforant pathway for afferents to reach the hippocampal formation and we propose that this pathway be designated the *superficial presubicular pathway* (SPSP) as this name describes the location of the fiber bundle but avoids a commitment to any limited set of afferent or efferent origins and targets.

7.8. The Hippocampal Commissures

In the rat there are extensive commissural connections linking the hippocampal formation and periarchicortical areas of both hemispheres and these connections pass through a dorsal hippocampal commissure located beneath the splenium of the corpus callosum and a ventral hippocampal commissure located immediately posterior to the septum and ventral to the body of the fornix (e.g., Blackstad, 1956; Wyss *et al.*, 1980). We have recently demonstrated in the rhesus monkey the existence of both dorsal and ventral hippocampal commissures that are basically homologous to the corresponding structures of the rodent brain (Demeter *et al.*, 1985). Nevertheless, there are several significant differences. Along with Amaral *et al.* (1984), we observed that unlike the rodent, most of the main body of the monkey hippocampal formation lacks detectable commissural connections. In addition, we demonstrated that some commissural fibers from the proisocortical and neocortical parts of the posterior parahippocampal gyrus pass through the angular bundle and into the alveus where they then pass caudally to ascend with the fimbria and cross the midline in the dorsal hippocampal commissure. Furthermore, we have also described a group of fibers unique to the monkey brain that cross the midline obliquely between the levels of the dorsal hippocampal and ventral hippocampal commissures. Since these fibers originate from the hippocampal formation but terminate in the contralateral septal area and not the contralateral hippocampal formation, we have designated them the *hippocampal decussation*. Since each of these systems overlaps with the next, for convenience we proposed that the entire system of crossing fibers including the dorsal hippocampal commissure, the hippocampal decussation, and the ventral hippocampal commissure be referred to as the *hippocampal commissure*. All of these components are illustrated in Fig. 41 and artistic reconstructions of these in the median sagittal plane and from above are presented in Figs. 42 and 43.

8. Immunohistochemistry

The recent growth in applying immunocytochemical procedures to studies of the CNS has provided an additional way to study the histochemical characteristics of the hippocampal formation. The value of this technique lies in the fact that any substance that can be purified and isolated from the CNS can potentially be used as an antigen to stimulate the production of specific antibodies that can be used to identify and localize the antigen in tissue. Such antigenic substances may be enzymes for which no reliable or specific enzyme histochemical procedures are available, e.g., choline acetyltransferase (ChAT), the synthetic enzyme for the putative neurotransmitter acetylcholine (ACh), and glutamic acid decarboxylase (GAD), the synthetic enzyme for the putative neurotransmitter GABA. Other antigenic substances may be neuropeptides such as the enkephalins, vasoactive intestinal polypeptide, and somatostatin, or neuroendocrine substances such as vasopressin, or even neurotransmitters themselves such as GABA or ACh. The list of substances for which an antibody is available grows almost weekly and many of these have been applied to investigations of the hippocampal formation where they reveal neurochemical properties of specific cell types and in some cases the neurochemical properties of different fiber plexuses. In reviewing this literature, several potential problems must be considered. First, the sensitivity of immunocytochemical methods is generally unknown and not amenable to quantification. Thus, positive results most often consist of the demonstration of intensely staining neuronal cell bodies while smaller and/or less intensely reactive processes such as proximal dendrites, the

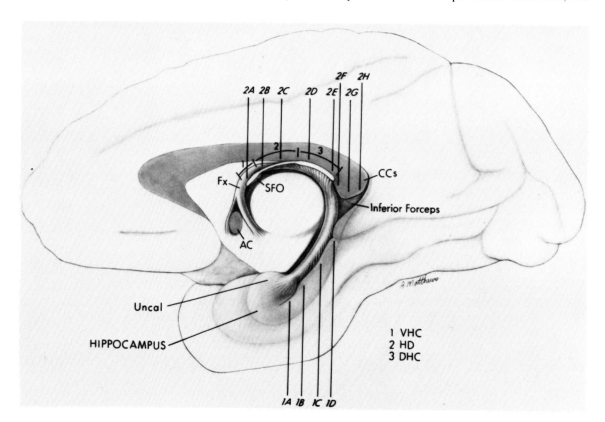

Figure 42. Relationship of the fimbria, fornix, and hippocampal commissure viewed from the medial side of the hemisphere. The levels of the sections shown in Figs. 40 and 41 are indicated by the designations 1A–1D for Fig. 40 and 2A–2H for Fig. 41. (From Demeter *et al.*, 1985.)

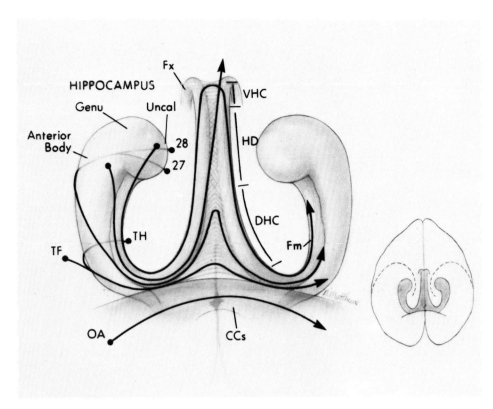

Figure 43. Summary of the origin and course of the different projection systems that cross the midline in the three components of the hippocampal commissural system and contrasts of these with the fibers in the inferior forceps of the splenium. (From Demeter *et al.*, 1985.)

entire dendritic tree, the axon, and the axon terminal field are less frequently demonstrated. Among the factors that influence the sensitivity of immunocytochemical labeling are: different antibodies to the same antigen prepared in different laboratories or by different manufacturers, different batches of antibody from the same source; the species from which the tissue was taken, how the tissue was fixed, or how the immunocytochemical reaction was performed. As a consequence, negative results (i.e., the failure to demonstrate the presence of an antigen in any given situation) are difficult to interpret and interspecies comparative studies are almost impossible to interpret. An additional limitation of these immunocytochemical studies that may be due in part to problems of sensitivity is the difficulty of identifying specific immunoreactive cells as the source of immunoreactive axons or terminal fields, although combining the immunocytochemical labeling with labeling using a retrograde tracer can help to resolve this issue. Hence, despite the large number of immunocytochemical studies describing the distribution of different substances in the hippocampal formation of the rat, only those pertinent to the few studies available in the monkey will be reviewed here.

In a unique comparative study of neuropeptides, Roberts *et al.* (1983) demonstrated the presence of six different peptides in fibers of the fimbria–fornix of the rat, the marmoset (New World) monkey, and the human. These peptides were cholecystokinin, (CCK), methionine-enkephalin (ME), neurotensin (NT), somatostatin (SOM), substance P (SP), and vasoactive intestinal polypeptide (VIP). These investigators reported that immunoreactive cell bodies for four of these peptides (CCK, NT, SOM, VIP) were observed within the CA subfields or subiculum of the hippocampal formation. While ME- and SP-immunoreactive fibers were observed in the fornix, no neurons immunoreactive for either of these neuropeptides were found in the hippocampal formation. These observations suggest that the ME- and SP-positive fibers in the fornix represent hippocampal afferents while CCK-, NT-, SOM-, and VIP-positive fibers could be extrinsic efferents leaving the hippocampal formation, afferents to the hippocampal formation, or both. In a later study in the rat, Roberts *et al.* (1984) reported that most of the SOM-positive neurons were located in the hilus of the dentate gyrus and in the stratum oriens of the CA3, CA2, and CA1 subfields while CCK-, and VIP-positive somata were located in the stratum moleculare and stratum radiatum of the CA3, CA2, and CA1 subfields as well as the molecular layer of the dentate gyrus. Leranth and Frotscher (1983) reported VIP-positive neurons in the stratum radiatum and stratum moleculare of the rat hippocampal formation but unlike Roberts *et al.* (1984), also found VIP-positive neurons in the stratum oriens. In all these layers, Leranth and Frotscher (1983) reported that by morphological criteria these VIP-positive neurons were all nonpyramidal cells and hence were likely to be local circuit neurons. If this were the case, then the VIP-positive fornix fibers would be solely afferents.

Greenwood *et al.* (1981) reported in the rat CCK immunoreactive fibers as well as perikarya that appeared to be CA3 and CA1 pyramidal cells and interneurons in the hilus of the dentate gyrus and all layers of the hippocampus proper. Handelmann *et al.* (1981) reported that immunoreactive fibers were solely derived from CCK-immunoreactive interneurons since lesions of extrinsic afferents (dorsal fornix and entorhinal cortex) failed to reduce CCK content as measured by radioimmunoassay. More recently, Harris *et al.* (1985) reported that CCK immunoreactivity in the CA1 region of the rat was found in interneurons in all layers but not in pyramidal cells.

These observations suggest that CCK, SOM, and VIP immunoreactivity may be largely limited to local circuit neurons involved in intrinsic projections rather than projection neurons. However, none of these neuropeptides appears to be specifically localized in or limited to neurons that give rise to any of the four major intrinsic circuits (dentate gyrus association pathway, mossy fiber pathway, Schaffer collateral pathway, or ammonic–subicular pathway). On the other hand, there is some evidence that leucine-enkephalin (LE) and/or ME may be specifically associated with the mossy fiber pathway even though ME was not observed to be intrinsic to the hippocampal formation by Roberts *et al.* (1983). Thus, investigations in the rat (LE and ME: Gall *et al.*, 1981) and tree shrew (LE: Fitzpatrick and Johnson, 1981) have reported enkephalin immunoreactivity in dentate gyrus granule cells and their mossy fiber efferents, suggesting that this peptide may be important in this intrinsic fiber pathway. The latter authors also report unpublished observations of LE immunoreactivity in the mossy fibers of the owl monkey, suggesting that this may be a phylogenetically stable feature of this pathway.

The distribution of SOM immunoreactivity in the monkey hippocampal formation has been investigated by Bakst *et al.* (1985). These investigators reported that the distribution of SOM-positive cells and fibers in both cynamolgus and squirrel monkeys was similar to that reported in the rat but was "more striking." Whether this reflects an actual increase in the density of SOM-positive neurons and/or fibers in the monkey hippocampal formation or reflects increased technical sophistication and immunohistochemical sensitivity is unclear. Nevertheless, it is interesting that like the rat, SOM-positive nonpyramidal cells were found most frequently in the hilus of the dentate gyrus as well as in the stratum oriens and stratum pyramidale of the CA3, CA2, and CA1 subfields and stratum pyramidale of the subiculum. These investigators were also able to demonstrate a very strong SOM-immunoreactive fiber plexus in the outer two-thirds of the molecular layer of the dentate gyrus as well as in the molecular layer of the ammonic subfields, loci where the principal extrinsic hippocampal afferents terminate. While SOM-positive fibers were observed in other layers of the hippocampal formation, none of these terminal fields could be specifically identified with the SOM-immunoreactive local circuit neurons in the hippocampal formation. However, Bakst *et al.* (1985) also reported SOM-positive cells in the entorhinal cortex where the perforant path input to the molecular layers of the dentate gyrus and ammonic subfields originates (Van Hoesen and Pandya, 1975), but relatively few of the SOM-positive cells were located in layers 2 and 3 of the entorhinal area where the cells of origin for the hippocampal projection are located. In addition, these authors report that they were unable to confirm these cells as even a partial origin of the SOM-positive projection in a double-label experiment using retrograde transport of HRP from the hippocampal formation. Thus, like CCK and VIP, SOM immunoreactivity appears to be localized in nonpyramidal cells that are probably local circuit neurons as well as in some specific layers of termination but it is not yet possible to determine if this immunoreactivity is associated with specific intrinsic efferent or extrinsic afferent systems.

In a similar investigation of neuropeptide Y (NPY) immunoreactivity in both rat and cynomolgus monkey, Kohler *et al.* (1986) reported the presence of NPY-immunoreactive cells in the hilus of the dentate gyrus and stratum oriens of the ammonic subfields and NPY-immunoreactive fibers and apparent terminals in the outer third of the molecular layer of the dentate gyrus and the molecular layer of the ammonic subfields. Like the investigations of CCK, VIP, and SOM within the hippocampal formation, NPY is localized to nonpyramidal cells and like SOM the greatest density of immunoreactive fibers is in the zone of termination of the extrinsic perforant path terminals. These investigators also reported unpublished observation of similar staining in the human hippocampal formation.

The presence of these various neuropeptides in nonpyramidal neurons of the hippocampal formation in rat, monkey, and man indicates that they are a stable feature of the mammalian hippocampal formation and suggests that they may play a significant role in hippocampal function. One possibility suggested by the presence of immunoreactive fibers in the molecular layer where extrinsic afferents terminate is that these neuropeptides participate in regulation of hippocampal afferent input. If such a neuromodulatory function exists, it would be important to determine if the immunoreactive fibers originate from the immunoreactive intrinsic neurons or if they are themselves extrinsic afferents. Since some extrinsic hippocampal efferents originate from nonpyramidal cells such as the septal projection of the fusiform neurons of the stratum oriens (e.g., Chronister and DeFrance, 1979) and the commissural projection of the dentate gyrus polymorphic neurons (e.g., Berger *et al.*, 1981) and both *classes* of neurons show neuropeptide immunoreactivity, the function of some of the extrinsic projections of the hippocampal formation may involve neuropeptides. However, determination of whether these nonpyramidal projection neurons are also immunoreactive for any of these neuropeptides or if they also give rise to additional intrinsic projections remains to be determined with appropriate double- or triple-labeling experiments. Until the specific intrinsic or extrinsic connections of neuropeptide-immunoreactive nonpyramidal neurons as well as the origin of the different immunoreactive axon terminal fields within the hippocampal formation are determined, it is not possible to draw firm conclusions about the potential role of these neuropeptides in hippocampal function.

9. Functional Considerations

It is impossible to provide a complete discussion of the many studies of hippocampal function that have been conducted over the years. However, some recent studies in monkeys as well as some in humans are important in light of our hypothesis that the primate hippocampal formation is a progressive structure and that progressive morphological development goes hand in hand with increased functional potential. Thus, it is not surprising that over the years, studies of hippocampal function in experimental animals, especially the rat, have generally failed to demonstrate memory deficits equivalent to those observed in humans with hippocampal damage. There have been several explanations for this observation. First, it has been postulated that the hippocampal lesions produced in experimental animals do not adequately mimic the lesions in humans, especially because there is almost always involvement of other structures as well. Second, it has been postulated that the behavioral tests of memory function in animals are not equivalent to those used in humans. Weiskrantz (1977) has pointed out that an alternative approach is to apply the forced choice recognition tasks used in animals to humans and indeed this appears to be a very useful approach (Moss *et al.*, 1986). A corollary of this notion is that the behavioral repertoire of some experimental animals may not include behaviors that allow memory function to be tested in an equivalent way regardless of the tasks employed. If our hypothesis is substantially correct and the human hippocampal formation has progressive morphological features, including connections with other parts of the forebrain that are not present in experimental animals and constitute the morphological basis for increased functional potential, then in a real sense both hypotheses would be true. That is, the lesion in the human, even if completely limited to the hippocampal formation, could not be duplicated in animals because the "progressive" morphological features are not there to damage and behavioral tests could not assess the effects of damage on the functions associated with these features. From this perspective one would postulate that some of the progressive morphological features of the primate hippocampal formation demonstrated by anatomical investigations in the monkey, may provide the morphological basis for the type of mnemonic functions involved in human memory. To the extent that the hippocampal formation of the monkey has some of these progressive morphological features, then behavioral investigations should be able to demonstrate functions and/or dysfunctions similar to those observed in humans with hippocampal lesions even though studies in rats would not. Of course, it is also likely that progressive morphological features and associated functions have developed that are unique to the human hippocampal formation and have no functional equivalent in any experimental animal. However, it is the contention of this review that there are striking morphological similarities between the hippocampal formation of monkey and man that clearly demonstrate that the primate hippocampal formation is likely to have some similar functional potentials in both species that may be quite different from that of the rat. This view is supported by recent neuropsychological investigations of both the monkey and man.

In this light it is of interest that in the past decade a variety of behavioral studies in monkeys as well as additional human neurological studies indicate that the monkey may indeed provide a good model for studying the contribution of the hippocampal formation and other limbic system structures to memory function. Thus, Mishkin (1978) demonstrated that combined hippocampal and amygdaloid lesions in monkeys produced an impairment in recognition memory that was similar in some respects to the amnestic syndrome described in the original reports on humans with medial temporal lobe lesions (Scoville and Milner, 1957; Penfield and Milner, 1958). It is clear that in most of these cases in addition to hippocampal damage there was also damage to the amygdala. While the devastating effect on memory in monkeys of these combined lesions is clear, there is ample evidence that the hippocampal formation alone makes a significant contribution to memory function (e.g., Mahut *et al.*, 1982) and indeed Mishkin (1982) has suggested that the amygdala and hippocampal formation may function as parallel and somewhat independent systems (Saunders *et al.*, 1984). In humans there is also striking evidence that pathology in the entorhinal area, the principal afferent input to the hippocampal formation as well as a major cortical target of hippocampal efferent projections, may be critical in some aspects of the human amnestic syndrome (McLardy, 1970; Hyman *et al.*, 1984). Since there is evidence in humans (Woolsey and Nelson, 1975) and in monkeys (Moss *et al.*, 1981) that destruction of the fornix does not produce memory deficits equivalent to hippocampal damage, it seems likely that the extensive cortical efferents of the primate hippocampal formation may be critical to the participation of the hippocampal formation in memory function. Mishkin (1982) argued that since behavioral tasks requiring simple habit formation can be learned in both monkeys and humans with temporal lobe limbic system damage, there may be an additional "primitive" memory system independent of the temporal lobe structures. The organization of the hippocampal formation presented in this review is compatible with this hypothesis but suggests that the primitive memory system may differ from the memory system of the temporal lobe limbic system in its independence from the connections of the hippocampal formation with the cerebral cortex.

10. Abbreviations

Ab	Angular bundle
AB	Accessory basal nucleus of the amygdala
AC	Anterior commissure
AChE	Acetylcholinesterase-reacted section
AD	AChE-free part of inner third of dentate gyrus molecular layer
AF	AChE-dense part of inner third of dentate gyrus molecular laye
Amyg	Amygdala
al	Alveus
APS	Anterior perforated substance
Assoc	Dentate gyrus association pathway
C	Caudal direction
Ant Body	Anterior level of the main body of the hippocampal formation
CA1,2,3,4	Cornu Ammonis 1, 2, 3, 4: subfields of Lorente de Nó (1934)
CC	Corpus callosum
CCb	Body of the corpus callosum
CCs	Splenium of the corpus callosum
CD	Caudate nucleus
CDh	Head of the caudate nucleus
CDt	Tail of the caudate nucleus
CE	Central nucleus of the amygdala
Cg	Cingulum bundle
CiS	Cingulate sulcus
Cl	Claustrum
cls	Callosal sulcus
CN	Cortical nucleus of the amygdala
Cort Amyg	Cortical nucleus of the amygdala
cs	Calcarine sulcus
CTA	Corticoamygdaloid transition area
D	Dorsal direction
DG	Dentate gyrus
DHC	Dorsal hippocampal commissure
Ento	Entorhinal cortex; also 28
F	Fusiform neuron of stratum oriens
fdf	Fimbriodentate fissure
Fm	Fimbria
Fx	Fornix
gc	Granule cell layer of the dentate gyrus
GCT	Geniculocalcarine tract
HATA	Hippocampal–amygdaloid transition area
Hb	Habenular nucleus
HD	Hippocampal decussation
HDB	Horizontal nucleus of the diagonal band
hf	Hippocampal fissure
IG	Induseum griseum
Inf Frp	Inferior forceps or inferior part of the forceps major
it	Inner third of the molecular layer of the dentate gyrus
L	Lateral direction
LB	Lateral basal nucleus of the amygdala
LMN	Lateral mammillary nucleus
lpe	Lamina principalis externa of the presubiculm
lpi	Lamina principalis interna of the presubiculum
LT	Lateral nucleus of the amygdala
LV	Lateral ventricle
M	Medial direction

MB	Medial basal nucleus of the amygdala
MC	Mammillary complex
MD	Medial dorsal thalamic nucleus
ME	Medial nucleus of the amygdala
Mid Body	Middle level of the main body of the hippocampal formation
ml	Molecular layer of hippocampal formation
mf	Mossy fiber layer (stratum lucidum) of the hippocampal formation
MMN	Medial mammillary nucleus
MMNpM	Medial mammillary nucleus par medialis
MMNpB	Medial mammillary nucleus pars basalis
MMNpL	Medial mammillary nucleus pars lateralis
mos	Medial orbital sulcus
MS	Medial septal nucleus
mt	Middle third of the molecular layer of the dentate gyrus
MMT	Mammillothalamic tract
NB	Nucleus basalis of Meynert
OA	Cortical area OA of von Bonin and Bailey (1947); also area 19
or	Stratum oriens of the hippocampal formation
ot	Outer third of the molecular layer of the dentate gyrus
OT	Optic tract
ots	Occipitotemporal sulcus
ott	Outer two-thirds of the molecular layer of the dentate gyrus
P	Pyramidal neuron of the CA1 subfield
ParaS	Parasubiculum
pm	Polymorph cell layer of the dentate gyrus
Post Body	Posterior level of the main body of the hippocampal formation
Post Column	Posterior column of the fornix
Pr1	Prorhinal 1 area of Van Hoesen and Pandya (1975)
PreS	Presubiculum; also 27
ProS	Prosubiculum
PHN	Posterior hypothalamic nucleus
PMN	Paramammillary nucleus
Pt	Putamen
Pul	Pulvinar
py	Pyramidal cell layer of the hippocampal formation
R	Rostral direction
rd	Stratum radiatum of the hippocampal formation
rs	Rhinal sulcus
RSplg	Retrosplenial granular cortex
S	Splenial direction
SCS	Supracallosal subiculum
Sept	Septal area or nuclei
SFO	Subfornical organ
SI–NB	Substantia innominata–nucleus basalis
SM	Stria medullaris
SPSP	Superficial presubicular pathway
Sub	Subiculum
T	Temporal direction
TF	Cortical area TF of von Bonin and Bailey (1947)
TH	Cortical area TH of von Bonin and Bailey (1947)
Thal	Thalamus
TMN	Tuberomammillary nucleus
V	Ventral direction
VDB	Vertical nucleus of the diagonal band
VHC	Ventral hippocampal commissure
27	Presubiculum (PreS)
28	Entorhinal cortex (Ento)

28L,I,M,S	Subdivisions of area 28 after Saunders and Rosene, 1987
35	Perirhinal cortex of Brodmann
49	Parasubiculum

ACKNOWLEDGMENTS. This research was supported by NIH Grants NS 19416 and PO1 AG 00001 (D.L.R.), and NS 14944 and PO1 NS 19632 (G.V.H.). We wish to thank Dr. Thomas Kemper for providing some of the human material and our collaborators Jeffery Ekstein, Dr. Mark Moss, Dr. Steven Demeter, and Dr. Richard Saunders for their contributions to the experimental observations. We also thank Nancy Roy, Kathleen Barry, Paige Bracci, and Cindy Fingado for technical assistance in preparing the monkey and rat material. Special thanks are also due to Paige Bracci for assistance in the preparation of the illustrations.

11. References

Aggleton, J. P., Desimone, R., and Mishkin, M., 1986, The origin, course and termination of the hippocampothalamic projections in the macaque, *J. Comp. Neurol.* **243**:409–421.

Alonso, A., and Kohler, C., 1982, Evidence for separate projections of hippocampal pyramidal and non-pyramidal neurons to different parts of the septum in the rat brain, *Neurosci. Lett.* **31**:209–214.

Amaral, D. G., 1978, A Golgi study of cell types in the hilar region of the hippocampus in the rat, *J. Comp. Neurol.* **182**:851–914.

Amaral, D. G., and Cowan, W. M., 1980, Subcortical afferents to the hippocampal formation in the monkey, *J. Comp. Neurol.* **189**:573–591.

Amaral, D. G., and Dent, J. A., 1981, Development of the mossy fibers of the dentate gyrus. I. A light and electron microscopic study of the mossy fibers and their expansions, *J. Comp. Neurol.* **195**:51–86.

Amaral, D. G., and Kurz, J., 1985, An analysis of the origins in the cholinergic and noncholinergic septal projections to the hippocampal formation in the rat, *J. Comp. Neurol.* **240**:37–59.

Amaral, D. G., Insauati, R., and Cowan, W. M., 1984, The commissural connections of the monkey hippocampal formation, *J. Comp. Neurol.* **224**:307–336.

Andersen, P., Bliss, T. V. P., and Skrede, K. K., 1971, Lamellar organization of hippocampal excitatory pathways, *Exp. Brain Res.* **13**:222–238.

Azmitia, E. C., and Segal, M., 1978, An autoradiographic analysis of the differential ascending projections of the dorsal median raphe nuclei in the rat, *J. Comp. Neurol.* **179**:641–668.

Bakst, I., and Amaral, D. G., 1984, The distribution of acetylcholinesterase in the hippocampal formation of the monkey, *J. Comp. Neurol.* **225**:344–371.

Bakst, I., Morrison, J. H., and Amaral, D. G., 1985, The distribution of somatostatin-like immunoreactivity in the monkey hippocampal formation, *J. Comp. Neurol.* **236**:423–442.

Berger, T. W., Swanson, G. W., Milner, T. A., Lynch, G. S., and Thompson, R. F., 1980, Reciprocal anatomical connections between hippocampus and subiculum in the rabbit: Evidence for subicular innervation of regio superior, *Brain Res.* **183**:265–276.

Berger, T. W., Semple-Rowland, S., and Basset, J. L., 1981, Hippocampal polymorph neurons are the cells of origin for ipsilateral association and commissural afferents to the dentate gyrus, *Brain Res.* **215**:329–336.

Blackstad, T. W., 1956, Commissural connections of the hippocampal region in the cat, with special reference to their mode of termination, *J. Comp. Neurol.* **105**:417–537.

Blackstad, T. W., Brink, K., Hem, J., and Jeune, B., 1970, Distribution of hippocampal mossy fibers in the rat: An experimental study with silver impregnation methods, *J. Comp. Neurol.* **138**:433–450.

Blumberg, B., 1984, Allometry and evolution of tertiary hominoids, *J. Hum. Evol.* **13**:613–676.

Brodal, A., 1947, The hippocampus and sense of smell: A review, *Brain* **70**:179–222.

Campbell, C. B. G., 1982, Some questions and problems related to homology, in: *Primate Brain Evolution* (E. Armstrong and D. Falk, eds.), Plenum Press, New York, pp. 1–11.

Carpenter, M. B., 1976, *Human Neuroanatomy*, 7the ed., Williams & Wilkins, Baltimore.

Carpenter, M. B., and Sutin, J., 1983, *Human Neuroanatomy*, 8th ed., Williams & Wilkins, Baltimore.

Cassell, M. D., and Brown, M. W., 1984, The distribution of Timm's stain in the nonsulphide-perfused human hippocampal formation, *J. Comp. Neurol.* **222**.461–471.

Chronister, R. B., and DeFrance, J. F., 1979, Organization of projection neurons of the hippocampus, *Exp. Neurol.* **66**:509–523.

Claiborne, B. J., Amaral, D. G., and Cowan, W. M., 1986, A light and electron microscopic analysis of the mossy fibers of the rat dentate gyrus, *J. Comp. Neurol.* **246**:435–458.

Cotman, C. W., and Nadler, J. V., 1978, Reactive synaptogenesis in the hippocampus, in: *Neuronal Plasticity* (C. W. Cotman, ed.), Raven Press, New York, pp. 227–271.

Crutcher, K. A., Madison, R., and Davis, J. N., 1981, A study of the rat septohippocampal pathway using anterograde transport of horseradish peroxidase, *Neuroscience* **6**:1961–1973.

Demeter, S., Rosene, D. L., and Van Hoesen, G. W., 1985, Interhemispheric pathways of the hippocampal formation, presubiculum, entorhinal and posterior hippocampal cortices in the rhesus monkey: The structure and function of the hippocampal commissures, *J. Comp. Neurol.* **233**:30–47.

DeVito, J., 1980, Subcortical projections to the hippocampal formation in squirrel monkey (Saimiri sciureus), *Brain Res. Bull.* **5**:285–289.

Divac, I., 1975, Magnocellular nuclei of the basal forebrain project to neocortex, brain stem, and olfactory bulb: Review of some functional correlates, *Brain Res.* **93**:385–398.

Edinger, H. M., Kramer, S. Z., Weiner, S., and Krayniak, P. F., 1979, The subicular cortex of the cat: An anatomical and electrophysiological study, *Exp. Neurol.* **63**:504–526.

Ekstein, J., and Rosene, D. L., 1987, Topography of the fornix trajectory and mammillary body termination of efferents from the subiculum, the supracallosal subiculum, and the hippocampal–amygdaloid transition area in the rhesus monkey, *J. Comp. Neurol.* submitted for publication.

Filimonoff, I. N., 1947, A rational subdivision of the cerebral cortex, *Arch. Neurol. Psychiatry* **58**:296–311.

Finch, D. M., Nowlin, N. L., and Babb, T. L., 1983, Demonstration of axonal projections of neurons in the rat hippocampus and subiculum by intracellular injection of HRP, *Brain Res.* **271**:201–216.

Finlay, B. L., and Slattery, M., 1983, Local differences in the amount of early cell deaths in neocortex predict adult specializations, *Science* **219**:1349–1351.

Fitzpatrick, D., and Johnson, R. P., 1981, Enkephalin-like immunoreactivity in the mossy fiber pathway of the hippocampal formation of the tree shrew (Tupaia glis), *Neuroscience* **6**:2485–2494.

Fricke, R., and Cowan, W. M., 1978, An autoradiographic study of the commissural and ipsilateral hippocampo-dentate projections in the adult rat, *J. Comp. Neurol.* **181**:253–270.

Frotscher, M., and Leranth, C., 1985, Cholinergic innervation of the rat hippocampus as revealed by choline acetyltransferase immunocytochemistry: A combined light and electron microscopic study, *J. Comp. Neurol.* **239**:237–246.

Frotscher, M., and Leranth, C., 1986, The cholinergic innervation of the rat fascia dentata: Identification of target structures on granule cells by combining choline acetyltransferase immunocytochemistry and Golgi impregnation, *J. Comp.Neurol.* **243**:58–70.

Frotscher, M., and Zimmer, J., 1986, Intracerebral transplants of the rat fascia dentata: A Golgi/electron microscope study of dentate granule cells, *J. Comp.Neurol.* **246**:181–190.

Gall, C., Brecha, N., Karten, H. J., and Chang, K. -J., 1981, Localization of enkephalin-like immunoreactivity to identified axonal and neuronal populations of the rat hippocampus, *J. Comp. Neurol.* **198**:335–350.

Geneser-Jensen, F. A., 1972, Distribution of acetylcholinesterase in the hippocampal region of the guinea pig. II. Subiculum and hippocampus, *Z. Zellforsch. Mikrosk. Anat.* **124**:546–560.

Gertz, S. D., Lindenberg, R., and Pavis, G. W., 1972, Structural variations in the rostral hippocampus, *Johns Hopkins Med. J.* **130**:367–376.

Goldman-Rakic, P. S., Selemon, L. D., and Schwartz, M. L., 1984, Dual pathways connecting the dorsolateral prefrontal cortex with the hippocampal formation and parahippocampal cortex in the rhesus monkey, *Neuroscience* **12**:719–743.

Gottlieb, D. I., and Cowan, W. M., 1973, Autoradiographic studies of the commissural and ipsilateral association connections of the hippocampus and dentate gyrus of the rat. I. The commissural connections, *J. Comp. Neurol.* **149:**393–421.

Greenfield, S., 1984, Acetylcholinesterase may have novel functions in the brain, *Trends in Neuroscience,* **7:**364–368.

Greenwood, R. S., Godar, S. E., Reaves, T.A., Jr., and Hayward, J. N., 1981, Cholecystokinin in hippocampal pathways, *J. Comp. Neurol.* **203:**335–350.

Gudden, A., 1881, Beitzrag zur kenntniss des corpus mammillare und der Sogenannten Schekel des fornix, *Arch. Psychiatr. Nervenkr.* **11:**428–452.

Haglund, L., Swanson, L. W., and Kohler, C., 1984, The projection of the supramammillary nucleus to the hippocampal formation: An immunohistochemical and anterograde transport study with the lectin PHA-L in the rat, *J. Comp. Neurol.* **229:**171–185.

Hamilton, C. R., 1983, Lateralization for orientation in split brain monkeys, *Behav. Brain Res.* **10:**399–403.

Handelmann, G. E., Meyer, D, K., Beinfeld, M. C., and Oertel, W. H., 1981, CCK-containing terminals in the hippocampus are derived from intrinsic neurons: An immunohistochemical and radioimmunological study, *Brain Res.* **224:**180–184.

Harris, K. M., Marshall, P. E., and Landis, D. M. D., 1985, Ultrastructural study of cholecystokinin-immunoreactive cells and processes in area CA1 of the rat hippocampus, *J. Comp. Neurol.* **233:**147–158.

Haug, F.-M. S., 1967, Electron microscopical localization of the zinc in the hippocampal mossy fibre synapses by a modified sulfide silver procedure, *Histochemie* **8:**355–368.

Haug, F.-M. S., 1973, Heavy metals in the brain. A light microscope study of the rat with Timm's sulphide silver method. Methodological considerations and cytological and regional staining pattern, *Adv. Anat. Embryol. Cell Biol.* **47:**7–71.

Haug, F.-M. S., Blackstad, T. W., Simonsen, A. H., and Zimmer, A. J., 1971, Timm's sulphide silver reaction for zinc during experimental anterograde degeneration of hippocampal mossy fibers, *J. Comp. Neurol.* **142:**23–31.

Herkenham, M., 1978, The connections of the nucleus reuiens thalami: Evidence for a direct thalamo-hippocampal pathway in the rat, *J. Comp. Neurol.* **177:**589–610.

Hjorth-Simonsen, A., 1971, Hippocampal efferents to the ipsilateral entorhinal area: An experimental study in the rat, *J. Comp. Neurol.* **142:**417–438.

Hjorth-Simonsen, A., 1972, Projections of the lateral part of the entorhinal area to the hippocampus and fascia dentata, *J. Comp. Neurol.* **146:**219–232.

Hjorth-Simonsen, A., 1973, Some intrinsic connections of the hippocampus in the rat: An experimental analysis, *J. Comp. Neurol.* **147:**145–161.

Hjorth-Simonsen, A., and Jeune, B., 1972, Origin and termination of the hippocampal perforant path in the rat studied by silver impregnation, *J. Comp. Neurol.* **144:**215–232.

Hjorth-Simonsen, A., and Laurberg, S., 1977, Commissural connections of the dentate area in the rat, *J. Comp. Neurol.* **174:**591–606.

Hyman, B. J., Van Hoesen, G. W., Damasio, A. R., and Barnes, C. L., 1984, Alzheimer's disease: Cell specific pathology isolates in the hippocampal formation, *Science* **225:**121–122.

Kohler, C., 1985, Intrinsic projections of the retrohippocampal region in the rat brain. I. The subicular complex, *J. Comp. Neurol.* **236:**504–522.

Kohler, C., Erisson, L., Davies, L., and Chan-Palay, V., 1986, Neuropeptide Y innervation of the hippocampal region in the rat and monkey brain, *J. Comp. Neurol.* **244:**384–400.

Kosel, K. C., Van Hoesen, G. W., and Rosene, D. L., 1983, A direct projection from the perirhinal cortex to the subiculum in the rat, *Brain Res.* **269:**347–351.

Krayniak, P. F., Siegel, A., Meibach, R. C., and Fruchtman, D., 1979, Origin of the fornix system in the squirrel monkey, *Brain Res.* **160:**401–411.

Krettek, J. E., and Price, J. L., 1977, Projections from the amygdaloid complex and adjacent olfactory structures to the entorhinal cortex and to the subiculum in the rat and cat, *J. Comp. Neurol.* **172:**723–752.

Laatsch, R. H., and Cowan, W. M., 1966, Electron microscopic studies of the dentate gyrus in the rat. I. Normal structure with special reference to synaptic organization, *J. Comp. Neurol.* **128:**359–396.

Laurberg, S., 1979, Commissural and intrinsic connections of the rat hippocampus, *J. Comp. Neurol.* **184:**685–708.

Leichnetz, G. R., and Astruc, J., 1975, Preliminary evidence for a direct projection of the prefrontal cortex to the hippocampus in the squirrel monkey, *Brain Behav. Evol.* **355:**355–364.

Leranth, C., and Frotscher, M., 1983, Commissural afferents to the rat hippocampus terminate on vasoactive intestinal polypeptide like immunoreactive non-pyramidal neurons: An EM immunocytochemical degeneration study, *Brain Res.* **276:**357–361.

Lewis, F. T., 1923, The significance of the term hippocampus, *J. Comp. Neurol.* **35:**213–230.

Lewis, P. R., Shute, C. C. D., 1967, The cholinergic limbic system: Projections to the hippocampal formation medial cortex, nuclei of the ascending cholinergic reticular system and subfornical organ and supra-optic crest, *Brain* **90:**521–542.

Lorente de Nó, R., 1934, Studies on the structure of the cerebral cortex. II. Continuation of the study of the ammonic system, *J. Psychol. Neurol.* **46:**113–177.

Loy, R., Koziell, D. A., Lindsey, J. D., and Moore, R. Y., 1980, Noradrenergic innervation of the adult rat hippocampal formation, *J. Comp. Neurol.* **189:**699–710.

Lynch, G., Matthews, D. A., Mosko, S., Parks, T., and Cotman, C. W., 1972, Induced acetylcholinesterase-rich layer in the rat dentate gyrus following entorhinal lesions. *Brain Res.* **42:** 311–318.

Lynch, G., Rose, G., and Gall, C., 1978, Anatomical and functional aspects of the septo-hippocampal projections. *Ciba Found. Symp.* **58:**5–24.

McLardy, T., 1955, Observations in the fornix of the monkey. II. Fiber studies, *J. Comp. Neurol.* **103:**327–343.

McLardy, T., 1963, Some cell and fiber peculiarities of the uncal hippocampus, *Prog. Brain Res.* **3:**71–88.

McLardy, T., 1970, Memory function in hippocampal gyri but not in hippocampi, *Int. J. Neurosci.* **1:**113–118.

McLardy, T., 1974, Hippocampal presubicular temporo-ammonic non-perforant path: Histological studies in man and macaques, *International Research Communications System.* **2:**1421.

Mahut, H., Zola-Morgan, S., and Moss, M., 1982, Hippocampal resections impair associative learning and recognition memory in the monkey, *J. Neurosci.* **2:**1214–1229.

Martin, R. D., 1982, Allometric approaches to the evolution of the primate nervous system, in: *Primate Brain Evolution* (E. Armstrong and D. Falk, eds.), Plenum Press, New York, pp. 39–56.

Meibach, R. C., and Siegel, A., 1975, The origin of fornix fibres which project to the mammillary bodies in the rat: A horseradish peroxidase study, *Brain Res.* **88:**508–512.

Meibach, R. C., and Siegel, A., 1977a, Efferent connections of the hippocampal formation in the rat, *Brain Res.* **124:**197–224.

Meibach, R. C., Siegel, A., 1977b, Subicular projections to the posterior cingulate cortex in rats, *Exp. Neurol.* **57:**264–274.

Mellgren, S. I., and Srebro, B., 1973, Changes in acetylcholinesterase and distribution of degenerating fibres in the hippocampal region after septal lesions in the rat, *Brain Res.* **52:**19–36.

Mesulam, M.-M., Mufson, E. J., Levey, A. I., and Wainer, B. H., 1983, Cholinergic innervation of cortex by the vasal forebrain: Cytochemistry and cortical connections of the septal area, diagonal band nuclei, nucleus basalis (substantia innominata), and hypothalamus in the rhesus monkey, *J. Comp. Neurol.* **214:**170–197.

Milner, B., 1970, *Biology of Memory*, Academic Press, New York, pp. 29–50.

Milner, T. A., Loy, R., and Amaral, D. G., 1983, An anatomical study of the development of the septo-hippocampal projection in the rat, *Dev. Brain Res.* **8:**343–371.

Mishkin, M., 1978, Memory in monkeys severely impaired by combined but not by separate removal of amygdala and hippocampus, *Nature* **273:**297–298.

Mishkin, M., 1982, A memory system in the monkey, *Philos. Trans. R. Soc. London B Ser.* **298:**85–95.

Mosko, S., Lynch, G., and Cotman, C. W., 1973, The distribution of septal projections to the hippocampus of the rat, *J. Comp. Neurol.* **152:**163–174.

Moss, M., and Rosene, D. L., 1984, A perfusion-fixation procedure for the concurrent demonstration of Timm's, horseradish peroxidase (HRP) and acetylcholinesterase (AChE) histochemistry. *J. Histochem. Cytochem.* **32:**113–116.

Moss, M. B., and Rosene, D. L., 1987, Acetylcholinesterase in the hippocampal formation of the rhesus monkey: A quantitative histochemical study. *J. Comp. Neurol.* submitted for publication.

Moss, M., Mahut, H., and Zola-Morgan, S., 1981, Concurrent discrimination learning of monkeys after hippocampal, entorhinal, or fornix lesions, *J. Neurosci.* **1:**227–240.

Moss, M., Albert, M. S., Butters, N., and Payne, M., 1986, Differential patterns of memory loss among patients with Alzheimer's disease, Huntington's disease, an alcoholic Korsakoff's syndrome, *Arch. Neurol.* **43:**239–246.

Moss, M. B., Rosene, D. L., and Mahut, H., 1987, Developmentally related changes in acetylcholinesterase in the hippocampal formation of the rhesus monkey following transections of the fornix. *J. Comp. Neurol.* submitted for publication.

Nomina Anatomica, 1983, 5th ed., Williams & Wilkins, Baltimore.

Nowakowski, R. S., and Davis, T. L., 1985, Dendritic arbors and dendritic excrescences of abnormally positioned neurons in area CA3c of mice carrying the mutation "hippocampal lamination deficit," *J. Comp.Neurol.* **239:**267–275.

Otsuka, N., Kishimoto, T., and Nagita, T., 1976, Histochemical studies on zinc of the hippocampal formation in the monkey. *Acta Histochem. Cytochem.* **9:**107–110.

Ottersen, O., 1982, Connections of the amygdala of the rat. IV. Corticoamygdaloid and intraamygdaloid connections as studied with axonal transport of horseradish peroxidase, *J. Comp. Neurol.* **205:**30–48.

Pandya, D. N., Van Hoesen, G. W., and Mesulam, M.-M., 1981, Efferent connections of the cingulate gyrus in the rhesus monkey, *Exp. Brain Res.* **42:**319–330.

Penfield, W., and Milner, B., 1958, Memory deficit produced by bilateral lesions in the hippocampal zone, *Arch. Neurol. Psychiatry* **79:**475–497.

Poletti, C. E., and Creswell, G., 1977, Fornix system efferent projections in the squirrel monkey: An experimental degeneration study, *J. Comp. Neurol.* **175:**101–128.

Pribram, K. H., 1961, Limbic system, in: *Electrical Stimulation of the Brain*, (D. E. Sheer, ed.), University of Texas Press, Austin, pp. 311–320.

Pribram, K. H., and Kruger, L., 1954, Functions of the olfactory brain, *Ann. N. Y. Acad. Sci.* **58:**109–138.

Price, J. L., 1981, *The Amygdaloid Complex*, Elsevier, Amsterdam, pp. 121–132.

Radinsky, L. B., 1969, Outlines of canine and felid brain evolution, *Ann. N.Y. Acad. Sci.* **167:**277–287.

Radinsky, L., 1982, Some cautionary notes on making inferences about relative brain size, in: *Primate Brain Evolution* (E. Armstrong and D. Falk, eds.), Plenum Press, New York, pp. 29–37.

Raisman, G., Cowan, W. M., and Powell, T. P. S., 1966, An experimental analysis of the efferent projection of the hippocampus, *Brain* **80:**83–108.

Ramón y Cajal, S., 1968, *The Structure of Ammon's Horn* (L. M. Kraft, transl.), Thomas, Springfield, Ill.

Rawlins, J. N. P., and Green, K. F., 1977, Lamellar organization in the rat hippocampus, *Exp. Brain Res.* **28:**335–344.

Reh, T., and Kalil, K., 1982, Development of the pyramidal tract in the hamster. II. An electron microscopic study, *J. Comp. Neurol.* **205:**77–88.

Riss, W., Halpern, M., and Scalia, F., 1969, Anatomical aspects of the evolution of the limbic and olfactory systems and their potential significance for behavior, *Ann. N.Y. Acad. Sci.* **159:**1096–1111.

Roberts, G. W., Allen, Y., Crow, T. J., and Polak, J. M., 1983, Immunocytochemical localization of neuropeptides in the fornix of the rat, monkey and man, *Brain Res.* **263:**151–155.

Roberts, G. W., Woodhams, P. L., Polak, J. M., and Crow, T. J., 1984, Distribution of neuropeptides in the limbic system of the rat: The hippocampus, *Neuroscience* **11:**35–77.

Rose, G., and Schubert, P., 1977, Release and transfer of [^{3}H]adenosine derivatives in the cholinergic septal system, *Brain Res.* **121:**353–357.

Rosene, D. L., and Van Hoesen, G. W., 1977, Hippocampal efferents reach widespread areas of the cerebral cortex and amygdala in the rhesus monkey, *Science* **198:**315–317.

Ruth, R. E., Collier, T. J., and Routtenberg, A., 1982, Topography between the entorhinal cortex and the dentate septotemporal cortex in rats. I. Medial and intermediate entorhinal projecting cells, *J. Comp. Neurol.* **209:**69–78.

Saunders, R. C., and Rosene, D. L., 1987, A comparison of efferents from the amygdala and the hippocampal formation in the rhesus monkey. I. Convergence in the entorhinal, prorhinal and perirhinal cortices, *J. Comp. Neurol.* submitted for publication.

Saunders, R. C., Murray, E. A., and Mishkin, M. 1984, Further evidence that the amygdala and hippocampus contribute equally to recognition memory, *Neuropsychologia* **22**:785–796.

Saunders, R. C., Rosene, D., and Van Hoesen, G. W., 1987, A comparison of the efferents of the amygdala of the hippocampal formation in the rhesus monkey. II. Reciprocal and non-reciprocal connections, *J. Comp. Neurol.* submitted for publication.

Schwerdtfeger, W. K., 1979, Direct efferent and afferent connections of the hippocampus with the neocortex in the marmoset monkey, *Am. J. Anat.* **156**:77–83.

Scoville, W. B., and Milner, B., 1957, Loss of recent memory after bilateral hippocampal lesions, *J. Neurol. Neurosurg. Psychiatry* **20**:11–21.

Sibley, C. G., and Ahlquist, J. E., 1984, The phylogeny of the hominid primates as indicated by DNA–DNA hybridization, *J. Mol. Evol.* **20**:2–15.

Siegel, A., Oghami, S., and Edinger, H., 1975, Projections of the hippocampus to the septal area in the squirrel monkey, *Brain Res.* **99**:247–260.

Simpson, D. A., 1952, The efferent fibres of the hippocampus in the monkey, *J. Neurol. Neurosurg. Psychiatry* **15**:79–92.

Sorensen, K. E., 1980, Ipsilateral projection from the subiculum to the retrosplenial cortex in the guinea pig, *J. Comp. Neurol.* **193**:893–911.

Sorensen, K. E., and Shipley, M. T., 1979, Projections from the subiculum to the deep layers of the ipsilateral presubicular and entorhinal cortices in the guinea pig, *J. Comp. Neurol.* **188**:313–334.

Stephan, A., 1963, Vergleichend-anatomische untersuchungen am uncus bei insectivoren und primaten, in: *The Rhinencephalon and Related Structures,* Vol. 3, (W. Bargman and J. P. Shade, eds.), Elsevier, Amsterdam, pp. 111–121.

Stephan, H., and Andy, O. J., 1970, The allocortex in primates, in: *The Primate Brain,* (C. R. Noback and W. Montagna, eds.), Appleton–Century–Crofts, New York.

Steward, O., 1976, Topographic organization of the projections from the entorhinal area to the hippocampal formation in the rat, *J. Comp. Neurol.* **167**:285–314.

Steward, O., and Scoville, S. A., 1976, Cells of origin of entorhinal cortical afferents to the hippocampus and fascia dentata of the rat, *J. Comp. Neurol.* **169**:347–370.

Swanson, L. W., 1981, A direct projection from Ammon's horn to prefrontal cortex in the rat, *Brain Res.* **217**:150–154.

Swanson, L. W., and Cowan, W. M., 1977, An autoradiographic study of the organization of the efferent connections of the hippocampal formation in the rat, *J. Comp. Neurol.* **172**:49–84.

Swanson, L. W., and Cowan, W. M., 1979, The connections of the septal region in the rat, *J. Comp. Neurol.* **186**:621–656.

Swanson, L. W., and Cowan, W. M., 1975, Hippocampal–hypothalamic connections: Origin in subicular cortex, not Ammon's horn. *Science* **189**:303–304.

Swanson, L. W., Wyss, J. M., and Cowan, W. M., 1978, An autoradiographic study of the organization of intra-hippocampal association pathways in the rat, *J. Comp.Neurol.* **181**:681–716.

Templeton, A. R., 1983, Phylogenetic inference from restriction endonuclease cleavage site maps with particular reference to the evolution of humans and the apes, *Evol.* **37**:221–244.

Van Hoesen, G. W., and Pandya, D. N., 1975, Some connections of the entorhinal (area 28) and perirhinal (area 35) cortices of the rhesus monkey. III. Efferent connections, *Brain Res.* **95**:39–59.

Van Hoesen, G. W., Rosene, D. L., and Mesulam, M.-M., 1979, Subicular input from temporal cortex in the rhesus monkey, *Science* **205**:608–610.

Veazy, R. B., Amaral, D. G., and Cowan, W. M., 1982, The morphology and the connections of the posterior hypothalamus in the cynomolgus monkey (Macaca Fasicularis). II. Efferent connections, *J. Comp. Neurol.* **207**:135–156.

Vogt, B. A., 1976, Retrosplenial cortex in the rhesus monkey: A cytoarchitectonic and Golgi study, *J. Comp. Neurol.* **169**:63–98.

Voneida, T. J., Vardaris, R. M., Fish, S. E., and Reiheld, T., 1981, The origin of the hippocampal commissure in the rat, *Anat. Rec.* **201**:91–103.

Weiskrantz, L., 1977, Trying to bridge some neurophysiological gaps between monkey and man, *Br. J. Psychol.* **68**:431–445.

West, J. R., Van Hoesen, G. W., and Kosel, K. C., 1982, A demonstration of hippocampal mossy fiber axon morphology using anterograde transport of horseradish peroxidase, *Exp. Brain Res.* **48**:209–216.

White, L. E., Jr., 1965, A morphologic concept of the limbic lobe, *Int. Rev. Neurobiol.* **8**:1–34.

Woolsey, R. M., and Nelson, J. S., 1975, Asymptomatic destruction of the fornix in man, *Arch. Neurol.* **32**:566–568.

Wyss, J. M., 1981, An autoradiographic study of the efferent connections of the entorhinal cortex in the rat, *J. Comp. Neurol.* **199**:495–512.

Wyss, J. M., Swanson, L. W., and Cowan, W. M., 1979, Evidence for an input to the molecular layer and stratum granulosum of the dentate gyrus from the supramammillary region of the hypothalamus, *Anat. Embryol.* **156**:165–176.

Wyss, J. M., Swanson, L. W., and Cowan, W. M., 1980, The organization of the fimbria, fornix, and ventral hippocampal commissure in the rat, *Anat. Embryol.* **158**:303–316.

Index

457